The Clinical Practice of Stem-Cell Transplantation

Volume 2

The Clinical Practice of Stem-Cell Transplantation

Volume 2

Edited by

John Barrett
Chief, Bone-Marrow Transplant Unit, Hematology Branch, National Heart Lung and Blood Institute National Institutes of Health, 9000 Rockville Pike, Bethesda MD 20892, USA

Jennifer G. Treleaven
Consultant Haematologist, Leukaemia Unit, Department of Medical Oncology, The Royal Marsden NHS Trust, Downs Road, Sutton, Surrey SM2 5PT, UK

ISIS
MEDICAL
MEDIA

Oxford

© 1998 by Isis Medical Media Ltd.
59 St Aldates
Oxford OX1 1ST, UK

First published 1998

All rights reserved. No part of this publication
may be reproduced, stored in a retrieval system,
or transmitted in any form or by any means, electronic,
mechanical, photocopying, recording or otherwise
without the prior permission of the copyright owner.

The Authors have asserted their right under the
Copyright, Designs and Patents Act, 1988,
to be identified as the Authors of this work.

British Library Cataloguing in Publication Data.
A catalogue record for this title is available from
the British Library.

ISBN 1 899066 70 5

Barrett, J (John)
The Clinical Practice of Stem-Cell Transplantation
John Barrett, Jennifer G. Treleaven (eds)

This book was edited by John Barrett and Jennifer Treleaven in their
private capacity. No official support or endorsement by the NHLBI or
NIH is intended and none should be inferred.

Always refer to the manufacturer's Prescribing
Information before prescribing drugs cited in this book.

Publisher: Dr Jonathan Gregory
Editorial Controller: Maren White
Production Manager: Julia Savory

Typeset by
Creative Associates, Oxford, UK

Colour reproduction by
Track Direct, UK

Produced by Phoenix Offset, HK
Printed in China

Distributed in USA by
Mosby-Year Book Inc.
11830 Westline Industrial Drive
St Louis MO 63146, USA

Distributed by
Plymbridge Distributors Ltd.
Estover Road
Plymouth
PL6 7PY, UK

Contents

Volume 1

Cover and chapter opening slides — ix
Contributors — x
Foreword — xvii
Preface — xix
Acknowledgements — xxi

Part 1
THE PLACE OF STEM-CELL TRANSPLANTATION IN THE TREATMENT OF MALIGNANT AND NON-MALIGNANT DISORDERS

Chapter 1	Introduction *Jennie Treleaven and John Barrett*	1
Chapter 2	Theoretical aspects of dose intensity and dose scheduling *Charlotte Rees, Phillip Beale, Ian Judson*	17
Chapter 3	Acute myeloid leukaemia *Helen Jackson, Lisa Robinson and Alan Burnett*	31
Chapter 4	Chronic myeloid leukaemia *John Goldman*	47
Chapter 5	Adult acute lymphoblastic leukaemia *John Barrett*	63
Chapter 6	Paediatric leukaemias *Pat Dinndorf*	83
Chapter 7	The myelodysplastic syndromes and acute myeloid leukaemia following myelodysplastic syndrome *Theo de Witte*	99
Chapter 8	Multiple myeloma *Noopur Raje and Ray Powles*	109
Chapter 9	Hodgkin's disease *Andrew J. Peniket and David C. Linch*	129
Chapter 10	Non-Hodgkin's lymphoma *Ama Rohatiner and Stephen Kelsey*	151
Chapter 11	Solid tumours in children *Simon Meller and Ross Pinkerton*	173
Chapter 12	Breast cancer *Pablo J. Cagnoni and Elizabeth.J. Shpall*	191
Chapter 13	Solid tumours in adults (excluding breast and germ cell) *Mark Hill and Martin Gore*	205
Chapter 14	Germ-cell tumours *Alan Horwich*	213

Chapter 15	Immunodeficiency diseases *Alain Fischer*	223
Chapter 16	Aplastic anaemia *Judith Marsh and Ted Gordon-Smith*	237
Chapter 17	Fanconi anaemia *Eliane Gluckman*	259
Chapter 18	Thalassaemia *Caterina Borgna-Pignatti*	267
Chapter 19	Sickle cell anaemia *Christiane Vermylen and Guy Cornu*	277
Chapter 20	Lysosomal storage diseases *Peter M. Hoogerbrugge and Dinko Valerio*	285
Chapter 21	Chronic lymphocytic leukaemia *Mauricette Michallet*	297
Chapter 22	Autoimmune disorders *Sally Killick*	305

Part 2
PRACTICAL ASPECTS OF STEM-CELL TRANSPLANTATION

Chapter 23	Pre-transplant evaluation of the patient and donor *Jayesh Mehta and Seema Singhal*	315
Chapter 24	HLA matching and compatibility testing *M Tevfik Dorak and Christopher H. Poynton*	325
Chapter 25	Searching the Registry for an unrelated donor *Susan Cleaver*	351
Chapter 26	Unrelated donor bone-marrow transplantation *Jacqueline Cornish, Nicholas Goulden and Michael Potter*	363
Chapter 27	Allogeneic related partially mismatched transplantation *P. Jean Henslee-Downey*	391
Chapter 28	Venous access *Claire Nightingale and Jacqueline Filshie*	419
Chapter 29	Marrow collection and processing *Michele Cottler-Fox*	433
Chapter 30	Use of cord blood *Hal E. Broxmeyer*	441
Chapter 31	Peripheral blood stem cells for autologous and allogeneic transplantation *Nigel H. Russell and Gail Miflin*	453

Volume 2

Part 2 continued

| Chapter 32 | T-cell depletion of allogeneic stem cell grafts
Adrian P. Gee and Carlos Lee | 473 |

Chapter 33	Purging tumour from autologous stem-cell grafts *Adrian P. Gee*	507
Chapter 34	Total body irradiation for bone-marrow transplant recipients *Chris Parker and Diana Tait*	537
Chapter 35	Preparative regimens for allogeneic bone-marrow transplantation *John Barrett*	549
Chapter 36	High dose regimens for autologous stem-cell transplantation *N. Claude Gorin*	571

PART 3
PROBLEMS AFTER TRANSPLANTATION

A. Graft-versus-host disease

Chapter 37	Acute graft-versus-host disease *Gérard Socié and Jean-Yves Cahn*	595
Chapter 38	Chronic graft-versus-host disease *Adriana Seber and Georgia B. Vogelsang*	619
Chapter 39	The histopathology of graft-versus-host disease *Keith P. McCarthy*	635

B. Take, rejection and relapse

Chapter 40	Graft failure: diagnosis and management *Jayesh Mehta and Seema Singhal*	645
Chapter 41	Minimal residual disease in acute leukemia *Jacques J.M. van Dongen, Tomasz Szczepanski and Marja J. Pongers-Willemse*	659
Chapter 42	Relapse and its management *Hans-Jochem Kolb and Johann Mittermüller*	677

C. Infection

Chapter 43	Bacterial infections *Unell Riley*	690
Chapter 44	Cytomegalovirus *Grant Prentice, Jane E. Grundy and Pearl Kho*	697
Chapter 45	Other viral infections *Diana Westmoreland*	709
Chapter 46	Fungal infections *Rosemary A. Barnes*	723
Chapter 47	Other infections *Rosemary A. Barnes*	741
Chapter 48	Reimmunisation after transplantation *Seema Singhal and Jayesh Mehta*	745
Chapter 49	General infection prophylaxis *Unell Riley*	757

D. Other important aspects

Chapter 50	Complications in the early post-transplant period *Nicola J. Philpott and Edward J. Kanfer*	767

Chapter 51	Neurological aspects of stem-cell transplantation *Paul V. Marks*	787
Chapter 52	Blood transfusion support *Mahes de Silva, Marcela Contreras and Ruth Warwick*	795
Chapter 53	Nutritional support *Louise Henry and Virginia Souchon*	811
Chapter 54	Readaptation to normal life *Michael A. Andrykowski and Richard P. McQuellon*	827

E. Late effects of transplantation

Chapter 55	Paediatric problems *Sally E. Kinsey*	839
Chapter 56	Endocrine and reproductive dysfunction in adults *Stephen M. Shalet*	849
Chapter 57	Fertility *Eric Simons and Kamal Ahuja*	855

PART 4
OTHER CONSIDERATIONS

Chapter 58	Setting up the transplant unit *Sarah Hart*	869
Chapter 59	Nursing management in the BMT unit *Helen Porter*	879
Chapter 60	Outpatient management *James A. Russell*	889
Chapter 61	Multicenter observational databases in bone-marrow transplantation *Philip A. Rowlings, Kathleen A. Sobocinski, Mei-Jie Zhang, John P. Klein and Mary M. Horowitz*	895
Chapter 62	Ethnic considerations *James Smith*	921
Index		941

Cover and chapter opening slides Volume 2

Part 2 continued

Cover
Eosinophilic blast crisis of chronic myeloid leukaemia — Sudan black stain

Chapter openings
Chapter 32	T-cell lymphocytes surrounded by magnetic microspheres (indirect immunofluorescence)
Chapter 33	Electron micrograph of magnetic microspheres
Chapter 34	Chronic lymphocytic leukaemia and prolymphocytic leukaemia — Giemsa stain
Chapter 35	Some of the alkylating agents currently in use for conditioning therapy prior to stem-cell Transplantation
Chapter 36	Howell-Jolly bodies in red cells after splenic damage

Part 3

Chapter 37	Acute graft-versus-host disease of the skin
Chapter 38	Spherocytosis seen in the peripheral blood in bacterial septicaemia in a patient with severe chronic graft-versus-host disease
Chapter 39	Liver fibrosis in veno-occlusive disease of the liver associated with graft-versus-host disease
Chapter 40	Supravital stain for reticulocytes
Chapter 41	FISH: 15:17 translocation in acute promyelocytic leukaemia
Chapter 42	Relapsed acute myeloid leukaemia (M5) — PAS stain
Chapter 43	Blood culture containing Cl. Perfringens organisms
Chapter 44	Cytomegalovirus inclusion bodies as seen on lung biopsy
Chapter 45	Red cell auto-autoagglutination occuring in association with systemic infection
Chapter 46	Candida hyphae
Chapter 47	Encapsulated cryptococcus — Nigrosin stain
Chapter 48	The septate hyphae of Aspergillus sp. showing acute angle branching
Chapter 49	PneumocystIs carinii
Chapter 50	Red cell fragmentation induced by cyclosporin
Chapter 51	Extramedullary haemopoiesis (spleen) in chronic myeloid leukaemia
Chapter 52	Blood grouping plate
Chapter 53	Ammonium oxalate crystals
Chapter 54	A bone marrow osteoclast
Chapter 55	Marrow involvement by rhabdomyosarcoma
Chapter 56	Electron micrograph of eosinophilic leukaemia cell
Chapter 57	Drawing of an embryo in the uterus, by Leonardo da Vinci, circa 1510, Windsor, Royal Library

Part 4

Chapter 58	A cell line stained with a supravital stain (bisbenzimide) and viewed under ultraviolet light
Chapter 59	Extramedullary erythropoiesis involving the liver
Chapter 60	Target cells and "tear drop" red cells as seen in the peripheral blood in the presence of bone-marrow fibrosis
Chapter 61	Bone marrow appearance in Nieman Pick disease
Chapter 62	Urate crystals

Contributors

Kamal Ahuja PhD
Scientific Director, IVF and Fertility Centre, The Cromwell Hospital, Cromwell Road, London SW5 0TU, UK

Michael A. Andrykowski PhD
Professor of Behavioural Science, Department of Behavioural Science, College of Medicine Office Building, University of Kentucky College of Medicine, Lexington, KY 40536-0086, USA

Rosemary A. Barnes MA MSc MD MRCP MRCPath
Senior Lecturer, Department of Medical Microbiology, University of Wales College of Medicine, Heath Park, Cardiff CF4 4XN, UK

John Barrett MD MRCP FRCPath
Professor, National Institute of Health, National Heart Lung and Blood Institute Bone Marrow Transplant Unit Rm 7N248, Building 10 Room 7C103, 9000 Rockville Pike, Bethesda MD 20892, USA

Philip Beale BSc FRACP
Institute of Cancer Research, Royal Marsden NHS Trust, Downs Road, Sutton, Surrey SM2 5PT, UK

Caterina Borgna-Pignatti MD
Istituto di Pediatria, Universita degli Studi di Ferrara, Via Savonarola 9, 44100 Ferrara, Italy

Hal E. Broxmeyer PhD
Chairman and Mary Margaret Walther Professor of Microbiology and Immunology, Scientific Director, Walther Oncology Center, Indiana University School of Medicine, 1044 W Walnut Street, Building R4, Room 302, Indianapolis, Indiana 46202-5121, USA

Alan K. Burnett MD FRCP FRCPath
Professor, Department of Haematology, University Hospital of Wales, Heath Park, Cardiff CF4 4XN, UK

Pablo J. Cagnoni MD
Assistant Professor of Medicine, University of Colorado Bone Marrow Transplant Program, University of Colorado Cancer Center, Denver, CO 80220, USA

Jean-Yves Cahn MD
Professor of Hematology, Service de Hématologie, Hôpital Jean Minjoz, Besancon, France

Susan A. Cleaver BSc
Technical Director, Anthony Nolan Bone Marrow Trust, The Royal Free Hospital, Pond Street, Hampstead, London NW3 2QG, UK

Marcela Contreras MD MRCPath FRCP(Edin)
Executive Director, NBS London and South East Zone Blood Centre, Colindale Avenue, London, NW9 5BG, UK

Jacqueline M. Cornish MB ChB
Associate Director, Paediatric Haematology/Oncology and Bone Marrow Transplantation Unit, Royal Hospital for Sick Children, St. Michael's Hill, Bristol BS2 8BJ, UK

Guy Cornu MD
Service d'Hématologie Pédiatrique, Cliniques Universitaires St. Luc, Avenue Hippocrate 10, 1200 Brussels, Belgium

Michele Cottler-Fox MD
Medical Director, Stem Cell Transplant Laboratory, University of Maryland Cancer Center, 22 South Greene Street, Baltimore, MD 21201-1595, USA

Mahes De Silva DCH FRCPath
Lead Consultant Immunohaematology, NBS London and South East Zone Blood Centre, Colindale Avenue, London NW9 5BG, UK

Contributors

Theo J.M. de Witte MD PhD
Professor of Internal Medicine, Division of Hematology, St Radboud University Hospital, Nijmegen, 8 Geert Grooteplein, 6525 GA Nijmegen, The Netherlands

Patricia A. Dinndorf MD
Professor of Pediatrics, GW University School of Medicine; Department of Hematology and Oncology, Children's National Medical Center, 111 Michigan Avenue NW, Washington DC 20010, USA

Tevfik T. Dorak MD
Lecturer in Haematology, Department of Haematology, University Hospital of Wales, Heath Park, Cardiff CF4 4XW, UK

Jacqueline Filshie MBBS FFARCS
Consultant Anaesthetist, Department of Anaesthetics, Royal Marsden NHS Trust, Downs Road, Sutton, Surrey SM2 5PT, UK

Alain Fischer MD PhD
Professor of Pediatric Immunology, Institute Federatif de Recherche Enfants-Malades, INSERM U 429, 149 Rue de Sevres, 75743 Paris Cedex 15, France

Adrian Gee MIBiol PhD
Professor of Medicine, Section of Blood and Marrow Transplantation, Department of Hematology, University of Texas M.D. Anderson Cancer Center, Box 24, 1515 Holcombe Boulevard, Houston, Texas 77030, USA

Eliane Gluckman MD
Professor of Hematology, Head, Bone Marrow Tranplant Unit, Hôpital St. Louis, 1 Avenue Claude Vellefaux 75475 Paris Cedex 10, France

John M. Goldman DM FRCP FRCPath
Professor, Department of Haematology, Imperial College School of Medicine, Hammersmith Hospital, Du Cane Road, London W12 0NN, UK

Edward C. Gordon-Smith MA MSc FRCP FRCPath
Professor of Haematology, Division of Haematology, St George's Hospital Medical School, Cranmer Terrace, Tooting, London, SW17 ORE, UK

Martin Gore PhD FRCP
Department of Medicine, Royal Marsden NHS Trust, Fulham Road, London SW3 6JJ, UK

N. Claude Gorin MD
Professor, Service des Maladies du Sang, CHU Saint-Antoine, 184 Rue du Faubourg St-Antoine 75012 Paris, France

Nicholas Goulden MB ChB MRCP
Lecturer/Senior Registrar in Haematology, Great Ormond Street Hospital, London WC1, UK

Jane Grundy PhD MRCPath
Reader in Viral Immunology, Department of Clinical Immunology, Royal Free Hospital School of Medicine, Rowland Hill Street, London NW3 2PF

Sarah M. Hart MSc BSc RGN FETC
Clinical Nurse Specialist, Infection Control, The Royal Marsden NHS Trust, Downs Road, Sutton, Surrey SM2 5PT, UK

Louise Henry MSc BSc SRD
Dietician, The Royal Marsden NHS Trust, Downs Road, Sutton, Surrey SM2 5PT, UK

P. Jean Henslee-Downey MD
Director, Division of Transplantation Medicine and Professor of Medicine and Pediatrics, University of South Carolina and Richland Memorial Hospital, Center for Cancer Treatment and Research, 7 Richland Medical Park, Columbia SC 29203, USA

Mark Hill MRCP
Consultant Medical Oncologist, Department of Medical Oncology, Royal Marsden NHS Trust, Fulham Road, London SW3 6JJ, UK

Peter M. Hoogerbrugge MD
Department of Pediatrics, Leiden University Hospital, PO Box 960, 2300 RC Leiden, and Sophia Children's Hospital, dr Molewaterplein 60, 3015 GJ Rotterdam, The Netherlands

Mary M. Horowitz MD MS
Professor of Medicine Haematology/Oncology, Scientific Director IBMTR/ABMTR North America, Medical College of Wisconsin, Milwaukee WI 53226, USA

Alan Horwich FRCP, FRCR, PhD
Professor of Radiotherapy, Honorary Consultant in Clinical Oncology, Department of Radiotherapy and Oncology, Royal Marsden NHS Trust, Down's Road, Sutton, Surrey SM2 5PT, UK

Helen Jackson BSc MRCP Dip MRCPath
Specialist Registrar, Department of Haematology, University Hospital of Wales, Heath Park, Cardiff CF4 4XW, UK

Ian Judson MA MD FRCP
Institute of Cancer Research, Block E, 15 Cotswold Road, Belmont, Sutton, Surrey SM2 5NG, UK

Edward J. Kanfer FRCP MRCPath
Senior Lecturer in Haematology, Hammersmith Hospital, Du Cane Road, London W12 0NN, UK

Steven M. Kelsey MD MRCP MRCPath
Consultant Haematologist, St Bartholomew's and Royal London School of Medicine and Dentistry, London E1 2AD

Pearl Kho PhD
Quintiles, Glaxo-Wellcome, Beckenham, Kent, UK

Sally Killick MRCP
Specialist Registrar in Haematology, Department of Haematology, Royal Marsden NHS Trust NHS Trust, Downs Road, Sutton, Surrey, SM2 5PT, UK

Sally Kinsey MD MRCP MRCPath FRCPCh
Consultant Paediatric Haematologist, Bone Marrow Transplant Unit, St. James' University Hospital, Beckett Street, Leeds, UK

John P. Klein PhD
Statistical Director, IBMTR/ABMTR North America, Statistical Center, International Bone Marrow Transplant Registry, Medical College of Wisconsin, Milwaukee, WI 53226, USA

Hans-Jochem Kolb MD
Professor of Medicine, Ludwig-Maximilians-Universität München, Klinikum Grosshadern Med. Klinik III, Marchioninistasse 17, Postfach 70 12 60, 8000 München 70, Germany

Carlos Lee BSc
Associate Director, Stem Cell Processing Laboratory, Division of Transplantation Medicine, Center for Cancer Treatment and Research, Richland Memorial Hospital and the University of South Carolina, USA

David Linch BA MB FRCP FRCPath
Professor, Department of Haematology, University College London Medical School, 98 Chenies Mews, London WC1 6HX

Paul Marks LLM MD FRCS
Consultant Neurosurgeon, Department of Neurosurgery, Leeds General Infirmary, Great George Street, Leeds LS1 3EX, UK

Judith C.W. Marsh BSc MBChB MRCP MRCPath MD
Senior Lecturer and Honorary Consultant Haematologist, Department of Haematology, St. George's Hospital Medical School, Cranmer Terrace, Blackshaw Road, Tooting, London SW17 0RE, UK

Keith P. McCarthy MB BS, MD, MRCPath
Consultant Histopathologist, Department of Pathology, Cheltenham General Hospital, Sandford Road, Cheltenham, Gloucestershire GL53 7AN, UK

Contributors

Richard McQuellon PhD
Director, Psychosocial Oncology, Bowman Gray School of Medicine, Wake Forest University, Medical Centre Boulevard, Winston Salem NC 27157-1082, USA

Jayesh Mehta MD
Associate Professor of Medicine, Division of Hematology/Oncology, University of Arkansas Center for Medical Sciences, 4301 West Markham, Mail slot 508, Little Rock, Arkansas 72205-9985, USA; Leukaemia Unit, Royal Marsden NHS Trust, Downs Road, Sutton, Surrey SM2 5PT, UK

Simon T. Meller FRCP DCH
Consultant Paediatrician and Paediatric Oncologist, Children's Department, Royal Marsden NHS Trust, Down's Road, Sutton, Surrey SM2 5PT, UK

Mauricette Michallet MD
Head of the Bone Marrow Transplantation Unit, Department of Haematology, Pavilion E, Hôpital Edouard Herriot, Place d'Arsonval, 69437 Lyon Cedex 03, France

Gail Miflin MRCP
LRF Fellow, Department of Haematology, Nottingham City Hospital NHS Trust, Hucknall Road, Nottingham NG5 1PB, UK

Johann Mittermueller MD
Ludwig-Maximilians-Universität München, Klinikum Grosshadern, Med. Klinik III, Marchioninistrasse 15, 81377 München, Germany

Claire E. Nightingale FRCA
Senior Registrar in Anaesthetics, c/o Dr J. Filshie, Department of Anaesthetics, Royal Marsden NHS Trust, Downs Road, Sutton, Surrey SM2 5PT, UK

Christopher C. Parker BA MRCP FRCR
Registrar in Clinical Oncology, Radiotherapy Department, Royal Marsden NHS Trust, Downs Road, Sutton SM2 5PT, UK

Andrew Peniket MRCP
Bone Marrow Transplant Fellow, Department of Haematology, University College London Medical School, 98 Chenies Mews, London WC1 6HX, UK

Nicola Philpott MRCP DipRCPath
Specialist Registrar in Haematology, Haematology Department, Hammersmith Hospital, DuCane Road, London W2 0NN, UK

Ross Pinkerton DCH MD FRCP
Professor, Children's Department, Royal Marsden NHS Trust, Downs Road, Sutton, Surrey SM2 5PT, UK

Helen Porter RGN Onc Cert MSc
Clinical Nurse Specialist, Haemato-oncology Unit, Royal Marsden NHS Trust, Down's Road, Sutton, Surrey SM2 5PT, UK

Michael N. Potter MA MB PhD MRCP MRCPath
Consultant/ Senior Lecturer in Haematology, Department of Haematology and Bone Marrow Transplantation, Royal Free Hospital, Pond Street, London NW3 2QG, UK

Ray Powles MD FRCP FRCPath
Physician in charge, Leukaemia Unit, Royal Marsden NHS Trust, Down's Road, Sutton, Surrey SM2 5PT, UK

Chris Poynton MDS FRCP MRCPath
Consultant Haematologist, Department of Haematology, University Hospital of Wales, Heath Park, Cardiff CF4 4XW, UK

Grant Prentice FRCP FRCPath
Professor, Department of Haematology, Royal Free Hospital, Pond Street, London NW3 2QG, UK

Noopur Raje MD
Division of Hematologic Malignancies, Dana Farber Cancer Institute and Department of Medicine, Harvard Medical School, Boston MA 02215 USA and Myeloma Unit, Royal Marsden NHS Trust, Downs Road, Sutton SM2 5PY

Charlotte Rees BSc MRCP
Institute of Cancer Research, Royal Marsden NHS Trust, Downs Road, Sutton, Surrey SM2 5PT, UK

Unell Riley MRCPath
Consultant Microbiologist, Microbiology Department, Royal Marsden NHS Trust, Down's Road, Sutton, Surrey SM2 5PT, UK

Lisa Robinson BSc MRCP MRCPath
Clinical Lecturer in Haematology, University of Wales, College of Medicine, Heath Park, Cardiff CF4 4XN

Ama Rohatiner MD FRCP
Reader in Medical Oncology and Consultant Physician, Department of Medical Oncology, St. Bartholomew's Hospital, 45 Little Britain, West Smithfield, London EC1A 7BE, UK

Philip A. Rowlings MBBS MS FRACP FRCPA
Assistant Professor of Medicine, Hematology/Oncology, Assistant Scientific Director IBMTR/ABMTR-North America, Medical College of Wisconsin, 8701 Watertown Plank Road, Milwaukee, Wisconsin 53226, USA

James A. Russell FRCP (Edin)
Clinical Professor of Medicine, University of Calgary; Director, Alberta Bone Marrow Tranplant Program, Tom Baker Cancer Center, 1331 29th Street NW, Calgary, Alberta T2N 4N2, Canada

Nigel H. Russell MD FRCP FRCPath
Reader in Haematology, University of Nottingham; Consultant in Haematology, Department of Haematology, Nottingham City Hospital NHS Trust, Hucknall Road, Nottingham NG5 1PB, UK

Adriana Seber MD
The Johns Hopkins University, 600 N. Wolfe St., Oncology Center Room 3-127, Baltimore, Maryland 21287-8985, USA

Stephen M. Shalet MD FRCP
Professor of Endocrinology, Holt Radium Institute, Christie Hospital NHS Trust, Wilmslow Road, Withington, Manchester M20 4BX, UK

Elizabeth J. Shpall MD
Director, Stem Cell Engineering Laboratory and Apheresis Program, Associate Director Bone Marrow Transplant Program, University of Colorado Health Sciences Center, Box B-190, 4200 East 9th Avenue, Denver CO 80262, USA

Eric G. Simons FRCOG
Clinical Director, Consultant Surgeon, IVF and Fertility Centre, The Cromwell Hospital, Cromwell Road, London SW5 0TU, UK

Seema Singhal MD
Assistant Professor of Medicine, Division of Haematology/Oncology, University of Arkansas for Medical Sciences, 4301 West Markham, Mail Slot 508, Little Rock, Arkansas 72205-9985, USA; Leukaemia Unit, Royal Marsden NHS Trust, Downs Road, Sutton, Surrey SM2 5PT, UK

James Smith MA STh SRN RMN
Former Chaplain, Royal Marsden NHS Trust; Retired, 22 Thrift Close, Stalbridge, Sturminster Newton, Dorset DT10 2LE, UK

Kathleen A. Sobocinski MS
Associate Statistical Director, IBMTR/ABMTR-North America, Medical College of Wisconsin, Milwaukee WI 53226, USA

Gerard Socié MD PhD
Associate Professor of Hematology, Service d'Hematologie– Greffe de Moelle, Hôpital St. Louis, 1 Avenue Claude Vellefaux, 75475 Paris Cedex 10, France

Virginia Souchon BScSRD
Dietician, Royal Marsden NHS Trust, Down's Road, Sutton, Surrey SM2 5PT, UK

Tomasz Szczepanski MD
Department of Pediatrics and Hematology, Silesian Medical School, Zabrze, Poland

Jennifer G. Treleaven MD FRCP FRCPath
Consultant Haematologist, Leukaemia Unit, The Royal Marsden NHS Trust, Downs Road , Sutton, Surrey SM2 5PT, UK

Diana Tait MD MRCP FRCR
Consultant in Radiotherapy, Radiotherapy Department, Royal Marsden NHS Trust, Down's Road, Sutton, Surrey SM2 5PT, UK

Dinko Valerio PhD
Department of Molecular Cell Biology, University of Leiden, The Netherlands and INTROGENE, PO Box 2048, 2301 CA Leiden, The Netherlands

Christiane G. Vermylen MD PhD
Service d'Hématologie Pédiatrique, Cliniques Universitaires Saint.-Luc, Avenue Hippocrate 10, 1200 Brussels, Belgium

Jack van Dongen MD PhD
Department of Immunology, University Hospital Dijkzigt, Erasmus University Rotterdam, P.O. Box 1738, 3000 DR Rotterdam, The Netherlands

Georgia B. Vogelsang MD
The Johns Hopkins University, 600 N. Wolfe Street, Oncology Center Room 3-127 Baltimore, Maryland 21287-8985, USA

Ruth M. Warwick MRCP FRCPath
Head Consultant, North London Blood Transfusion Centre, Colindale Avenue, London NW9 5BG, UK

Diana Westmoreland BM BS MA MSc DPhil FRCPath
Consultant Virologist, Department of Medical Microbiology and Public Health Laboratory, University Hospital of Wales, Heath Park, Cardiff CF4 4XW, UK

Marja Willemse PhD
Department of Immunology, University Hospital Dijkzigt, Erasmus University Rotterdam, PO Box 1738, 3000 DR Rotterdam, The Netherlands

Mei-Jie Zhang PhD
Statistician, IBMTR/ABMTR-North America, Medical College of Wisconsin, Milwaukee WI 53226, USA

Foreword

It is an honour and privilege for the President of the European Blood and Marrow Transplantation Group (EBMT) to introduce this book on clinical practice of stem-cell transplantation. It appears at a fascinating and challenging time for this form of treatment. Within a span of 30 years, bone marrow transplantation, once an experimental venture, has become established practice and forms an integral part of the treatment plan for many disease categories. It is estimated that over 30,000 transplants worldwide, at least 14,000 of which were carried out in Europe, took place in 1996 from various donor types and sources. Numbers of transplants are still increasing. Cord blood has recently been introduced as an additional donor source, and new indications such as autoimmune disorders, are on the horizon. The decrease in treatment-related mortality observed over the last few years indicates that there will be an expansion to disease categories not necessarily associated with a lethal outcome.

This period of rapid expansion and change, shown by the shift within a few years from bone marrow to peripheral blood as donor source, produces confrontation between health care and health management. Medical procedure is no longer at the discretion of individual physicians. Budget constraints, cost efficiency considerations and standard operating procedures dictate plans for treatment. It is essential to have tools for coping with this situation. Cooperative national and international groups are one way, a textbook providing a solid background of the latest information another. I hope this book will be useful for all those involved in clinical blood or marrow transplantation for dealing with interactions between basic research, laboratory, nursing care and clinical medicine. The reward will be the well-being of the patients.

Alouis Gratwohl, 1997

Preface

A prerequisite for successful stem-cell transplantation is a coordinated team approach. Procedures are complex, and require haematological, general medical, surgical, psychological, nursing and laboratory input. Management is very interventive, both in terms of diagnosis and treatment, and requires a high degree of understanding between care team and patient.

In recent years, there has been a rapid expansion in the use of stem-cell transplantation worldwide, with new transplant teams coming into being each year. New specialists and new teams need practical information about the application of stem-cell transplantation in clinical practice, and the procedures involved. It is not always easy to obtain such information quickly and concisely. The indications for stem-cell transplantation have expanded considerably, and its place in treatment programmes is now much better defined. As these refinements have occurred and the procedure has become safer, more disease categories have become amenable to stem cell transplantation as a treatment approach, for example, chronic lymphocytic leukaemia, breast cancer, and autoimmune diseases. Also, patients are now better informed about treatment options. Treatment decisions have to be made very rapidly, and there are still many areas of controversy. Protocol books can help, but by their nature they rarely contain reference to the reasons behind the practice laid down. It is also difficult to keep protocol books either up-to-date, complete, or easy to locate on the unit.

With these considerations in mind, we have compiled this book which represents current transplantation practice across the entire discipline. It covers autologous and allogeneic transplantation using marrow, peripheral blood stem cells and cord blood, for the treatment of malignant and non-malignant conditions. There are four main sections: the first covers the place of stem cell transplantation in the treatment of the various malignant and non-malignant conditions. The second deals with the practical aspects of transplantation of relevance prior to the transplant, and the third section deals with practical issues occurring after the transplant. Finally, the fourth section is concerned with more general issues such as out-patient management and setting up transplant units. All of the contributors have had first-hand experience in clinical BMT, in the USA, Europe and Great Britain. We hope that with our broad choice of experts, we have succeeded in avoiding bias relating to a particular unit and that, as far as possible, the views presented reflect those generally accepted.

The aim of this book is to update the reader on advances in these fields and to provide an overview of the relevant literature. It is also to give an easy-to-find and easy-to-comprehend outline of the major problems which may be encountered, and their investigation, diagnosis and treatment, which are largely presented in the form of tables.

The book will be of use to healthcare workers in the field of bone-marrow transplantation, and particularly to those who have hands-on responsibility for patients, including doctors, nurses, pharmacy staff and many others. It is hoped that students of Medicine will also find it readable, and that it will afford them some insight into the complexities which now face us when dealing with patients undergoing these intensive forms of treatment.

Jennifer Treleaven and John Barrett
May 1998.

Acknowledgements

We wish to thank the many colleagues who have kindly provided clinical photographs for this book and, in particular, Peter Mortimer, David Swirsky, Lynn Hiorns, Daniel Catovsky, Nazar Al–asiri and Alison Leiper. We are also very grateful to Ben Hilditch, who uncomplainingly redrew many of the figures to a very high standard, and to Ray Stuckey and Dennis Underwood for their excellent photographic skills, always applied with such good humour. Finally, we thank all of our patients who, by bearing with our errors and successes, have made the procedure of stem-cell transplantation a viable therapeutic option.

Practical aspects of stem-cell transplantation

Part 2 continued

T-cell depletion of allogeneic stem-cell grafts

Purging tumour from autologous stem-cell grafts

Total body irradiation for bone-marrow transplant recipients

Preparative regimens for allogeneic bone-marrow transplantation

High-dose regimens for autologous stem-cell transplantation

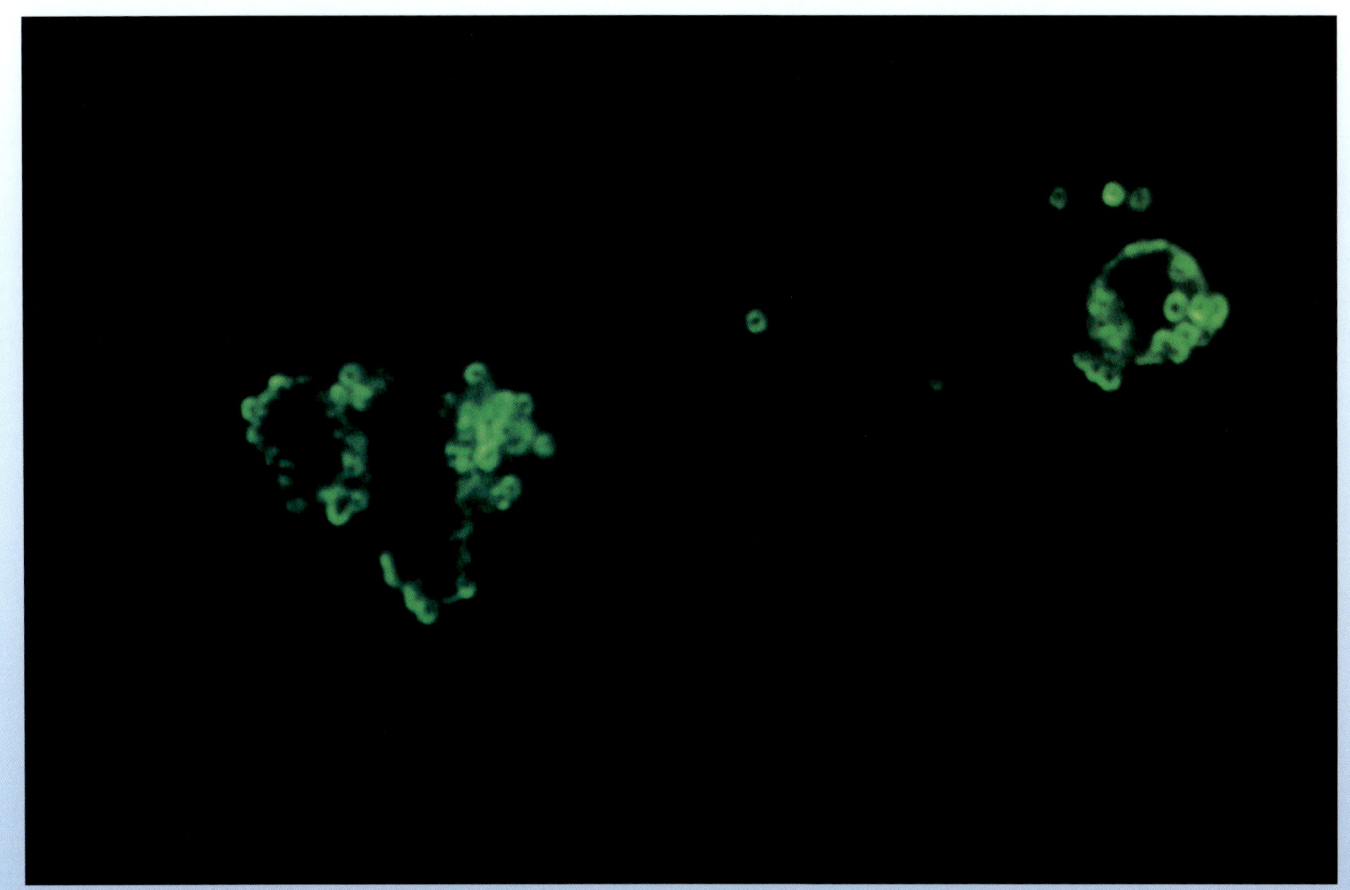

Chapter 32

T-cell depletion of allogeneic stem-cell grafts

Adrian P. Gee and Carlos Lee

Introduction

Graft-versus-host disease (GvHD) occurs when immunocompetent cells within the haematopoietic progenitor cell graft recognize and react to antigenic differences expressed by normal tissues and cells of the recipient [1,2]. The antigens involved in triggering GvHD are primarily those of the human leukocyte antigen (HLA) system and are encoded by genes on chromosome six in humans [3]. Early attempts to transplant marrow grafts, prior to the discovery of the HLA system, resulted in fatal GvHD in the majority of recipients, and threatened to put an end to bone-marrow rescue following myeloablative therapy [4]. HLA matching of related donors and potential recipients at the HLA-A, -B and D/DR loci has been shown, however, to reduce the incidence and severity of GvHD dramatically [3], although 30–50% of these patients will still develop the disease, which will be severe in about 25% of cases [5]. Recent reports suggest that matching at the HLA-C locus may prove to be of additional benefit [3].

Graft-versus-host disease was not seen in animal transplantation models in which foetal cells were used as the source of haematopoietic stem cells [6]. These grafts were inherently devoid of mature T-cells, suggesting that T-lymphocytes may be mediators of GvHD, and that *ex vivo* depletion of these cells from marrow grafts may be valuable as prophylaxis. Elimination of T-cells from grafts using either antilymphocyte or antithymocyte antibodies, alone or in combination with complement (C') [7,8], or by agglutination with soybean lectin [9] was shown to prevent GvHD in mouse and dog transplant models, and to result in long-term stable chimaeric engraftment. These results stimulated the development of a number of clinical trials in which T-cell depletion of the marrow graft was examined [10]. A variety of techniques were tested; however, for many years the most popular method involved debulking the graft of the majority of mature cell populations by incubation with the lectin soybean agglutinin (SBA), rosetting the remaining T-cells with sheep erythrocytes and removal of these rosettes by centrifugation on a density cushion [11]. This approach was used successfully to prepare HLA-mismatched grafts from parents for transplantation to children with leukaemia [12] or severe combined immunodeficiency [13]. The discovery of monoclonal antibody (MAb) technology and the production of many of these reagents with specificity towards pan-T-cell antigens, or antigens expressed by various T-cell subsets, led to the development of a number of protocols for antibody-mediated T-cell depletion of marrow grafts [10].

Although these trials often achieved their main goal of decreasing the incidence and severity of GvHD [14], this was usually associated with an approximately tenfold increase in engraftment failure [14] (Figure 32.1), and a fivefold increase in leukaemic relapse in HLA-matched sibling donor transplants [14], particularly in patients with chronic myelogenous leukaemia [15]. As a result, there was no overall improvement in survival when T-cell depleted grafts were used in this context.

The finding that T-cell depletion and the abrogation of GvHD resulted in increased disease relapse supported the concept that there was a beneficial graft-versus-leukaemia (GvL) effect that was associated with the development of GvHD [16]. Considerable effort has been expended to determine whether GvL and GvHD are mediated by the same effector cells, with the aim of engineering grafts to enhance the former, while removing cells that produce the latter [17]. In parallel, there have been many claims that GvHD may also be mediated by other cell types, e.g. natural killer (NK) cells [18] or specific T-cell subsets [1], and attempts have been made to improve clinical outcomes by removing these cells from haematopoietic grafts. The results have been variable, and have generally supported the proposal that effective GvHD prophylaxis is dependent upon many factors of which T-cell depletion is but one component. The nature of the disease, the degree of HLA incompatibility, the method of conditioning the patient, the technique used to engineer the graft, and the post-transplant immunomodulation therapy are all important factors in determining outcome.

Attempts to use unmanipulated grafts from donors other than HLA-matched siblings have generally resulted in an increase in both the incidence and severity of GvHD [3–5]. In the case of matched unrelated donor (MUD) transplants, GvHD is believed to be induced by mismatches at both minor HLA loci and non-HLA antigens [19]. In partially-mismatched related donor transplants there is an increased likelihood of matching at these loci; however, there are

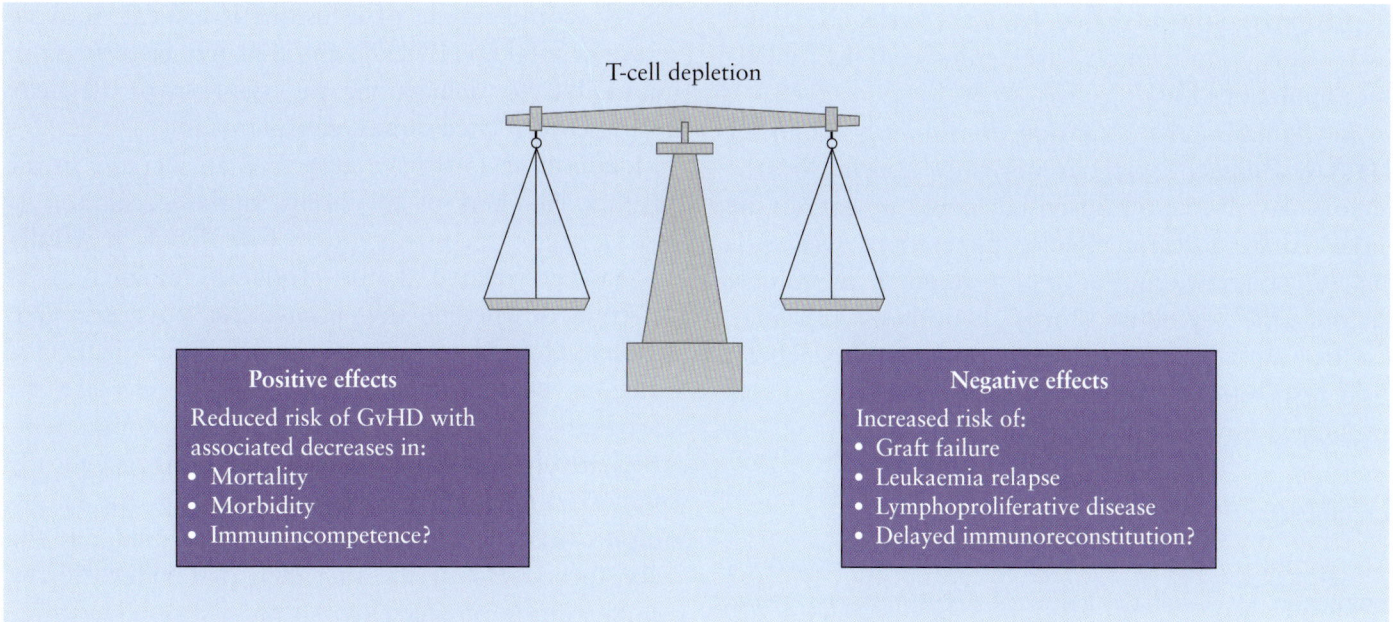

Figure 32.1 The T-cell depletion balance.

now varying degrees of mismatch of the major HLA antigens [20; see also Chapter 27]. This has led to the widespread use of T-cell depletion of grafts from alternative donors, with the aim of reducing the risk of GvHD, while ensuring adequate engraftment and retention of the GvL response [21,22].

Initial clinical results achieved using allogeneic grafts derived from other sources, for example, mobilized peripheral blood and placental/umbilical cord blood, raised the hope that there was a reduced risk of acute GvHD associated with these types of transplants [23–25]. Allogeneic peripheral blood progenitor cell transplants do not appear to have the very high incidence of acute GvHD that might have been anticipated based solely upon the mature T-cell content of the grafts (although there is still a significant incidence of acute GvHD [26,27]), but the incidence and severity of chronic GvHD is higher than with marrow grafts [28]. Similarly, as clinical experience in cord blood transplantation increases, it is clear that these grafts cannot be used as a source of generic stem cells and that histocompatibility differences will have an important effect on clinical outcome [29]. Initial fears that these grafts could not be manipulated *ex vivo* without unacceptable cell losses have been laid to rest, and a number of studies have now shown that it is possible to T-cell deplete cord blood grafts for allogeneic transplantation [30].

Mechanisms of graft-versus-host disease

Graft-versus-host disease is primarily triggered by T-lymphocytes in the graft responding to histocompatibility differences with the recipient cells [1–3]. In HLA-matched sibling transplants, these differences are between minor HLA antigens which are expressed on recipient cells and presented either directly to donor T-cells, or via antigen-presenting cells, such as dendritic cells or macrophages [31]. Direct presentation of the antigen in the context of major histocompatibility complex (MHC) class I molecules (HLA-A, B, C) triggers $CD8^+$ T-cells. Antigen processed by antigen-presenting cells and presented in the context of MHC class II and the appropriate co-stimulatory molecules results in activation of $CD4^+$ cells, which will in turn stimulate $CD8^+$ cytotoxic cells. Histo-incompatibilities at class I or class II (HLA D/DR) loci are thought to preferentially stimulate clonal expansion of $CD8^+$ or $CD4^+$ cells respectively, and such a system has been demonstrated in rodents [32]. In most murine models for HLA-matched, minor antigen-mismatched human transplants, depletion of the $CD8^+$ T-cell populations from the graft prevents, or reduces, GvHD in the recipients [33,34]. The situation is, however, less straightforward than these findings would suggest since, in certain donor–recipient strain combinations, GvHD is predominantly mediated by CD4+ cells [35], and GvL and engraftment are enhanced by CD8+ subpopulations [36].

In humans, the situation is similarly complex [31,37]. Clinical GvHD is not only affected by the factors described previously, but could potentially be mediated by different effector populations (NK cells [18,38]) directly, and/or via a number of soluble factors (the 'cytokine storm' hypothesis [39–41]). Control must be achieved while retaining a beneficial GvL response, without knowing whether the effects are indeed functionally separable.

Graft-versus-leukaemia

Abrogation of the GvL effect in chronic myelogenous leukaemia by T-cell depletion of *HLA-matched grafts* substantially increases the risk of disease relapse, thereby negating any benefit achieved by preventing GvHD [15]. Use of a T-cell depleted matched or mismatched *unrelated graft* has been shown to compensate for this reduction in GvL [42]. Although the GvL mechanism is incompletely understood, its close association with the development of GvHD, and its restoration by increasing the degree of allodisparity suggests that alloreactive responses may be involved, in which MHC antigens are the targets [16]. This cannot, however, be the only mechanism, since many freshly-isolated leukaemia cells lack MHC class I and II antigens [43], although their expression can be stimulated by treatment with tumour necrosis factor and/or interferon [44]. An alternative GvL pathway may involve the targeting of minimal residual disease via:
- minor histocompatibility antigens [45];
- tissue specific antigens, e.g. CD13 and CD33 [17]; and/or
- leukaemia-associated antigens, e.g. the p210 fusion protein resulting from the t9:22 translocation of the Philadelphia chromosome in chronic myelogenous leukaemia [46].

T-cell clones with specificity towards leukaemic cells have been generated *ex vivo* [47,48], and attempts have been made to activate T-cells in grafts with the aim of generating a GvL effect *in vivo* [49]. *In vivo* demonstrations of GvL have, however, predominantly come from the use of post-transplant infusions of donor leukocytes (donor leukocyte infusions) to treat relapsed disease in animals [50] and humans [17,51].

The dose and timing of infusions is critical to avoid severe or fatal GvHD [52], and this may be difficult or impossible to achieve in the context of partially mismatched related donor transplants [53].

Lamb *et al.* [54] have described an increase in the absolute numbers of $\gamma\delta^+$ T-cells in the circulation of disease-free recipients of T-depleted partially mismatched related donor grafts. It remains to be determined whether this population possesses GvL activity. However, fractionation of donor leukocyte infusions before infusion may help to increase the specificity of their antileukaemia component. Alternatively, effector T-cell populations genetically engineered to contain a suicide gene, e.g. the herpes simplex thymidine kinase gene, could be used, and the cells 'turned off' at the first sign of GvHD [55] by administration of ganciclovir.

In reality, the GvL response is probably multifactorial, involving multiple pathways, effectors and mediators. Although originally described in, and still predominantly associated with, chronic myelogenous leukaemia [16], a similar effect has been described in acute leukaemias [56].

Failures of graft engineering to achieve complete prophylaxis of GvHD while promoting a GvL response are largely due to our lack of ability to identify the appropriate effector cell populations, rather than failure of the graft engineering technology *per se*. As more is understood about the mediators of these responses, the cell-separation methodology is probably already available to achieve the desired clinical outcome.

Graft failure

T-cell depletion is associated with an increased risk of graft failure [14,57], from about 2% in recipients of unmanipulated matched sibling donor grafts to >10% in T-depleted graft recipients [14, 58]. This may take the form of:
- failure to engraft, which appears to be predominantly an immunological phenomenon;
- initial engraftment followed by pancytopenia;
- late graft failure [58], which has been primarily attributed to recurrence of disease [59].

Graft rejection is thought to be mediated by residual immunocompetent cells in the recipient [60]. These are predominantly suppressor T-cells (CD3+8+57+) in recipients of matched sibling donor grafts and cytotoxic T-cells (CD3+8+57−HLA-DR+) in patients rejecting grafts from matched unrelated donors [61,62]. Both patterns have been seen in recipients of grafts from partially mismatched grafts from related donors [63], where the Vβ expression by the effector cells appeared to be restricted. Strategies for overcoming rejection include intensification of immunosuppression and increasing the inoculum of donor T-cells or facilitator cells (see later) within the graft.

Ex vivo engineering of an allogenic graft can, therefore, have a major impact on successful engraftment, control of GvHD and maintenance or stimulation of a GvL response (Figure 32.1).

T-cell depletion technology

Traditionally, T-cell depletion has been achieved by negative selection, in which the T-cells, or T-cell subsets, have been specifically targeted and eliminated from the graft. Recently, positive selection has been examined as an alternative [64,65]. In this procedure the haematopoietic stem cells are enriched, usually using a selection technology based upon their expression of the CD34 antigen and the T-cells are discarded within the CD34-negative population. Clinical experience using positive selection on allogeneic grafts is increasing, but is still somewhat limited [65,66].

Negative selection from bone marrow

It has been estimated that up to 90% of cellular mass in a bone-marrow harvest represents contaminating peripheral blood collected during the harvest procedure [67]. As a result, the T-cell content of a marrow harvest may vary widely depending on the experience of the harvester and the volume of material collected. There is a law of diminishing returns with larger harvests, such that in an attempt to collect more cells to compensate for anticipated losses during the T-cell depletion procedure, contamination by blood increases, and the T-cell content of the harvest rises in parallel (Table 32.1). In a study of T-cell phenotype and distribution in initial aspirates obtained during marrow harvesting (i.e. when the peripheral blood contamination was minimal) we generated the information shown in Figure 32.2.

Table 32.1 Bone-marrow harvest problem

- Up to 90% of cellular mass in a bone-marrow harvest represents contaminating peripheral blood
- T-cell content of a marrow harvest may thus vary widely
- With larger harvests, contamination by blood increases, and the T-cell content of the harvest rises in parallel

Although the level of depletion desired will depend on the clinical application and a number of other factors, Kernan *et al.* have indicated that the final graft should contain a T-cell dose of $<1 \times 10^5$ T-cells/kg recipient body weight to prevent GvHD in recipients [68]. This was confirmed in a study of 70 matched sibling donor transplants in which a fixed dose of 1×10^5 T-cells/kg was administered [69]. There were no graft failures, and GvHD was limited to grades I–II skin involvement, although chronic GvHD occurred in 31%, but was again was predominantly limited to the skin. There was an 8% incidence of relapse in standard risk leukaemias, with a projected five-year survival of 80%, and a procedure-related mortality of 11%. If the T-cell dose is decreased further, the risk of both graft failure and disease relapse will generally increase, as discussed previously. Many *ex vivo* procedures are capable of achieving these 'clinically relevant' levels of depletion (Table 32.2), although T-cell add-back [70] or stem-cell supplementation [71] may sometimes be required to compensate in cases of overdepletion.

Negative T-cell selection may be achieved either by destroying the cells within the graft or by their physical removal from the cell mixture (Table 32.2). In both cases, the procedure may or may not involve the use of T-cell-directed monoclonal antibodies. Non antibody-mediated techniques have predominantly used either sheep erythrocyte rosetting and SBA or centrifugal elutriation.

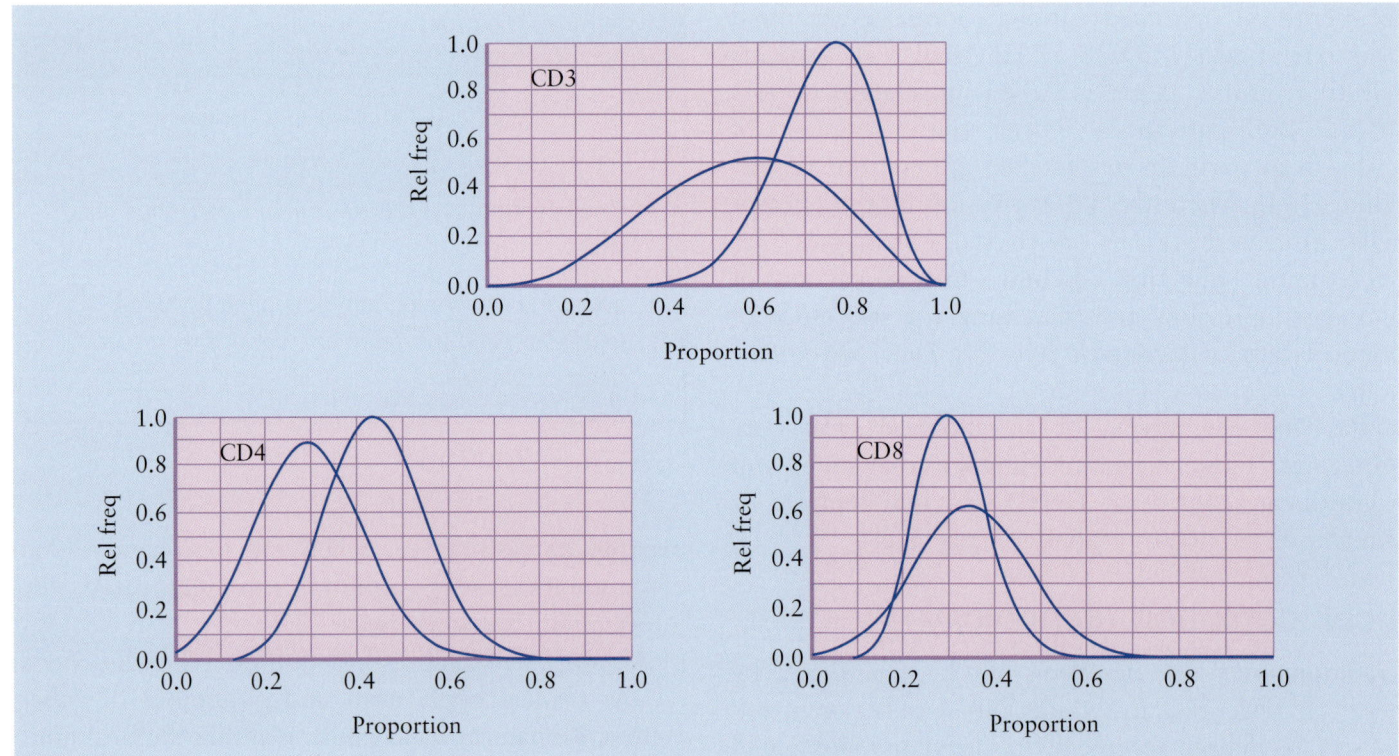

Figure 32.2 Frequency distributions of T-cells and T-cell subpopulations in peripheral blood and bone marrow. Bone-marrow samples were obtained from the initial aspirates collected for a bone-marrow harvest. T-cells were enumerated by flow cytometric analysis. Data are presented from 56 normal individuals.

Table 32.2 Methods for T-cell depletion of allogeneic stem-cell grafts		
Method	Removed	Destroyed *in situ*
Non-antibody mediated	Density gradients Centrifugal elutriation E-rosetting Soybean lectin	Cytotoxic drugs – AraG etc.
Antibody-mediated	Panning Magnetic microspheres Magnetic colloids Floating beads Immunorosettes Immunoaffinity columns CD34-based stem-cell selection	Antibody + complement Immunotoxins

E-rosetting and lectin treatment

SBA binds to and agglutinates cells bearing N-acetyl-D-galactosamine which is expressed on all mature blood elements, including T-cells, but not by pluripotent haematopoietic progenitor cells [72]. As a result, the majority of the non-stem cells are crosslinked to form aggregates. These are separated on a gradient of 5% bovine serum albumin [11]. Alternatively, the lectin can be coated onto a plastic surface which is then used to remove SBA-positive cells by panning [73]. Agglutination used alone achieves a 1.26 ± 0.34 log depletion of T-cells (measured by E-rosette formation;

$n = 87$) [11], with preferential removal of CD4+ cells [74], and enrichment of CD34+ cells, colony-forming cells of the granulocyte–macrophage lineage (CFU-GM) and blast forming units – erythroid(BFU-E) [11].

The post-lectin graft contains a $>1 \times 10^5$ T-cell/kg dose associated with a 50% probability of producing grade I or greater GvHD in HLA-matched transplants [68]. These can be removed by rosetting with erythrocytes or by panning over plastic surfaces coated with anti-T-cell antibodies.

E-rosetting

T-lymphocytes possess the CD2 antigen which acts as a receptor for sheep red blood cells. The physiological relevance of this phenomenon is unknown. However, when mixed with sheep erythrocytes, CD2-positive T-cells will form rosettes. This technique was initially used as a method of quantitating T-cells within peripheral blood. Rosette formation changes the size and density of the T-cell population which can then be specifically depleted by sedimentation or density-gradient centrifugation. For additional depletion of SBA-treated grafts, the erythrocytes are pretreated with 2-aminoethylisothiouronium bromide (AET) and irradiated (3000 rads) [11]. The SBA-negative graft cells are mixed with AET-treated erythrocytes, pelleted and incubated on ice for one hour. The gently resuspended rosetted cells are layered onto a Ficoll-Hypaque density cushion and spun at $600\,g \times 25$ minutes. The interface cells are collected and washed prior to infusion [11]. These depletion steps ultimately result in a graft that contains $6.6 \pm 3.6\%$ of the harvested nucleated cells, giving an infused cell dose of $4.4 \pm 6.2 \times 10^7$/kg. There is an overall 2.4 ± 0.5 log depletion of clonable T-cells, translating to a T-cell dose of $0.6 - 32.8 \times 10^4$/kg [11].

Transplantation of 87 grafts processed using the soybean agglutinin–erythrocyte method into 61 HLA-matched and 26 HLA-mismatched recipients resulted in a 3% incidence of grades I–II GvHD in 58 evaluable matches and a 16% incidence in the 25 evaluable mismatches [11]. Results for specific indications have been reported separately [12,13].

Panning

An alternative method for depleting residual T-cells in lectin-treated grafts is panning on a plastic surface coated with antibodies to CD5 and CD8 [75]. A device for this purpose was developed by Applied Immune Sciences (now part of RPR GenCell). SBA-depleted cells are preincubated in 0.1% heat-inactivated gammaglobulin solution (to reduce non-specific binding to the plastic surfaces) and 5×10^8 cells in a final volume of 100 ml in buffered saline containing antibiotics and 1 mM EDTA. Following a one hour incubation, the non-adherent cells are drained into a second device (together with washings from the first device) and incubated for an additional hour. The supernatant cells are then collected, washed and infused.

The overall nucleated cell recovery for this technique is greater than with rosetting, but the frequency of clonable T-cells is similar [11]. This results in a lower overall T-cell depletion and the distribution of CD4+ and CD8+ cells is different. This device has been used in a double-blind trial of T-cell depletion in 57 patients undergoing mismatched related or unrelated transplantation [75]. Methotrexate, cyclosporin and steroids were used for prophylaxis. The study was still blinded at the time of this report. However, in 54 evaluable patients, there were 4 (7%) primary graft failures and 6 patients had no engraftment data. Seventeen have died within 60 days of transplant and 16 (30%) had grade III acute GvHD. Actuarial 100-day survival for all the evaluable patients was $52 \pm 14\%$. These devices are still in clinical trials and are not therefore commercially available.

As an alternative, the SBA-negative fraction can be further depleted using immunomagnetic techniques described later, resulting in a slightly higher overall depletion (3.0–3.5 logs) [76].

The original SBA–erythrocyte rosetting procedure took in excess of 18 hours to complete. However, modifications have now reduced this to seven to ten hours [11]. Improved recoveries of early precursor cells have been described when a triple depletion with neuraminidase-treated erythrocytes was used [77]. Substitution of *Sambucus nigra* agglutinin for soybean agglutinin has also been claimed to improve progenitor cell recovery and decrease graft processing time [78], as has a simplified rosetting procedure [79].

The major concern is the use of animal serum and cells (bovine serum albumin and sheep erythrocytes) in the procedure, as this is now actively discouraged by regulatory agencies. Approval for their use requires extensive testing of lots which can be prohibitively expensive. Nonetheless, there is widespread clinical experience using this method, particularly for transplantation of haplo-identical donors in severe combined immunodeficiency and leukaemia.

Centrifugal elutriation

Centrifugal elutriation separates cells on the basis of their size and density. In this technique, the cells enter a spinning chamber and separate under the influence of the centrifugal force. The effects of this force can be balanced using an opposing force of fluid flow into the spinning chamber, such that when these two forces are in balance, the cells will segregate by their size and density. They may then be harvested sequentially from the chamber by altering the speed of the centrifuge or the fluid flow rate [80,81].

Although this technique has been used to purge tumour cells from autologous bone-marrow grafts [82], the primary application has been in T-cell depletion of allogeneic grafts. The procedure is relatively simple and can be computer assisted [80]. However, the separation hardware is somewhat intimidating and requires an experienced operator. Initially only small-volume elutriation chambers were available, but this is no longer the case, and an adult-sized graft can now be easily processed within eight hours. Since none of the fractions is lost during the procedure and the system is closed, it is possible to recombine the fractions, if required, to achieve the desired T-cell content within the final graft.

One difficulty associated with certain elutriation protocols has been loss of smaller stem cells in the fraction that is to be transplanted [83]. However, this problem has not been seen in all elutriation procedures [84]. The CD34-positive cell population ends up being approximately equally divided between the T-cell depleted and enriched fractions. The depleted fraction contains predominantly the larger CD34-positive committed progenitor population, whereas the T-cell enriched fraction contains the smaller, more primitive stem cells [85]. This has caused concerns about an additional risk of delayed engraftment and graft failure [86] and the solution has been to recover stem cells from the T-cell enriched (small cell) fraction using a CD34-based enrichment technique, and to add these cells back to the T-cell-depleted fraction [83,85]. This results in an engineered cell graft containing a CD34-positive and CFU-GM dose similar to that in the starting marrow, but a T-cell dose of ~6×10^5/kg [85].

The elutriation procedure itself takes approximately four hours from receipt of the unfractionated marrow, and the combined technique with CD34-positive cell addback takes five to six hours. The advantages are the use of a closed system, lack of requirement for biological agents (in the simplified protocol) and the ability to computerize the procedure, including data collection. The disadvantages are the depletion of stem cells, requiring a supplementary procedure involving a biological agent and additional time and expense.

Clinical results obtained using the combined elutriation/positive selection approach have revealed the critical interdependence of *in vitro* and *in vivo* immunomodulation [85]. It was found that CD34-positive cell add-back appeared to overcome allograft rejection mechanisms, with the result that minimal post-bone-marrow transplant (BMT) suppression was required to prevent graft rejection [85]. Patients who received grafts that were T-cell depleted by elutriation alone required a six-month course of cyclosporin A [87]. In contrast, rapid and sustained engraftment, with minimal (<10%) or no acute or chronic GvHD, was achieved using the combined method for graft engineering, and only 80 days of cyclosporin A prophylaxis in a study of 30 patients receiving marrow grafts from matched related donors [88]. It remains to be seen whether similar results can be achieved using only the positive selection step for T-cell depletion.

Extended cycle elutriation has been described for depletion of HLA-disparate grafts [89]. In this procedure, $0.5–0.75 \times 10^5$ T-cells/kg were added back to elutriated harvests from 10 patients with haematopoietic malignancies to promote engraftment and a GvL effect. Double-cycle elutriation was employed to deplete >3 logs of T-cells. The patients received combination chemotherapy, total body irradiation and pre- and post-BMT immunosuppression. All engrafted, but 5 (50%) developed grade II or III GvHD and 2 (20%) subsequently developed chronic GvHD. Two patients (20%) have relapsed at a median of 206 days (46–1035 days) and 4 (40%) have died of BMT-related complications.

Drug-mediated techniques

The use of cytotoxic drugs to engineer grafts has been largely restricted to tumour purging in autologous transplantation. Some methods have been developed for purging T-cell acute lymphoblastic leukaemias and lymphomas and it has been proposed that these could be used for T-cell depletion of allografts [90,91]. The combination of the two nucleosides 2′-deoxycoformycin (dCF) (Pentostatin) and 2′-deoxyadenosine (dAdo) has been shown to exhibit selective toxicity towards T-cells in normal bone marrow [90]. By careful optimization and timing of the incubation procedures, 1.5–2.5 log depletions can be achieved, without significant toxicity towards normal myeloid and erythroid progenitors. Ficoll Hypaque-separated cells with a final haematocrit of <5% are initially incubated with dCF for 30–60 minutes at 37°C in medium containing irradiated plasma. To this mixture is added the dAdo and the cells are incubated for 18 hours at 37°C on a shaker/rocker. The cells are then washed extensively prior to infusion.

9-Beta-D-arabinofuranosylguanine (araG), a nucleoside analogue, has been used *in vivo* for the treatment of T-cell leukaemias and for purging autologous grafts in murine models [91]. In T-cells it is converted to its corresponding arabinosylguanine nucleotide triphosphate, which results in inhibition of DNA synthesis. Incubation of freshly isolated T-leukaemia cells or lymphoblastoid cell lines with 100 μM araG for 18 hours eliminated 6 logs of clonogenic T-cells. Under the same conditions, committed myeloid and erythroid colony-forming cells were not significantly inhibited.

L-Leucyl-L-leucine methyl ester (LLME) is a lysosomotropic agent that is selectively toxic to human and murine precursor and effector cytotoxic cells including T-cells, NK cells and monocytes [92,93]. In animal studies [92], pre-incubation of allogeneic marrow and spleen cells with LLME completely protected 30 recipients from lethal GvHD, and engraftment was improved compared to that seen in antibody and complement-treated grafts. Incubations of human cells with 50–250 μM LLME resulted in ablation of NK cell effectors, lymphokine activated killer (LAK) precursors and effectors and alloantigen specific cytotoxic T-cells, although resistant T-cells were seen in some individuals. Concentrations of 100–250 μM partially or completely inhibited colony formation by committed myeloid, erythroid and monocyte progenitor cells [93]. Transplants have been performed with LLME-treated grafts with successful engraftment in the recipients (A. Pecora, personal communication). However, these data have yet to be published.

Monoclonal antibodies

T-cell identification and subsetting was greatly facilitated by the development of monoclonal antibodies (MAb) directed against cell-surface antigens. Numerous antibodies are now available which distinguish T-cells from other leukocytes (pan T-cell antibodies) and which differentiate between subsets of T-cells. These antibodies are frequently directed against antigens with biological activity, and therefore may potentially be used to alter the functional integrity of the graft to achieve a particular clinical outcome. It is also true, as a consequence, that these antigens cannot be regarded simply as inert and passive markers. Their use to mediate cell separation may trigger a functional response within the cell, which may affect the separation procedure itself, or even the activity of other cells within the graft. The most commonly used CD targets include CD2, 3, 5 and 6 for pan T-cell depletion and CD4 and 8 for T-cell subset depletion (see later). The choice of marker will also depend upon the method used to eliminate the antibody-sensitized cells, for example IgG_{2a} or IgM mouse MAb must be used for C′-mediated depletions [94], and we have found that mouse-anti-CD3 IgG antibodies cannot be used effectively with paramagnetic microspheres [95]. Although a variety of antibodies have been used clinically, by far the greatest experience has been with the CAMPATH series [96].

Monoclonal antibodies and complement

The ability of cell-bound MAb to fix and activate C′ has been widely used for *ex vivo* T-cell depletion. Complement, in the form of unfractionated animal serum, or autologous serum or plasma, represents an efficient physiological method of lysing cells, through the assembly and insertion of an attack complex of C′ component proteins into the membrane, with resulting colloid osmotic lysis of the cell [94]. Efficient activation of the C′ cascade requires crosslinkage of the C1q component by a doublet of IgG molecules or a single IgM antibody molecule. Cells with low expression of the target antigen will therefore tend to escape complement-mediated lysis initiated by IgG molecules [97,98]. This can be an advantage for T-cell depletion applications, where a small number of residual cells is believed to facilitate engraftment. Antibody sensitization is performed in the cold (4°C), or at ambient temperature depending upon the lability and motility of the target antigen, whereas incubation with the C' source is carried out at ambient temperature or at 37°C. In most cases xenogeneic whole serum is used, although certain rat MAb (e.g. CAMPATH-1 antibodies) are capable of fixing human C' [96]. In these cases, *ex vivo* treatment with the MAb, followed by infusion into the patient can achieve adequate levels of T-cell depletion, mediated through the presence *ex vivo* of residual C' proteins in the harvested graft, and/or by patient C' *in vivo* [99]. When animal serum is used as the C' source, the treated graft is extensively washed prior to infusion [96]. In addition, it is necessary to screen multiple batches of C' to find one with low levels of non-specific (direct) toxicity towards haematopoietic cells. Commercial sources are available (e.g. from Pel-Freez, Brown Deer, Wisconsin and from C-Six Diagnostics, Mequon, Wisconsin, USA). These reagents should be used under an investigational new drug exemption (IND) from the Food and Drug Administration.

We have found that non-specific toxicity may become apparent when incubation temperatures are increased beyond 22–24°C (unpublished observations). In certain grafts, excessive clumping of cells may occur during incubation with MAb and C', primarily due to lysis of T-cells and release of DNA into the cell suspension. Addition of DNase to the incubation mixture can reverse this effect, and highly purified and recombinant forms of this enzyme are now available [100].

There are, in addition, a number of anticomplementary factors that may interfere with T-cell lysis [101]. These range from a decay-accelerating factor associated with nucleated marrow cells [101,102], to the presence of heparin and heparin fragments [103]. These are generally adequately diluted out during the preparation of the mononuclear cell suspension. Chelating anticoagulants such as anticoagulant citrate dextrose-A (ACD-A) can completely inhibit C' activity and should be avoided, or removed by extensive washing prior to incubation with MAb and C'.

Control of C'-mediated lysis is virtually impossible, and in most applications excess concentrations of both the MAb and C' are added to the reaction mixture, which is allowed to go to the reaction end-point. Surprisingly, this can achieve remarkably reproducible levels of T-cell depletion in a well-characterized system. However, since the target cells are lysed in the process, this approach does not permit recovery and analysis of the T-cell population. The presence of dead or dying target cells and of cell debris can make the analysis of depletion by flow cytometry difficult to interpret. Incubation of samples for an additional hour at 37°C can facilitate analysis, as can the use of vital stains, such as 7-amino actinomycin D (7-AAD).

The Food and Drug Administration discourages the use of animal sera for human therapeutic procedures, and requires that C' meets the same testing standards as are currently mandated for MAb products intended for intravenous infusion [104]. Several manufacturers are striving to meet this goal. However, it is likely that other Mab-mediated methods for T-cell depletion will ultimately replace the use of C'.

CAMPATH antibodies

The CAMPATH series of rat MAb are directed against a glycoprotein that is attached to the lymphocyte membrane via a lipid anchor [105]. These antibodies efficiently activate the human C' cascade and have therefore found widespread use for T-cell depletion (Table 32.3).

The majority of antibodies in the initial CAMPATH-1 series were IgM or IgG_{2c} monoclonals, although a single IgG_{2a} was also isolated [106]. These antibodies bound to virtually all human T- and B-cells, in addition to macrophages and monocytes [96], and to most lymphoid leukaemic cells, but to only a

Table 32.3 CAMPATH series of rat monoclonal antibodies

- Directed against a glycoprotein attached to the lymphocyte membrane via a lipid anchor
- Activate the human C' cascade and have found widespread use for T-cell depletion
- Majority of antibodies in the initial CAMPATH-1 series were IgM or IgG_{2c} monoclonals, although a single IgG_{2a} was also isolated

minority of myeloid leukaemias [107]. The antigen identified by these antibodies has been designated as CDw52 [108], and is not expressed significantly by normal colony-forming haematopoietic progenitor cells (Table 32.4). Variable levels of expression on primate leukocytes and on cells of the erythroid lineage have also been described [96]. The CAMPATH antigen is thought to be a 12 amino acid glycoprotein with a single N-linked carbohydrate and a glycosyl-phosphatidyl anchor at the C-terminus [109].

CAMPATH-1M (the IgM monoclonal) has been used in combination with donor serum to purge T-cells from HLA-matched grafts and was found in a series of 11 patients to be effective for preventing GvHD, even in the absence of post-transplant immunosuppression. However, graft failure was reported in 3 patients [110]. This was thought to be primarily due to immunological rejection. In a subsequent analysis of patients transplanted for malignant diseases [111], the incidence of acute GvHD greater than grade I was 17% and greater than grades III–IV was 7%. The incidence of graft failure was ~20% but could be reduced to ~13% by the use of cyclosporin A, and combined use of cyclosporin A and total lymphoid irradiation (TLI) further reduced the incidence to ~4% in a small cohort of patients.

In an attempt to reduce the incidence of graft failure further, CAMPATH-1G (IgG$_{2b}$) was administered to patients at a dose of 5–10 mg/day for five days before starting chemotherapy [96]. The protocol used to T-cell deplete the graft was left unchanged, and the patients did not receive other GvHD prophylaxis. *In vivo* administration of the MAb was shown by limiting dilution analysis to produce T-cell depletions equivalent to those achieved using total body irradiation or busulfan plus cyclophosphamide [112]. Using this approach in HLA-matched transplants, the incidence of graft failure was reduced to ~9%, there was only 2% severe acute GvHD with no severe chronic GvHD, and leukaemia-free survival was improved [96].

Based upon these data, CAMPATH-1G was used to opsonize T-cells within the graft [99,113], with the intent that these cells would be lysed when infused into the patients, and was also administered *in vivo* to the recipients at or around the time of transplant. Use of CAMPATH-1G to treat the graft without addition of C′ resulted in a low incidence of severe GvHD and graft failure, and improvements in transplant-related mortality and leukaemia-free survival in patients who predominantly received TLI without post-transplant immunosuppression. Lysis of cells within the graft is achieved within ~30 minutes in the presence of residual donor plasma, but can also occur when grafts are separated on Ficoll and washed prior to addition of the antibody [96]. When the MAb was administered *in vivo* to patients who received no other post-BMT immunosuppression [114], the incidence of severe acute GvHD was increased to ~17% (although better than would be expected without GvHD prophylaxis). However, there was higher severe chronic GvHD and substantial transplant-related mortality.

When *ex vivo* and *in vivo* use was combined in a small study of 28 patients, none suffered from GvHD, but there was a 25% incidence of graft failure [96]. This may, in part, be due to the delay of about five days in engraftment that was seen in patients who received CAMPATH-1G *in vivo* [111]. This effect was thought to be due to the possible elimination of a lymphocyte subset(s) that facilitates engraftment [96].

In a review of the use of CAMPATH antibodies for *in vitro* and *in vivo* T-cell depletion in matched sibling transplants [96] with a ten-year follow-up, the risk of relapse in acute myelogenous leukaemia and acute lymphoblastic leukaemia plateaued at ~30%, whereas in chronic myelogenous leukaemia the risk of relapse continued for at least five years and plateaued at ~60% at seven years. This confirms the importance of a GvL effect in chronic myelogenous leukaemia. Attempts to produce such an effect in patients with acute leukaemia, following transplantation of CAMPATH-

---

Table 32.4 CAMPATH antibodies

- Bind to:
  Virtually all human T- and B-cells
  Macrophages and monocytes
  Most lymphoid leukaemic cells
  Only a minority of myeloid leukaemias

- The antigen identified by these antibodies has been designated as CDw52 and is not expressed significantly by normal colony-forming haematopoietic progenitor cells

treated matched sibling grafts, by the administration of graded increments of donor leukocytes, were associated with clinically significant GvHD and with a decreased relapse rate, which was most apparent in patients with acute lymphoblastic leukaemia [56].

An analysis of the use of CAMPATH-1 antibodies in 180 non-HLA identical transplants (MUD and partially mismatched related donor transplants) [96] showed that there was a 14% incidence of severe acute GvHD in evaluable patients. However, the incidence of graft failure was 51% in patients who did not receive the antibody *in vivo*. In those who died, the incidence was reduced to 24%. These results were not substantially altered by the use of conventional GvHD prophylaxis.

The incidence of lymphoproliferative disorders or secondary lymphomas following the use of CAMPATH antibodies has been very small (10 cases out of 1529 transplants) [115], and there has been no evidence of increased fatal infections compared to other forms of GvHD prophylaxis, although slow T-cell recovery and a high incidence of cytomegalovirus (CMV) viremia have been described [96].

These results are consistent with the pan T-cell depletion achieved with CAMPATH antibodies and improvements may be achieved by adding back T-cells or T-cell subsets to the graft and/or to the patients post-transplant.

Other monoclonal antibodies and complement

The majority of other MAb used for graft manipulation have been derived from mouse hybridomas and do not fix human C′ efficiently (Table 32.5). For this reason they are primarily used *ex vivo* and C′, usually in the form of whole baby rabbit serum, is added exogenously.

Anti-CD3

The anti-CD3 MAb OKT3 was the first MAb approved by the Food and Drug Administration in the United States for therapeutic applications. It is approved for *in vivo* administration for treatment of acute renal allograft rejection and for steroid-resistant acute cardiac and hepatic allograft rejection [116]. In these applications, it binds to and blocks the function of the 20 000 dalton CD3 antigen receptor. Binding of the MAb results in early mitogenic activation of T-cells, leading to release of cytokines [117], and myeloid colony-stimulating factors (e.g. GM-CSF) [118] and

Table 32.5 Other monoclonal antibodies used with complement for graft manipulation

- Pan T-cell antibody combinations (anti-CD2 + CD3 and anti-CD2 + CD5 + CD7)
- Anti-CD2
- Anti-CD3
- Anti-CD6
- Anti-$\alpha\beta$

blocking of cellular function. The antibody has been infused to treat steroid-resistant GvHD [119] and used to activate T-cells *in vitro* for potential use in adoptive anticancer immunotherapy [120,121].

Early *in vitro* studies indicated that, in combination with C′, it eliminated >90% of T-cells, but that combinations of MAb were required to achieve >99% depletion [122]. OKT3 opsonization of marrow cells from histocompatible sibling donors was studied in ten patients with haematological malignancies [123]. Concentrated nucleated marrow cells were incubated with 1 mg OKT3 for 30 minutes at 4°C prior to infusion. All recipients engrafted in a mean of 22 days, and 9 of the 10 survived for more than 100 days. However, 5 recipients developed acute GvHD. Addition of neonatal rabbit C′ to the opsonized cells resulted in a 96% reduction in the mitogenic response of the cells [123]. Using a similar opsonization protocol (but incubation at ambient temperature), 17 patients received OKT3 treated HLA-matched or minor mismatched grafts in a protocol that included prophylactic methotrexate [124]. Three recipients developed grade II GvHD or greater, which was fatal in 2 cases when complicated by CMV infection. One patient developed transient grade I GvHD and the remainder showed no evidence. The overall incidence of GvHD was 18% in this study, in comparison to an historical incidence of 79%. In this study it was anticipated that the opsonized T-cells would be lysed recipient C′. However, it has been demonstrated that OKT3-sensitized cells are not effectively lysed by fresh human autologous C′ [125].

Anti-CD3 MAb and C′ have been used to T-cell deplete one- to three-antigen mismatched related or closely-matched unrelated marrow grafts for transplantation to 6 children with juvenile chronic myelogenous leukaemia [126]. All engrafted granulocytes and platelets within 21 days, and developed grade II or less GvHD. Two died of infection, 1 relapsed at day 177 and died at day 939 and 3 were alive and well at the time of the report, at 180–2400 days.

We have also used anti-CD3 MAb [OKT3] for *ex vivo* T-cell depletion of related partially-mismatched allografts [127]. In an attempt to develop a 'Food and Drug Administration-friendly' procedure, we substituted OKT3, in an off-label indication, for T10B9 [127] (see later). Using a closed system, mononuclear marrow cells were separated on Ficoll Hypaque from heparinized harvests obtained from donors mismatched at one to three major HLA loci. These cells were resuspended at 3×10^7/ml in lactated Ringer's solution containing 0.5% v/v plasma protein fraction (PPF), and incubated for 30 minutes on ice with 10 μg OKT3/ml. Screened baby rabbit C' was added to give a final 50% v/v concentration and the mixture was rotated at ambient temperature for 90 minutes. The cells were then washed, adjusted to a concentration of 5×10^7/ml, in a final volume of 50–200 ml, and re-infused into the recipients. This method resulted in a median of a 2.49 log depletion (range 1.51–3.97, $n = 110$) of T-cells, as determined by limiting dilution analysis. Patients received a median T-cell dose of 4.63×10^4/kg (range 3.34–58.2) and a median total nucleated cell dose of 8.7×10^7/kg (range 0.24–3.21). The probability of engraftment was 98%, with a median of 15 days to a neutrophil count of 1000/μl. The incidence of acute GvHD of grades II–IV was 32% and of grades III–IV was 16% ($n = 109$). These early clinical results compare very favourably with those that we have previously obtained using an anti-αβ MAb (T10B9; see later) and C'. In spite of the lower infused T-cell dose, due to the pan specificity of OKT3 stable engraftment was achieved with a comparably low incidence of GvHD.

OKT3 has been used in combination with anti-CD2 (OKT11) to purge T-cells from matched sibling donor grafts in 10 patients with poor-prognosis haematological diseases, who received post-BMT methotrexate (MTX) for 11–100 days. Use of the two antibodies resulted in depletion of 88.3% ± 11.8% of T-cells with 75.8 ± 12.2% recovery of myeloid progenitors. All patients engrafted (23.3 ± 5.1 days to 500 granulocytes/μl) and no GvHD was observed. At the time of the report, 7 of the 10 were alive and well in continuous remission at 2–10 months post-BMT [128].

In a mouse model for matched unrelated donor transplantation for leukaemia [129], depletion of $CD3^+$ cells using antibody and C' resulted in a decrease in death due to GvHD (from 37 to 6%), but an increase in disease relapse (from 30 to 62%). In contrast, depletion with anti-CD5 MAb and C' had no effect on relapse or GvHD, but significantly increased graft failure and thereby decreased overall survival.

Anti-CD2
Anti-CD2 antibodies, predominantly the CT-2 MAb, have also been used in combination with C' in early T-cell-depletion studies. Treatment of grafts results in 99% depletion of T-cells, as assessed by E-rosette formation and flow cytometry [130]. In a prospective, randomized double-blind trial of 40 patients with leukaemia [131], the incidence of acute GvHD was reduced from 65% in those receiving T-replete grafts, to 15% in those infused with CT-2-treated marrow. There were no graft failures in the non-manipulated graft recipients, but a 12.5% incidence of graft failure with T-cell-depleted grafts. There was a higher, but not statistically different rate of relapse in patients receiving the T-depleted grafts (7 patients in the CT-2-treated group versus 2 patients in the control group), and residual leukaemia was detected by cytogenetics in 5 other patients in the experimental arm. Overall survival was similar in both groups. Using the same MAb in a study of 8 histocompatible and 15 non-histocompatible transplants, prompt engraftment with minimal GvHD was seen in 7 of the 8 histocompatible cases, in spite of no post-BMT GvHD prophylaxis. In contrast, 11 of the 15 non-histocompatible recipients failed to engraft, and grades II–IV GvHD were seen in 2 of the 4 who did engraft [130]. Clinical outcomes could not be related to the results of *in vitro* analyses of the T-cell-depleted grafts.

Anti-CD6
Anti-CD6 MAb recognize an antigen that is present on mature T-cells, but not B-cells, NK cells or myeloid precursors. In a study of 112 HLA-identical sibling donor transplants for haematological malignancies,

grafts were purged with three cycles of anti-CD6 MAb (anti-T12) antibody and rabbit C′ (with no prophylactic post-BMT immunosuppression) [132]. Eighteen percent of patients developed grades II–IV GvHD and 8 patients suffered chronic GvHD. Three of 112 (2.7%) patients failed to engraft and 1 patient developed late graft failure associated with CMV infection. In a subgroup of 50 good-risk patients, the probability of three-year disease-free survival was estimated at 50% with a 44-month median follow-up.

In a subsequent ten-year review of the use of this antibody for T-cell depletion of 171 HLA-matched grafts [133], initial engraftment was 98%, with 96% achieving stable haematological reconstitution. Fifteen percent of patients developed acute GvHD, while 5% experienced chronic GvHD, and transplant-related mortality was 17%. The authors suggest that administration of interleukin-2 (IL-2) post-BMT expands the numbers of circulating NK cells and may be associated with a decrease in disease relapse rates.

A combination of anti-CD6 and anti-CD8 with C′ has been used to treat the grafts of 31 HLA-matched donor–recipient pairs [134]. Grafts were processed on a COBE 2991 cell processor, incubated with a combination of MAb, and treated with two rounds of rabbit C′. One patient died too early for evaluation, 1 failed to engraft and of the 29 remaining evaluable patients, 22 (76%) had no acute GvHD at a minimum of 60 days post-BMT, 6 (21%) had grade I and 1 had grade III acute GvHD. Again, there was no clear correlation between the T-cell content of the graft and clinical outcome.

A subsequent review of 37 HLA-matched transplants using grafts depleted with this combination of MAb showed that the recipients regained low normal numbers of CD8$^+$ cells at 60 days post-BMT, but that reconstitution of CD4$^+$ cells required $\geq$150 days. In previous studies where efficient T-cell depletion was not achieved, there was an overshoot of CD8$^+$ cells during the first 60 days [135].

T-cell depletion using anti-CD6 + anti-CD8 and C′ was compared to GvHD prophylaxis with cyclosporin A and methotrexate (four doses) in a randomized trial in 46 leukaemia patients receiving HLA-identical sibling transplants [136]. All but 1 patient engrafted, although the pace of engraftment was faster in recipients of T-depleted marrows. These patients had a higher incidence of grades II–III acute GvHD (23% versus 12%) and of chronic GvHD (51% versus 23%). Relapse was the primary cause of death in this study. At four years, the cumulative incidence was 39% for recipient of T-depleted grafts and 54% in the cyclosporin A + methotrexate group.

Anti $\alpha\beta$

T10B9.1A31, an IgM MAb which reacts with the $\alpha\beta$ heterodimer of the T-cell receptor, has been extensively used to treat kidney allograft rejection [137], and for T-cell depletion of allogeneic marrow grafts from matched sibling [42], closely-matched unrelated donors [138,139] and partially mismatched related donors [22,140].

In a study of 48 chronic myelogenous leukaemia patients, 28 of whom were mismatched at one or more major HLA loci, who received T10B9-treated grafts and post-BMT cyclosporin A, 94% achieved durable engraftment, and the actuarial probability of developing grades II–IV GvHD and grades III–IV were 39.6% and 8.3% respectively [139]. There was no difference in the incidence of grades II–IV GvHD between those receiving matched (36.8% incidence) or mismatched grafts (41.4%). The probability of two-year disease-free survival was 49% in the former group and 51% in the latter. As described previously, in a subsequent comparative analysis of the relapse rates in patients receiving T10B9-depleted HLA-identical sibling donor grafts compared to those transplanted with similarly processed grafts from unrelated donors, there was a lower relapse rate in the unrelated donor group [42]. This was attributed to a GvL effect associated with the increased HLA disparity [42].

We have used T10B9 to purge T-cells from grafts obtained from partially mismatched related donors [127]. Mononuclear marrow cells were resuspended at 3×10^7/ml in lactated Ringer's solution containing 0.5% v/v PPF and incubated for 30 minutes on ice with 10 µg T10B9/ml. Screened baby rabbit C′ was added to give a final 50% v/v concentration, and the mixture rotated at ambient temperature for 90 minutes. The cells were then washed, adjusted to a concentration of 5×10^7/ml and re-infused into the recipients. This method resulted in a median 1.85 log depletion (range 1.15–4.48, $n = 98$) of T-cells, as determined by limiting dilution analysis (LDA). Patients received a median T-cell dose of 6.77×10^4/kg (range 1.5–60.0) and a nucleated cell dose of 1.42×10^8/kg (range 0.54–3.65).

The probability of engraftment in these patients was 90%, with a median of 18 days to a neutrophil count of 1000/μl. The incidence of grades II–IV GvHD was 21% and of grades III–IV was 11% ($n = 98$).

Pan T-cell antibody combinations
Combinations of pan T-cell antibodies (anti-CD2 + CD3 and anti-CD2 + CD5 + CD7) have been used together with C' to treat HLA-identical grafts in a study of 51 patients with various acute leukaemias or chronic myelogenous leukaemia, the majority of whom were given total body irradiation plus cyclophosphamide as conditioning therapy, and did not receive post-BMT immunosuppressive prophylaxis. Ten patients (19.1%) either failed to engraft or suffered graft failure, and 12 patients (23%) died within three months of 'graft-related' complications. Graft failure was found to be associated with the number of CFU-GM and the dose of T-cells infused.

The observation that the combination of MAb to CD2, 5 and 7 spares normal long-term colony-forming cells in human marrow has been taken to indicate that these graft failures are not attributable to direct toxicity towards stem cells [141]. A later multicentre study used this antibody combination and a single round of C' to treat the HLA-matched grafts for 62 consecutive patients with poor prognosis haematological malignancies. Twenty-six patients received post-BMT GvHD prophylaxis with either MTX or cyclosporin A. The mean T-cell dose was $0.66 \pm 0.56 \times 10^6$ cells/kg. In agreement with the previous study, the incidence of graft failure was 19%, but there was only one case of greater than grade II acute GvHD. Graft failure was attributed primarily to lack of radiotherapy in the conditioning regimen, fractionation of the total body irradiation and patient age >30 years. In contrast, the dose of nucleated cells or T-lymphocytes did not seem to influence engraftment [142].

Immunotoxins
Rather than using a generic agent to destroy MAb-sensitized T-cells, a toxic moiety can be directly conjugated to each antibody molecule to create an immunotoxin. This provides a highly specific method for delivering the killing agent to the target cell surface. However, it must then be translocated through the membrane to reach its primary site of action. Although a variety of toxins have been tested, the initial experience was mainly with ricin, a plant toxin derived from the castor bean. The issues associated with the synthesis and use of ricin-based immunoconjugates are discussed more fully in the chapter on autologous stem cell purging. In brief, the toxic activity is associated with the A chain of the molecule, whereas the B chain facilitates transport into the cell, but also binds to galactosyl residues on the cell surface. When the intact toxin molecule is used, therefore, it is necessary to block this non-antibody-directed binding by adding fluid-phase lactose during incubation with the cells. Although the problem can be overcome by using A chain immunotoxins, these tend to be less potent, necessitating the addition of lysosomotropic amines or carboxylic ionophores to improve transport to the site of action within the cytoplasm.

Several MAb have been conjugated to ricin for T-cell depletion, including anti-CD3, 5, 6, 4 and 8 [143]. The CD3 and CD5 antigens would appear to be particularly suitable targets since they cap and internalize once bound by the antibody, facilitating incorporation of the toxin into the target cell. Both the intact ricin molecule and the A chain have been used in conjugates with intact antibody molecules or with the F[ab']$_2$ fragment.

Early studies using an anti-CD3 MAb conjugated to ricin A chain to treat HLA-identical grafts produced disappointing results [144]. Treatment with the immunotoxin achieved a 3 log depletion of CD3$^+$ cells, and prevention of acute GvHD without the use of post-BMT immunosuppression; however, there was a 25% incidence (2 of 8) of graft failure. In an attempt to prevent the anti-CD3 MAb activating the T-cells, conjugates have been prepared using the F[ab']$_2$ fragment coupled to deglycosylated ricin A chain [145]. In animal studies, this immunotoxin produced >95% inhibition of T-cell mitogenesis *in vitro*, and when administered *in vivo* in an aggressive acute GvHD murine model it depleted ~80% of T-cells in the recipients and was beneficial in the treatment of established GvHD.

The majority of reported clinical studies have, however, focused on the use of anti-CD5-based immunotoxins. Ricin A chain conjugates prepared with the F[ab']$_2$ fragment of an anti-CD5 MAb (T101) were found to be two orders of magnitude more effective for T-cell depletion than those made with the intact antibody, and this activity was increased further by carrying out incubation with the marrow cells at pH 7.8 [146]. In an early clinical study using this approach [147], 99.5% depletion of T-cells was achieved, with a 9.1% actuarial rate of acute GvHD; however, there was an 18% incidence of graft failure in this study.

An anti-CD5 IgG$_{2a}$/ricin A-chain immunotoxin was used by Antin and colleagues [148] to purge the grafts of 55 patients (38 HLA matched and 17 mismatched) with acute or chronic leukaemia ($n = 53$) or myelodysplastic syndrome ($n = 2$). Patients were conditioned using cytosine arabinoside, cyclophosphamide and total body irradiation. Mononuclear cells were enriched from the harvested marrow, washed in Hank's balanced salt solution containing 0.5% human serum albumin (HSA) and resuspended in RPMI-1640 containing 5% human serum albumin, with L-glutamine and without sodium bicarbonate. The cell concentration was adjusted to achieve a final concentration of 2×10^7/ml and a haematocrit <3% during incubation with the immunotoxin. The immunotoxin was added to the incubation mixture, which also contained 20mM ammonium chloride and 5% tromethamine (at a final pH of 7.8 ± 0.15 at ambient temperature) to a final concentration of 10^{-8}M ricin A chain. Incubation was performed in transfer packs on a rocker for two hours at 37°C. The pH at the end of the reaction was typically 7.6 ± 0.1. The treated grafts were infused without filtering over the course of 30 minutes. T-cell depletion efficiency was assessed using assays for proliferation and function of the cells, rather than viability after treatment, since cytotoxicity requires division of the cells.

In this study, four assays were used: flow cytometric analysis after a five-day incubation with phytohaemagglutinin and interleukin-2, T-cell proliferation, limiting dilution analysis and colony assays for committed haematopoietic progenitor cells. This protocol routinely depleted >95% T-cells resulting in an average T-cell dose of $6.2 \pm 4.9 \times 10^5$/kg (as measured by LDA). The grafts were enriched for γδ T-cells, B-cells and NK cells. Treatment had no effect on normal colony-forming cells. All patients engrafted at a median of 18 days (12–33 day range) to 500 granulocytes/ml. Platelet engraftment (>50 000/μl) was achieved in 31 days (14–82 days) for the matched patients and 29 days (14–122 days) for the mismatched recipients. Late graft failures occurred in 2 of the matched cases (5.2%; both myelodysplastic syndromes) and 1 of the mismatched cases (4.2%; a patient with CMV hepatitis at the time of failure). Of the HLA-matched transplants evaluable for GvHD, grades II–III acute GvHD occurred in 10 of 39 (26%) and all responded to methylprednisolone. There were no cases of grade IV GvHD or deaths from GvHD. Four patients subsequently developed lymphoproliferative disorders at days 60–118 post-transplant. Three of these patients died, and although the lymphoma in the fourth responded to donor buffy-coat infusions, the patient died from grade IV acute GvHD. Four of 30 patients (13%) developed chronic GvHD. In the mismatched group, grades II–IV acute GvHD was seen in 7 of 17 patients (41%) and 3 died of grade IV GvHD. No chronic GvHD was seen in 9 evaluable cases.

An anti-CD5-ricin immunotoxin was also used to T-cell deplete histocompatible marrow grafts in a study of 29 patients with advanced leukaemia [149]. Donor cell engraftment was documented in all but 1 case. Increasing the dose of immunotoxin used from 300 to 1000 ng resulted in a statistically significant reduction in the incidence of acute GvHD (from 100 to 34%). There was no correlation between the dose of T-cells infused, as determined by LDA, and subsequent GvHD. However, a correlation was observed with the presence of viable CD5$^-$ T-cells in samples of the T-depleted graft that had been cultured for 16 days with Interleukin-2 (IL-2).

Depletion of specific T-cell subsets has been used in an attempt to eliminate cells mediating GvHD, while retaining those responsible for a GvL response. In murine marrow models, it has been shown that depletion of CD8$^+$ cells is sufficient to reduce or prevent GvHD following transplantation of grafts that were matched at major histocompatibility loci but mismatched at minor loci [33,34]. This approach has been examined in clinical trials using grafts depleted of CD8$^+$ cells by immunomagnetic separation (see later) and potentially suitable immunotoxins have been prepared using anti-CD4 and anti-CD8 MAb [150]. These were capable of killing at least 3 logs of T-cells and inhibited clonal proliferation in a dose-dependent manner with minimal effects on normal myeloid and erythroid colony-forming cells.

The IL-2 receptor has also been used as the target for immunotoxin-mediated T-cell depletion [151,152]. In laboratory studies, Cavazzana-Calvo et al. [153] activated host blood and marrow T-cells by exposure to recipient cells in a two-day mixed leukocyte culture, and were able to show that incubation with the anti-IL-2 ricin immunotoxin destroyed IL-2 receptor-positive T-cells and completely inhibited a primary MLC and cytotoxic activity, with minimal effect on alloreactivity towards a third party's cells. The treatment produced a 20–50-fold reduction in antihost activity without affecting normal colony-forming progenitor cells. A similar approach was used by Chaudhary et al. [154], who developed a recombinant single-chain immunotoxin composed of the variable regions of an anti-Tac MAb and truncated diphtheria toxin. This showed specific cytotoxicity towards cells bearing the p55 subunit of the IL-2 receptor and killed activated human T-cells generated in a mixed leukocyte reaction.

Attempts to target the leukocyte function antigen LFA1, which is present on cytolytic T-cells, NK cells and monocytes, were made in a murine model [155] using an anti-LFA1–ricin A-chain immunotoxin. Incubation of marrow cells with the immunotoxin for two hours in the presence of ammonium chloride reduced cytolytic T-cell activity by 2 logs, significantly reduced NK-cell activity and was capable of preventing GvHD in certain recipient–donor mouse strain pairs. A significant incidence of allo-engraftment failure was seen and attributed to removal of stem cells or essential accessory cell populations, which may require supplementation by addback of positively selected cells.

Although most studies have used ricin as the toxic moiety, a number of other toxins have been tested. These include pokeweed antiviral protein (PAP), diphtheria toxin and various enzymes [156]. A 3-log depletion of marrow T-cells was described using an anti-CDw52 pan-leukocyte MAb coupled to glucose oxidase and lactoperoxidase [157]. The two conjugates act synergistically by producing toxic hydrogen peroxide and halides. In order to do so, they are first incubated with marrow cells, which are then washed and incubated with the specific substrates for the enzymes in the immunotoxins. This treatment did not affect normal myeloid or erythroid precursors. PAP is a hemitoxin which depurinates ribosomes. The toxin lacks the B chain and its associated non-specific binding properties. Immunotoxins have been prepared using PAP and used predominantly for purging tumour cells from autologous marrow grafts [158].

T-cell-directed immunotoxins (predominantly directed against the CD5 antigen) have also been used *in vivo*, with variable success, to prevent or treat acute GvHD, alone or in combination with T-cell depletion of the graft [22,159–161].

Immunomagnetic T-cell depletion
Microspheres
Antibody-sensitized T-cells can be captured onto a solid phase, which can then be separated from the cell mixture. This provides a method for physically separating the T-cells from the graft, thereby avoiding the addition of potentially toxic agents, and the release of cellular contents from dead or dying cells. One of the most convenient solid phases for effecting this type of separation is the paramagnetic particle. This material can be reacted either directly with the anti T-cell MAb, or with an anti-immunoglobulin antibody, as a second-step reagent. The types of particles, their advantages and disadvantages, collection methods, etc. are discussed in detail in the chapter on purging tumor cells from autologous grafts. The most widely clinically used particle is the superparamagnetic microsphere manufactured by Dynal. These have been extensively employed for tumour purging, but are equally suitable for T-cell depletion of allografts. For tumour purging applications, where the aim is complete capture of all target cells, it is necessary to use multiple tumour-directed MAb for identification of the target population, which is then interacted with anti-immunoglobulin antibody-coated beads. In the case of T-cell depletion, we and others have shown that effective depletions can be achieved using a one-step procedure (direct immunomagnetic separation) [95]. In this technique, the anti-T-cell MAb can be passively adsorbed to the polystyrene beads, in the case of IgM MAb, or the anti-Ig coated microspheres can be reacted with IgG anti-T-cell MAb. The washed beads are stable for long periods and can be added directly to a mononuclear cell preparation of the graft. Rosettes of beads and T-cells are formed rapidly (although an incubation time of 1–2 hours at 4°C, with continuous gentle mixing is usually recommended), and these can be removed by exposure of the treated graft to a magnetic field generated by externally placed permanent magnets. Separation is usually accomplished by two exposures to the magnets. In the first, the transfer pack containing the cells is placed

onto the magnets and a static separation is performed. The non-rosetted cells are then drained or pumped from the pack and passed in continuous flow over a second magnetic array, to capture any free beads and rosetted T-cells that escaped the first separation.

In our hands, anti-CD3 MAb are not suitable for immunomagnetic T-cell depletion using microspheres [95]. During separation, breakages occurred at various points between the cell and the beads. This may be partly due to activation of the T-cells and capping and internalization of the antigen antibody complex. Attempts to resolve this problem by using anti-CD3 coated anti-Ig beads, and by increasing the bead to T-cell ratio were only partially successful, and superior results were routinely achieved using anti-CD2 or anti-CD-5 MAb [95].

Clinical studies using indirect immunomagnetic separation and anti-CD3 (OKT3) have, however, been described [162], in which residual T-cells were quantitated by flow cytometry. A 1.7-log depletion of CD3$^+$ cells was described, which correlated significantly with the depletion of CD5$^+$ cells. The median infused dose of CD3$^+$, CD4$^+$ and CD8$^+$ cells was 0.49, 0.68 and 1.18×10^6/kg, respectively. Primary engraftment was achieved in 96% of a group of HLA-matched unrelated ($n = 36$) or one-antigen mismatched related donors ($n = 10$). Three patients had late graft failure, which occurred more frequently in patients who received $< 1 \times 10^6$ CD33$^-$34$^+$ cells. The rate of grades II–IV GvHD was 37% and was significantly higher in patients receiving $>0.4 \times 10^6$ CD3$^+$ cells/kg. These data are somewhat difficult to interpret, due to the analysis technique used to detect residual T-cells. It is not clear whether these were assayed by multidimensional analysis, the preferred technique, or by staining with single MAb. The antigens that are described could either be blocked by the MAb used for depletion, or are also present on non-T-cell in marrow. As indicated in the report, there is also not a one-to-one correlation between T-cells detected by immunophenotyping and by limiting dilution analysis.

In small-scale laboratory experiments, Vartdal et al. [163] used anti-CD2/CD3 MAb linked to anti-Ig-coated microspheres, at a 10:1 bead-to-nucleated cell ratio, to deplete >99.98% of T-cells, as assessed by LDA. Recoveries of non-T-cells ranged from 43–74% (median 58%, which increased to 85% in large-scale preliminary experiments) with viabilities of 99% and retention of both colony-forming activity by committed progenitor cells and stroma-forming cells. Similar results were obtained on blood and marrow by Gee et al. [164] using anti-CD2 and anti-CD3, alone and in combination, by an indirect separation technique. Response to mitogens was reduced by 92–95%, and could be decreased further by adding anti-CD8 MAb to the depletion cocktail. Subset depletion of CD8$^+$ and CD4$^+$ cells was also shown to be highly efficient using this technique.

Knobloch et al. [165] compared immunomagnetic separation using anti-CD2 with SBA–erythrocyte rosetting and found that the former depleted up to 2.76 logs of T-cells with 82% recovery of haematopoietic cells, whereas the lectin protocol depleted 3.39 logs with a 59% recovery. A similar comparison was described by Collins et al. [166,167] for depletions using CAMPATH-1 plus C', ricin A chain immunotoxin and SBA agglutination alone and combined with E-rosetting or immunomagnetic separation with anti-CD2/3/8 beads. SBA alone gave a 1 log depletion, while CAMPATH and immunotoxin gave 2 logs, whereas, in contrast to Knobloch's findings, SBA–erythrocyte rosetting gave 2.9 logs and SBA/immunomagnetic separation gave 3.2 logs.

Wang et al. [168] used anti-CD2 MAb, but substituted anti-CD5 and anti-CD7 for anti-CD3, and used an indirect separation technique to deplete malignant T-cells seeded into bone-marrow samples using a 50:1 bead-to-target T-cell ratio. They achieved a 3.3–3.6 log depletion using individual MAb, which increased to 4 logs when all three were combined and to 5 logs when two treatment cycles were used. Two autologous grafts were purged using this technique, with complete removal of T-cells, as judged by an immunocytochemical technique, and multilineage stable engraftment.

Anti-CD6 MAb was tested with magnetic microspheres by Egeland et al. [169] in laboratory experiments using an indirect technique and a 40:1 bead-to-target cell ratio. This resulted in 2–3 log depletions. However, significant numbers of CD2$^+$ and CD3$^+$ cells remained after the separations and these responded to phytohaemagglutinin, IL-2 and allogeneic cells. Using this technique, the depletion of mitogen and IL-2-responsive cells was reduced by only 1–2 logs. The authors speculated that this may be due to failure to deplete T-cells with low expression of

CD6, rather than modulation of the antigen during separation. They contrasted these findings with the efficient control of GvHD in HLA-identical transplants that had been achieved using anti-CD6 MAb and C'[170]. In our experience, this difference is unlikely to be due primarily to target antigen density, since immunomagnetic separation is usually more efficient than C' at eliminating cells with a low expression of antigen [97,171].

In an attempt to retain a GvL effect while abrogating GvHD, selective depletion of CD8+ cells from HLA-matched sibling donor grafts has been tested using MAb in combination with either C' or Dynal magnetic microspheres [172]. Patients received grafts depleted of 1.5–2.0 logs of CD8+ cells together with post-BMT cyclosporin A. In a randomized study, patients showed a reduced rate of GvHD without an increase in leukaemia relapse [173]. Jansen et al. used direct immunomagnetic depletion of CD8+ cells in marrow grafts from HLA-identical siblings ($n = 20$) or alternative donors ($n = 9$) [174]. The procedure removed >95% of the target T-cells, resulting in a dose of $1.4 \pm 2.7 \times 10^5$ CD8+ cell/kg. Recoveries of normal committed colony-forming progenitors were >100%. GvHD prophylaxis included cyclosporin starting at day –1. All but 1 patient engrafted (500 granulocytes/μl) in a median of 17 days (range 12–23 days). Four patients (20%) receiving HLA-identical grafts developed grade II or greater GvHD, whereas this was seen in 5 of the 8 (63%) receiving grafts from alternative donors. Interestingly, nearly all patients developed fevers around day 7, accompanied by fluid overload, mild skin rashes and shortness of breath, and required treatment with steroids.

Nanoparticles and colloids

Paramagnetic nanoparticles have been primarily used for the enrichment of stem cells from marrow and mobilized peripheral blood. However, early laboratory studies showed that this system is also suitable for T-cell depletion. In one configuration [175], T-cells were reacted with anti-T-cell MAb and incubated with biotinylated F[ab']$_2$ fragments of goat anti-mouse IgG. These complexes were then linked to biotin-coated dextran-ferrite nanoparticles using fluoresceinated streptavidin. The rosetted T-cells were then removed by passage over a column of steel wool placed in a magnetic field. Using this method to separate T-cells from 1×10^8 mononuclear marrow cells, a 2.1 log depletion of clonable T-cells was achieved with one passage over the column. This increased to 2.3 logs after a second passage. Depletion with a single anti-CD3 MAb was as effective as separations employing a mixture of anti-CD2/CD5/CD7. The recovery of non-T-cells was 79% after the first passage and 61% after the second, with BFU-E and CFU-GM recoveries of 70% and 51%, respectively.

In contrast to results with paramagnetic *microspheres*, we have found that paramagnetic *nanoparticles* can be used for effective T-cell depletion with anti-CD3 MAb [176]. This is probably due in part to the very rapid reaction kinetics between the MAb-sensitized cells, and the possibility that these very tiny particles could be internalized by the target cells and still render them susceptible to collection in the magnetic field. In these studies, the aim was to achieve a level of T-cell depletion with OKT3 anti-CD3 and nanoparticles similar to that achieved using the same antibody and complement. This had achieved a high incidence of stable engraftment with a low incidence of acute GvHD in a series of more than 100 patients receiving partially mismatched grafts from related donors [127]. The efficiency of high-gradient immunomagnetic separation, combined with the variability in the T-cell burden in marrow grafts, prompted us to use a standardized dose of nanoparticles per fixed number of CD3+ cells, determined prior to the *ex vivo* treatment. At this fixed ratio (50 μl nanoparticles/10^7 CD3+ cells), it was possible to achieve very reproducible depletions of T-cells (2.30 ± 0.04 logs by LDA, $n = 3$), with excellent recoveries of CD34+ progenitors ($71.7 \pm 5.4\%$, $n = 9$) and colony-forming cells ($77.9 \pm 7.5\%$ for CFU-GM and $84.3 \pm 15.2\%$ for BFU-E; $n = 3$) [176].

In a clinical study, 47 patients with leukaemia or myelodysplastic syndrome received unrelated donor grafts depleted of CD3+ cells using tetrameric anti-CD3/antidextran antibody complexes and submicron immunomagnetic particles [70]. High incidences of graft failure and disease relapse following the first 27 transplants necessitated modifying the protocol to include addback of T-cells to a dose of 2×10^5/kg, and addition of cyclosporin A for prophylaxis. The mean T-cell depletion was 3.64 ± 0.67 logs with $74.7 \pm 21\%$ recovery of CD34+ cells. Forty-three percent of patients receiving T-depleted grafts without addback had grade II or greater GvHD and 18% suffered grade III or greater GvHD, compared to 85% and 54%, respectively, in those whose grafts were supplemented by T-cells. There were 4 (15%) GvHD-related deaths in the former group and 6 (46%) deaths in the latter cohort. The incidence of graft failure was 22% in patients receiving the heavily-depleted grafts versus 8% in those transplanted with T-cell supplemented grafts. Relapse mortality was 41% (11 patients) in the first group and there were no relapses in the second group. The actuarial probability of survival at one year was 25% (range 10–44%) in the T-depleted group and 54% (range 25–76%) in the T-supplemented group. The authors concluded that the antibody that was used (anti-CD3) may activate clonal T-cells, or that in the absence of T-cells, NK cells may initiate GvHD. They also observed that infusion of as few as 1×10^3 T-cells could result in clinically significant GvHD in some patients. The strategy of T-cell addback, either directly to the graft [69], or by infusion within 15 minutes of the graft [177], has been used by others, with variable success.

Magnetic colloids as the cell capture matrix have also been described [167,178–180]. These have the advantage that their binding capacity for antibodies is so high that it is not necessary to remove unbound anti-target cell MAb from the reaction mixture before addition of the anti-immunoglobulin colloid. The difficulties with this approach have mainly related to the production of stable colloids and the development of large-scale separation devices. Yau *et al.* [167] used an avidin-based cobalt colloid to separate T-cells in a two-step procedure. In the first step, marrow cells were incubated with a panel of anti-CD2/CD3/CD4/CD8 MAb, washed and reacted with biotinylated, affinity-purified IgG fraction of goat antimouse immunoglobulins. In the second step, the cells were incubated with the avidin-based colloid, and the colloid-coated T-cells separated on high-gradient separation column. The procedure depleted ~1.7 logs of target cells, with a 45% recovery of haematopoietic colony-forming progenitors. In clinical applications this would translate to a T-cell dose of ~5×10^5/kg.

T-cell depletion of allogeneic peripheral blood progenitor cell (PBPC) grafts

There is currently considerable interest in the use of drug/growth factor-mobilized peripheral blood as a source of the allograft [181]. These grafts routinely contain about tenfold the number of T-cells found in a bone-marrow harvest [182]. However, this has not translated into a directly proportional increase in the incidence or severity of acute GvHD in the recipients [23], although chronic GvHD incidence may be higher in these patients [26,28]. In a study of 55 recipients of allogeneic HLA-matched related PBPC grafts who received FK506 pretransplant and methylprednisolone on days 5–28 followed by a tapered dose, the incidence of grades II–IV GvHD was 30% and of grades III–IV was 8% [27]. This was reduced to zero by the addition of 5 mg/m^2 MTX on days 1, 3 and 6, although this resulted in a two-day delay in the median time to 500 neutrophils/µl.

In a five-centre European study of HLA-matched related PBPC transplants [183], acute GvHD occurred in 27 of 49 evaluable patients (55%), the majority of whom received cyclosporin plus short-course MTX as prophylaxis, and was grade II or greater in 24%. Chronic GvHD occurred in 18 of 39 patients (46%) and was extensive in 7 of these. It remains to be determined whether T-cell depletion of the apheresis products can provide additional prophylaxis of GvHD.

Technically, these products can be depleted using the majority of the methods developed for marrow manipulation [184,185]. They have a different cellular composition, both in terms of T-cell content, and of phagocytic cells and platelets, which may pose a challenge to some separation systems. At present, an adequate graft usually requires the collection of more than one apheresis product, which will necessitate multiple depletion procedures, or the storage and pooling of several collections. There are data that suggest that collections may be held for up to 72 hours without harm [186,187]. The conditions for optimal storage have not been rigorously established. However, colony-forming units appear to be maintained adequately at 4°C, when the cell concentration is kept below 5×10^7/ml and the pH is kept above 7.0.

Depletion can be achieved by either negative or positive selection [184,185,188]. Dreger *et al.* [185] compared positive selection using the CellPro biotinylated anti-CD34/avidin column Ceprate SC system and the Baxter Isolex anti-CD34 immunomagnetic bead method, with negative selection using CAMPATH-1 Mab and C'. Negative selection resulted in a 2.16 log depletion of CD3$^+$ cells and recovery of 39% of the NK and 56% of the CD34+ cells. Positive selection resulted in a 4.04 log CD3+ using the Isolex device, versus a 3.12 log depletion with the Ceprate system. There was a 5.0 versus 3.27 log depletion of NK cells and a 36 versus 27% recovery of CD34+ cells, respectively. The CD34+ cell purity in the negatively-selected preparation was 1.7% compared to 94% and 65% in the positively-selected products.

We have compared T-cell depletion achieved by CD34+ selection using high gradient imunomagnetic selection with nanoparticles (Figures 32.3 and 32.4) and using an immunoaffinity column (Figure 32.5). In both cases, clinically appropriate levels of T-cell removal could be obtained on a small scale.

Bensinger et al. [188,189] used the Ceprate SC and Isolex systems to enrich CD34+ cells from HLA-matched PBPC for transplantation to older patients with advanced haematological malignancies. In the first study [188], using the CellPro device, collections were made from 10 donors and the CD34+ were enriched and infused daily for four consecutive days. Prophylaxis included cyclosporin alone (5 patients) or in combination with MTX (5 patients). The median dose of CD34+ cells was 10.1×10^6/kg, with a CD3+ cell dose of 0.90 (range $0.5–2.5 \times 10^6$/kg). Patients engrafted 500 granulocytes/μl at a median of 14 days (range 9–20); however, 3 patients died at days 54, 63 and 72 with granulocyte but not platelet recovery. Acute GvHD was seen in all patients, and was grade II or greater in 9, and grade III or greater in 5 cases. Six patients were alive at days 79–276 post-transplant.

In the second study [189], the Isolex device was used to process PBPC from 20 HLA-identical sibling donors. A 3.9 log depletion of T-cells was achieved, with a median dose of 0.08 (range 0.01–1.12, $\times 10^6$ CD3+ cells/kg and 6.4 (range 2.4–10.2) $\times 10^6$ CD34 cells/kg. Patients received cyclosporin as part of GvHD prophylaxis and no growth factors were given. All patients engrafted neutrophils in a median of 13 days and achieved an unsupported platelet count of 20 000/μl in a median of 9 days. Acute GvHD developed in 16 patients (73%) and was grade II or greater in 9 cases. However, no grade IV disease was seen and there were no GvHD-related deaths. Donor chimaerism was seen in all 16 evaluable patients. There were 6 transplant-related deaths and 8 patients were alive at the time of the report at 52–460 days post-transplant.

Link et al. [66] used the Ceprate SC system to deplete HLA-identical sibling PBPC grafts of 2–3 logs of T-cells (median CD3+ cell dose/kg = 1.2×10^6). When transplanted to 10 patients with haematological malignancies who received cyclosporin with or without MTX for additional prophylaxis, all engrafted neutrophils within 15 days, and achieved a stable

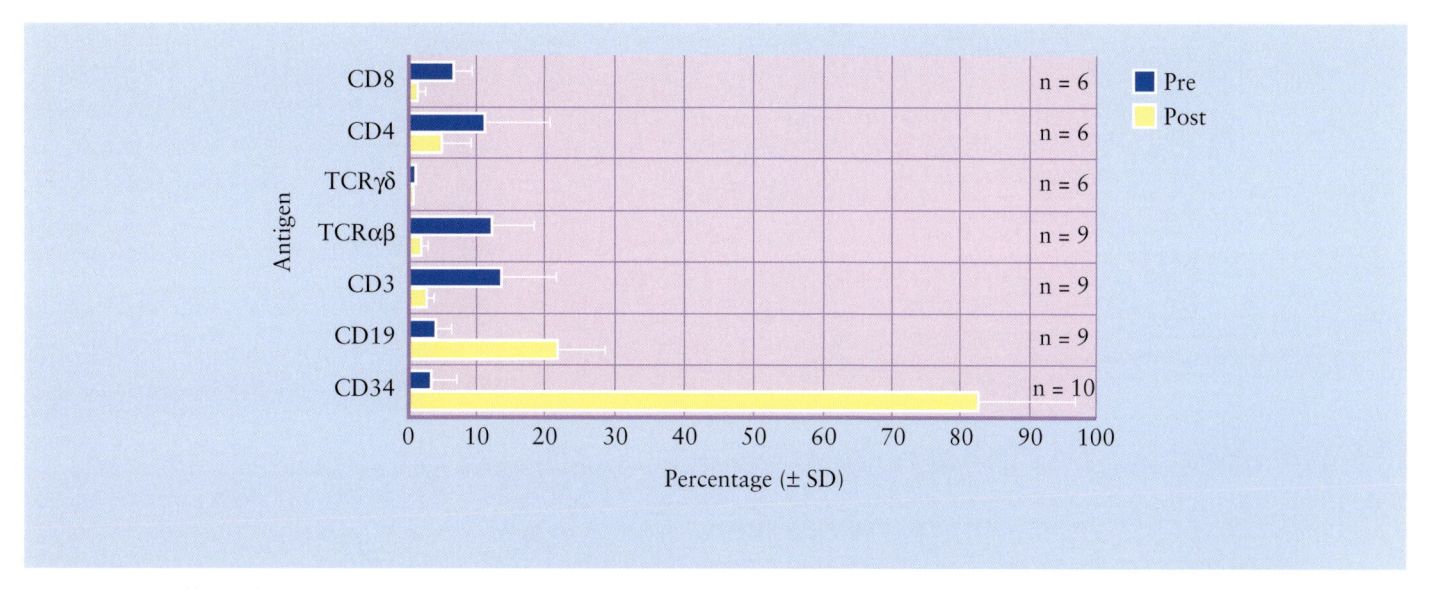

Figure 32.3 Effect of immunomagnetic CD34+ cell selection on residual lymphocyte subpopulations. Bone-marrow samples were depleted of CD34+ cells by high gradient immunomagnetic separation using paramagnetic nanoparticles (the MACS system). Residual lymphocyte subpopulations were quantitated by flow cytometry.

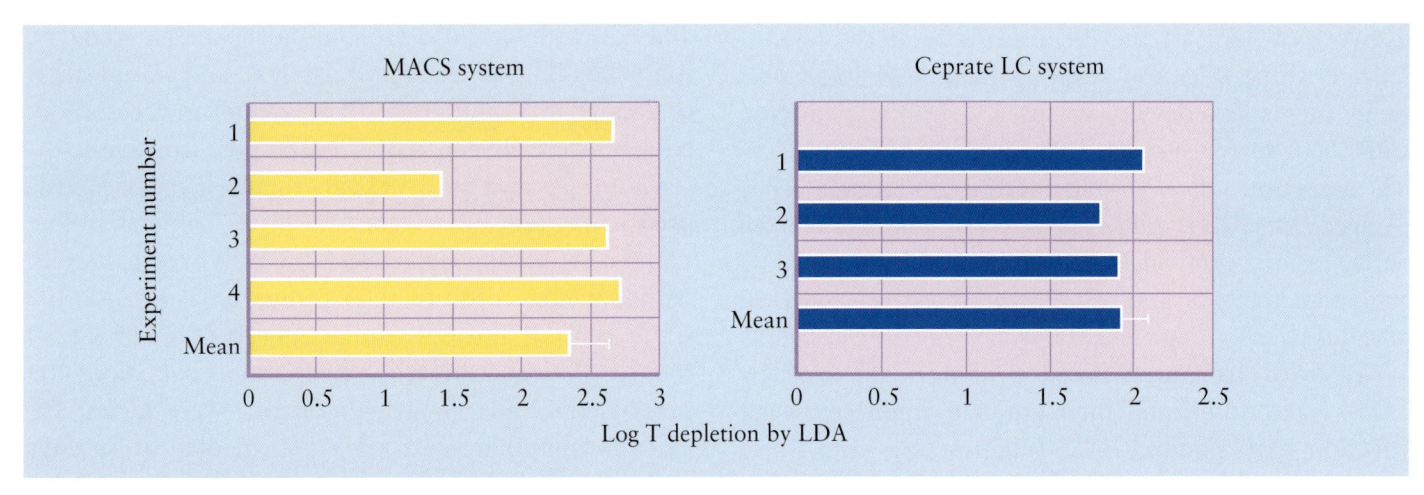

Figure 32.4 Comparison of two methods of CD34⁺ cell selection on T-cell content of bone marrow. Bone-marrow samples were depleted of CD34⁺ cells by immunomagnetic separation using paramagnetic nanoparticles (MACS system) or by an immunoaffinity method (Ceprate LC system). Residual T-cells in the positively selected fraction were quantitated by limiting dilution analysis.

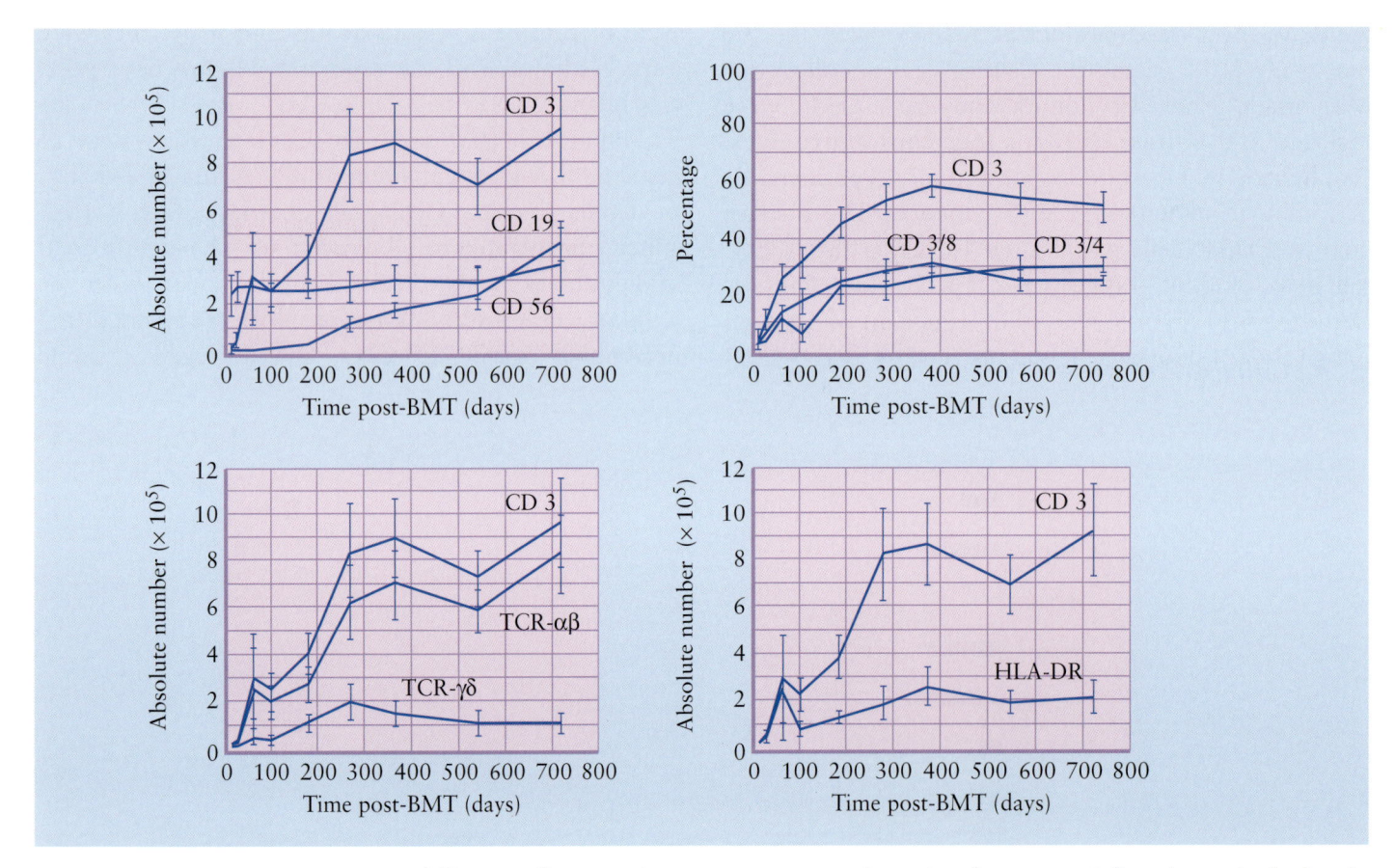

Figure 32.5 Immunoreconstitution following allogeneic bone-marrow transplantation from a partially-mismatched related donor. The pattern of reconstitution is shown for T-cells, B-cells and NK cells (upper left), helper and suppressor T-cells (upper right), αβ and γδ T-cells (lower left) and for class II-positive lymphocytes (lower right). Data were obtained from 25 patients who remained disease-free throughout evaluation. See Lamb et al. [211] for details.

donor haematopoiesis. Two of the 3 patients who received cyclosporin alone died of GvHD (median of grade III disease), whereas those who received MTX in addition developed primarily grade I disease, but 2 have relapsed.

T-cell depletion by positive selection

A number of methods are available for enriching CD34+ cells from haematopoietic grafts (see Chapter 33 on autologous graft purging). In small-scale experiments, de Wynter et al. [190] compared fluorescence-activated cell sorting (FACS), panning on CELLector flask, immunomagnetic separation using microspheres (IMS) and nanoparticles (MACS), and immunoaffinity separation (IAS) to enrich CD34+ cells from marrow, peripheral and cord blood. They concluded that the most effective techniques were FACS and MACS, although IAS gave good purities, but lower yields of colony-forming cells. They emphasize that these results may change as the systems are scaled up for clinical use, and they do not indicate their effect on the T-cell content of the preparations.

As has been indicated above, it is possible to achieve clinically useful levels of T-cell depletion in PBPC grafts by positive selection of cells bearing the CD34 antigen [189]. This is also true for marrow grafts. Cottler-Fox et al. [64] used the Ceprate SC immunoaffinity column to enrich CD34+ cells from eleven mobilized PBPC and ten bone-marrow collections that were made for autologous transplantation and gene-marking studies. The CD3+ T-cell content of the samples was reduced by approximately 3 logs, with a mean CD34+ cell purity of $53.3 \pm 27.9\%$ in the PBPC preparations and of $65.4 \pm 10.9\%$ in the marrow samples. By calculation, this would translate to infusion of 3.4×10^4 bone-marrow T-cells/kg and 1.2×10^5 T-cells/kg/apheresis.

The Isolex system was used to enrich CD34+ cells in a study of 14 patients with leukaemia or myelodysplastic syndrome who received marrow grafts from HLA-identical sibling donors [65]. Grafts were depleted of $2.7 + 0.1$ logs of T-cells, representing an infused dose of $8.93 \pm 1.7 \times 10^6$ CD3+ cells/kg and $1.21 \pm 0.20 \times 10^6$ CD34+ cells/kg. Granulocyte engraftment (500/µl) was achieved in a median of 10.5 days, with platelet engraftment (>20 000/µl) in 27 days. There was no grade III or IV GvHD. However, the incidence of grade II or lower disease was not reported.

Cord blood manipulation

Cord blood represents a rich source of stem cells and has been used successfully to engraft adult recipients [25]. The majority of these transplants have been performed using HLA-matched or one-antigen mismatched grafts, and the incidence of acute GvHD was originally reported to be lower than expected with marrow grafts [24]. This has encouraged transplantation of cord blood across increasingly disparate HLA barriers, and even in one case, infusion of a mixture of non-HLA typed cells (JE Wagner, personal communication). The true incidence and severity of GvHD that accompanies cord blood transplantation should become apparent as numbers and follow-ups on patients increase. Initial reports indicated that *ex vivo* manipulation of these grafts resulted in excessive losses of stem cells. However, a number of investigators have now demonstrated that T-cell depletion can be achieved by both positive and negative selection. Laver et al. [30] achieved a 2.2 log T-cell depletion using T10B9 and C′, whereas CD34 enrichment using the Ceprate LC system resulted in a 3.6 log depletion of T-cells and a recovery of 10.3% of CD34+ cells at a purity of $60 \pm 5.5\%$. In contrast, MAb and C′ treatment resulted in recovery of $75 \pm 19\%$ of CD34+ cells and improved recoveries of committed colony-forming cells.

The Isolex-50 immunomagnetic system [191] achieved CD34+ enrichment purities of $82.4 \pm 1.1\%$ (range $43.4 - 94.7$, $n = 33$) and yields of $63.6 \pm 6.6\%$. These data did not indicate the level of T-cell depletion obtained.

Laboratory evaluation of T-cell depletion

Depletion of T-cells can be quantitated by immunophenotyping and/or by functional assays. Immunophenotyping is generally performed by flow cytometry using panels of MAb directed against antigens other than those that are used for the depletion. The accuracy of this approach is facilitated by careful selection of the components of the antibody panel and by the use of rare-event analysis. Accurate results can be obtained when T-cells have been physically removed from the graft. However, when they are eliminated *in situ*, it is important to include a viability stain, such as 7-AAD during the analysis to exclude dead or dying cells. Even under these circumstances the presence of cell debris, and delayed expression of cell death (for example, when using MAb plus C′ or immunotoxin) may make interpretation difficult. For these reasons, most centres use a functional assay to detect T-cells that are capable of proliferation. Since not every T-cell in the graft will proliferate under *ex vivo* culture conditions, the numbers detected will be lower than those measured by immunophenotyping.

Samples of the graft, pre- and post-depletion are cultured for 4–16 days under conditions that stimulate T-cell proliferation. The T-cells, or T-cell subsets [192], in these cultures may then be enumerated by immunofluorescence techniques, or by scoring colonies visually or by uptake of tritiated thymidine, under limiting dilution conditions [193–195]. In general, these assays give only crude information with respect to prediction of clinical outcome. In gross terms, the T-cell content of the graft may correlate with the presence or absence of acute GvHD. However, this relationship is often weak, undoubtedly reflecting our lack of knowledge of:

- the cells involved in initiating and sustaining GvHD;
- our inability to reproduce the events occurring *in vivo* in an *in vitro* assay system.

This situation may be improved by the use of more sophisticated assays for the frequency of cytotoxic T-cell precursor populations that respond specifically to alloantigens on recipient cells [196–198]. A similar approach can be used to quantitate T-cells that may express antileukaemia activity, in order to determine the potential for a GvL effect [196,199].

Immune reconstitution

Quantitative and functional immunodeficiency is characteristic of all patients who have received stem-cell transplants. Depending on the source of the graft, the type of *ex vivo* manipulation of the graft, post-transplant immunosuppressive therapy, the incidence and severity of GvHD, post-transplant infections and so on, this may last for months to years and may be expressed as a quantitative and qualitative deficit. The impact of using a T-cell-depleted graft may be double-edged, in that prevention of GvHD can enhance immunoreconstitution [200], while reconstitution of normal T-lymphocyte numbers [201] and function [202] may be additionally delayed.

The general pattern of reconstitution in recipients regardless of the type of graft is the early appearance of NK cells [203] two to three weeks post-transplant. B-cell recovery to normal numbers is within two to three months and may overshoot at six to eight months post-transplant [204,205] in recipients of allogeneic grafts. Functional activity, as measured by proliferative responses, was normal by two to three months and then remained elevated from four to 18 months, and, although normal IgM synthesis was seen at four to six months, recipients of T-cell-depleted grafts did not show normal production of IgG until 13–15 months post-BMT – about six months later than recipients of non-manipulated grafts [201,204, 206,207].

The first T-cell phenotype to be seen is usually $CD3^+/8^+$ with decreased numbers of $CD4^+$ cells for about six months in all recipients [201,208]. T-cell depletion of the graft delays recovery of this subpopulation, which normally occurs at seven to nine months, by about three months. Differences in the patterns of reconstitution between recipients of non-depleted and CAMPATH-depleted HLA-identical grafts have been described [209]. In recipients of unmanipulated grafts, repopulation is predominantly of donor origin, whereas in T-depleted graft recipients residual patient $CD8^+$ T-cells could also be detected. The mixed population expanded rapidly for two months post-BMT, and in the majority of patients, this was followed by the appearance of a wave of donor T-cells at about nine months, which corrected the previously inverted CD4/CD8 ratio.

Responses to phytohaemagglutinin recovered by about five months in recipients of unmanipulated grafts and by about one year in recipients of T-depleted marrow [201,210]. The latter also showed lower frequencies of precursors for proliferating and cytotoxic T-cells for the first six months [202], and although the differences between the two groups then resolved, the numbers remained subnormal. There was no significant effect of T-cell depletion on helper precursor frequencies. A similar pattern of reconstitution has been described in recipients of T-cell-depleted partially mismatched related donor grafts [211,212] (Figure 32.5).

Reports of the effects of T-cell depletion on immunoreconstitution must, however, be interpreted with caution when attempting to determine the effects of *ex vivo* manipulation. Few studies [201,209] have examined reconstitution in comparable groups of patients and interpretation is further complicated by the use of different types of graft manipulation, post-transplant therapeutic interventions, development of GvHD and so on.

New approaches

There is little doubt that T-cell depletion of HLA-matched and partially mismatched grafts can provide effective prophylaxis against GvHD. At the same time, it is recognized that this is achieved at a potentially increased risk for graft failure, disease relapse, lymphoproliferative disease and delayed immunoreconstitution. This has prompted investigation of other types of graft manipulation. In particular, there is interest in:

- use of stem-cell supplementation to overcome histocompatibility barriers;
- *ex vivo* depletion of the T-cell subpopulation that specifically recognizes antigenic differences expressed on the recipient's cells; and
- the role of facilitating cell populations to enhance engraftment of haematopoietic stem cells and solid organs in allodisparate transplants.

Aversa *et al.* [71] described the use of combined T-cell depleted (E-rosetting with or without SBA) marrow and PBPC haplo-identical grafts to transplant 17 leukaemia patients. These infusions contained a tenfold higher number of committed colony-forming cells than in marrow alone. Patients were conditioned using total body irradiation, antithymocyte globulin, cyclophosphamide and thiotepa. All but 1 patient (94%) engrafted and 1 died of grade IV GvHD (6%). However, 9 of the 16 engrafted patients (56%) died of transplant-related toxicity within 18–180 days after transplant. The protocol was modified to treat 24 patients with advanced leukaemia [213] by T-depleting the marrow using SBA and the PBPC using E-rosetting and CD34$^+$ cell selection, to produce a final graft containing a mean of 1.3×10^7 CD34$^+$ cells/kg and 3×10^4 CD3$^+$ cells/kg. Fludarabine was also substituted for cyclophosphamide to reduce the toxicity of the conditioning regimen. Twenty-two patients engrafted (92%) and 1 other achieved secondary engraftment. At the time of the report (one to nine months post-transplant; median six months), <5% had developed acute GvHD and there was no chronic GvHD. There were 8 non-haematological deaths (29%) and 1 patient has relapsed. Immune recovery was characterized by the presence and persistence of CD3$^+$/8$^+$ cells which co-expressed inhibitory NK receptors for HLA-C alleles and which functioned like NK cells, and could lyse fresh leukaemia cells.

These early findings support the finding in animal models [214] that increasing the stem-cell dose can be of value in crossing histocompatibility barriers. In a much larger patient group with longer follow-up, Henslee-Downey *et al.* have achieved comparable results using T-cell-deleted two- and three-antigen mismatched marrow alone [22,140].

The specific depletion of T-cells that recognize antigens on the recipient's normal cells offers the possibility of abrogating GvHD while retaining the potential for a GvL response. Rencher *et al.* [215] cultured donor T-cells with host-derived lymphoblastoid cell lines. This induced activation by mismatched host HLA, and these cells were removed by fluorescence activated cell sorting, based upon their size and expression of multiple activation markers. The residual cells retained helper and cytotoxic responses to foreign antigens but not to HLA antigens. A similar strategy has been examined by Barrett *et al.* [17,45] who have eliminated recipient-responsive cells by a 2–4 hour exposure to immunotoxins directed against T-cell activation markers. The practicality of using this approach to deplete grafts, rather than donor leukocyte infusions, remains to be established.

Ildstad and co-workers [216,217] have described a subpopulation (0.4%) of marrow cells which express a characteristic CD8$^+$/3$^+$/45$^+$/Thy 1$^+$, class II$^{dim/intermediate}$/$\alpha\beta^-$/$\gamma\delta^-$ phenotype. As few as 30 000 of the cells could facilitate engraftment of purified murine allogeneic bone marrow or foetal liver [216] stem cells in an MHC-specific manner. This would be of particular value as a supplement to heavily T-cell-depleted grafts, such as those obtained by positive selection or highly efficient immunomagnetic techniques.

Conclusions

The technology for depleting subpopulations of cells from haematopoietic stem-cells grafts has developed dramatically within a short period. Cells may be positively or negatively selected with relatively high efficiencies and on a clinically-appropriate scale. These advances have not, however, been similarly paralleled by developments in our understanding of the aetiology and control of GvHD. A complex picture is emerging of multiple possible effector cells, humoral mediators and positive and negative regulators, which suggests that most approaches to prevention and/or control could be easily circumvented. Added to this complexity is the issue of separability of GvHD and GvL responses. Recent data from functional depletion experiments, and from donor leukocyte infusions used to treat relapsed disease in HLA-matched graft recipients, suggest that separation of these effects may indeed be possible. In practical terms, in spite of so many unanswered questions, it is somewhat chastening to realize that effective control of GvHD can be achieved by the relatively simple technique of subtotal T-cell depletion. It is to be hoped that an improved understanding of the complex reactions occurring between the graft and its recipient will ultimately translate into relatively simple modifications of current graft engineering techniques to achieve improved clinical outcomes.

Acknowledgements

The authors express their sincere thanks to colleagues in the Division of Transplantation Medicine at the University of South Carolina, Columbia, and, in particular, to Drs Lawrence Lamb, Zhou Ye and Jean Henslee-Downey. Thanks also to Aretta Talbert and Gloria Todd for their secretarial assistance.

References

1. Hakim F and Mackall CL. The immune system: effector and target of graft-versus-host disease. In: *Graft-vs-Host Disease*, 2nd edn. JL Ferrara, HJ Deeg and SJ Burakoff (eds), 1996: 257–290 (New York: Marcel Dekker).
2. Billingham RE. The biology of graft-versus-host reactions. In: *The Harvey Lectures*, 1967; **62**: 21–78 (New York: Academic Press).
3. Beatty P. Role of histocompatibility antigens in the development of graft-versus-host disease. In: *Graft-vs-Host Disease*, 2nd edn. JL Ferrara, HJ Deeg and SJ Burakoff (eds), 1996: 607–614 (New York: Marcel Dekker).
4. Thomas ED. The evolution of the scientific foundation of marrow transplantation based on human studies. In: *Bone Marrow Transplantation*. SJ Forman, KG Blume and ED Thomas (eds), 1994: 12–15 (Cambridge, MA: Blackwell Scientific Publications).
5. Beatty PG. The immunogenetics of bone marrow transplantation. *Transfus Med Rev* 1994; **8**: 45–58.
6. Bortin MM and Saltzstein EC. Graft-versus-host inhibition: fetal liver and thymus cells minimize secondary disease. *Science* 1969; **164**: 316–318.
7. Kolb HJ, Reider I, Rodt H et al. Anti-lymphocyte antibodies and bone marrow transplantation. VI. Graft versus host tolerance in DLA-incompatible dogs following *in vitro* treatment with bone marrow with absorbed antithymocyte globulin. *Transplantation* 1979; **27**: 242–245.
8. Rodt H, Thierfelder S and Eulitz M. Anti-lymphocyte antibodies and marrow transplantation. III. Effects of heterologous anti-brain antibodies in acute secondary diseases in mice. *J Immunol* 1974; **4**: 25–29.
9. Reisner Y, Itsicovitch L, Meshorer A and Sharon N. Hematopoietic stem cell transplantation using mouse bone marrow and spleen cells fractionated by lectins. *Proc Natl Acad Sci USA* 1978; **75**: 2933–2936.
10. Gale RP. T cells, bone marrow transplantation and immunotherapy: use of monoclonal antibodies. *Ann Intern Med* 1987; **106**: 257–274.
11. Collins NH, Kernan NA, Bleau SA and O'Reilly RJ. T-cell depletion of allogeneic human bone marrow grafts by soybean lectin agglutination and either sheep red blood cell rosetting or adherence on the CD5/CD8 CELLector. In: *Bone Marrow Processing and Purging: A Practical Guide*. AP Gee (ed.), 1992: 201–12 (Boca Raton, FL: CRC Press).
12. Reisner Y, N, Kirkpatrick D et al. Transplantation for acute leukemia with HLA-A and B, nonidentical parental marrow cells fractionated with soybean agglutinin and sheep red blood cells. *Lancet* 1981; **ii**: 327–331.
13. Reisner Y, Kapoor N, Kirkpatrick D et al. Transplantation for severe combined immunodeficiency with HLA-A, B, D, DR incompatible parental marrow cells fractionated with soybean agglutinin and sheep red blood cells. *Blood* 1983; **61**: 341–348.
14. Marmont AM, Horowitz MM, Gale RP et al. T-cell depletion of HLA-identical transplants in leukemia. *Blood* 1991; **78**: 2120–2130.
15. Goldman JM, Gale RP, Horowitz MM et al. Bone marrow transplantation for chronic myelogenous leukemia in chronic phase: increased risk for relapse associated with T-cell depletion. *Ann Intern Med* 1988; **108**: 806–814.
16. Horowitz MM, Gale RP, Sondel PM et al. Graft-versus-leukemia reactions after bone marrow transplantation. *Blood* 1990; **75**: 555–562.
17. Barrett AJ. Strategies to enhance the graft-versus-malignancy effects in allogenic transplants. *Ann NY Acad Sci* 1995; **770**: 203–212.
18. MacDonald GC and Gartner JG. Prevention of acute lethal graft-versus-host disease in F1 hybrid mice by pretreatment of the graft with anti-NK-1.1 and complement. *Transplantation* 1992; **54**: 147–151.
19. Martin PJ. Increased disparity for minor histocompatibility antigens as a potential cause of increased GvHD risk in marrow transplantation from unrelated donors compared with related donors. *Bone Marrow Transplant* 1991; **8**: 217–223.
20. Henslee-Downey PJ. Choosing an alternative bone marrow donor among available family members. *Am J Pediatr Hematol Oncol* 1993; **15**: 150–161.
21. Ash RC, Horowitz MM, Gale RP et al. Bone marrow transplantation from related donors other than HLA-identical

siblings: effect of T cell depletion. *Bone Marrow Transplant* 1991; **7**: 443–452.
22. Henslee-Downey PJ, Parrish RS, MacDonald JS *et al.* Combined *in vitro* and *in vivo* T lymphocyte depletion for the control of graft-versus-host disease following haploidentical marrow transplant. *Transplantation* 1996; **61**: 738–745.
23. Bensinger WI, Buckner CD, Demirer T *et al.* Transplantation of allogeneic peripheral blood stem cells. *Bone Marrow Transplant* 1996; **17**(Suppl 2): S56–S57.
24. Wagner JE, Kernan NA, Steinbach M *et al.* Allogeneic sibling cord blood transplantation in forty-four children with malignant and non-malignant disease. *Lancet* 1995; **346**: 214–219.
25. Kurtzberg J, Laughlin M, Graham M *et al.* Placental blood as a source of hematopoietic stem cells for transplantation into unrelated recipients. *New Engl J Med* 1996; **335**: 157–166.
26. Urbano-Ispizua A, Garcia-Conde J, Brunet S *et al.* High incidence of chronic graft-vs-host disease after allogeneic peripheral blood progenitor cell transplantation from matched related donors. *Blood* 1996; **88**(Suppl 1): 617 (abstr).
27. Przepiorka D, Ippoliti C, Khouri I *et al.* Microdose methotrexate vs. methylprednisolone in combination with tacrolimus for prevention of acute graft-vs-host disease GvHD after allogeneic blood stem cell transplantation. *Blood* 1996; **88**(Suppl 1): 418a.
28. Champlin RE, Andrellini P, Przepiorka D *et al.* Allogeneic transplantation of peripheral blood progenitor cells. In: *Proceedings of the Fourth International Symposium on Blood Cell Transplantation*, 18.4 abst., 1996.
29. Goldman S, Sweetman R, Suen Y *et al.* A high incidence of severe acute graft vs host disease (aGvHD) following unrelated cord blood transplants UCBT: HLA mismatching, but not serum soluble IL-2 receptor levels are predictive. *Blood* 1996; **88**(Suppl 1): 422a.
30. Laver J, Traycoff CM, Abdel-Mageed A *et al.* Effects of CD34+ selection and T cell immunodepletion on cord blood hematopoietic progenitors: relevance to stem cell transplantation. *Exp Haematol* 1995; **23**: 1492–1496.
31. Barrett AJ. Graft-vs-host disease. In: *Bone Marrow Transplantation in Practice*. JG Treleaven and AJ Barrett (eds), 1992: 257–272 (Edinburgh: Churchill Livingstone).
32. Sprent J, Schaefer M, Lo D *et al.* Properties of purified T cell subsets. II. *In vivo* responses to class I vs class II H-2 differences. *J Exp Med* 1986; **163**: 998–1011.
33. Korngold R and Sprent J. Variable capacity of LE T4 + T cells to cause lethal graft-versus-host disease across minor histocompatibility barriers in mice. *J Exp Med* 1987; **165**: 52–64.
34. Korngold R and Sprent J. T cell subsets and graft-versus-host disease. *Transplantation* 1987; **44**: 335–339.
35. Sykes M and Abraham VS. IL-2 reduces graft vs host disease and preserves a graft vs leukemia effects by selectively inhibiting CD4+ T cell activity. *J Immunol* 1993; **150**: 197–205.
36. Palathumpat V, Dejbakhsh-Jones S and Strober S. The role of purified CD8+ T cells in graft-versus-leukemia activity and engraftment after allogeneic bone marrow transplantation. *Transplantation* 1995; **60**: 355–361.
37. Ferrara JL, Deeg HJ and Burakoff SJ (eds). *Graft-vs-Host Disease*, 2nd edn, 1996 (New York: Marcel Dekker).
38. Johnson BD and Truitt RL. A decrease in graft-vs-host disease without loss of graft-vs-leukemia reactivity after MHC-matched bone marrow transplantation by selective depletion of donor NK cells *in vivo*. *Transplantation* 1992; **54**: 104–112.
39. Ferrara JLM. Cytokine dysregulation as a mechanism of graft versus host disease. *Curr Opin Immunol* 1993; **5**: 794–799.
40. Krenger W and Ferrara JLM. Dysregulation of cytokines during graft-versus-host disease. *J Haematother* 1996; **5**: 3–14.
41. Jadus MR and Wepsic HT. The role of cytokines in graft-versus-host reactions and disease. *Bone Marrow Transplant* 1992; **10**: 1–14.
42. Hessner MJ, Endean DJ, Casper JT *et al.* Use of unrelated marrow grafts compensates for reduced graft-versus-leukemia reactivity after T-cell-depleted allogeneic marrow transplantation for chronic myelogenous leukemia. *Blood* 1995; **86**: 3987–3996.
43. Garrido F, Cabrera T, Concha A *et al.* Natural history of HLA expression during tumor development. *Immunology Today* 1993; **14**: 491–499.
44. Seong D, Sims S, Johnson *et al.* Activation of class I HLA expression by TNF alpha and gamma interferon is mediated through protein kinase C-dependent pathway in CML cell lines. *Br J Haematol* 1991; **78**: 359–367.
45. Datta AR, Barrett AJ, Jiang YZ *et al.* Distinct T-cell populations distinguish chronic myeloid leukemia cells from lymphocytes in the same individual: a model for separating GvHD from GvL reactions. *Bone Marrow Transplant* 1994; **14**: 517–524.
46. Bocchia M, Korontavit T, Xu Q *et al.* Specific cellular immunity to *bcr–abl* oncogene-derived peptides. *Blood* 1996; **87**: 3587–3592.
47. Falkenberg JH, Faber LM, van den Elshout M *et al.* Generation of donor-derived antileukemic cytotoxic T cell responses for treatment of relapsed leukemia after allogeneic HLA-identical bone marrow transplantation. *J Immunother* 1993; **14**: 305–309.
48. Van Lochem E, de Gast B and Goulmy E. *In vitro* separation of host-specific GvH and GvL cytotoxic T cell activities. *Bone Marrow Transplant* 1992; **10**: 181–183.
49. Verma UN, Areman EM, Sacher RA and Mazumder A. *In vitro* activation of peripheral blood stem cells with interleukin-2. *Progr Clin Biol Res* 1994; **389**: 245–255.
50. Johnson BD, Drobyski WR and Truitt RL. Delayed infusion of normal donor cells after MHC-mismatched bone marrow transplantation provides an anti-leukemia reaction without graft-versus-host disease. *Bone Marrow Transplant* 1993; **11**: 329–337.
51. Kolb HJ; Mittermuller J, Clemm Ch *et al.* Donor leukocyte transfusions for treatment of recurrent chronic myelogenous leukemia in marrow transplant patients. *Blood* 1990; **76**: 2462–2465.
52. Mackinnon S, Papadopoulos EB, Carabasi MH *et al.* Adoptive immunotherapy evaluating escalating doses of donor leukocytes for relapse of chronic myeloid leukemia after bone marrow transplantation: separation of graft-versus-leukemia responses from graft-versus-host disease. *Blood* 1995; **86**: 1261–1268.
53. Pati A, Henslee-Downey PJ, Godder K *et al.* Donor leukocyte infusions as immunotherapy following partially mismatched related donor PMRD bone marrow transplant BMT to prevent relapse in high risk patients PTS. In: *Blood Cell and*

Bone Marrow Transplants – The Sixth Biennial Sandoz-Keystone Symposium on Bone Marrow Transplantation, 1996: 60(Abstr).

54. Lamb LS, Henslee-Downey PJ, Parrish RS et al. Increased frequency of TCR gd+ T-cells in disease-free survivors following T cell depleted partially mismatched related donor bone marrow transplantation for leukemia. *J Haematother* 1996; **5**: 503–510.

55. Gallot G, Hallet M-M, Gaschet J et al. Human HLA-specific T cell clones with stable expression of a suicide gene: a possible tool to drive and control a graft-versus-host – graft-versus-leukemia reaction? *Blood* 1995; **83**: 1098–1103.

56. Naparstek, Or R, Nagler A et al. T cell depleted allogeneic bone marrow transplantation for acute leukemia using Campath-1 antibodies and post-transplant administration of donor's peripheral blood lymphocytes for prevention of relapse. *Br J Haematol* 1995; **89**: 506–513.

57. Patterson J, Prentice HG, Brenner MK et al. Graft rejection following HLA matched T lymphocyte-depleted bone marrow transplantation. *Br J Haematol* 1986; **63**: 221–230.

58. Kernan NA, Bordignon C, Heller G et al. Graft failure after T cell-depleted human leukocyte antigen identical marrow transplants for leukemia: I. Analysis of risk factors and results of secondary transplants. *Blood* 1989; **74**: 2227–2232.

59. Kernan NA. T cell depletion for prevention of graft-versus-host disease. In: *Bone Marrow Transplantation*. SJ Forman, KG Blume and ED Thomas (eds), 1994: 124–135 (Boston, MA: Blackwell Scientific Publications).

60. Butturini A, Seeger RC and Gale RP. Recipient immune-competent T lymphocytes can survive intensive conditioning for bone marrow transplantation. *Blood* 1986; **68**: 954–956.

61. Donohue J, Homge M and Kernan NA. Characterization of cells emerging at the time of graft failure after bone marrow transplantation from an unrelated marrow donor. *Blood* 1993; **82**: 1023–1029.

62. Kernan NA. Graft failure following transplantation of T cell depleted marrow. In: *Graft-versus-Host Disease: Immunology, Pathophysiology and Treatment*. HJ Deeg, SF Burakoff, JLM Ferrara and K Atkinson (eds), 1990: 557–570 (New York: Marcel Dekker).

63. Lamb LS, Szafer F, Henslee-Downey PJ et al. Characterization of acute graft rejection in T cell-depleted partially mismatched related donor bone marrow transplantation. *Exp Hematol* 1995; **23**: 1595–1600.

64. Cottler-Fox M, Cipolone K, Yu M et al. Positive selection of CD34+ hematopoietic cells using an immunoaffinity column results in T-cell deletion equivalent to elutriation. *Exp Haematol* 1995; **23**: 320–322.

65. Cornetta K, Mills B, Hanna M et al. Allogeneic bone marrow transplantation using CD34 enriched cells. *Blood* 1996; **88**(Suppl 1): 483a.

66. Link H, Arseniev L, Bähre O et al. Transplantation of allogeneic CD34+ blood cells. *Blood* 1996; **87**: 4903–4909.

67. Holdrinet RSG, von Egmond JV, Wessels JMC and Haanen C. A method for quantification of peripheral blood admixture in bone marrow aspirates. *Exp Haematol* 1980: **8**: 103–107.

68. Kernan NA, Collins NH, Juliano L et al. Clonable T lymphocytes in T-cell depleted bone marrow transplants correlate with development of graft versus host disease. *Blood* 1986; **68**: 770–773.

69. Verdonck LF, Dekker AW, de Gast GC et al. Allogeneic bone marrow transplantation with a fixed low number of T cells in the marrow graft. *Blood* 1994; **83**: 3090–3096.

70. Simpson DR, Phillips GL, Thomas TE et al. Ex vivo depletion of T lymphocytes by immunomagnetic beads to decrease graft-versus-host disease after unrelated donor marrow transplantation. *Blood* 1996; **10**(Suppl 1): 420a (Abstr).

71. Aversa F, Tabilio A, Terenzi A et al. Successful engraftment of T cell depleted haploidentical 'three loci' incompatible transplants in leukemia patients by addition of recombinant human granulocyte colony-stimulating factor-mobilized peripheral blood progenitor cells to bone marrow inoculum. *Blood* 1994; **84**: 3948–3955.

72. Reisner Y, Kapoor N, Hodes MZ et al. Enrichment for CFU-C from murine and human bone marrow using soybean agglutinin. *Blood* 1982; **59**: 360–363.

73. Lebkowski J, Schain L, Harvey M et al. Isolation and culture of human CD34+ hematopoietic stem cells using AIS CELLectors. In: *Hematopoietic Stem Cells – The Mulhouse Manual*. E Wunder, H Sovalat, PR Hénon and S Serker (eds), 1994: 215–230 (Dayton, OH: Alpha Med Press).

74. Reisner Y, Pahwa S Chian JW et al. Separation of antibody helper and antibody suppressor human T cells using soybean agglutinin. *Proc Natl Acad Sci USA* 1980; **77**: 6778–6782.

75. Gajewski J, Wall D, Adkins D et al. A randomized double blind trial of T cell depletion TCD with CD5/8 CELLector in addition to cyclosporine (CSA), methotrexate (MTX) and steroids for acute graft versus host disease (aGvHD) prevention in HLA mismatched (MM) bone marrow transplants. *Blood* 1996; **88**(Suppl 1): 253a.

76. Frame JN, Collins NH, Cartagena T et al. T cell depletion of human bone marrow. Comparison of Campath-1 plus complement, anti-T cell ricin A chain immunotoxin, and soybean agglutinin alone or in combination with E or immunomagnetic beads. *Transplantation* 1989; **47**: 984–988.

77. Woolfrey AE, Neudorf S and Filipovich AH. Comparison of two immuno-mechanical methods of T-cell depletion of human bone marrow for prevention of graft-versus-host disease: soybean lectin agglutination and sheep erythrocyte depletion versus triple rosette depletion. *Thymus* 1985; **7**: 327–334.

78. Mumcuoglu M, Manor D and Slavin S. Enrichment for CFU-GM from human marrow using *Sambucus nigra* agglutinin: potential application to bone marrow transplantation. *Exp Haematol* 1986; **14**: 946–950.

79. Reisner Y, Friedrich W and Fabian I. A shorter procedure for preparation of E-rosette-depleted bone marrow for transplantation. *Transplantation* 1986; **42**: 312–315.

80. Noga SJ, Davis JM, Thoburn CJ and Donnenberg AD. Lymphocyte dose modification of the bone marrow allograft using elutriation. In: *Bone Marrow Processing and Purging: A Practical Guide*. AP Gee (ed.), 1992: 175–200 (Boca Raton, FL: CRC Press).

81. Almici C, Donnenberg AD and Rizzoli V. Counterflow centrifugal elutriation: experimental and clinical applications. *J Haematother* 1992; **1**: 279–288.

82. Slaper-Cortenbach ICM, de Vries van Rossen A, Huijbens RJF et al. Neuroblastoma purging by immunorosette depletion. *Progr Clin Biol Res* 1991; **377**: 147–162.

83. Noga SJ, Davis JM, Schepers K et al. The clinical use of elutriation and positive stem cell selection columns to engineer

the lymphocyte and stem cell composition of the allograft. *Prog Clin Biol Res* 1994; **389**: 317–324.
84. Preijers F, Ruijs P, Schattenberg A and de Witte T. T-cell depletion from allogeneic bone marrow by counterflow centrifugation is not associated with a substantial loss of CD34-positive cells. *Prog Clin Biol Res* 1994; **389**: 339–344.
85. Noga SJ and Civin CI. Positive stem cell selection of hematopoietic transplantation. In: *Graft-vs-Host Disease*, 2nd edn. JL Ferrara, HJ Deeg and SJ Burakoff (eds), 1996: 717–731 (New York: Marcel Dekker).
86. Wagner JE, Santos GW, Noga SY et al. Lymphocyte depletion of donor bone marrow by counterflow centrifugal elutriation: results of a phase I–II clinical trial. *Blood* 1990; **75**: 1370–1377.
87. Noga SJ and Hess AD. Lymphocyte depletion in bone marrow transplantation: will modulation of graft-versus-host disease prove to be superior to prevention? *Semin Oncol* 1993; **20**: 28–33.
88. Noga S, Vogelsang G, Seber A et al. The incidence of GvHD, but not engraftment is affected by cyclosporine A CSA duration following transplantation with CD34+ augmented/elutriated A/E marrow. *Blood* 1995: **86**(Suppl 1): 395a.
89. Quinones RR, Gutierrez RH, Dinndorf PA et al. Extended-cycle elutriation to adjust T-cell content in HLA-disparate bone marrow transplantation. *Blood* 1993; **82**: 307–317.
90. Haleem A, Kurtzberg J, Olsen GA et al. Combined chemoseparation and immunoseparation of clonogenic T lymphoma cells from human bone marrow using 2'-deoxycoformycin, deoxyadenosine, 3A1 monoclonal antibody and complement. *Cancer Res* 1987; **47**: 4608–4612.
91. Hebert ME, Greenberg ML, Chaffee S et al. Pharmacologic purging of malignant T cells from human bone marrow using 9-β-D-arabinofuranosylguanine. *Transplantation* 1991; **52**: 634–640.
92. Blazar BR, Thiele DL and Vallera DA. Pretreatment of murine donor grafts with L-leucyl-L-leucine methyl ester: elimination of graft-versus-host disease without detrimental effects on engraftment. *Blood* 1990; **75**: 798–805.
93. Pecora AL, Bordignon C, Fumagalli L et al. Characterization of the *in vitro* sensitivity of human lymphoid and hematopoietic progenitors to L-leucyl-L-leucine methyl ester. *Transplantation* 1991; **51**: 524–531.
94. Gee AP. Antibody and complement-mediated cell separation. In: *Cell Separation Methods and Applications*. D Recktenwald (ed.), 1996 (Cambridge, MA: Marcel Dekker) In press.
95. Gee AP, Mansour V and Weiler M. T cell depletion of human bone marrow. *J Immunogen* 1989; **16**: 103–115.
96. Hale G and Waldmann H. CAMPATH-1 monoclonal antibodies in bone marrow transplantation. *J Haematother* 1994; **3**: 15–32.
97. Janssen WE, Lee C, Gross S and Gee AP. Low antigen density leukemia cells: selection and comparative resistance to antibody-mediated marrow purging. *Exp Haematol* 1989; **17**: 252–257.
98. Gee AP, Mansour VH and Weiler MB. Effects of target antigen density on the efficacy of immunomagnetic cell separation. *J Immunol Methods* 1991; **142**: 127–133.
99. Jacobs P, Wood L, Fullard L et al. T cell depletion by exposure to CAMPATH-1G *in vitro* prevents graft-versus-host disease. *Bone Marrow Transplant* 1994; **13**: 763–769.
100. Rowley SD. Recombinant human deoxyribonuclease for hematopoietic stem cell processing. *J Haematother* 1995; **4**: 99–104.
101. Gee AP, Bruce KM, Morris TD and Boyle MDP. Evidence for an anti-complementary associated with human bone marrow cells. *J Nat Cancer Inst* 1985; **75**: 441–445.
102. Zhong RK, Kozii R and Ball ED. Homologous restriction of complement-mediated cell lysis can be markedly enhanced by blocking decay-accelerating factor. *Br J Haematol* 1995; **91**: 269–274.
103. Weiler JM, Edens RE, Linhardt RJ and Kapelanski DP. Heparin and modified heparin inhibit complement activation *in vivo*. *J Immunol* 1992; **148**: 3210–3216.
104. Points to consider in the manufacture and testing of monoclonal antibody products for human use. *Fed Reg* 1994; **56**: 148.
105. Xia M-Q, Hale G, Lifely MR et al. Structure of the CAMPATH-1 antigen, a GPI-anchored glycoprotein which is an exceptionally good target for complement lysis. *Biochem J* 1993; **293**: 633–640.
106. Hale G, Clark MR and Waldmann H. Therapeutic potential of rat monoclonal antibodies: isotype specificity of antibody-dependent cell-mediated cytotoxicity with human lymphocytes. *J Immunol* 1985; **134**: 3056–3061.
107. Hale G, Swirsky D, Waldmann H and Chan LC. Reactivity of the monoclonal antibody CAMPATH-1 with human leukemia cells and its possible application for autologous bone marrow transplantation. *Br J Haematol* 1985; **60**: 41–48.
108. Hadam MR. Cluster report: CDw52. In: *Leucocyte Typing IV*. W Knapp, B Dorken, WR Gilks, EP Rieber, RE Schmidt, H Stein and AEG von dem Borne (eds), 1989: 670 (Oxford: Oxford University Press).
109. Hale G, Xia M-Q, Tighe HP et al. The CAMPATH-1 antigen CDw52. *Tissue Antigens* 1990; **35**: 118–127.
110. Waldmann H, Or R, Hale G et al. Elimination of graft versus host disease by *in vitro* depletion of alloreactive lymphocytes using monoclonal rat anti-human lymphocyte antibody CAMPATH-1. *Lancet* 1984; **2**: 483–486.
111. Hale G and Waldmann H. Control of graft-versus-host disease and graft rejection by T cell depletion of donor and recipient with CAMPATH-1 antibodies. Results of matched sibling transplants for malignant diseases. *Bone Marrow Transplant* 1994; **13**: 597–611.
112. Theobald M, Hoffman T, Bunjes D and Heit W. Comparative analysis of *in vivo* T cell depletion with radiotherapy, combination chemotherapy, and the monoclonal antibody CAMPATH-1G, using limiting dilution methodology. *Transplantation* 1990; **49**: 553–559.
113. Naparstek E, Hardan I, Ben-Shahar H et al. A new method for prevention of graft versus host disease GvHD. *Exp Haematol* 1989; **17**: 723(Abstr).
114. Willemze R, Richel DJ, Falkenberg JHF et al. *In vivo* use of CAMPATH-1G to prevent graft-versus-host disease and graft rejection after bone marrow transplantation. *Bone Marrow Transplant* 1992; **9**: 255–261.
115. Simon M, Bartram CR, Friedrich W et al. Fatal B-cell lymphoproliferative syndrome in allogeneic marrow graft recipient. A clinical, immunobiological and pathological study. *Virchow's Arch B Cell Pathol* 1990; **60**: 307.
116. Ortho Multicenter Transplant Study Group. A randomized clinical trial of OKT3 monoclonal antibody for acute rejection

of cadaveric renal transplants. *New Engl J Med* 1985; **313**: 337–342.
117. Swinnen LJ and Fisher RI. OKT3 monoclonal antibodies induce interleukin-6 and interleukin-10: a possible cause of lymphoproliferative disorders associated with transplantation. *Curr Opin Nephrol Hypertension* 1993; **2**: 670–678.
118. Platzer E, Rubin BY, Lu L et al. OKT3 monoclonal antibody induces production of colony-stimulating factors. for granulocytes and macrophages in cultures of human T lymphocytes and adherent cells. *J Immunol* 1985; **134**: 265–271.
119. Gleixner B, Kolb HJ, Holler E et al. Treatment of aGvHD with OKT3: clinical outcome and side effects associated with release of TNF-alpha. *Bone Marrow Transplant* 1991; **8**: 93–98.
120. Ueda M, Joshi ID, Dan M et al. Preclinical studies for adoptive immunotherapy in bone marrow transplantation. Generation of anti-CD3 activated cytotoxic T cells from normal donors and autologous bone marrow transplant candidates. *Transplantation* 1993; **56**: 351–356.
121. Bianchi A, Montacchini L, Barral P et al. CD3-induced T cell activation in the bone marrow of myeloma patients: major role of CD4+ cells. *Br J Haematol* 1995; **90**: 625–632.
122. Granger S, Janossy G, Francis G et al. Elimination of T lymphocytes from human bone marrow with monoclonal T antibodies and cytolytic complement. *Br J Haematol* 1982; **50**: 367–374.
123. Filipovich AH, McGlave P, Ramsay NK et al. Treatment of donor bone marrow with OKT3 pan-T monoclonal antibody for prophylaxis of graft-vs-host disease (GvHD) in histocompatible allogeneic bone marrow transplantation. *J Clin Immunol* 1982; **2**(Suppl 3): 154S–7S.
124. Prentice HG. OKT3 incubation of donor marrow for prophylaxis of acute graft-vs-host disease (GvHD) in allogeneic bone marrow transplantation. *J Clin Immunol* 1982; **2**(Suppl 3): 148S–53S.
125. Filipovich AH, McGlave PB, Ramsay NK et al. Pretreatment of donor bone marrow with monoclonal antibody OKT3 for prevention of acute graft-versus-host disease in allogeneic histocompatible bone marrow transplantation. *Lancet* 1982; **i**: 1266–1269.
126. Bunnin, NJ, Casper JT, Lawton C et al. Allogeneic marrow transplantation using T cell depletion with juvenile chronic myelogenous leukemia without HLA-identical siblings. *Bone Marrow Transplant* 1992; **9**: 119–122.
127. Lee C, Henslee-Downey PJ, Brouillette M et al. Comparison of OKT3 and T10B9 for *ex vivo* T cell depletion of partially mismatched related bone marrow transplants BMT. *Blood* 1995; **86**(Suppl 1): 625a.
128. Herve P, Flesch M, Cahn JY et al. Removal of marrow T cells with OKT3-OKT11 monoclonal antibodies and C' to prevent acute graft-versus-host disease. A pilot study in ten patients. *Transplantation* 1985; **39**: 138–143.
129. OKunewick JP, Kociban DL, Machen LL and Buffo MJ. Comparison of the effects of CD3 and CD5 donor T cell depletion on graft-versus-leukemia in a murine model for MHC-matched unrelated donor transplantation. *Bone Marrow Transplant* 1994; **13**: 11–17.
130. Kohler PC, Erickson C, Finlay JL et al. *In vitro* analysis of donor bone marrow following monoclonal antibody treatment for the prevention of acute graft-versus-host disease. *Cancer Res* 1986; **46**: 5413–5418.
131. Mitsuyasu RT, Champlin RE, Gale RP et al. Treatment of donor bone marrow with monoclonal anti-T cell antibody and C' for the prevention of graft-versus-host disease. A prospective, randomized, double-blind trial. *Ann Intern Med* 1986; **105**: 20–26.
132. Soiffer RJ, Murray C, Mauch P et al. Prevention of graft-versus-host disease by selective depletion of CD6-positive T lymphocytes from donor marrow. *J Clin Oncol* 1992; **10**: 1191–1200.
133. Soiffer RJ and Ritz J. Selective T-cell depletion of donor allogeneic marrow with anti-CD6 monoclonal antibody, rationale and results. *Bone Marrow Transplant* 1993; **12**(Suppl 3): 7S–10S.
134. Gilmore MJ, Patterson J, Ivory K et al. Standardization of T-cell depletion in HLA matched bone marrow transplantation. *Br J Haematol* 1986; **64**: 69–75.
135. Janossy G, Prentice HG, Grob JP et al. T lymphocyte regeneration after transplantation of T cell depleted allogeneic bone marrow. *Clin Exp Immunol* 1986; **63**: 577–586.
136. Ringden O, Pihlstedt P, Markling L et al. Prevention of graft-versus-host disease with T cell depletion or cyclosporin and methotrexate. A randomized trial in adult leukemic marrow recipients. *Bone Marrow Transplant* 1991; **7**: 221–226.
137. Waid TH, Lucas BA, Amlot P et al. T10B9.1A31 anti-T cell monoclonal antibody: Preclinical studies and clinical treatment of solid organ allograft rejection. *Am J Kidney Dis* 1989; **14**: 61–70.
138. Ash RC, Casper JT, Chitambar CR et al. Successful allogeneic transplantation of T cell depleted bone marrow from closely HLA-matched unrelated donors. *New Engl J Med* 1990; **322**: 485–494.
139. Drobyski WR, Ash RC, Casper JT et al. Effect of T-cell depletion as graft-versus-host disease prophylaxis on engraftment and disease-free survival in unrelated marrow transplantation for chronic myelogenous leukemia. *Blood* 1994; **83**: 1980–1987.
140. Henslee-Downey PJ, Abhyankar SH, Parrish RS et al. Use of partially mismatched related donors extends access to allogeneic marrow transplant. *Blood* 1997; **89**: 3864–3872.
141. Rio B, Bernier C, Andreu G et al. T cell depletion does not affect long-term human bone marrow culture. *Bone Marrow Transplant* 1987; **1**: 311–315.
142. Racadot E, Herve P, Beaujean F et al. Prevention of graft versus host disease in HLA-matched bone marrow transplantation for malignant diseases: a multicentric study of 62 patients using 3 pan-T monoclonal antibodies and rabbit C'. *J Clin Oncol* 1987; **5**: 426–435.
143. Uckun FM and Myers DE. Allografts and autograft purging using immunotoxins in clinical bone marrow transplantation for hematologic malignancies. *J Haematother* 1993; **2**: 155–163.
144. Martin PJ, Hansen JA, Torok-Storb B et al. Effects of treating marrow with CD3-specific immunotoxin for prevention of acute graft-versus-host disease. *Bone Marrow Transplant* 1988; **3**: 437–444.
145. Vallera DA, Taylor PA, Panoskaltsis-Mortari A and Blazar BR. Therapy for ongoing graft-versus-host disease induced across the major or minor histocompatibility barrier in mice with anti-CD3 Fab'.2-ricin toxin A chain immunotoxin. *Blood* 1995; **86**: 4367–4375.

146. Casellas P, Rauel S and Bourrie B. T lymphocyte killing by T101-ricin A chain immunotoxin: pH dependent potentiation with lysosomotropic amines. *Blood* 1988; **72**: 1197–1202.
147. Laurent G, Maraninchi D, Gluckman E et al. Donor bone marrow treatment with T101 Fab fragment ricin A-chain immunotoxin prevents graft-versus-host disease. *Bone Marrow Transplant* 1989; **4**: 367–371.
148. Antin JH, Weinstein HJ, Bouloux C and Bierer BE. Immunotoxin-mediated depletion of CD5+ T cells from bone marrow for graft-versus-host disease prophylaxis. In: *Bone Marrow Processing and Purging: A Practical Guide*. AP Gee (ed), 1991: 213–230 (Boca Raton, FL: CRC Press).
149. Filipovich AH, Vallera D, McGlave P et al. T cell depletion with anti-CD5 immunotoxin in histocompatible bone marrow transplantation. The correlation between residual CD5 negative T cells and subsequent graft-versus-host disease. *Transplantation* 1990; **50**: 410–415.
150. Uckun FM, Myers DE, Ledbetter JA et al. Cell-type specific cytotoxicity of anti-CD4 and anti-CD8 ricin immunotoxins against human alloreactive T cell clones. *Blood* 1989; **74**: 2445–2454.
151. Ghetie MA and Vitteta ES. Recent developments in immunotoxin therapy. *Curr Opin Immunol* 1994; **6**: 707–714.
152. Youle RJ. Mutations in diphtheria toxin to improve immunotoxin selectivity and understand toxin entry into cells. *Semin Cell Biol* 1991; **2**: 39–45.
153. Cavazzanna-Calvo M, Fromont C, Le Diest F et al. Specific elimination of alloreactive T cells by an anti-interleukin 2 receptor B chain specific immunotoxin. *Transplantation* 1990; **50**: 1–7.
154. Chaudhary VK, Gallo MG, Fitzgerald D and Pastan I. A recombinant single-chain immunotoxin composed of anti-Tac variable regions and a truncated diphtheria toxin. *Proc Natl Acad Sci USA* 1990; **87**: 9491–9494.
155. Blazar BR, Carroll SF and Vallera DA. Prevention of murine graft versus host disease and bone marrow alloengraftment across the major histocompatibility barrier after donor graft preincubation with anti-LFA1 immunotoxin. *Blood* 1991; **78**: 3093–3102.
156. Ito H, Morizet J, Coulombel L and Stanislawski M. T cell depletion of human marrow using an oxidase–peroxidase enzyme immunotoxin. *Bone Marrow Transplant* 1990; **6**: 395–398.
157. Ito HO, Morizet J, Coulombel L et al. An immunotoxin system intended for bone marrow purging composed of glucose oxidase and lactoperoxidase coupled to monoclonal antibody 097. *Bone Marrow Transplant* 1989; **4**: 519–527.
158. Irvin JD and Uckun FM. Pokeweed antiviral protein: ribosome inactivation and therapeutic applications. *Pharmacol Ther* 1992; **55**: 279–302.
159. Przepiorka D, LeMaistre CF, Huh YO et al. Evaluation of anti-CD5 ricin A chain immunoconjugate for prevention of acute graft-vs-host disease after HLA-identical marrow transplantation. *Ther Immunol* 1994; **1**: 77–82.
160. Koehler M, Hurwitz CA, Krance RA et al. Xomazyme-CD5 immunotoxin in conjugation with partial T cell depletion for prevention of graft rejection and graft-versus-host disease after bone marrow transplantation from matched related donors. *Bone Marrow Transplant* 1994; **13**: 571–575.
161. Weisdorf D, Filipovich AH, McGlave P et al. Combination graft-versus-host disease prophylaxis using immunotoxin anti-CD5-RTA Xomazyme-CD5 plus methotrexate and cyclosporine or prednisone after unrelated donor marrow transplantation. *Bone Marrow Transplant* 1993; **12**: 531–536.
162. Przepiorka D, Huh YO, Khouri I et al. Graft failure and graft-vs-host disease after subtotal T-cell-depleted marrow transplantation: correlations with marrow hematopoietic and lymphoid subsets. *Prog Clin Biol Res* 1994; **389**: 557–563.
163. Vartdal F, Kvalheim G, Lea TE et al. Depletion of T lymphocytes from human bone marrow. *Transplantation* 1987; **43**: 366–371.
164. Gee AP, Lee C, Sleasman JW et al. T lymphocyte depletion of human peripheral blood and bone marrow using monoclonal antibodies and magnetic microspheres. *Bone Marrow Transplant* 1987; **2**: 155–163.
165. Knobloch C, Spadinger U, Rueber E and Friedrich W. T cell depletion from human bone marrow using magnetic beads. *Bone Marrow Transplant* 1990; **6**: 21–24.
166. Collins NH, Gee AP and Henslee-Downey PJ. T-cell depletion of allogeneic bone marrow transplants by immunologic and physical techniques. In: *Stem Cell and Marrow Processing for Transplantation*. L Lasky and P Warkentin (eds), 1994: 149–168 (Bethesda, MD: American Association of Blood Banks).
167. Yau JC, Reading CL, Thomas MW et al. Purging of T lymphocytes with magnetic affinity colloid. *Exp Haematol* 1990; **18**: 219–222.
168. Wang MY, Kvalheim G, Kvaløy S et al. An effective immunomagnetic method for bone marrow purging in T cell malignancies. *Bone Marrow Transplant* 1992; **9**: 319–323.
169. Egeland T, Albrechtsen D, Martin PJ and Hansen JA. Immunomagnetic depletion of CD6+ cells from bone marrow and peripheral blood. *Bone Marrow Transplant* 1990; **5**: 193–198.
170. Bosserman LD, Murray C, Takvorian T et al. Mechanism of graft failure in HLA-matched and HLA-mismatched bone marrow transplant recipients. *Bone Marrow Transplant* 1989; **4**: 239–245.
171. Boyle MDP and Gee AP. Low antigen density tumor cells – an obstacle to effective autologous bone marrow purging? *Cancer Invest* 1987; **5**: 113–118.
172. Champlin R, Giralt S, Przepiorka D et al. Selective depletion of CD8-positive T-lymphocytes for allogeneic bone marrow transplantation: engraftment, graft-versus-host disease and graft versus leukemia. *Prog Clin Biol Res* 1992; **377**: 385–398.
173. Nimer SD, Giorgi J, Gajewski JL et al. Selective depletion of CD8+ cells for prevention of graft-versus-host diseases after bone marrow transplantation: a randomized controlled trial. *Transplantation* 1994; **57**: 82–87.
174. Jansen J, Hanks S, Akard L et al. Selective T cell depletion with CD8-conjugated magnetic beads in the prevention of graft-versus-host disease after allogeneic bone marrow transplantation. *Bone Marrow Transplant* 1995; **15**: 271–278.
175. Kögler G, Bru Capdeville A, Hauch M et al. High efficiency of a new immunological magnetic cell sorting method for T cell depletion of human bone marrow. *Bone Marrow Transplant* 1990; **6**: 163–168.
176. Arpaci F, Gee AP, Brouillette M et al. Controllable T cell depletion by high gradient magnetic separation. *Exp Haematol* 1996; **24**: 626(Abstr).

177. Gingrich RD, Lee C-K, Hohl RD *et al*. Graded incremental donor T cell addback GIAB following allogeneic bone marrow transplantation Al-BMT. *Blood* 1995; **86**(Suppl 1): 625a.
178. Kemshead JT, Hancock J and Liberti P. Immunomagnetic colloids for the enrichment of tumor cells from peripheral blood and bone marrow: a model system. *J Haematother* 1994; **3**: 51–57.
179. Fletcher RC and Picolli SP. Capacity of colloidal goat anti-mouse IgG ferrofluid to negatively deplete cells. *Prog Clin Biol Res* 1994; **389**: 79–87.
180. Bieva C, Vander Drugghen FJ and Stryckmans PA. Malignant leukemic cell separation by iron colloid immunomagnetic adsorption. *Exp Haematol* 1989; **17**: 914–920.
181. Gratwohl A and Schmitz N. First International Symposium on Allogeneic Peripheral Blood Precursor Cell Transplants. *Bone Marrow Transplant* **17**(Suppl 2): S1–3.
182. Dreger P, Haferlacht T, Eckstein V *et al*. G-CSF-mobilized peripheral blood progenitor cells for allogeneic transplantation: safety, kinetics of mobilization and composition of the graft. *Br J Haematol* 1994; **87**: 609–613.
183. Miflin G, Russell NH, Hutchinson RM *et al*. Allogeneic PBSCT – an evaluation of engraftment kinetics and GvHD risk. *Blood* 1996; **88**(Suppl 1): 616a.
184. Suzue T, Kawano Y, Takaue Y and Kuroda Y. Cell processing protocol for allogeneic peripheral blood stem cells mobilized by granulocyte colony-stimulating factor. *Exp Haematol* 1994; **22**: 888–892.
185. Dreger P, Viehmann K, Steinmann J *et al*. G-CSF-mobilized peripheral blood progenitor cells for allogeneic transplantation. Comparison of T cell depletion strategies using different CD34+ selection strategies or CAMPATH-1. *Exp Haematol* 1995; **23**: 147–154.
186. Jestice HK, Scott MA, Ager S *et al*. Liquid storage of peripheral blood progenitor cells for transplantation. *Bone Marrow Transplant* 1994; **14**: 991–994.
187. Ruiz Arguelles GJ, Ruiz Arguelles A, Perez Romano B *et al*. Filgrastim mobilized peripheral blood stem cells can be stored at 4°C and used in autografts to rescue high-dose chemotherapy. *Am J Hematol* 1995; **48**: 100–103.
188. Bensinger WI, Buckner CD< Rowley S *et al*. Transplantation of allogeneic CD34+ peripheral blood stem cells PBSC in patients with advanced hematologic malignancies. *Bone Marrow Transplant* 1996; **17**(Suppl 2): S38–9.
189. Bensinger WI, Rowley S, Lilleby K *et al*. Reduction in graft-versus-host disease GvHD after transplantation of CD34 selected allogeneic peripheral blood stem cells PBSC in older patients with advanced malignancies. *Blood* 1996; **88**(Suppl 1): 421a.
190. de Wynter EA, Coutinho LH, Pei X *et al*. Comparison of purity and enrichment of CD34+ cells from bone marrow, umbilical cord and peripheral blood primed for apheresis using five separation systems. *Stem Cells* 1995; **13**: 524–532.
191. Ishizawa L, Burgess J, Hardwick A *et al*. Selection of human CD34+ cells using indirect immunomagnetic procedures and a magnetic cell separation system. In: *Hematopoietic Stem Cells: The Mulhouse Manual*. E Wunder, H Sovalat, PR Hénon and S Serke (eds), 1994: 171–182 (Dayton, OH: Alpha Medical Press).
192. Kawanishi Y, Flomenberg N, Cook-Craig A *et al*. A new limiting dilution culture system for detection of T cell subsets in T-cell depleted marrow grafts. *J Haematother* 1996; **5**: 485–496.
193. Kernan NA, Flomenberg N, Collins NH *et al*. Quantitation of T lymphocytes in human bone marrow by limiting dilution assay. *Transplantation* 1985; **40**: 317–322.
194. Marciniak E, Romond EH, Thompson JS *et al*. Laboratory control in predicting clinical efficacy of T cell depletion procedures used for prevention of graft-versus-host disease: importance of limiting dilution analysis. *Bone Marrow Transplant* 1988; **3**: 589–598.
195. Hazlett L, Lee C, Brouillette M *et al*. Improving limiting dilution assay methods for evaluating T cell content in bone marrow. *J Haematother* 1995, **4**: 206(Abstr).
196. Hoffman T, Theobald M, Bunjes D *et al*. Frequency of bone marrow T cells responding to HLA-identical non-leukemic and leukemic stimulator cells. *Bone Marrow Transplant* 1993; **12**: 1–8.
197. Bishara A, Brautbar C, Nagler A *et al*. Prediction by a modified mixed leukocyte reaction assay of graft-versus-host disease and graft rejection after allogeneic bone marrow transplantation. *Transplantation* 1994; **57**: 1474–1479.
198. Spencer A, Brookes PA, Kaminski E *et al*. Cytotoxic T lymphocyte precursor frequency analyses in bone marrow transplantation with volunteer unrelated donors. *Transplantation* 1995; **59**: 1302–1308.
199. Salomo M, Steinman J, Glass B *et al*. Leukemia-specific allogeneic donor T cells: quantification by limiting dilution assay. *Bone Marrow Transplant* 1995; **15**: 179–186.
200. Noel DR, Witherspoon RP, Storb R *et al*. Does graft-versus-host disease influence the tempo of immunologic recovery after allogeneic human bone marrow transplantation? *Blood* 1978; **51**: 1087–1105.
201. Keever CA, Small TN, Weiner-Fedus S *et al*. Immune reconstitution following bone marrow transplantation. Comparison of recipients of T cell depleted marrow with recipients of conventional marrow grafts. *Blood* 1989; **73**: 1340–1350.
202. Daley JP, Rozans MK, Smith BR *et al*. Retarded recovery of functional T cell frequencies in T-cell depleted bone marrow transplant recipients. *Blood* 1987; **70**: 960–964.
203. Rooney CM, Wimperis JZ, Brenner MK *et al*. Natural killer cell activity following T-cell depleted allogeneic bone marrow transplantation. *Br J Haematol* 1986; **62**: 413–420.
204. Small TN, Keever CA, Weiner-Fedus S *et al*. B-cell differentiation following autologous, conventional or T-cell depleted bone marrow transplantation: a recapitulation of normal B-cell ontogeny. *Blood* 1990; **76**: 1647–1656.
205. Ault KA, Antin JH, Ginsburg D *et al*. Phenotype of recovering lymphoid cell populations after marrow transplantation. *J Exp Med* 1985; **161**: 1483–1502.
206. Brenner MK, Wimperis JZ, Reittie JE *et al*. Recovery of immunoglobulin isotypes following T cell depleted allogeneic bone marrow transplantation. *Br J Haematol* 1986; **64**: 125–132.
207. Wimperis JZ, Prentice HG, Karayiannis P *et al*. Transfer of a functioning humoral immune system in transplantation of T lymphocyte depleted bone marrow. *Lancet* 1986; **i**: 339–343.
208. Janossy G, Prentice HG, Grob JP *et al*. T lymphocyte regeneration after transplantation of T cell depleted allogeneic bone marrow. *Clin Exp Immunol* 1986; **63**: 577–586.

209. Roux E, Helg C, Dumont-Girard F et al. Analysis of T-cell repopulation after allogeneic bone marrow transplantation: significant differences between recipients of T cell depleted and unmanipulated grafts. *Blood* 1996; **87**: 984–992.
210. Soiffer RJ, Bosserman L, Murray C et al. Reconstitution of T cell function after CD6-depleted allogeneic bone marrow transplantation. *Blood* 1990; **75**: 2076–2084.
211. Lamb LS, Parrish RS, Walker M et al. Peripheral lymphocyte reconstitution during the first year following bone marrow transplantation from a partially mismatched related donor. *J Haematother* 1995; **4**: 239(Abstr).
212. Kook H, Goldman F, Padley D et al. Reconstruction of the immune system after unrelated or partially matched T cell depleted bone marrow transplantation in children: immunophenotypic analysis and factors affecting the speed of recovery. *Blood* 1996; **88**: 1089–1097.
213. Martelli MF, Aversa F, Velardi A et al. New tools for crossing the HLA barrier: fludarabine and megadose stem cell transplants. *Blood* 1996; **88**: 484a.
214. Bachar-Lustig E, Rachamim N, Li H-W et al. Megadose of T cell depleted bone marrow overcomes MHC barriers in sublethally irradiated mice. *Nature Medicine* 1995; **1**: 1268–1273.
215. Rencher SD, Houston JA, Lockey TD and Hurwitz JL. Eliminating graft-versus-host potential from T cell immunotherapeutic populations. *Bone Marrow Transplant* 1996; **18**: 415–420.
216. Galnes BA, Colson YL, Kauffman CL and Ildstad ST. Facilitating cells enable engraftment of purified fetal liver stem cells in allogeneic recipients. *Exp Haematol* 1996; **24**: 902–913.
217. Kaufman CL, Colson YL, Wren SM et al. Phenotypic characterization of a novel bone marrow-derived cell that facilitates engraftment of allogeneic bone marrow stem cells. *Blood* 1994; **84**: 2436–2446.

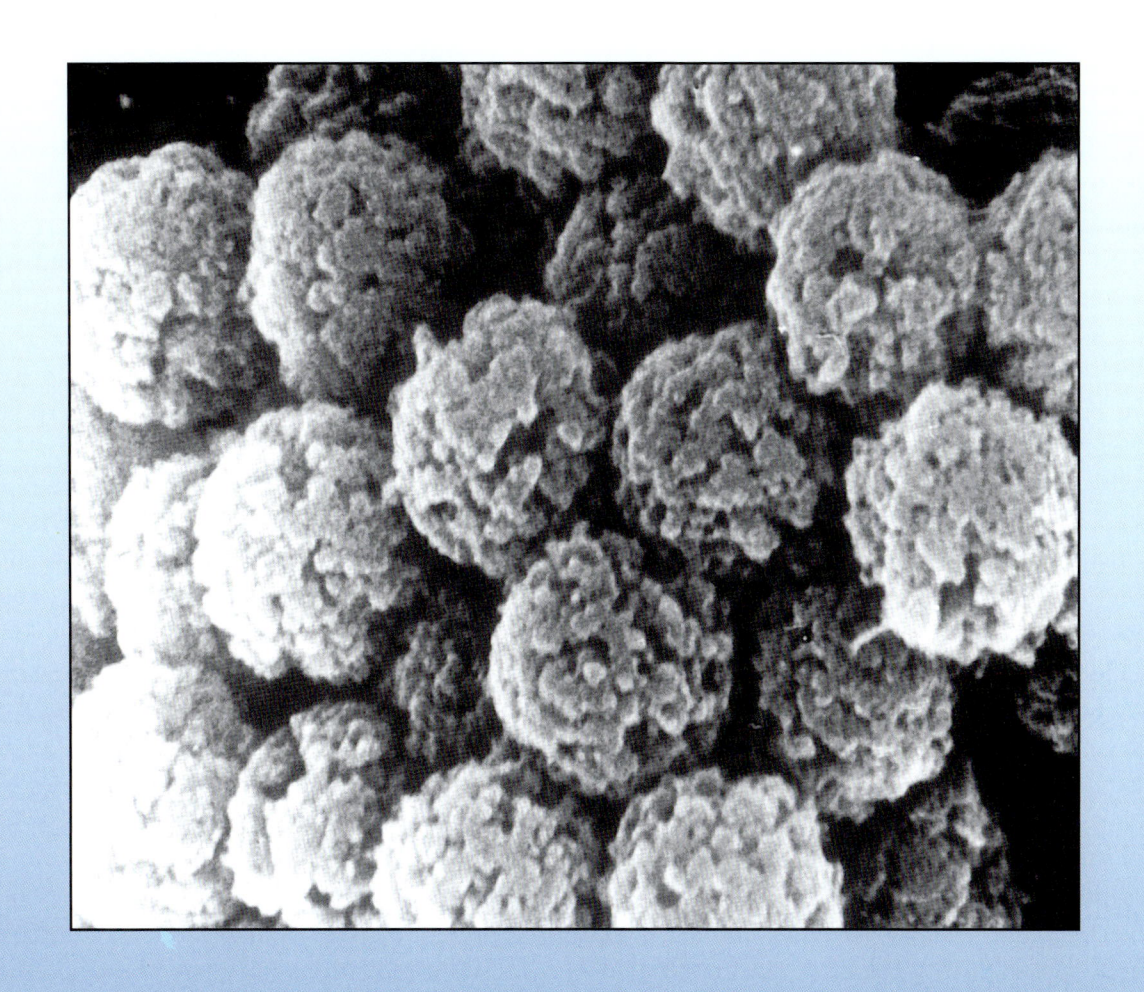

Chapter 33

Purging tumour from autologous stem-cell grafts

Adrian P. Gee

Introduction

Access to stem-cell transplantation has been limited, historically, by the availability of histocompatible sibling donors [1]. Attempts to overcome this problem have included the use of matched unrelated [2] and partially mismatched related donors [3]; however, the most widely used alternative graft is autologous stem cells [4]. Of the 10 450 stem-cell transplants performed in Europe in 1994, 6811 were autologous, whereas ten years earlier, allogeneic transplants outnumbered autologous by nearly two to one [4]. This dramatic shift has been accompanied by a similar change in the source of the autologous graft. In 1991, 90% of autologous grafts were obtained from bone marrow, whereas in 1994, 65% consisted of mobilized peripheral blood progenitor cells [4]. These changes have certainly improved access to stem-cell transplantation and have overcome the problems of graft-versus-host disease and graft rejection associated with allogeneic transplantation; however, a continuing concern has been infusion of occult tumour cells in the graft [5]. Improvements in the sensitivity of methods for the detection of minimal residual disease have demonstrated that many autologous grafts contain tumour cells [6–8] that have clonogenic activity *in vitro* [9,10] and may, therefore, be capable of initiating disease relapse *in vivo*. The true clinical significance of infusing these cells with the graft remains to be established by formal randomized trials. These studies are complex, require accrual and follow-up of large numbers of patients for a prolonged period, and have raised ethical concerns about knowingly infusing viable tumour cells into patients. As a result, proponents of removing, or purging, these cells from the graft have relied upon indirect evidence to support their position. This has been drawn from a number of sources. A retrospective analysis of clinical outcomes in 263 acute myelogenous leukaemia (AML) patients transplanted in first remission [11] concluded that the 69 patients who received grafts purged with mafosfamide showed an increase in leukaemia-free survival and a decreased probability of relapse. This difference was most apparent in the patients who were autografted within six months of achieving complete remission. In a subsequent update of 919 autografts [12], these findings were confirmed, and purging was also found to be of value for patients who had received total body irradiation as part of their conditioning regimen. A decreased incidence of late relapses in AML patients who received grafts treated with 4-hydroperoxycyclophosphamide (4HC) has been attributed to the effects of purging [13]. Analysis of 31 grafts infused into patients with advanced stage breast cancer revealed that six contained tumour cells detected by immunocytochemistry (ICC), and these patients showed a trend towards decreased overall survival, when compared to the patients receiving ICC-negative grafts [14].

In contrast, several investigators have not seen any advantages to the use of purged grafts in lymphoma [15], high-risk acute lymphoblastic leukaemia [16], neuroblastoma [17] and non-Hodgkin's lymphoma [18]. These studies were not, however, designed to evaluate the role of graft purging. The observation that relapse post-transplant also occurs predominantly at sites of previous disease [19] has been taken to indicate that it is due to failure of the high-dose regimen, rather than infusion of tumour in the graft. Likewise, isolated cases of atypical sites of early recurrence, such as in the lungs in non-Hodgkin's lymphoma, have been interpreted to be the result of graft contamination [20]. Long-term remissions have been reported, however, in patients who have received tumour cells in the graft [21], suggesting that occurrence, site and probability of relapse are modulated by many factors other than the simple presence of the tumour cells. It has been estimated in leukaemia that the risk of relapse arising from occult cells in the graft is less than 10% [22].

Some of the strongest evidence for the clinical benefits of purging come from studies in which patients with B-cell non-Hodgkin's lymphoma, at a single centre, received purged marrow grafts in which residual tumour could or could not be detected by the highly sensitive polymerase chain reaction (PCR) [23]. Patients receiving efficiently purged (PCR-negative) grafts showed a highly significant increase in disease-free survival, and the authors concluded that the inability to purge residual lymphoma cells was the most important prognostic indicator in predicting relapse. It has been argued, however, that the ability to purge the graft to PCR negativity may simply be a surrogate marker for two clinically different subsets of patients [24].

When tumour cells were infused with the marrow they became rapidly detectable in the peripheral blood in the immediate post-transplant period [25] and could subsequently be detected in the marrow. The majority of these patients subsequently relapsed; however, in 19 of 134 patients, the marrow became PCR-negative [26]. This re-emphasizes that the simple presence of tumour cells in the graft does not guarantee a poor prognosis, since these cells may either be eliminated *in vivo* by immune mechanisms or have been irreversibly damaged by prior therapy. This may be resolved by taking serial marrow aspirates post-transplant, although in such a study in children with acute lymphoblastic leukaemia who engrafted with purged PCR-positive marrow, there was no correlation between the PCR status of marrow aspirates post-transplant and subsequent relapse of disease [27]. These contrasting findings may be due to differences in the nature of the diseases, the study design and size and technical variables in the PCR assays.

The other main source of data in support of the value of graft purging has come from gene-marking studies [28]. In these studies, AML and neuroblastoma cells in autologous marrow grafts have been retrovirally transfected with the neomycin-resistance gene which provides a method for detecting and tracking the cells post-transplant. Gene-marked tumour cells detected at the site of relapse can only have originated from the autologous graft. Initial reports in AML [29], and subsequently in neuroblastoma [30], demonstrated that relapse in the majority of patients was associated with the appearance of marked tumour cells. Currently, 4 of 12 AML patients have relapsed and 3 of these showed marked tumour; 5 of 9 neuroblastoma patients have relapsed and marked cells were detected in 4 cases. In a second-generation study in AML patients who received purged grafts, 1 of 14 has relapsed and did not show marked cells; however, relapse occurred two months post-transplant and was felt to originate from endogenous disease (H. Heslop, personal communication). Analysis of tumour-cell DNA for discrete marker-gene integration sites has suggested that, in these gene-marker studies, at least 200 clonogenic tumour cells must have been infused in the graft. Given the relatively low efficiency of transduction (0–23.5%, mean 10.5% [28]), these small numbers of tumour cells would appear to have potent tumourigenic potential compared to the presumably much larger number of cells that survive high-dose therapy *in vivo*. This is supported both by the gene-marking studies and by the improvement in disease-free survival seen in lymphoma patients who received grafts purged to PCR negativity [23,26]. If this hypothesis is correct, the clinical importance of purging these cells would be significantly greater than their numbers suggest.

Alternatively, the gene-marked tumour cells may be functionally identical to those remaining in the patient, but they selectively 'homed' to a site that is particularly favourable for proliferation and the initiation of relapse, in the same way that pluripotent haematopoietic cells migrate to marrow spaces. Purging these cells from the graft would not be expected to provide substantial clinical benefit and would simply tip the balance in favour of relapse arising from residual cells in the patient. Ultimately, the importance of purging autologous grafts can only be resolved in a controlled randomized clinical trial, and efforts are underway in Europe to conduct such a study in non-Hodgkin's lymphoma. The development of highly effective purging modalities should not, in itself, be expected to transform outcomes in autologous transplantation. The results from identical-twin transplants may be used as the benchmark for what can be achieved, and further improvements will require improved strategies for the treatment of minimal residual disease, including induction of an autologous graft-versus-disease response and the use of post-transplant immunotherapy.

Tumour detection

In the absence of definitive data on the clinical value of stem-cell purging, the philosophy among its advocates has been to develop and use a variety of techniques, as long as these can be documented to remove tumour cells effectively *ex vivo*, without compromising the engraftment potential of the stem-cell preparation. Central to the development of these methods is the use of highly sensitive assays to quantitate tumour cells and to monitor their removal [7,31]. Conventional histological methods are of limited value for this purpose, since they rarely detect infiltrations of <1% tumour cells. This is already at the upper limit of tumour burden for most purging techniques, and even inefficient purging results in a graft that is tumour-free by histology.

Major improvements in the sensitivity of detection have been made possible by the advent of monoclonal antibody and molecular biology technology [7,9,10,31]. Many tumours contain cells with a characteristic pattern of antigen expression. This may be in the form of overexpression or absence of antigens found on normal cells of the same histological type, expression of antigens found normally only during foetal development, or expression of unique antigens that appear to be specific to the tumour [7]. Monoclonal antibodies directed against these antigens are now widely available and have been used in both flow cytometric analysis and immunocytochemical staining.

Flow cytometry offers the advantages of speed and the ability to analyze very large numbers of cells. Although the size and granularity of the cell populations can be discriminated by forward and orthogonal light-scatter characteristics, this approach does not permit direct examination of the morphology of the cells, which can usually resolve problems of non-specific staining of non-cancer cells. Non-specific binding of antibodies, for example through the Fc receptor, is a major complication to the use of flow cytometry to detect small numbers of tumour cells. It can often be prevented by pre-incubation of the sample with normal serum, and by the use of multiple antibodies to improve discrimination between cancer cells and normal cell populations. Multiparameter analysis [32], which combines information on light-scatter properties and staining characteristics, can further enhance the sensitivity of this technique. In some cases, further improvements can be achieved by adding to the stained sample known numbers of highly fluorescent beads with unique light-scatter properties. Gating strategies are then used to collect only information from the beads and the stained tumour cells [33]. The number of normal, unstained cells passing through the cytometer can then be back-calculated from the number of cells represented by each bead. Fluorescence-activated cell sorting is also a useful method for enriching tumour-cell populations for subsequent morphological and molecular analysis [34].

Immunocytochemical staining is able to provide additional important information on the morphology of the stained cells, which can reduce the incidence of false-positives [7,9,31]. The technique is somewhat labour-intensive, requires a thorough knowledge of histopathology and in-depth characterization of the sample preparation method, so that accurate quantitation is possible [7]. This method is, however, capable of providing sensitivities of 1 tumour cell in 100 000–250 000 [7,31,35] which makes it the most suitable antibody-mediated method for monitoring purging efficiency [31]. It should be recognized, however, that even at its most sensitive, this technique would fail to detect 40 000 tumour cells in an average graft infused into a 100 kg patient.

Molecular techniques offer improvements in sensitivity [10,22,31]. The most widely used method is the PCR, which permits detection of one tumour cell in $1-10 \times 10^6$ normal cells [36]. The technique is based upon repeated cycles of duplication of a nucleotide sequence containing a marker that is characteristic of the tumour cell. Scrupulous laboratory technique must be used to achieve reliable results and the technique is, at present, only semiquantitative, and is normally used only to indicate presence or absence of the marker within the limits of detection of the assay system. In several clinical studies a correlation has been reported between PCR-negativity of the graft and clinical outcome post-transplant [22], although this has not been a universal finding [21]. At present, PCR offers the highest sensitivity for determining purging efficiency; however, extremely careful experimental technique is essential, and in purging methods where the tumour cells are destroyed *in situ*, nuclear material is released from dying target cells into the medium and may be amplified to give a PCR-positive signal. This can be overcome by treating the purged sample with DNase before performing the PCR assay [37]. At a maximal sensitivity of 1 cell in 10^7, a PCR-negative graft may still contain 10 000 tumour cells and it is not known whether this inoculum would be sufficient to initiate relapse post-transplant. In animal models for leukaemia, injection of as few as 10 cells can result in lethal disease in all animals and, by extrapolation from these models in AML, it has been suggested that the ED_{50} for the human disease is 1000–10 000 cells [38].

Purging techniques

Elimination of tumour cells from a bone-marrow graft may be achieved either by destruction or physical removal of the tumour cell (negative selection) or by enrichment of the haematopoietic stem-cell population required to reconstitute the recipient (positive selection) [39]. While there are a number of techniques available for purging (Table 33.1), positive selection methods are based on the use of antibodies directed against the CD34 antigen which is expressed on a variety of early committed progenitor cells, including pluripotent stem cells [40], as well as high capillary endothelial cells [41] and possibly even on some tumour-cell populations [42].

Physical methods

Unit gravity sedimentation, density-gradient centrifugation and centrifugal elutriation have all been used as tumour-purging modalities [43]. In most cases, the differences in size and density between normal and tumour cells are insufficient to use any of these techniques alone to achieve effective purging; however, they can provide a useful up-front debulking prior to using more specific approaches. Sedimentation under unit gravity is of value for debulking tumours that tend to occur as aggregates or clumps within the marrow, for example, neuroblastoma [44]. Allowing these cells to settle under gravity followed by aspiration of the supernatant cell suspension, can result in a 1 log depletion of the tumour [45].

Although density gradient, or density cushion centrifugation is widely used as a method to enrich mononuclear cell populations from blood and marrow, it can actually serve to enrich tumour cells, which tend to collect in the light density fraction (unpublished observations). Centrifugation of blood or marrow seeded with tissue-cultured human breast cancer or neuroblastoma cells, on a Ficoll Hypaque density cushion ($d = 1.077$ g/ml), usually results in a doubling of the initial seeding level when the mononuclear cell fraction is examined. This is accompanied, however, by a parallel two- to fivefold enrichment of CD34-positive progenitor cells within the same fraction, resulting in no overall change, or a slight improvement in the stem cell:tumour cell ratio. Further improvements can be achieved by changing the density or type of the separation material. Percoll cushions [46] of various densities can be used to enrich stem-cell populations and deplete tumour cells and/or T-lymphocytes from bone marrow.

Centrifugal elutriation is a sophisticated form of centrifugation in which the centrifugal force on cells in

Table 33.1 Tumour purging techniques

	Removed	Destroyed in situ
Non-antibody mediated	Density gradients Centrifugal elutriation Sedimentation	Cytotoxic drugs Photoactive agents Alkyl lysophospholipids Hyperthermia/freezing Antisense oligonucleotides Ribozymes Selective cell culture Cytotoxic effector cells
Antibody mediated	Panning – negative selection Magnetic microspheres Magnetic 'colloids' Floating beads Immunorosettes Immunoaffinity columns High-speed cell sorting CD34-based +ve selection	Antibody + complement Immunotoxins Radioimmunoconjugates

a spinning chamber is balanced by an opposing fluid flow into the chamber [47]. Under steady-state conditions, cells within the chamber will segregate based upon their size and density. They can then be sequentially eluted from the chamber, either by changing the speed of the rotor or the fluid flow. This method has been used most extensively for depleting T-cells from allogeneic marrow grafts [48]; however, it results in a significant loss of smaller CD34-positive cells, which must be recovered from another eluted fraction and added back to the graft [49]. The differences in size and density between most tumour cells and normal haematopoietic progenitors is probably insufficient to allow this method to be used as a primary purging technique. In addition, the heterogeneity in physical properties of tumour cells from different patients will make it difficult to standardize.

In an attempt to institute a more uniform technique, methods have been developed to alter the density of the target cells by attachment of particles, such as beads and erythrocytes [50]. Tetrameric antibody complexes, consisting of an antitumour monoclonal antibody linked to an anti-red-cell antibody by two rat anti-mouse immunoglobulin antibody molecules, have been used to rosette neuroblastoma and leukaemia cells in marrow with erythrocytes. These rosetted cells were then separated by centrifugal elutriation with limited success [50].

Biophysical methods

Temperatures above 42°C have been reported to eradicate up to 2 logs of human clonogenic leukaemia cells while sparing 65% of colony-forming cells of the granulocyte–macrophage lineage (CFU-GM) [51]. At 44°C, this differential effect is lost. The effects of heat appear to be most damaging to late-committed progenitors, whereas long-term repopulating cells are relatively resistant [52]. In model experiments, exposure to 42°C for 2 hours resulted in destruction of 4–6 logs of leukaemic cells but only 50% of CFU-GM [53]. Treatment of human marrow and peripheral blood stem cells for 1 hour at 42°C did not impair engraftment and had no significant effect on the CFU-GM content [54]. Combining hyperthermia with drugs [55] and/or cytokines [56], or alkyl-lysophospholipids [57], has been reported to increase tumour-cell kill. Leukaemic progenitors have also been reported to be more sensitive to cryopreservation than their normal committed counterparts, suggesting that freezing the graft may contribute to purging [58] although this has not been confirmed in studies on cryopreserved marrow from patients with AML [59].

Culture purging

In vitro culture of grafts has been used as a purging technique for both acute and chronic myeloid leukaemia (CML) [60] and has been proposed for use in myeloma [61]. Similar results have also been reported in acute lymphoblastic leukaemia (ALL), where culture of the marrow for 4–10 weeks resulted in disappearance of leukaemic cells in about half of the cultures [62]. Culture of ALL marrows under serum-containing and serum-free conditions for three weeks resulted in the disappearance of *bcr–abl*-positive cells in 5 of 5 and 2 of 5 cultures respectively [63], although the production of CFU-GM was similar in both cases. In a study of 31 cases of acute leukaemia and myelodysplastic syndromes [64], culture resulted in normal cellular morphology in 15 of 25 leukaemia patients, but in only 1 of 6 myelodysplastic marrows. Cytogenetic analysis showed that culture resulted in complete or partial replacement of acute leukaemia cells by normal cells in *de novo* acute leukaemia, and by Philadelphia chromosome-positive cells in CML in blast crisis, indicating that multiple outcomes are possible using this purging approach [64]. An examination of non-adherent cells from CML marrow cultures has indicated that the disappearance of Ph^1-positive cells in this fraction may be largely fortuitous, since Ph^1-positive cells were still likely to be present in the adherent stroma at the end of the three- to four-week culture period [65]. Others have reported differences in purging efficiency depending on whether the cultures are established from blood or marrow [66]. In a single patient report, blood samples from a patient with chronic granulocytic leukaemia could be cultured within four weeks to *bcr–abl*-negativity, whereas those from marrow could not.

The efficacy of long-term culture as a purging modality depends on the ability to demonstrate both removal of the tumour to the limits of detection of the most sensitive assay available, and retention of engraftment potential by the cultures. Considerable effort is currently being devoted towards *ex vivo* expansion of pluripotent and early committed progenitor cells using combinations of recombinant growth factors, serum-free media and current good manufacturing practices. It remains to be determined whether the optimal conditions for haematopoietic cell culture will achieve effective removal of tumour cells. If a graft can be expanded from a small blood or marrow aspirate, the number of malignant cells in the initial culture can be minimized, and this approach may become a routine purging option, provided that repeated replication does not 'burn-out' pluripotent stem cells [67]. Until that time, culture purging of large grafts is laborious, expensive, may risk failure to engraft and is probably not a viable alternative when compared to other techniques.

Purging by cytotoxic effector cells

The use of various autologous cytotoxic cells for graft purging has been proposed in a number of diseases. Lymphokine activated killer (LAK) cells, generated by incubation of lymphocytes with interleukin-2 (IL-2), have been shown to deplete 2–3 logs of leukaemia cells from marrow without affecting normal committed colony-forming cells, haematological recovery or survival in laboratory experiments with human cells and in animal models [68,69]. Autologous bone- marrow cells can also be stimulated by IL-2 to show cytolytic activity towards leukaemia cells, and this activity is potentiated by the addition of IL-1, tumour necrosis factor-α (TNF-α), and γ-interferon (IFN-γ) [70], although these cytokines may also suppress generation of CFU-GM [71]. Marrow cells cultured with IL-2 generate predominantly CD3/CD8-positive T-cells [71,72] and CD56-positive natural killer cells, and IL-6, TNF-α, and IFN-γ appear to be generated in the culture supernatants [72]. The generation of cytotoxic activity requires at least six days [72]. Large-scale culture systems have been described for the generation of activated killer cells for either *ex vivo* or *in vivo* therapeutic procedures [73]. A seven-day culture of light-density cells seeded at 1×10^6 ml in medium containing foetal bovine serum and 1000μ/ml IL-2 resulted in activated cells that showed cytotoxicity towards tissue-cultured leukaemic targets, and maintenance of normal long-term culture-initiating cells [73].

An alternative approach is to culture the marrow in the presence of IL-2 and allow endogenously-generated killer cells to purge the tumour *in situ* [74]. Ten-day incubation in the presence of 1000μ/ml IL-2 resulted in Ph^1-negative cultures in 4 patients with CML; however, the number of normal colony-forming progenitors decreased after the first 7 days. This approach has been tested clinically in 5 patients with ALL whose marrow was cultured for ten days with 1000UmL IL-2 [75]. Increases in both LAK and natural killer (NK) activity were seen following incubation, when patients received $0.64–1.56 \times 10^8$ nucleated cells ($1.87–44.8 \times 10^4$ CFU-GM). Four patients engrafted with counts of 0.5×10^9 granulocytes/litre on days 22–36, and platelet counts of 50×10^9/litre on days 25–42. One patient remained thrombocytopenic until relapse and 1 died on day 12 post-transplant.

Cytokine-activated cells may be targeted to the tumour cells by using bispecific antibodies including anti-CD3 × anti-CD13 for AML [76,77], or by the addition of the anti-CD3 monoclonal antibody OKT3 [78] which binds to AML cells via CD64, the high-affinity Fc receptor. More complex activation procedures have been proposed for the generation of cytokine-induced killer (CIK) effectors. These include sequential incubation with IFN-γ on day 0, and IL-1, IL-2 and anti-CD3 on day 1 [79]. The resulting CD56-positive cells were able to lyse up to 3 logs of autologous and allogeneic CML cells, while reducing CFU-GM by only 25% [79]. Monocytes activated by IFN-γ have also been proposed as cytotoxic effectors and were capable of a 2-log reduction of AML cells with little effect on committed colony-forming progenitors (CFU-GM, CFU-E and BFU-E) [80]. Recently, a human, lethally-irradiated major histocompatibility complex (MHC)-non-restricted cytotoxic T-cell line was shown to be extremely effective for purging both lysis-sensitive and lysis-resistant leukaemia cells in a model system. The former reverted to PCR and culture negativity, while the latter were devoid of tumourigenic activity when transplanted into severe combined immunodeficient SCID-hu mice 9 [81].

The ability to generate tumour-directed cytotoxic effector cells is now being exploited clinically for both *ex vivo* and *in vivo* therapy and has produced promising results, particularly in the allogeneic setting where the predominant mechanism of action may be entirely different. For purging applications, the efficacy of this approach should be further confirmed by the use of state-of-the-art assays for residual tumour cells.

Cytotoxic drugs

A variety of cytotoxic agents have been used for purging, including chemotherapeutic drugs, photoactive agents and alkyl-lysophospholipids. The most widely used drugs have been 4HC [82] and mafosfamide (a sulphoethylthio derivative), which are cyclophosphamide derivatives that do not require *in vivo* activation to exert their effects. Inside the cell 4HC is activated to phosphoramide mustard, which is the active metabolite for cyclophosphamide [83]. In addition, incubation with the drug produces internucleosomal DNA fragmentation that is characteristic of apoptosis [84]. These drugs have been used extensively for purging in acute myelogenous leukaemia [85,86], acute lymphocytic leukaemia [87], multiple myeloma [88] and, with variable success, in chronic myelogenous leukaemia [89,90], breast cancer [91,92], and acute myelogenous leukaemia secondary to myelodysplastic syndromes [93]. The procedure is technically simple, involving incubation of mononuclear marrow cells with the drug at a fixed dose [83,86], or at a concentration previously determined for each individual patient in small-scale experiments [94]. In the latter case, there was, however, often a poor correlation between the results of the small-scale test and the large-scale marrow purge [94], and there has been no demonstrated direct correlation between the effects of the drug on normal and leukaemic cells [83]. The treated cells are then washed and cryopreserved for later infusion.

Careful preparation of the nucleated cell fraction for drug treatment is particularly important [95] since aldehyde dehydrogenase, which is present in erythrocytes, can interfere with the cytotoxic action of 4HC. It has also been reported that the nucleated cell concentration during incubation affects sensitivity to 4HC [96], and that autologous and allogeneic plasma contain a factor that may increase the cytotoxicity of mafosfamide towards normal progenitor cells [97]. Prolonged engraftment times are characteristic of 4HC-treated grafts, since the drug destroys many committed progenitor cells [83], such as CFU-GM, but spares pluripotent progenitors in a hierarchical dose–response relationship [98]. Interestingly, *in vitro* studies suggest that delayed platelet engraftment, frequently seen with 4HC-purged grafts, may not be due to loss of CFU-Megakaryocyte [99].

At purging doses of 60 µg/ml, 4HC destroys 4–5 logs of T-cells, and almost completely eliminates both LAK and NK cell activity [100], which may impair the function of lymphocytes in the mature graft. In a clinical study, however, increased numbers of CD16-positive cells post-transplant correlated with a significant increase in cytotoxicity towards the NK-sensitive K562 leukaemia cell line, and the effects persisted for at least one year post-transplant [101].

Protective agents, such as amifostine [92,102], have been used to spare early- and late-committed progenitors, while preserving the anti-leukaemic effects of 4HC. Alternatively, administration of recombinant growth factors post-transplant can be used to accelerate haematopoiesis and reduce hospital stay [92,103].

Clinical results obtained using 4HC and mafosfamide-purged grafts in AML have been taken to indicate the importance of purging in improving outcome [11,12], and in particular in reducing the risk of late relapse of disease, notably for patients who are transplanted within six months of achieving complete remission [13]. 4HC has been combined with etoposide [104], doxorubicin [105], vincristine and methylprednisolone [106], nucleoside analogues [107], hyperthermia [55] and monoclonal antibodies [108]. Regulatory approval has not been obtained in the United States for 4HC [109], therefore access has been restricted to participants in an ongoing clinical trial.

Photoactive agents and alkyl-lysophospholipids

A variety of other agents have been used or proposed for purging either alone or in combination. These include marine alkaloids [110], lectins [111,112], steroids [113,114], phthalates [115], esters [116], HMG-CoA reductase inhibitors [117], adenosine triphosphate [118] and a variety of nucleoside analogues [107,119,120]. Of particular importance are photoactive drugs and alkyl-lysophospholipids. The former, represented predominantly by merocyanine (MC540) and porphyrin derivatives, e.g. pofimer sodium (Photofrin) and benzoporphyrin derivative monoacid ring A (BPD), exert their effects by sensitizing cells to the effects of light [121]. The mechanism of their cytotoxic action is not completely understood. The majority of clinically important photosensitizers exert their effects by type II reactions, in which highly reactive single molecular oxygen is formed. This, in turn, reacts with a variety of targets including lipids, nucleic acids, amino acids, proteins, purines, pyrimidines and carbohydrates. The selectivity towards certain tumour cells, particularly leukaemias, lymphomas and neuroblastomas is not fully understood [121,122], but can be affected by dose fractionation [123], post-irradiation conditions, especially temperature [124], changes in cellular repair mechanisms [125] and differences in intracellular concentration [121]. Killing can also be enhanced by the addition of salicylate [126,127] and the radioprotective agent, ethiofos [128]. Photofrin II and MC540 are roughly equivalent in their ability to kill leukaemia and lymphoma cells while sparing normal haematopoietic progenitors [122]. Under conditions which spare 50% of normal CFU-GEMM progenitors, MC540 eliminates 4–8 logs of clonogenic leukaemia and lymphoma cells [129]. In an animal model system [130], BPD killed 5–6 logs of L1210 leukaemia cells *in vitro*, while depleting less than 1 log of committed myeloid progenitors. *In vivo*, a purging dose of 100 ng/ml of BPD resulted in approximately 4-log depletion of tumour and successful haematopoietic engraftment of 50% of the animals. Differences in the effects of various photosensitizers on tumour cells expressing the multiple drug-resistance gene have also been described [131,132].

For purging with MC540, a washed, bone-marrow buffy coat with a haematocrit of 4% (since the absorption spectra of MC540 and haemoglobin substantially overlap [122]) is first prepared in HEPES-buffered α-modified Dulbecco's medium containing 1–2% AB serum and 100 U/ml heparin, and adjusted to 1×10^7 cells/ml (large grafts can be processed at 2×10^7/ml). MC540 (Kodak, Rochester, NY; stock solution contains 1 μg/ml in 50% ethanol) is added to give a final concentration of 15 μg/ml. Photoirradiation was achieved using a UVAR® photopheresis system (Therakos Inc., West Chester, PA). This device, which is approved in the United States for the palliative treatment of the skin manifestations of cutaneous T-cell lymphoma, consists of a Haemonetics-type blood centrifuge (which is used to prepare the buffy coat), a roller pump, which transfers the cells from one reservoir to another via an illumination cassette, and temperature sensors, to alert the operator if the temperature rises above 41°C. The illumination cassette (volume 190 ml) consists of six clear acrylic, double-walled cylinders that are used to pass a 2-mm thick cell suspension past tubular fluorescent bulbs (GTE Sylvania ~3.6 mW/cm^2). The cells are cooled during exposure by passage of air between the bulb and the inner wall of the chamber. The entire cassette including the bulbs is disposable. The cells are pumped through the system at 100 ml/min into the second reservoir, and then the direction of flow is reversed for the second exposure. Following treatment, the cells are pelleted, washed three times in buffer and cryopreserved. The dose of dye-mediated irradiation can be controlled either by changing the number of passages through the illumination cassette, or by reducing the concentration of serum in the illumination medium [133].

In a clinical study [133], 21 patients with acute leukaemia or lymphoma received MC540-purged grafts. Nine died early from infection or relapse and the majority of those who were evaluable engrafted late, taking 23–67 days to achieve an absolute neutrophil count of 500. Three patients received unpurged back-up grafts. The delayed engraftment was attributed primarily to poor marrow quality [133]. At the time of the report, there were two long-term survivors, at >45 months post-transplant, who were disease-free and haematologically and immunologically normal.

Alkyl-lysophospholipids are anticancer drugs that have the cell membrane as their primary site of action. They target enzymes involved in signal transduction, phospholipid synthesis and maintenance of membrane integrity [134]. They have also been found to inhibit tumour-induced angiogenesis, downregulate the expression of cell adhesion molecules [135] and show selective cytotoxicity towards neoplastic cells [136]. One of the compounds with the highest therapeutic index is edelfosine (1-O-octadecyl-2-O-methyl-*rac*-glycero-3-phosphocholine [ET-18-OCH$_3$]). In animal models, injection of purged marrow into lethally irradiated mice resulted in a dose-dependent increase in survival [137], and a similar differential effect was found *in vitro* for human marrow seeded with a leukaemic cell line [138]. Interestingly, the purging effect was augmented by cryopreservation of the treated samples [138,139], and a similar effect has been reported for breast cancer purging [140]. The differential effect of edelfosine on normal and leukaemic cells, and the dose and time-dependent nature of this effect have been confirmed in a number of *in vitro* experiments [141].

The clinical purging procedure is relatively simple [141,142]. Nucleated marrow cells are incubated at a concentration of 2×10^7/ml in RPMI 1640 medium containing 10% autologous plasma to which has been added edelfosine to give a final concentration of 50–100 µg/ml. Incubation is carried out for 4 hours at 37°C with shaking. The cells are then centrifuged at 258 g for 10 minutes, the supernatant aspirated, and the cells adjusted to a concentration of 8×10^7/ml before addition of an equal volume of freezing medium and cryopreservation.

In a clinical study, 29 patients with acute leukaemia in second or subsequent remission, early relapse, either with a history of extramedullary relapse, or requiring more than one round of induction to achieve remission, were transplanted with edelfosine-purged marrow [141,142]. Five patients died of infectious complications during aplasia. The median days to recovery of 500 granulocytes/µl were 26 (range 16–47 days) at an edelfosine dose of 50 µg/ml, and 39 days (range 18–66 days) at a dose of 75 µg/ml. Median days to recovery of 25 000 platelets/µl were 52 (range 24–178) and 49 days (range 12–125) respectively. The median survival was 555 days and median disease-free survival 237 days. At the time of the report 13 patients were alive, and 10 were disease-free, although one was still transfusion-dependent and another had a karyotypic abnormality. Only 1 of 10 patients purged at the lower dose remains in remission (at 1613 days). It has been suggested that combinations with other agents, such as the lipoidal amine CP-46.665 and hyperthermia [57,143], and reducing the concentration of serum during incubation [144] may further improve the efficacy of purging with ether lipids.

Molecular biology-based purging

A newly emerging category of purging techniques is those based on molecular biology. Genes have been identified that confer growth advantage to tumour cells and which can be used to target a tumour-cell population. It is possible to design antisense oligonucleotides to complement a region of a particular gene or messenger RNA and which would, therefore, potentially prevent replication of the tumour cells [145]. This may be achieved by a variety of mechanisms [146], including blocking of transcription through sequence-specific hybridization, preventing mRNA processing and/or transport from the nucleus to the cytoplasm, preventing attachment of the mRNA to the ribosome, inhibiting translation by the ribosomal complex and/or leading to mRNA degradation by RNase H [147].

The use of antisense oligonucleotides alone, or in combination with mafosfamide purging [148], has been proposed for purging in chronic myelogenous leukaemia [149] where the target is *bcr–abl*, in acute myelogenous leukaemia where expression of p53 tumour suppression gene is increased and can be targeted [150], and in various acute and chronic leukaemias where *c-myb* was targeted [151].

When co-cultures of normal marrow mononuclear cells and primary acute myelogenous leukaemia blasts were treated with *c-myb* antisense, only normal colonies could be identified. Similar results were obtained using CML blast co-cultures [146], and efficient destruction of the malignant cell clone has been confirmed in replating experiments [152]. Chemical modification of the oligomers is often carried out in order to provide increased resistance to nucleases and enhanced membrane solubility [146]; however, this can alter targeting efficiency, which may also be affected by the secondary structure of the targeted RNA sequence. In addition, improved purging efficiency of cultured CML by *bcr–abl*-directed antisense oligomers cells has been demonstrated using three repeated treatments of 24 hours, compared to a single treatment at the same, or double, the concentration. Neither treatment schedule had a significant effect on normal CFU-GM or more immature progenitors [149].

In early clinical studies, a 26-mer specific for the B2A2 junction of *bcr–abl* was used for purging marrow from a patient with CML in accelerated phase [153]. This resulted in a 24% reduction in CFU-GM and a 41% decrease in CD34-positive cells. The patient showed engraftment in 15 days, and reconstituted platelets in 17 days and neutrophils in 25 days. Philadelphia-negative cells were detected by fluorescence *in situ* hybridization post-transplant and the patient, at the time of the report, was in complete haematological remission nine months post-transplant.

Investigators at the University of Nebraska have used OL(1)p53, a 20-mer phosphorothioate oligonucleotide directed against p53 mRNA, for purging in patients with either AML or myelodysplastic syndrome [154]. Marrows were incubated with the 1 μM OL(1)p53 for 36 hours at 37°C in gas-permeable cell culture flasks, washed and cryopreserved until infusion. This treatment had no effect on the growth of myeloid or erythroid progenitor colonies. Eight patients have received oligonucleotide-purged grafts and engrafted to an absolute neutrophil count of $>0.5 \times 10^9$/litre in a median of 22 days. These studies are ongoing.

Ribozymes are specific RNA sequences that have the ability to cleave other RNA molecules in a catalytic fashion. The hammerhead ribozyme is composed of a catalytic hammerhead region and flanking oligonucleotides that bind specifically to targeted sequences [155]. Multi-unit ribozymes, which target several sites on *bcr–abl*, have been designed for purging in CML, and have been shown to be more efficient than single-unit ribozymes in cleaving *bcr–abl* substrate RNA. Ribozyme uptake by cultured CML cells was markedly enhanced both by liposome delivery using lipoectin, and by receptor-mediated delivery via the folate receptor; however, only receptor-targeted delivery or constitutive expression via retroviral vectors, resulted in reduced *bcr–abl* kinase levels [155]. In subsequent experiments using mouse myeloblasts transfected with the *bcr–abl* gene, treatment with multi-unit ribozymes targeted via the folate receptor, resulted in a 3-log reduction in the level of *bcr–abl* mRNA. Work is currently in progress to develop a clinical purging system based upon this approach.

Antibody-targeted purging

The exquisite specificity of monoclonal antibodies provides a method for both identifying and effecting the separation of target cells from stem-cell grafts. The antigen used for targeting need not be truly tumour-specific, but should not be expressed by other cells in the mixture. A number of effector mechanisms are available for the negative or positive selection of antibody-sensitized cells. These include, for negative selection, coupling of toxins or isotopes to the antibody, and incubation of sensitized cells with complement. Positive selection techniques using antibodies include immunorosetting, immunomagnetic separation with superparamagnetic particles and colloids, floating beads, immunoaffinity columns and panning.

Antibody and complement

One of the earliest and most widely used methods for purging was complement-mediated target-cell lysis [156]. This approach has the advantage that multiple monoclonal antibodies can be used to identify the target, which is then eliminated by the addition of complement in the form of whole serum. The target cells are destroyed by activation of the classical complement pathway [157] which is initiated by the C1q component of complement being activated when crosslinked by cell-bound antibody. This results in a cascade reaction involving binding and sequential activation of complement components, formation of a membrane attack complex and colloid osmotic lysis of the target cell [157].

The choice of antibodies is limited only by their ability to fix the complement source which, in the case of purging, is usually baby rabbit serum. IgM monoclonals fix complement efficiently since a single molecule of the antibody is able to bind and crosslink C1q through its subunits [157]. In contrast, a doublet of IgG molecules must be bound to the cell surface to achieve the same effect [158]. This does not present a problem when the cell expresses the target antigen at high or normal density. On cells with low surface expression of the antigen, IgG doublet formation is more difficult, and the complement cascade is not triggered. Escape from lysis due to target low antigen expression has been described in several experimental systems [159–161].

The heterogeneity in antigen expression shown by tumour cells within a patient and between different patients presents a challenge to effective purging when complement is used with a single monoclonal antibody [162]. This can be resolved by using panels of antibodies directed against a variety of independently expressed antigens; however, failure of complement-mediated purging using multiple antibodies has been described in clinical studies [23].

Many complement sources show non-specific toxicity towards human marrow cells, and it is usually necessary to screen several batches of serum in order to avoid this effect [163]. The selected batch is sterilized by membrane filtration and stored at −70°C until use. In the United States, pending regulatory requirements indicate that complement will also be required to meet the same standards of testing as monoclonal antibodies that are used in therapeutic procedures [164]. In some cases, autologous serum has been used as the complement source. This has been added to the antibody-sensitized cells *ex vivo*, or the cells have been infused into the patient to be eliminated by complement *in vivo* [165].

Complement-mediated cell lysis can be inhibited by a number of factors. Cation-chelating anticoagulants, such as EDTA, can sequester calcium ions that are required for effective complement activation [157]. In the cases where these anticoagulants have been used for harvesting, extensive washing of the cells before the addition of complement, and the use of calcium- and magnesium-containing buffers or media are strongly recommended. We have also shown, and others have recently confirmed, that an anticomplementary factor is associated with normal marrow cells [166,167]. This is a decay-accelerating factor which interferes with the ordered interaction of early complement components on the target-cell surface. Again, extensive washing of the cells prior to complement treatment can reduce this effect [166].

If the choice is made to use antibody and complement for clinical purging, the method is technically simple [168] (once optimization of the system has been carried out in preclinical experiments). A mononuclear cell fraction of the graft is preferred, due to the extensive downstream manipulation of the cells, during which granulocytes can be disrupted and release DNA into the cell suspension, resulting in 'gelling' of the cells. After washing, the cells are resuspended at high concentration in medium containing protein (e.g. plasma protein fraction) to which is added the monoclonal antibody mixture. The cells are incubated on ice with occasional mixing usually for 30–90 minutes. Opinions differ on whether it is necessary to remove fluid-phase antibody before the addition of complement. In our experience, this has not been necessary. The complement source is thawed immediately before use and added directly to the antibody-treated cell suspension. The action of complement is temperature-dependent [157]. A source that is ice-cold will not effectively lyse cells. It is important to ensure that the cell suspension rapidly reaches ambient temperature, or 37°C, upon the addition of complement. The temperature and time of incubation should be chosen based upon preclinical experiments. In most cases the end-point is reached within 90 minutes at ambient temperature. Continuous gentle mixing is recommended throughout the incubation period. Depending upon the system, the destruction of cells during this incubation can result in release of DNA into the suspension, with resulting aggregation and clumping of the graft. This can be reduced by the addition of DNase with the complement [169]. After incubation the cells are washed extensively (three or four times) to remove complement and nuclease, prior to cryopreservation and storage. An automated method for purging with antibody and complement has been described in which incubation and washing steps are performed in the bowl of a cell-separation centrifuge [170].

The analysis of complement-treated grafts is complicated by the fact that some target cells may retain membrane integrity immediately after treatment, but lose it subsequently. These cells may be detected by immunofluorescence procedures and represent 'false'-positives. These cells may be induced to undergo lysis by incubating the sample for at least 60 minutes at 37°C prior to analysis [168]. Where molecular detection techniques are employed [23,171], nucleic acids released by lysed cells can also give false-positive results, and incubation of the sample with DNase before analysis has been recommended [37].

For the reasons stated earlier, complement-mediated purging has generally fallen out of favour. Many investigators have shown that the same monoclonal antibodies used as immunotoxins or with magnetic microspheres produce superior results. The difficulty of sourcing and testing complement for therapeutic procedures has also contributed to the decline in its use. In spite of these limitations, complement continues to be used in clinical studies of autologous marrow purging [167] and the depletion of T-cells from allogeneic grafts [165,172]. It is particularly suited to the latter application, where it is important to retain a small number of residual T-cells in the graft to assist engraftment and potentially contribute to a graft-versus-leukaemia response.

Immunotoxins

An alternative method to complement for eliminating antibody-sensitized tumour cells from a graft is to use a toxin, such as ricin, abrin, gelonin or diphtheria toxin. These molecules cannot be added directly to the graft, but must be targeted by direct conjugation to a tumour-directed monoclonal antibody, or other tumour-directed agent, such as peanut agglutinin [173], or an agent which spares pluripotent stem cells, e.g. certain cytokines [174]. Conjugation may be achieved by chemical means [175] or by recombinant technology [174]. This adds a degree of complexity to the procedure, since conjugates must be prepared and quality controlled for each antibody in the panel, which can be hazardous and time-consuming. The conjugates are added in combinations which reflect the antigenic profile of the tumour. In contrast to complement, the use of multiple antibodies with toxins has not always produced superior results [176].

The most widely used toxin is ricin which is isolated from the castor bean (*Ricinis communis*). The molecule consists of two disulphide-linked chains. The short, toxic polypeptide A chain exerts its effects by enzymatically inactivating ribosomes by depurination, thereby inhibiting protein synthesis [177]. The longer B chain, which can bind to galactosyl residues on cells, facilitates transport of the A chain across the cell membrane and prevents its lysosomal transfer and degradation [178]. If the intact molecule is used to prepare the immunotoxin, it is necessary to block the lectin activity of the B chain, which would target the conjugate non-specifically by binding to sugars on non-target cells. This can be achieved by carrying out the incubations in buffers containing lactose, or by covalent attachment of affinity ligands to the B chain. An alternative approach is to prepare the conjugates with only the toxic A chain of ricin; however, these have generally been found to be less effective, due primarily to poor translocation into the cell. This can be improved by the addition of lysosomotropic amines, such as ammonium chloride or carboxylic ionophores [179]. Ricin-based immunotoxins have been proposed or used for purging acute leukaemias [177,180,181], breast cancers [182] and multiple myeloma [183].

Another toxin that has been used for graft manipulation is pokeweed antiviral protein (PAP), which is member of a family of single-chain, ribosome-inactivating proteins, known as hemitoxins [177]. PAP lacks the B chain with its non-specific binding properties and has been used to prepare immunotoxins for the treatment of lymphoid malignancies [184,185]. Other candidate toxins for the preparation of purging immunotoxins include gelonin [175], *Pseudomonas* exotoxin A [186] and diphtheria toxin lacking the binding domain and targeted to T-cells via the interleukin-2 receptor [187,188]. The availability of new toxins, the ability to engineer improved specificity [189] and to utilize other cell-surface targets, such as cytokine receptors, hold renewed promise for this form of purging.

Immunophysical purging
Panning

Linkage of the tumour-directed monoclonal antibody to a solid phase facilitates the physical separation of tumour cells from the graft. The solid phase can take a number of forms, ranging from a flat surface, through large beads and microspheres, to nanoparticles and colloids [43]. The configuration of the separation device is radically affected by the choice of the solid phase. Lansdorp has calculated that in order to immobilize a fixed amount of antibody, a flat surface area of $600\,cm^2$ would be required, whereas the same amount could be attached to a column of beads occupying a volume of less than 5 ml, to less than 1 ml bed volume of microspheres, or to several hundred microlitres of colloidal material [190]. A flat surface configuration, while requiring a relatively large surface, has the advantage of potentially lower non-specific trapping of cells that is characteristic of column separations. The antibody is usually attached to a polystyrene or chemically modified plastic surface, either by passive adsorption or chemical coupling, and non-coated surfaces are blocked by incubation with protein such as albumin.

Many factors affect the efficiency of antibody immobilization and are outside the scope of this review. In the case of purging applications where multiple monoclonal antibodies are used to optimize tumour-cell capture, it may be difficult to achieve adequate attachment of all of the antibodies in a manner which will compensate for the heterogeneity of antigen expression that is found between patients. As a result, panning applications in graft processing have predominantly focused on the removal of T-cells from allogeneic grafts [191,192] or the enrichment of normal haematopoietic progenitor cells expressing the CD34 antigen [193,194]. Given the low frequency of CD34-positive cells, a two-step procedure has been described to debulk the marrow of irrelevant cells prior to incubation on the immobilized anti-CD34 (Figure 33.1). In this first step, nucleated cells are incubated on

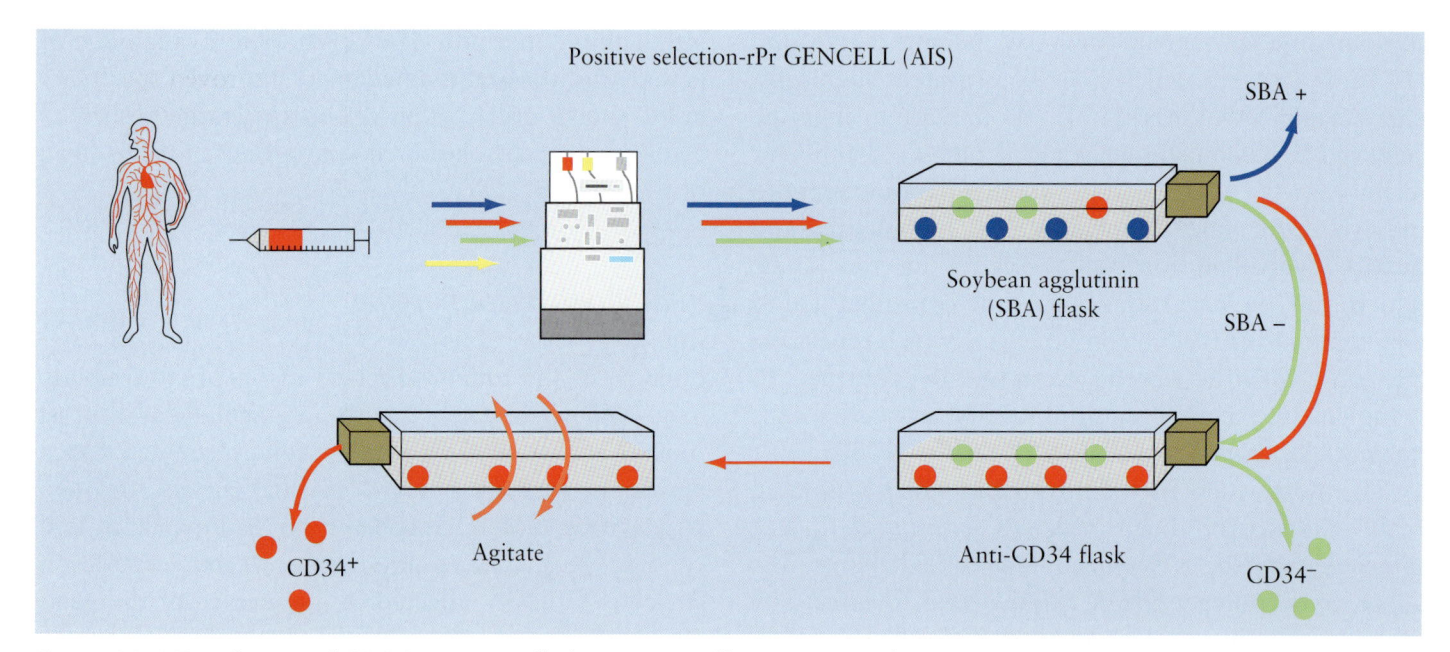

Figure 33.1 Enrichment of CD34-positive cells by immunoadherence using the GENCELL CELLector™ system. Haematopoietic progenitor cells are first incubated on a surface coated with soybean agglutinin (SBA). The SBA-negative cells are aspirated and incubated on an anti-CD34 monoclonal antibody-coated surface. The non-adherent cells are decanted and the CD34-positive cells recovered by physical detachment or by incubation.

plastic-immobilized soybean agglutinin (SBA) [195], which retains the majority of the population, but does not bind primitive haematopoietic cells. These are aspirated or decanted and incubated on the anti-CD34-coated surface, to which they adhere, and can be recovered, after aspirating the CD34-negative fraction, by shaking or tapping the plastic surface or by incubation of the device at 37°C for 3 hours [193]. This system was developed by Applied Immune Sciences (now rPr GENCELL) [193–195] and originally produced in two configurations, either as coated T flasks with a surface area of 25 cm^2, or as parallel large sheets of coated polystyrene enclosed within a chamber, providing a total surface area of 624 cm^2 [193]. The larger system is capable of handling ~5 $\times$ 10^8 SBA-negative cells, obtained from the large-scale, 3000 cm^2, SBA CELLector, which can process up to 4 $\times$ 10^9 erythrocyte-depleted cells. The purity of the final CD34-positive population, in small-scale experiments, ranged from 43.4% for non-mobilized peripheral blood to 81.5% for cytokine-stimulated blood, with bone marrow at 74.2% with a yield of 30% [193]. The SBA step achieves a 1-log depletion of tumour, while the combined steps result in a 3-log depletion overall [194].

Immunoaffinity columns

Use of beads as the solid phase allows configuration of the separation system into a column. This approach has been used by CellPro in the development of its CEPRATE devices [196] (Figure 33.2). As described above for panning, the choice was made to focus on the development of positive selection systems based on anti-CD34. Unlike the rPr GENCELL system, the target cells and antibody are reacted in fluid phase. Capture of the sensitized cells is achieved by using a biotinylated anti-CD34 which then reacts with the avidin coating on a column of beads. The target cells are retained on the column, from which non-target cells are eluted. The CD34-positive fraction can be recovered from the column by physical breakage of the link between the beads and the cells. In the small-scale device this is achieved by gently squeezing the column. Using this system for small-scale marrow separations, purities of 68.7 to 93.7% (n = 9) were achieved with yields of 23.1 to 46.4%.

In the clinical-scale separator (Figure 33.3), an impeller is built into the base of the column to stir the matrix gently and release the CD34-positive cells. Flow of cells and buffers over the column, and recovery of the various cell fractions in the clinical device is under

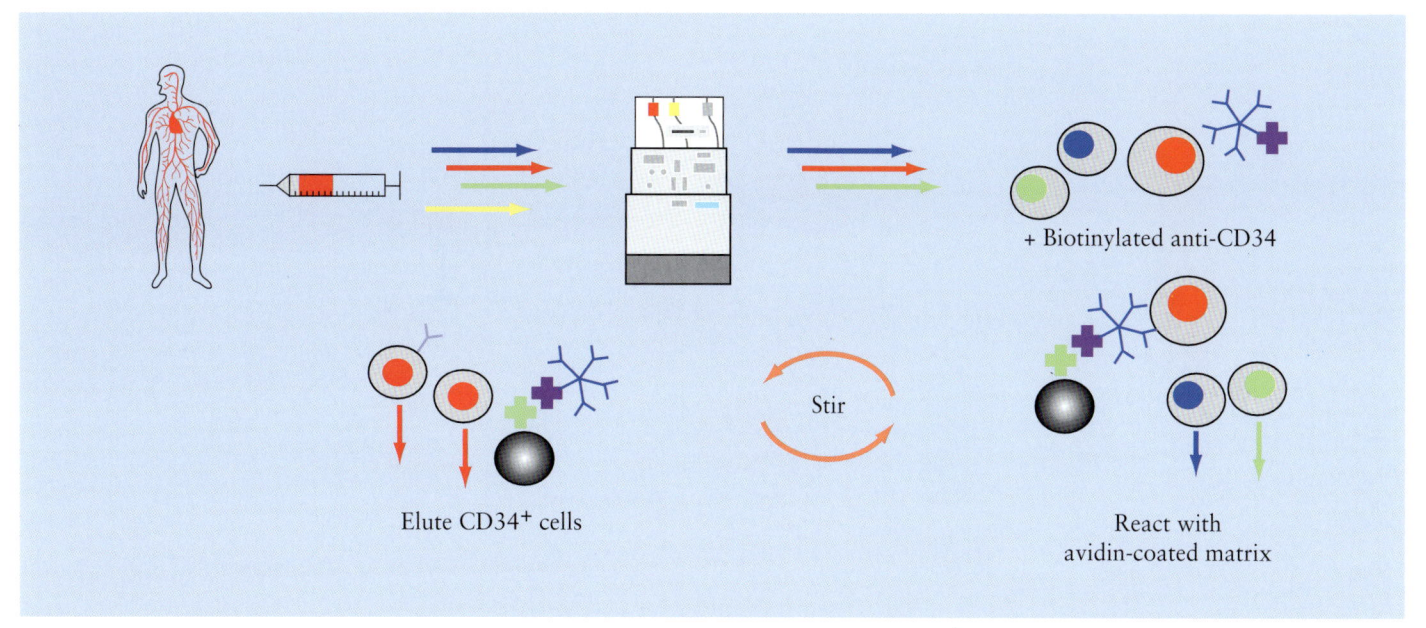

Figure 33.2 Enrichment of CD34-positive cells on the CellPro biotin avidin affinity column. Haematopoietic progenitor cells are incubated with a biotinylated anti-CD34 monoclonal antibody and then passed over a column of beads coated with avidin. The CD34-positive cells are eluted from the column by stirring the solid-phase matrix.

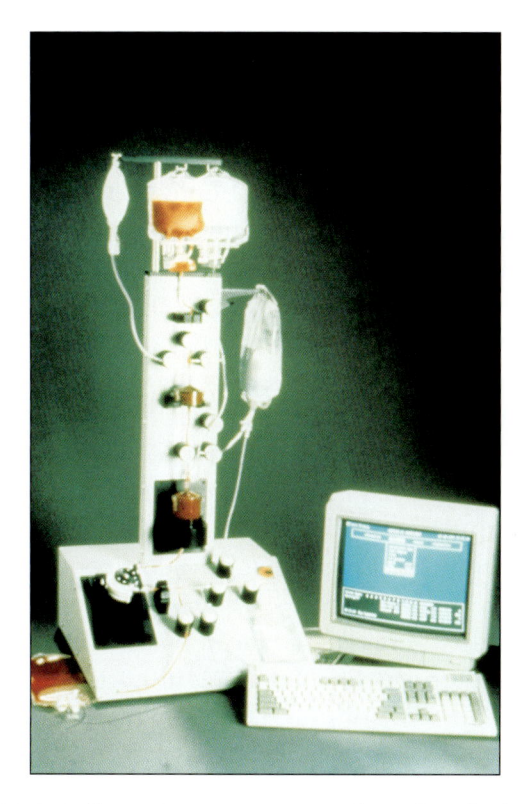

Figure 33.3 CellPro CEPRATE™ SC clinical-scale device. Haematopoietic progenitor cells are sensitized with biotinylated anti-CD34 monoclonal antibody and passed over the avidin-coated matrix under the control of a computer. The CD34-positive cells are detached from the column by stirring the matrix using an impeller located at the base. (Courtesy CellPro Inc.)

the control of a computer. The device has received regulatory approval in Europe and Canada, and approval is pending in the United States. It has been used extensively for enriching CD34-positive cells from both marrow [196] and mobilized peripheral blood progenitor cells [197,198].

Immunomagnetic separation

An alternative collection method is to use a solid-phase matrix that can be collected in a magnetic field. This is the principle behind immunomagnetic separation, which has been used both for positive and negative selection [199]. The matrix can be in the form of microspheres, microparticles, nanoparticles or a colloid. The size of the particles determines the method used for their collection. Microspheres and microparticles can be readily captured in a magnetic field generated by small rare-earth magnets, whereas nanoparticles and colloids, because of their size, must be collected using a high-gradient magnetic field (Figure 33.4). This can be produced by placing an array of metallic particles, wires or pins within a magnetic field produced by strong permanent magnets. The cell suspension that has been reacted with the magnetic matrix is then passed over the metallic array, which captures cells that are coated with the magnetic material. The non-target cells are unaffected by the array, and the target cells may be

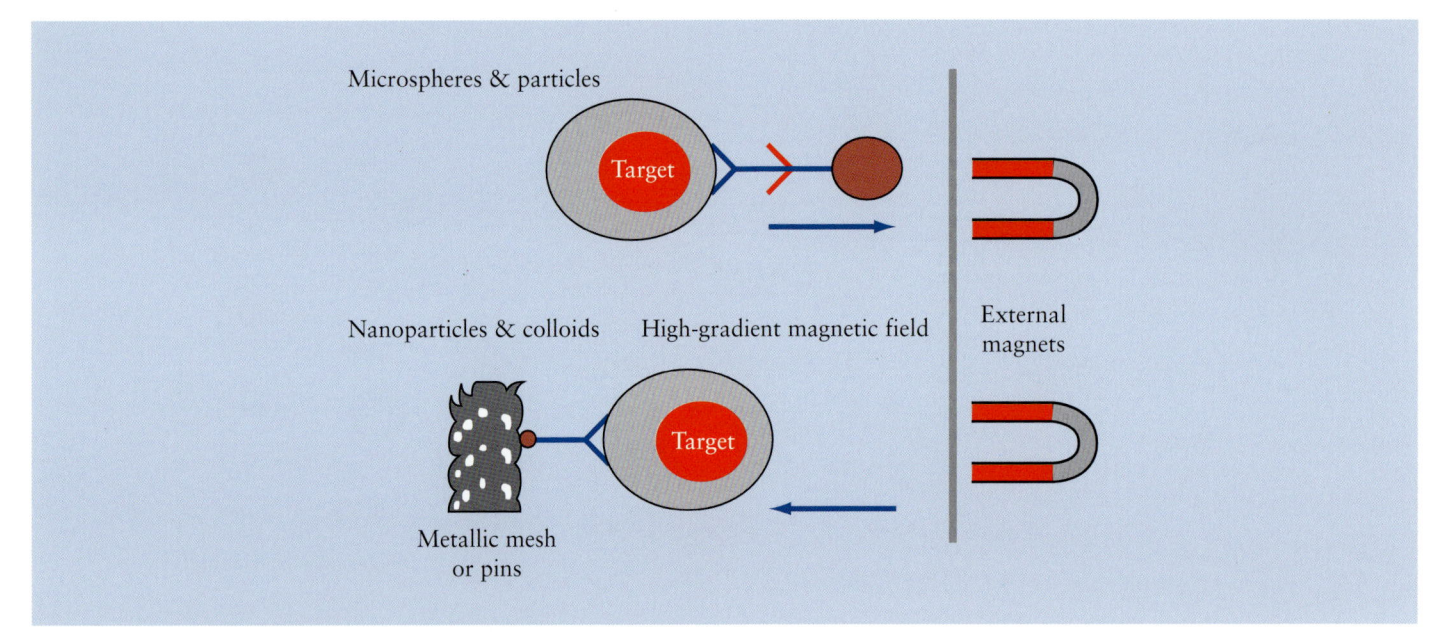

Figure 33.4 Immunomagnetic separation systems. (Top panel) *Target cells coated with paramagnetic microspheres or particles can be separated from a complex cell mixture by exposing the cell suspension to a magnetic field generated by externally placed permanent magnets. The target cells are attracted towards the magnets.* (Bottom panel) *Target cells coated with paramagnetic nanoparticles cannot be directly captured by attraction towards externally placed magnets due to the small size of the particles. The magnets are used to generate a high-gradient magnetic field in metallic wire or pins inside the collection vessel. The cells are retained on the wire and can be recovered by removing the vessel from the magnetic field.*

recovered by demagnetizing the array by simply removing it from the magnetic field [197].

For clinical stem-cell manipulation, microspheres have been most widely used, although microparticles have also been used for purging [200], and nanoparticles are in early clinical trials in Europe for positive selection applications. In most cases, an indirect method has been used in which the cell suspension is incubated with the monoclonal reagent(s) directed against the target cell(s), unbound antibody is washed out, and anti-immunoglobulin antibody (anti-Ig)-coated magnetic matrix is added. This approach provides easy saturation of all antibody-binding sites on the target cells, and allows use of multiple monoclonal antibodies to compensate for any heterogeneity in antigen expression by the target cells. The disadvantage is that fluid-phase antibody must then be removed prior to the addition of the anti-Ig-coated matrix in order to avoid blocking of the antibody-binding sites on the matrix. In the case of true magnetic colloids, the antibody-binding capacity is extremely large and colloids can absorb the fluid-phase antibody and still retain their ability to react with the target-cell-bound antibody [201]; therefore, it is unnecessary to wash out any unbound monoclonal antibody. Direct separations, in which the anti-target cell antibody is attached to the matrix can give satisfactory results when the target antigen is expressed universally and at high levels by the cells that are to be separate, for example, CD2 by T-cells [202]. In purging applications, this approach is not recommended.

The M450 superparamagnetic microspheres, manufactured by Dynal AS of Oslo, have been extensively used for purging in a variety of diseases, although microparticles produced by PerSeptive Biosystems (formerly Advanced Magnetics) have also been used for leukaemia purging in Europe [200]. The Dynal beads are uniform 4.5 μm diameter polystyrene spheres that contain magnetite dispersed throughout their volume (Figure 33.5). They are available uncoated, precoated with a variety of target-cell-directed antibodies, or with anti-Ig. As described above, for purging applications, an indirect technique using the anti-Ig particles is preferred. In most cases, a mononuclear cell (MNC) preparation of the graft material is required to reduce the proportion of

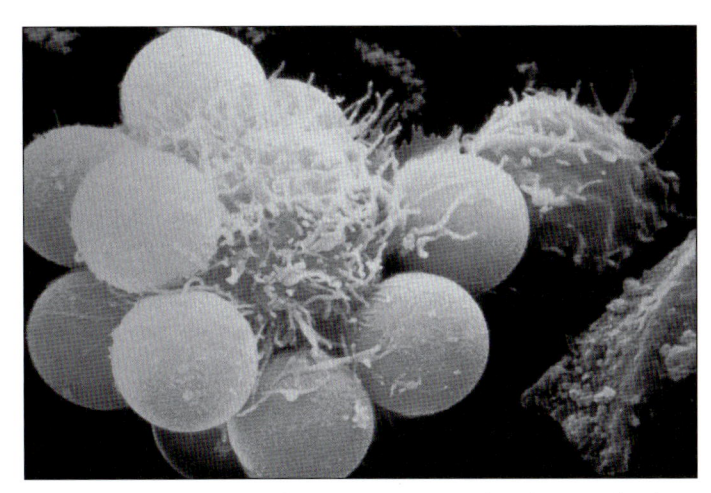

Figure 33.5 Scanning electron micrograph of an antibody-sensitized lymphoma cell rosetted with Dynal M450™ superparamagnetic microspheres. (Courtesy Dynal Inc.)

phagocytic cells which could non-specifically sequester the beads. The MNC are reacted, normally for 30–60 minutes, with the panel of monoclonal antibodies under conditions which favor sensitization of the target cells, i.e. high cell concentration, low reaction volume, buffered medium containing protein (e.g. plasma protein fraction), low temperatures (on ice or 4°C, to reduce antibody capping) and occasional mixing. The unbound antibody is then removed by washing. For efficient removal, three or four washes with 50–200 ml (depending on cell numbers) cold buffer is adequate. The anti-Ig-coated beads are then added at a bead:target cell ratio that has been determined to give optimal separation in preclinical experiments. In most cases, this is in the range of 50 to over 100 beads/tumour cell, which usually translates to one or two beads per nucleated cell. The incubation conditions should promote interaction of the beads with the antibody-sensitized target cells, i.e. low volume, slow continuous and gentle mixing for 30 to over 60 minutes. Prolonged or vigorous mixing at high bead:cell ratios can result in physical damage to the cells and should be avoided. Prior to exposure to the magnetic field, the volume of the reaction mixture can be increased by the addition of buffer. This reduces the cell concentration and reduces the chance of non-target cells being trapped by the beads as they are pulled towards the magnets.

Separation of the target cells from the mixture is usually achieved in two stages [199]. First the transfer pack containing the cells is exposed statically to a magnetic field which effects the bulk separation of target-cell–bead rosettes and free beads. This field should have high magnetic reach-out so that it penetrates the entire thickness of the cell suspension. The cells are then passed over a second array of magnets to capture any remaining target cells and beads. This secondary array consists of magnets with high holding force, so that once beads are attracted to the magnet surface, they are not dislodged by the flow of the cell suspension. For large-scale separations, a variety of separators have been described, either of the continuous flow design or using the combination approach [203,204]. A device (the MaxSep™) (Figure 33.6) was developed for research applications by Baxter Biotech [205].

It is important to emphasize that any immunomagnetic separation procedure must be carefully optimized if it is to achieve satisfactory performance [199,206]. Factors that should be addressed include selection of monoclonal antibodies, buffer systems, antibody concentration, incubation conditions, bead:cell ratio, mixing conditions, separation conditions (separator design, flow rate), assessment of purging efficiency and effects of system components on normal haematopoietic cells. These experiments are frequently complicated by the lack of availability of good model systems [207] and the issues associated with the detection of residual tumour cells.

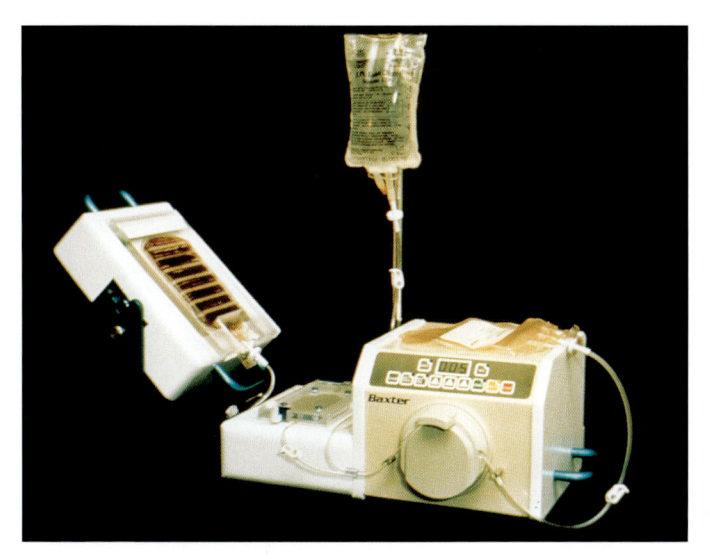

Figure 33.6 Baxter MaxSep™ large-scale separator for negative immunomagnetic separation. This device is not approved for sale for clinical applications. (Courtesy Baxter Biotech.)

Microsphere-based immunomagnetic separations are capable of depleting tumour cells to the limits of detection of most currently available assays, i.e. 4–6 logs removal [208,209]. They are unaffected by anticomplementary factors, do not require the prepreparation of antibody bead conjugates, and are more effective at capturing cells with low expression of a target antigen [159]. In some cases, certain antigens, e.g. CD3, do not seem suitable as targets for bead separations [210], and very high expression of an antigen may result in poor cell capture for steric reasons [211]. Improved performances have been reported when multiple rounds of bead treatment are performed [208,212], probably as a result of effectively increasing the bead:cell ratio upon each successive incubation, and the improvements are usually obtained at the expense of normal cell recovery. Nonetheless, immunomagnetic purging is generally regarded as the method of choice in many diseases, due to its high efficiency, low toxicity and adequate recovery of haematopoietic progenitor cells.

As an alternative to tumour purging by negative selection, immunomagnetic enrichment of CD34-positive cells has been described [198]. Systems have been developed based upon the Dynal microspheres (Figure 33.7) (the Baxter Biotech Isolex™ separators) (Figure 33.8)] [213] and the Miltenyi nanoparticles (Figure 33.9) (the Miltenyi MACS™ laboratory systems and the AmCell clinical scale separators) (Figure 33.10) [214,215]. As described previously, these two matrices require different approaches for their collection within a magnetic field. The Miltenyi MACS particles must be captured in a high-gradient magnetic field which is achieved by placing a column of metallic particles or wire between the poles of permanent magnets. The CD34-positive particle-coated cells are retained on the column, while non-target cells are recovered in the effluent. The target cells can then be eluted from the column by removal of the magnetic field.

The target-cell capture system has also had to be modified for the Dynal microspheres, since the target cells must now be recovered from the bead–cell rosettes, which in the case of negative selection are usually discarded. The rosettes are therefore collected using a different configuration of magnets and the separation chamber is now a solid walled chamber rather than a collapsible transfer pack [213]. Incubation of the anti-CD34 sensitized cells and beads is carried out in the chamber which is then exposed to the magnets. The collected rosettes and free beads are then washed in the chamber to remove non-target cells, the detachment reagent is then added, and by re-exposure of the

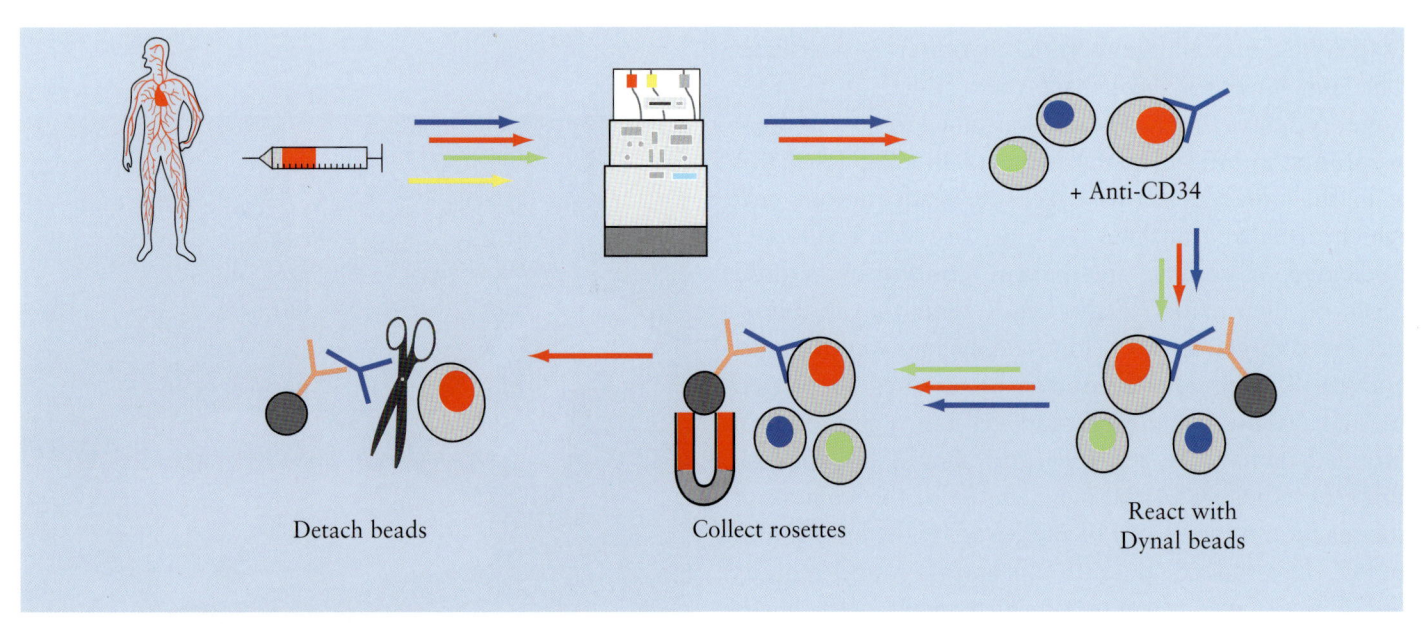

Figure 33.7 Immunomagnetic enrichment of CD34-positive cells using superparamagnetic microspheres (Baxter/Dynal). Haematopoietic progenitor cells are sensitized with anti-CD34 monoclonal antibody and incubated with Dynal M450 superparamagnetic microspheres coated with anti-immunoglobulin antibody. The rosetted cells are collected in a magnetic field. The beads can be detached from the CD34-positive cells by incubation with chymopapain, a competitive peptide or an anti-Fab antibody.

chamber to the magnetic field, the beads can be retained while the CD34-positive cells are recovered in the effluent. Baxter has developed semi-automated (Isolex™ 300) and fully automated (Isolex™ 300i (Figure 33.8)) versions of their positive selection devices, which are now in clinical trials in Europe and the United States. Separation of the CD34-positive cells from the beads is achieved by incubation either with the enzyme chymopapain (Chymocell™), which cleaves an epitope on the CD34 antigen that is recognized by the Baxter anti-CD34 monoclonal antibody [213] or by incubation with a peptide (PR34+ stem-cell releasing agent) [216] that competes with the CD34 epitope on the target cells for the binding site on the anti-CD34 antibody. The use of chymopapain, while effective, is complicated by its effects on other surface antigen on both the target cells and any tumour cells that may be present in the final product. Digestion of antigens on tumour cells which may be targeted in a negative selection procedure makes it impossible to purge the CD34-selected cell population, and combined procedures must be configured as a tumour purge followed by a positive

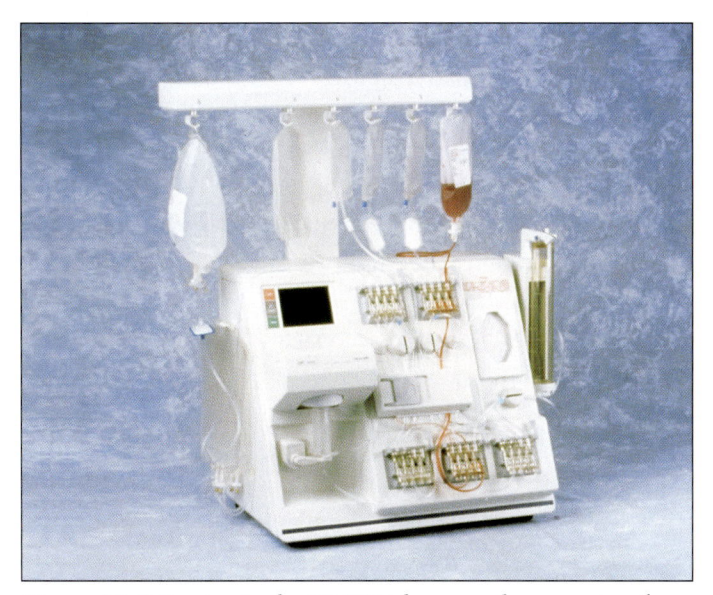

Figure 33.8 Baxter Isolex™ 300i large-scale separator for immunomagnetic enrichment of CD34-positive cells. Incubation of anti-CD34 sensitized cells and magnetic microspheres, separation of the rosetted cells, and detachment of the beads is achieved under computer control in the column shown at the right of the device. This device is not approved for sale in the United States for clinical applications. (Courtesy Baxter Biotech.)

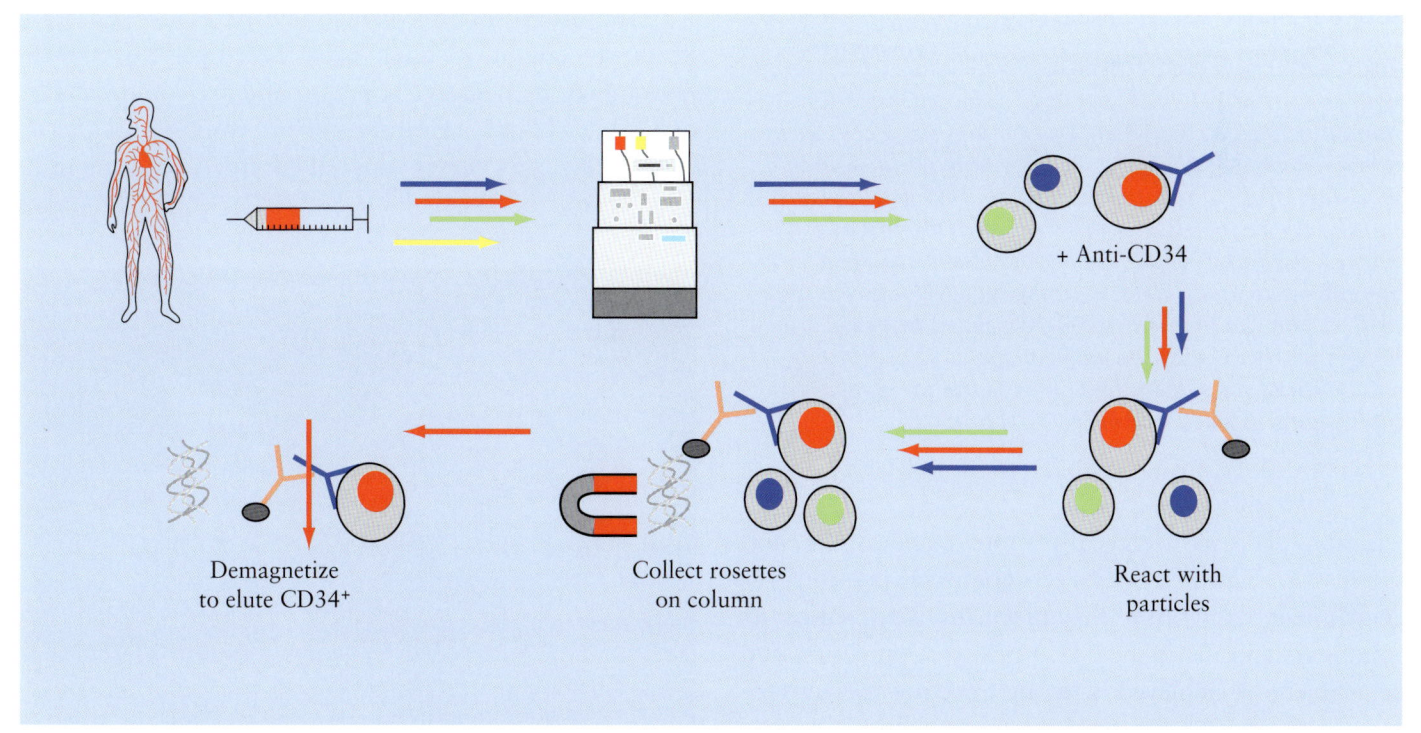

Figure 33.9 Immunomagnetic enrichment of CD34-positive cells using paramagnetic nanoparticles (Miltenyi/Amcell). Haematopoietic progenitor cells are sensitized with anti-CD34 monoclonal antibody and incubated with Miltenyi paramagnetic particles coated with anti-immunoglobulin antibody. Alternatively, the cells can be directly interacted with anti-CD34-coated particles. The rosetted cells are collected onto a column of metallic material placed in a high-gradient magnetic field. The CD34-positive cells are recovered from the column by removing it from the field. The particles can be detached from the CD34-positive cells by incubation MultiSort™ reagent.

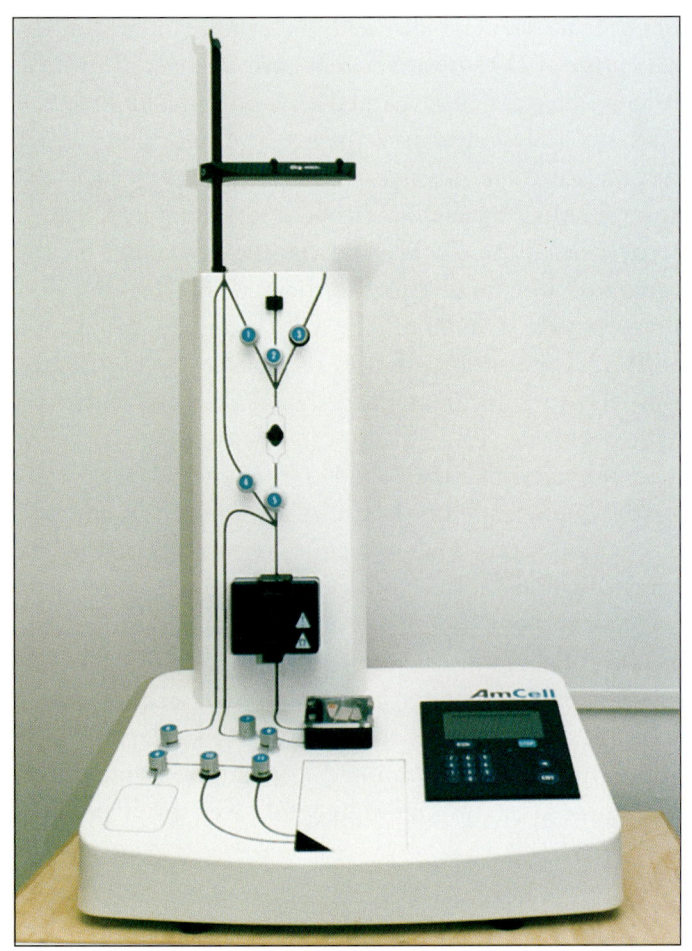

Figure 33.10 Miltenyi/Amgen large-scale separator for immunomagnetic enrichment of CD34-positive cells using paramagnetic nanoparticles. A disposable set (not shown), consisting of the separation column and tubing, is placed into the device which contains the externally-placed magnets used to generate the high gradient field, and computer-activated valves to control the flow of cells and buffers. The CD34-positive cells are eluted from the column by removal of the magnetic field. This device is not approved for sale in the United States for clinical applications. (Courtesy AmCell Corporation.)

The column configuration of the separator means that special attention must be paid to priming, loading and washing procedures to ensure good fluid flow and optimal separation performance. The clinical scale device, developed by AmCell (Figure 33.10), is an automated version in which many of these steps are under computer control. In model experiments, in which tissue-cultured breast cancer cells were seeded at 0.01 to 2.5% into buffy coats or normal leukapheresis products, depletions of 3.01 to 4.65 logs were obtained using this device [215]. The target cells that are recovered from the columns are coated with the nanoparticles (Figure 33.11). This does not interfere with their analysis by flow cytometry or their functional characteristics, as assessed by their ability to proliferate and differentiate in tissue culture. Clinical trials, now underway in Europe, will determine whether the particles have any effect on homing of the cells to the marrow spaces and subsequent engraftment of the patient. Recently, an enzymatic reagent (MultiSort™) [217] which detaches the particles from the cells was described. This detachment leaves the anti-CD34 antibody attached to the cell surface.

Laboratory systems using nanoparticles and high gradient separation have been developed for CD34 enrichment by negative selection and are commercially available [218]. Colloid-based immunomagnetic separation has been described for experimental selection. This is technically more cumbersome and expensive. The use of a competitive peptide for detachment overcomes this problem [216], since its actions are specific to the CD34-positive population and detachment is achieved without affecting the surface characteristics or function of the target cells.

The smaller size of the Miltenyi particles results in more rapid reaction kinetics and fewer effects of target antigen density on the separation performance. The procedure for preparing the cells for separation is very similar to that described for the microspheres [214].

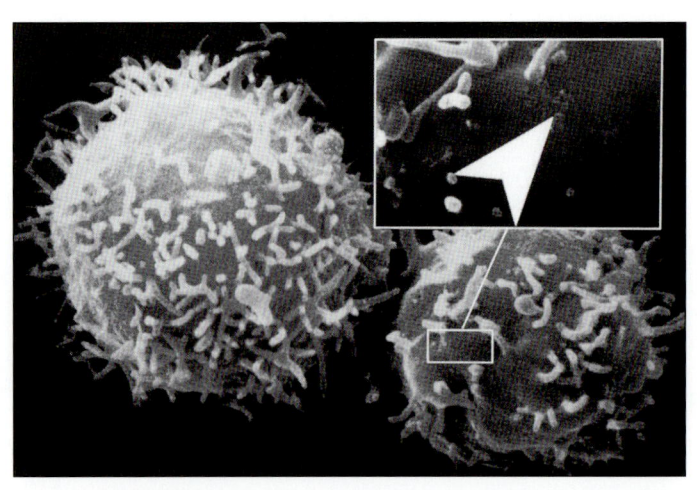

Figure 33.11 Scanning electron micrograph of target-cell coated with Miltenyi paramagnetic nanoparticles. The inset shows a high-power micrograph in which the nanoparticles are indicated by the arrow. Contrast the size of the particles with the microspheres shown in Figure 33.5. (Courtesy Miltenyi Biotec.)

separations but has not been used for clinical purposes at this time [201].

The performance of most positive selection systems is comparable and variable [219]. Under optimal conditions, separation purities of >90% with yields of >80% can be achieved by most of the commercially available separators. The major difficulties have been in achieving this level of performance for clinical-scale separations on a routine basis. The tremendous heterogeneity in the cellular composition of the starting material may, in part, be responsible for this problem. This may be reduced by using a carefully prepared mononuclear cell fraction and by the inclusion of preseparation steps in which non-specifically adherent or reactive cells are either removed by incubation with a 'dummy' solid phase, or blocked by treatment with buffers containing irrelevant immunoglobulin. In spite of these steps, occasional yields and purities of <20% have still been described for most systems.

The use of CD34 separation has also not solved the problem of tumour contamination of the graft [220]. The variable cell purity of the final product from these procedures has an associated risk of variable levels of tumour contamination of the preparation, and careful examination of the enriched fraction by immunocytochemistry has revealed the presence of tumour cells [35]. This has not been resolved by using mobilized peripheral blood progenitor cells (PBPC) as the starting material [220]. Although the level of infiltration of this material by tumour cells is routinely lower than with bone marrow [31], tumour can still be detected in CD34-enriched PBPC grafts, although, in some cases, these cells did not appear to be clonogenic [221]. There have also been reports that certain tumour cells may express the CD34 antigen [42], and would, therefore, be actively enriched by positive selection. This has stimulated interest in combining positive and negative selection to achieve maximal tumour depletion. The sequence of positive followed by negative selection would appear to be the most practical, since the CD34 selection procedure dramatically reduces the scale and cost of the subsequent purging step. The difficulty is that evaluation of the efficacy of this approach will be complicated by the very small number of cells available following each procedure, and by the potential for damage to the pluripotent stem cell by prolonged manipulation. These issues must also be addressed in the context of the additional cost of the procedure and the ultimate clinical benefit to the patient.

Summary

In summary, the clinical relevance of tumour purging in autologous haematopoietic stem-cell transplantation remains to be demonstrated definitively. Results from retrospective data analyses, gene-marking studies and non-randomized purging trials support the idea that the presence of tumour cells in the graft may contribute to relapse of disease post-transplant. The relative burden of tumour cells in the graft versus those surviving high-dose therapy in the patient would argue that the cells in the graft must represent a potent tumourigenic subpopulation if they are to be primarily responsible for relapse. If this is indeed the case, the development of effective purging methods may contribute to improved clinical outcome. Optimized purging by negative selection is capable of depleting tumour from grafts to the limits of currently available detection assays. Positive selection of CD34-positive cells is generally faster, less expensive and requires a single monoclonal antibody. The selected cells are capable of restoring haematopoiesis in the recipients; however, the separations have been extremely variable with respect to both yield and purity, and tumour cells have been detected in the positively-selected graft. The combination of positive and negative selection in certain diseases may improve purging efficiency and reduce the cost of the negative selection procedure by decreasing its scale. The value of any technology must be based on its clinical benefit and not on its availability. The relevance of purging may ultimately be determined from the clear demonstration that tumour cells within the marrow or blood present a risk to the patient that is out of proportion to their relative numbers, and/or the results from randomized clinical trials.

References

1. Doney K, Fischer L, Appelbaum F et al. Treatment of adult acute lymphoblastic leukemia with allogeneic bone marrow transplantation. Multivariant analysis of factors affecting acute graft-versus-host disease and relapse and relapse-free survival. Bone Marrow Transplant 1991; 7: 453–459.
2. Anasetti C and Hansen J. Bone marrow transplantation from HLA-partially matched related donors and unrelated volunteer donors. Bone Marrow Transplant SJ Forman, KG Blume and ED Thomas (eds) 1994 665–679 (New York: Marcel Dekker).
3. Henslee-Downey P. Choosing an alternative bone marrow donor among available family members. Am J Pediatr Hematol Oncol 1993; 15: 150–161.
4. Gratwohl A and Schmitz N. Introduction. First International Symposium on Allogeneic Peripheral Blood Precursor Cell Transplants. Bone Marrow Transplant 1996; 17(Suppl 3): S1–S3.
5. Sharp JG. Micrometastases and transplantation. J Haematother 1996; 5: 519–524.
6. Campana D and Pui C. Detection of minimal residual disease in acute leukemia: methodologic advances and clinical significance. Blood 1995; 85: 1416–1434.
7. Pantel K, Schlimok G, Angstwurm M et al. Methodological analysis of immunocytochemical screening for disseminated epithelial tumor cells in bone marrow. J Haematother 1994; 3: 165–173.
8. Moss T, Sanders DG, Lasky LC and Bostrom B. Contamination of peripheral blood stem cell harvests by circulating neuroblastoma cells. Blood 1990; 76: 1879–1883.
9. Ross AA, Cooper BW, Lazarus HM et al. Detection and viability of tumor cells in peripheral blood stem cell collections from breast cancer patients using immunohistochemical and clonogenic assay techniques. Blood 1993; 82: 2605–2610.
10. Chan WC, Wu GQ, Greiner TC et al. Detection of tumor contamination of peripheral stem cells in patients with lymphoma using cell culture and polymerase chain reaction technology. J Haematother 1994; 3: 175–184.
11. Gorin NC, Aegerter P, Auvert B et al. Autologous bone marrow transplantation for acute myelocytic leukemia in first remission: a European survey of the role of marrow purging. Blood 1990; 75: 1606–1614.
12. Gorin NC, Labopin M, Meloni G et al. Autologous bone marrow transplantation for acute myeloblastic leukemia in Europe: further evidence of the role of marrow purging by mafosfamide. European Co-operative Group for Bone Marrow Transplantation (EBMT). Leukaemia 1991; 5: 896–904.
13. Miller CB, Rowlings P, Jones RJ et al. In vitro treatment of grafts in AML. In: Blood Cell and Bone Marrow Transplants: the Sixth Biennial Sandoz–Keystone Symposium on Bone Marrow Transplantation, Abstract no. 003, 1996 (Silverthorne: Keystone Symposia).
14. Brockstein BE, Ross AA, Moss T et al. Tumor cell contamination of bone marrow harvest products: clinical consequences in a cohort of advanced stage breast cancer patients undergoing high-dose chemotherapy. J Haematother 1996; 5: 617–624.
15. Weisdorf DJ, Haake R, Miller WJ et al. Autologous bone marrow transplantation for progressive non-Hodgkin's lymphoma: clinical impact of immunophenotype and in vitro purging. Bone Marrow Transplant 1991; 8: 135–142.
16. Gilmore MJ, Hamon MD, Prentice HG et al. Failure of purged autologous bone marrow transplantation in high risk acute lymphoblastic leukemia in first complete remission. Bone Marrow Transplant 1991; 8: 19–26.
17. Garaventa A, Ladenstein R, Chauvin F et al. High-dose chemotherapy with autologous bone marrow rescue in advanced stage IV neuroblastoma. Eur J Cancer 1993; 29A: 487–491.
18. Schouten HC, Colombat P, Verdonck LF, Gorin NC et al. Autologous bone marrow transplantation for low-grade non-Hodgkin's lymphoma: the European Bone Marrow Transplant Group experience. EBMT Working Party for Lymphoma. Ann Oncol 1994; 5(Suppl 2): 147–149.
19. Matthay KK, Atkinson JB, Stram DO et al. Patterns of relapse after autologous purged bone marrow transplantation for neuroblastoma: a Children's Cancer Group pilot study. J Clin Oncol 1993; 11: 2226–2233.
20. Rossetti F, Deeg HJ and Hackman RC. Early pulmonary recurrence of non-Hodgkin's lymphoma after autologous marrow transplantation: evidence for reinfusion of lymphoma cells? Bone Marrow Transplant 1995; 19: 417–425.
21. Peters SO, Stockschlader M, Hegwisch-Becker S et al. Infusion of tumor contaminated bone marrow for autologous rescue after high-dose therapy leading to long-term remission in a patient with relapsed Philadelphia chromosome-positive acute lymphoblastic leukemia. Bone Marrow Transplant 1995; 15: 783–784.
22. Hagenbeek A. Leukemic cell kill in autologous bone marrow transplantation: in vivo or in vitro? Leukaemia 1992; 6(Suppl 4): 85–87.
23. Gribben JG, Freedman AS, Neuberg D et al. Immunologic purging of marrow assessed by PCR before autologous bone marrow transplantation for B-cell lymphoma. New Engl J Med 1991; 325: 1525–1533.
24. Lazarus HM, Rowe JM and Goldstone AH. Does in vitro marrow purging improve the outcome after autologous bone marrow transplantation? J Haematother 1993; 2: 457–466.
25. Gribben JG, Neuberg D, Barber M et al. Detection of residual lymphoma cells by polymerase chain reaction in peripheral blood as significantly less predictive for relapse than detection in bone marrow. Blood 1994; 83: 3800–3807.
26. Gribben JG, Neuberg D, Freedman AS et al. Detection by polymerase chain reaction of residual cells with the bcl-2 translocation is associated with increased risk of relapse after autologous bone marrow transplantation for B-cell lymphoma. Blood 1993; 81: 3449–3457.
27. Kiyoi H, Kojima S, Kato K et al. Detection of minimal residual disease in patients with childhood common acute lymphoblastic leukemia after autologous bone marrow transplantation with ex vivo purging and system IL-2 infusion: unsuccessful prediction of subsequent relapse. Bone Marrow Transplant 1995; 16: 437–442.
28. Rill DR, Moen RC, Buschle M et al. An approach for the analysis of relapse and marrow reconstitution after autologous marrow transplantation using retrovirus-mediated gene transfer. Blood 1992; 79: 2694–2700.

29. Brenner MK, Rill DR, Moen RC et al. Gene-marking to trace the origin of relapse after autologous bone marrow transplantation. *Lancet* 1993; **341**: 85–86.
30. Rill DR, Santana VM, Roberts WM et al. Direct demonstration that autologous bone marrow transplantation for solid tumors can return a multiplicity of tumorigenic cells. *Blood* 1994; **84**: 380–383.
31. Moss TJ. Detection of minimal residual disease in autologous grafts. *Immunomethods* 1994; **5**: 226–231.
32. Stelzer GT, Shults KE, Wormsley SB and Loken MR. Detection of occult lymphoma cells by multidimensional flow cytometry. *Prog Clin Biol Res* 1991; **377**: 629–635.
33. Simpson SJ, Vachula M, Kennedy MJ et al. Detection of tumor cells in the bone marrow, peripheral blood, and apheresis products of breast cancer patients using flow cytometry. *Exp Haematol* 1995; **23**: 1062–1068.
34. DeSombre K, Tyler CL, Silva O et al. A comparison of immunohistochemistry, two color immunofluorescence and flow cytometry with cell sorting for the detection of micrometastatic breast cancer in the bone marrow. *J Haemather* 1996; **5**: 57–62.
35. Shpall EJ, Jones RB, Bearman SI et al. Transplantation of enriched CD34-positive autologous marrow into breast cancer patients following high-dose chemotherapy: influence of CD34-positive peripheral blood progenitors and growth factors. *J Clin Oncol* 1994; **12**: 28–36.
36. Negrin RS. Use of the polymerase chain reaction for the detection of tumor cell involvement of bone marrow and peripheral blood: implications for purging. *J Haemather* 1992; **1**: 361–368.
37. Vervoordeldonk SF, Merle PA, Steenbergen EJ et al. The effects of DNase on the detection of residual malignant cells by polymerase chain reaction after immunologic purging of autologous bone marrow cells. *Prog Clin Biol Res* 1993; **389**: 601–612.
38. Hagenbeek A and Martens AC. Reinfusion of leukemic cells with the autologous marrow graft preclinical studies on lodging and regrowth of leukemia. *Leuk Res* 1985; **9**: 1389–1395.
39. Gee AP. Immunologically based methods for the elimination of tumor cells from autologous stem cell grafts. *Immunomethods* 1994; **5**: 232–242.
40. Civin CI, Trischmann TM, Fackler MJ et al. Summary of the CD34 cluster workshop. In: *Leucocyte Typing IV White Cell Differentiation Antigens*. W Knall, B Dorken and EP Ruber (eds), 1989: 818–825 (Oxford: Oxford University Press).
41. Sutherland DR and Keating A. The CD34 antigen: structure, biology and potential clinical applications. *J Haemather* 1992; **1**: 115–129.
42. Reading CL, Gazitt Y, Estrov Z and Juttnet C. Does CD34+ cell selection enrich malignant stem cells in B cell (and other) malignancies? *J Haemather* 1996; **5**: 97–98.
43. Gee AP. Malignant cell purging – Immunophysical techniques. In: *Stem Cell and Marrow Processing for Transplantation*. L Lasky and P Warkentin (eds), 1994: 83–102 (Bethesda, MD: American Association of Blood Banks).
44. Figdor CG, Voute PA, De Kraker J et al. Physical cell separation of neuroblastoma cells from bone marrow. In: *Advances in Neuroblastoma Research*. AE Evans, GJ D'Angio and RC Seeger (eds), 1985: 471 (New York: Alan R Liss).
45. Reynolds CP, Moss TJ, Seeger RC et al. Sensitive detection of neuroblastoma cells in bone marrow for monitoring the efficacy of marrow purging procedures, In: *Advances in Neuroblastoma Research*. AE Evans, GJ D'Angio and RC Seeger (eds), 1985: 425–442 (New York: Alan R Liss).
46. Schriber JR, Dejbakhsh-Jones S, Kusnierz-Glaz CR et al. Enrichment of bone marrow and blood progenitor (CD34+) cells by density gradients with sufficient yields for transplantation. *Exp Haematol* 1995; **23**: 1024–1029.
47. Almici C, Donnenberg AD and Rizzoli V. Counterflow centrifugal elutriation: experimental and clinical applications. *J Haematother* 1992; **1**: 279–288.
48. Noga SJ, Davis JM, Thoburn CJ and Donnenberg AD. Lymphocyte dose modification of bone marrow In: *Bone Marrow Processing and Purging: A Practical Guide*. AP Gee (ed.), 1991: 175–200 (Boca Raton FA: CRC Press).
49. Noga SJ, Davis JM, Schepers K et al. The clinical use of elutriation and positive stem cell selection columns to engineer the lymphocyte and stem cell composition of the allograft. *Prog Clin Biol Res* 1993; **389**: 317–324.
50. Slaper-Cortenbach ICM, de Vries van Rossen A, Huijbens RJF, van Leeuwen EF et al. Neuroblastoma purging by immunorosette depletion. *Prog Clin Biol Res* 1991; **377**: 147–162.
51. Moriyama Y, Nikkuni K, Saito H et al. Effect of hyperthermia on both primary proliferation and self renewal of human leukemic progenitor cells *in vitro*: its application to *in vitro* purging. *Leukaemia* 1991; **5**: 332–335.
52. Wierenga PK, Konings AW and Down JD. Studies on the hyperthermic sensitivity of the murine hematopoietic stem cell compartment. *Exp Haematol* 1995; **23**: 108–111.
53. Moriyama Y, Goto T, Hashimoto S et al. Prediction of the ability to purge clonogenic B cell lymphoma from normal BM *in vitro* by heat: their survival curves correspond to a curve reflecting mortality in humans. *Bone Marrow Transplant* 1993; **11**: 437–441.
54. Herrmann RP, O'Reilly J, Meyer BF and Lazzaro G. Prompt haemopoietic reconstitution following hyperthermia purged autologous marrow and peripheral blood stem cell transplantation in acute myeloid leukemia. *Bone Marrow Transplant* 1992; **10**: 293–295.
55. Gidali J and Feher I. The effect of combined purging with mafosfamide and hyperthermia on murine haematopoietic stem cells and leukaemogenic cells. *Bone Marrow Transplant* 1992: **10**: 479–483.
56. Osman Y, Moriyama Y and Shibata A. Enhanced elimination of Ph+ chromosome cells *in vitro* by combined hyperthermia and other drugs (AZT, IFN-alpha, TNF and quercetin): its application to autologous transplantation for CML. *Exp Haematol* 1995; **23**: 444–452.
57. Min W, Kim D, Lee J et al. Autologous bone marrow rescue for patients with acute myelogenous leukemia: purging with hyperthermia and ether lipid *in vitro*. *Prog Clin Biol Res* 1994; **389**: 197–203.
58. Allieri MA, Lopez M, Douay L et al. Clonogenic leukemic progenitor cells in acute myelocytic leukemia are highly sensitive to cryopreservation: possible purging effects for autologous bone marrow transplantation. *Bone Marrow Transplant* 1991; **7**: 101–105.
59. Zaheer HA, Gibson FM, Bagnara M et al. Differential sensitivity to cryopreservation of clonogenic progenitor cells

and stromal precursors from leukemic and normal bone marrow. *Stem Cells* 1994; **12**: 180–186.
60. Coutinho LH, Testa NG, Chang J et al. The use of cultured bone marrow cells in autologous transplantation. *Prog Clin Biol Res* 1990; **333**: 415–432.
61. Tarella C, Omede P, Boccadoro M et al. Early disappearance of murine plasmacytoma stem cells in long term bone marrow culture. *Leuk Res* 1992; **16**: 743–750.
62. Schiro R, Coutinho LH, Will A et al. Growth of normal versus leukemic bone marrow cells in long term culture from acute lymphoblastic and myeloblastic leukemias. *Blut* 1990; **61**: 267–270.
63. Ozsahin H, Fabrega S, Douay L et al. Application of serum-free liquid bone marrow cultures to bone marrow purging for autologous bone marrow transplantation in acute lymphoblastic leukemia. *Nouv Rev Fr Hematol* 1990; **32**: 353–355.
64. Firkin FC, Birner R, Russell SH and Garson OM. Contrasting patterns of neoplastic cell behavior in long-term culture of bone marrow from patients with acute leukaemia and myelodysplastic disorders. A survey of responses in 31 cases with cytogenetic determination of neoplastic status of cultured cells in 17 studies. *Br J Haematol* 1990; **75**: 476–484.
65. Santucci MA, Zaccaria A, Testoni N et al. Long-term culture of chronic myeloid leukemia bone marrow cells. *Haematologica* 1991; **76**: 357–362.
66. Smith MA, Mills KI and Smith JG. Long-term culture and molecular biological studies highlight differences in relative BCR-ABL expression levels in the peripheral blood and bone marrow of a patient with chronic granulocytic leukemia. *Br J Haematol* 1994; **88**: 406–408.
67. Haber DA. Clinical implications of basic research: Telomeres, cancer and immortality. *New Engl J Med* 1995; **332**: 955–956.
68. Long GS, Cramer DV, Harnaha JB and Hiserodt JC. Lymphokine-activated killer (LAK) cell purging of leukemia bone marrow: range of activity against different hematopoietic malignancies. *Bone Marrow Transplant* 1990; **6**: 169–177.
69. Gambacorti-Passerini C, Rivoltini L, Fizzotti M et al. Selective purging by human interleukin-2 activated lymphocytes of bone marrow contaminated with a lymphoma line or autologous leukemic cells. *Br J Haematol* 1991; **78**: 197–205.
70. Charak BS, Agah R, Gray D and Mazumder A. Interaction of various cytokines with interleukin-2 in the generation of killer cells from human bone marrow: application in purging of leukemia. *Leuk Res* 1991; **15**: 801–810.
71. Dickinson AM, Middleton SL, Latham J et al. Cytokine treatment of human bone marrow activates anti-leukaemia effector cells: monitoring of purging by polymerase chain reaction and DNA analysis. *Leukaemia* 1995; **9**: 444–449.
72. Klingemann HG, Neerunjun J, Schwulera U and Ziltener HJ. Culture of normal and leukemic bone marrow in interleukin-2: analysis of cell activation, cell proliferation and cytokine production. *Leukaemia* 1993; **7**: 1389–1393.
73. Klingemann HG, Deal H, Reid D and Eaves CJ. Design and validation of a clinically applicable culture procedure for the generation of interleukin-2 activated natural killer cells in human bone marrow autografts. *Exp Haematol* 1993; **21**: 1263–1270.
74. Verma UN, Bagg A, Brown E and Mazumder A. Interleukin-2 activation of human bone marrow in long-term cultures: an effective startegy for purging and generation of anti-tumor cytotoxic precursors. *Bone Marrow Transplant* 1994; **13**: 115–123.
75. Beaujean F, Bernaudin F, Kuentz M et al. Successful engraftment after autologous transplantation of 10 day cultured bone marrow activated by interleukin-2 in patients with acute lymphoblastic leukemia. *Bone Marrow Transplant* 1995; **15**: 691–696.
76. Kaneko T, Fusauchi Y, Kakui Y et al. A bispecific antibody enhances cytokine-induced killer-mediated cytolysis of autologous acute myeloid leukemia cells. *Blood* 1993; **81**: 1333–1341.
77. Kaneko T, Fusauch Y, Kakui Y et al. Cytotoxicity of cytokine-induced killer cells coated with bispecific antibody against acute myeloid leukemia cells. *Leukaemia Lymphoma* 1994; **14**: 219–229.
78. Notter M, Ludwig WD, Bremer S and Thiel E. Selective targeting of human lymphokine-activated killer cells by CD3 monoclonal antibody against the interferon-inducible high-affinity Fc gamma RI receptor (CD64) on autologous acute myeloid leukemic blast cells. *Blood* 1993; **82**: 3113–3124.
79. Scheffold C, Brandt K, Johnston V et al. Potential of autologous immunologic effector cells for bone marrow purging in patients with chronic myeloid leukemia *Bone Marrow Transplant* 1995; **15**: 33–39.
80. van de Loosdrecht AA, Ossenkoppele GJ, Beelen RH et al. In vitro purging of clonogenic leukemic cells from human bone marrow by interferon gamma-activated monocytes. *Cancer Immunol Immunother* 1994, **38**: 346–352.
81. Cesano A, Pierson G, Visonneau S et al. Use of a lethally irradiated major histocompatibility complex nonrestricted cytotoxic cell line for effective purging of marrows containing lysis-sensitive or -resistant leukemic targets. *Blood* 1996; **87**: 393–403.
82. Jones RJ. Purging with 4-hydroperoxycyclophosphamide. *J Haematother* 1992: **1**: 343–348.
83. Rowley SD and Davis JM. The use of 4-HC in autologous purging. In: *Bone Marrow Processing and Purging: A Practical Guide.* AP Gee (ed.), 1991: 247–262 (Boca Raton FA: CRC Press).
84. Bullock G, Tang C, Tourkina E et al. Effect of combined treatment with interleukin-3 and interleukin-6 on 4-hydroperoxycyclophosphamide-induced programmed cell death or apoptosis in human myeloid leukemia cells. *Exp Haematol* 1993; **21**: 1640–1647.
85. Yeager AM, Rowley SD, Kaizer H and Santos G. *Ex vivo* chemopurging of autologous bone marrow with 4-hydroperoxycyclophosphamide to eliminate occult leukemic cells. Laboratory and clinical observations. *Am J Pediatr Hematol Oncol* 1990; **12**: 245–256.
86. Yeager AM, Kaizer H, Santos GW et al. Autologous bone marrow transplantation in patients with acute non-lymphocytic leukemia: a study of *ex vivo* marrow treatment with 4-hydroperoxycyclophosphamide. *New Engl J Med* 1986; **315**: 141–147.
87. Laporte JP, Douay L, Lopez M et al. One hundred-twenty-five adult patients with primary acute leukemia autografted with marrow purged by mafosfamide: a ten-year single institution experience. *Blood* 1994; **84**: 3810–3818.
88. Reece DE, Barnett MJ, Connors JM et al. Treatment of multiple myeloma with intensive chemotherapy followed by

autologous BMT using marrow purged with 4-hydroperoxycyclophosphamide. *Bone Marrow Transplant* 1993; **11**: 139–146.
89. Carlo-Stella C, Mangoni L, Almici C et al. Autologous transplant for chronic myelogenous leukemia using marrow treated *ex vivo* with mafosfamide. *Bone Marrow Transplant* 1994; **14**: 425–432.
90. Nieborowska-Skorska M, Skorski T, Ratajczak MZ et al. Successful mafosfamide purging of bone marrow from chronic myelogenous leukemia (CML) cells. *Folia Histochem Cytobiol* 1993; **31**: 161–167.
91. Passos-Coelho J, Ross AA, Davis JM et al. Bone marrow micrometastases in chemotherapy-responsive advanced breast cancer: effect of *ex vivo* purging with 4-hydroperoxycyclophosphamide. *Cancer Res* 1994; **54**: 2366–2371.
92. Shpall EJ, Stemmer SM, Bearman SI et al. New strategies in marrow purging for breast cancer patients receiving high-dose chemotherapy with autologous bone marrow transplantation. *Breast Cancer Res Treat* 1993; **26**(Suppl): S19–23.
93. Laporte JP, Isnard F, Lesage S et al. Autologous bone marrow transplantation with marrow purged by mafosfamide in seven patients with myelodysplastic syndromes in transformation (AML-MDS): a pilot study. *Leukaemia* 1993; **7**: 2030–2333.
94. Gorin NC, Douay L, Laporte J et al. Autologous bone marrow transplantation using marrow incubated with Asta Z 7557 in adult acute leukemia. *Blood* 1986; **67**: 1367–1376.
95. Rowley SD, Davis JM, Piantadosi S et al. Density gradient separation of autologous bone marrow grafts before *ex vivo* purging with 4-hydroperoxycyclophosphamide. *Bone Marrow Transplant* 1990; **6**: 321–327.
96. Jones RJ, Zuehlsdorf M, Rowley SD et al. Variability in 4-hydroperoxycyclophosphamide activity during clinical purging for autologous bone marrow transplantation. *Blood* 1987; **70**: 1490–1494.
97. Giarratana MC, Gorin NC and Douay L. Plasma interacts with mafosfamide toxicity to normal haematopoietic progenitor cells: impact on *in vitro* marrow purging. *Nouv Rev Fr Hematol* 1995; **37**: 125–130.
98. Douay L, Giarratana MC, Labopin M et al. Characterization of late and early hematopoietic progenitor/stem cell sensitivity to mafosfamide. *Bone Marrow Transplant* 1995; **15**: 769–775.
99. Ratajczak MZ, Ratajczjak J, Kuczynski W et al. In vitro sensitivity of human hematopoietic progenitor cells to 4-hydroperoxycyclophosphamide. *Exp Haematol* 1993; **21**: 1663–1667.
100. Zhong RK, Donnenberg AD, Rubin J and Ball ED. Differential effects of 4-hydroperoxycyclophosphamide and anti-myeloid monoclonal antibodies on T and natural killer cells during bone marrow purging. *Blood* 1994; **83**: 2345–2351.
101. Almici C, Manoni L, Carlo-Stella C et al. Natural killer cell regeneration after transplantation with mafosfamide purged autologous bone marrow. *Bone Marrow Transplant* 1995; **16**: 95–101.
102. Douay L, Hu C, Giarratana MC and Gorin NC. Amifostine (WR-2721) protects normal haematopoietic stem cells against cyclophosphamide derivatives' toxicity without compromising their antileukaemic effects. *Eur J Cancer* 1995; **31A**(Suppl 1): S14–16.

103. Kennedy MJ, Davis J, Passos-Coelho J et al. Administration of human recombinant granulocyte colony-stimulating factor (filgrastim) accelerates granulocyte recovery following high-dose chemotherapy and autologous marrow transplantation with 4-hydroperoxycyclophosphamide-purged marrow in women with metastatic breast cancer. *Cancer Res* 1993; **53**: 5424–5428.
104. Gulati S, Acaba L, Yahalom J et al. Autologous bone marrow transplantation for acute myelogenous leukemia using 4-hydroperoxycyclophosphamide and VP-16 purged bone marrow. *Bone Marrow Transplant* 1992; **10**: 129–134.
105. Domenech J, Georget MT, Gihana E et al. Evaluation of doxorubicin in combination with mafosfamide for *in vitro* elimination of myeloid and lymphoid tumor cells from human bone marrow. *Bone Marrow Transplant* 1992; **9**: 101–106.
106. Rowley SD, Miller CB, Piantadosi S et al. Phase I study of combination drug purging for autologous bone marrow transplantation. *J Clin Oncol* 1991; **9**: 2210–2218.
107. Johnston JB, Verburg L, Shore T et al. Combination therapy with nucleoside analogs and alkylating agents. *Leukaemia* 1994; **8**(Suppl 1): S140–143.
108. Rubin J, Malley V and Ball ED. A combination of anti-CD15 monoclonal antibody PM-81 and 4-hydroperoxy-cyclophosphamide augments tumor cytotoxicity while sparing normal progenitor cells. *J Haematother* 1994; **3**: 121–127.
109. Rowley SD. Bone marrow purging, 4-hydroperoxy-cyclophosphamide and the FDA. *J Haematother* 1993; **2**: 289–292.
110. Einat M, Lishner M, Amiel A, Nagler A et al. Eilatin: novel marine alkaloid inhibits *in vitro* proliferation of progenitor cells in chronic myeloid leukemia patients. *Exp Haematol* 1995; **23**: 1439–1444.
111. Rhodes EG, Baker PK, Rhodes JM et al. Autologous bone marrow transplantation for myeloma patients using PNA and CD19-purged marrow rescue. *Bone Marrow Transplant* 1994; **13**: 795–799.
112. Kapelushnik J, Nagler A, Or R et al. Autologous bone marrow transplantation for stage IV neuroblastoma: the role of soybean agglutinin purging. *Transplant Proc* 1993; **25**: 2375–2376.
113. Juneja HS, Harvey WH, Brasher WK and Thompson EB. Successful *in vitro* purging of leukemic blasts from marrow by cortivazol, a pyrazolosteroid: a preclinical study for autologous transplantation in acute lymphoblastic leukemia and non-Hodgkin's lymphoma. *Leukaemia* 1995; **9**: 1771–1778.
114. Pineiro L, Fay J, Collins R and Herzig G. Bone marrow purging with etoposide/methylprednisolone in patients undergoing autologous bone marrow transplantation. *Prog Clin Biol Res* 1994; **389**: 17–21.
115. Wu C, Yang K, Pei X et al., Bone marrrow purging with dibutyl phthalate–experimental basis and preliminary clinical application. *Leuk Res* 1995; **19**: 557–560.
116. Rosenfeld CS. Potential of phenylalanine methylester as a bone marrow purging agent. *Blood* 1992; **80**: 2401–2405.
117. Newman A, Clutterbuck RD, DeLord C et al. The sensitivity of leukemic bone marrow to simvastatin is lost at remission: a potential purging agent for autologous bone marrow transplantation. *J Inv Med* 1995; **43**: 269–274.
118. Hatta Y, Aizawa S, Itoh T et al. Cytotoxic effect of extracellular ATP on L1210 leukemic cells and normal hemopoietic stem cells. *Leuk Res* 1994; **18**: 637–641.

119. Gravatt LC, Chaffee S, Hebert ME et al. Efficacy and toxicity of 9-beta-D-arabinofuranosylguanine (araG) as an agent to purge malignant T cells from murine bone marrow: application to an *in vivo* T-cell leukaemia model. *Leukaemia* 1993; **7**: 1261–1267.

120. Kurtzberg J. Guanine arabinoside as a bone marrow purging agent. *Ann NY Acad Sci* 1993; **685**: 225–236.

121. Levy JG, Dowding C, Mitchell D et al. Selective elimination of malignant stem cells using photosensitizers followed by light treatment. *Stem Cells* 1995; **13**: 336–343.

122. Sieber F. Phototherapy, photochemotherapy and bone marrow transplantation. *J Haematother* 1993; **2**: 43–62.

123. Qiu K and Sieber F. Merocyanine 540-sensitized photoinactivation of leukemia cells: effects of dose fractionation. *Photochem Photobiol* 1992; **56**: 489–493.

124. Yamazaki K and Sieber F. Effects of temperature on merocyanine 40-sensitized photoinactivation of leukemia and normal hematopoietic cells. *Blood* 1993; **82**: 655a.

125. Sieber F, Gaffney DK, Yamazaki T and Qiu K. Importance of cellular defense mechanisms in the photodynamic purging of autologous marrow grafts. *Prog Clin Biol Res* 1994; **389**: 147–154.

126. Anderson MS, Kalyanaraman B and Felix JB. Enhancement of merocyanine 540-mediated phototherapy by salicylate. *Cancer Res* 1993; **53**: 806–809.

127. Traul DL, Anderson GS, Bilitz JM et al. Potentiation of merocyanine 540-mediated photodynamic therapy by salicylate and related drugs. *Photochem Photobiol* 1995; **62**: 790–799.

128. Meagher RC, Rothman SA, Paul P et al. Purging of small cell lung cancer cells from human bone marrow using ethiofos (WR-2721) and light-activated merocyanine 540. *Cancer Res* 1989; **49**: 3637–3641.

129. Sieber F. Merocyanine 540. *Photochem Photobiol* 1987; **46**: 1035–1042

130. Jamieson C, Richter A and Levy JG. Efficacy of benzoporphyrine derivative, a photosensitizer in selective destruction of leukemia cells using a murine tumor model. *Exp Haematol* 1993; **21**: 629–634.

131. Gulati SC, Lemoli RM, Igarashi T and Atzpodien J. Newer options for treating drug resistant (MDR+) cancer cells using photoradiation therapy. *Leukaemia Lymphoma* 1994; **12**: 427–433.

132. Mulroney CM, Gluck S and Ho AD. The use of photodynamic therapy in bone marrow purging. *Semin Oncol* 1994; **21**(Suppl 15): 24–27.

133. Sieber F. Extracorporeal purging of bone marrow grafts by dye-sensitized photoirradiation. In: *Bone Marrow Processing and Purging: A Practical Guide*. AP Gee (ed.), 1991: 263–280 (Boca Raton FA: CRC Press).

134. Vogler WR. Bone marrow purging in acute leukemia with akyl-lysophospholipids: a new family of anti-cancer drugs. *Leukaemia Lymphoma* 1994; **13**: 53–60.

135. Candal FJ, Bosse DC, Vogler WR and Ades EW. Inhibition of angiogenesis in a human microvascular endothelial cell line by ET-18-OCH3. *Cancer Chemother Pharmacol* 1994; **34**: 175–178.

136. Andreesen R, Modolell M, Weltzien HU et al. Selective destruction of human leukemic cells by alkyl-lysophopholipids. *Cancer Res* 1978; **38**: 3894–3899.

137. Glasser L, Somberg LB and Vogler WR. Purging murine leukemic marrow with alkyl-lysophospholipids. *Blood* 1984; **64**: 1288–1291.

138. Okamoto S, Olson AC, Vogler WR and Winton EF. Purging leukemic cells from simulated human remission marrow with alkyl-lysophospholipid. *Blood* 1987; **69**: 1381–1387.

139. Verdonck LF, Heesbeen EC, van Heugten HG et al. The cytotoxicity of alkyl-lysophospholipid on clonogenic leukemia cells and on normal bone marrow progenitor cells is highly, but differentially, increased by cryopreservation. *Bone Marrow Transplant* 1992; **9**: 241–245.

140. Dietzfelbinger HF, Kuhn D, Zafferani M et al. Removal of breast cancer cells from bone marrow by *in vitro* purging with ether lipids and cryopreservation. *Cancer Res* 1993; **53**: 3747–3751.

141. Vogler WR and Berdel WE. Autologous bone marrow transplantation with alkyl-lysophospholipid-purged marrow. *J Haematother* 1993; **2**: 93–102.

142. Vogler WR, Berdel WE, Olson AC et al. Autologous bone marrow transplantation in acute leukemia with marrow purged with alkyl-lysophospholipid. *Blood* 1992; **80**: 1423–1429.

143. Okamoto S, Olson AC, Berdel WE and Vogler WR. Purging of acute myeloid leukemia cells by ether lipids and hyperthermia. *Blood* 1988; **72**: 1777–1783.

144. Heesbeen EC, Rijksen G, van Heugten HG and Verdonck LF. Influence of serum levels on leukemic cells destruction by the ether lipid ET-18-OCH3. *Leuk Res* 1995; **19**: 417–425.

145. Pierga JY and Magdelenat H. Applications of antisense oligonucleotides in oncology. *Cell Mol Biol* 1994; **40**: 237–261.

146. Hijiya N and Gewirtz AM. Oncogenes, molecular medicine and bone marrow transplantation. *J Haematother* 1992; **1**: 369–378.

147. Walder RY and Walder JA. Role of RNase H in hybrid-arrested translation by antisense oligonucleotids. *Proc Natl Acad Sci USA* 1988; **85**: 5011–5015.

148. Skorski T, Nieberowska-Skorska M, Barletta C et al. Highly efficient elimination of Philadelphia leukemic cells by exposure to *bcr/abl* antisense oligodeoxynucleotides combined with mafosfamide. *J Clin Inv* 1993; **92**: 194–202.

149. De Fabritiis P, Amadori S, Calabretta B and Mandelli F. Elimination of clonogenic Philadelphia-positive cells using bcr-abl antisense oligodeoxynucleotides. *Bone Marrow Transplant* 1993; **12**: 261–265.

150. Bishop MR, Warkentin PI, Jackson JD et al. Antisense oligonucleotide OL(1)p53 for *in vitro* purging of autologous bone marrow in acute myelogenous leukemia. *Prog Clin Biol Res* 1994; **389**: 183–187.

151. Calabretta M, Sims RB, Valtieri M et al. Normal and leukemic hematopoietic cells manifest differential sensitivity to inhibitory effects of c-*myb* antisense oligodeoxynucleotides: an *in vitro* study relevant to bone marrow purging. *Proc Natl Acad Sci USA* 1991; **88**: 2351–2355.

152. Ratajczak MZ, Hijiya N, Cantani L et al. Acute and chronic phase chronic myelogenous leukemia colony-forming units are highly sensitive to growth inhibitory effects of c-*myb* antisense oligodeoxynucleotides. *Blood* 1992; **78**: 1956–1961.

153. de-Fabritiis K, Amadori S, Petti MC et al. *In vitro* purging with *bcr-abl* antisense oligodeoxynucleotides does not prevent haematologic reconstitution after autologous bone marrow transplantation. *Leukaemia* 1995; **9**: 662–664.

154. Jackson JD, Tarantolo SR, Bayever E et al. Ex vivo treatment of bone marrow with phosphorothioate oligonucleotide OL(1)p53 for autologous transplantation in acute myeloblastic leukemia and myelodysplastic syndrome. *J Haematother* 1997; 441–446.
155. Leopold L, Shore SK, Newkirk T et al. Ribozyme mediated therapy for chronic myelogenous leukemia. *Prog Clin Biol Res* 1994; **389**: 175–182.
156. Gee AP and Boyle MDP. Purging tumor cells from bone marrow by antibody and complement: a critical appraisal. *J Nat Cancer Inst* 1988; **80**: 154–159.
157. Gee AP. Titration of components of the classical complement pathway. *Methods Enzymol* 1983; **93**: 339–374.
158. Borsos T. Immunoglobulin classes and complement-fixing activity. *Prog Immunol* 1971; **1**: 842.
159. Janssen WE, Lee C, Gross S and Gee AP. Low antigen density leukemia cells: selection and comparative resistance to antibody-mediated marrow purging. *Exp Haematol* 1989; **17**: 252–257.
160. Boyle MDP and Gee AP. Low antigen density tumor cells – an obstacle to effective autologous bone marrow purging? *Cancer Invest* 1987; **5**: 113–118.
161. Gee AP, Bruce KM, J. van Hilten J et al. Selective loss of expression of a tumor-associated antigen on a human leukemia cell line induced by treatment with monoclonal antibody and complement. *J Nat Cancer Inst* 1987; **78**: 25–29.
162. Taupier MA, Kearney JF, Liebson PJ et al. Nonrandom escape of tumor cells from immune lysis due to intraclonal fluctuation in antigen expression. *Cancer Res* 1983; **43**: 4050–4056.
163. Roy DC, Felix M, Cannady WG et al. Comparative activities of rabbit complements of different ages using an *in vitro* marrow purging model. *Leuk Res* 1990; **14**: 407–416.
164. 'Points to Consider in the Manufacture and Testing of Monoclonal Antibody Products for Human Use (1994)'. *Federal Register* 1994; **56**: 148.
165. Hale G and Waldmann H. CAMPATH-1 monoclonal antibodies in bone marrow transplantation. *J Haematother* 1994; **3**: 15–31.
166. Gee AP, Bruce KM, Morris TD and Boyle MDP. Evidence for an anti-complementary associated with human bone marrow cells. *J Nat Cancer Inst* 1985; **75**: 441–445.
167. Zhong RK, Kozii R and Ball ED. Homologous restriction of complement-mediated cell lysis can be markedly enhanced by blocking decay-accelerating factor. *Br J Haematol* 1995; **91**: 269–274.
168. Gee AP. Antibody and complement-mediated cell separation. In: *Cell Separation Methods and Applications*. D Recktenwald (ed.), 1996. (New York: Marcel Dekker). In press.
169. Rowley SD. Recombinant human deoxyribonuclease for hematopoietic stem cell processing. *J Haematother* 1995; **4**: 99–104.
170. Ball E. Monoclonal antibodies and complement for autologous marrow purging. In: *Bone Marrow Processing and Purging: A Practical Guide*. AP Gee (ed.), 1991: 281–292 (Boca Raton FA: CRC Press).
171. Negrin RS, Kiem HP, I.G. Schmidt-Wolf IG et al. Use of the polymerase chain recation to monitor the effectiveness of *ex vivo* tumor cell purging. *Blood* 1991; **77**: 654–660.
172. Godder K, Pati A, Abhyankar S, Gee AP, Parrish R, Lee C and Henslee-Downey PJ. Partially mismatched related donor transplants as salvage therapy for patients with refractory leukemia who relapse post-BMT. *Bone Marrow Transplant* 1996; **17**: 59–63.
173. Lazzaro GE, Meyer BF, Willis JI et al. The synthesis of a peanut agglutinin-ricin A chain conjugate: potential as an *in vitro* purging agent for autologous bone marrow in multiple myeloma. *Exp Haematol* 1995; **23**: 1347–1352.
174. Chan CH, Blazar BR, Eide CR et al. A murine cytokine fusion toxin specifically targeting the murine granulocyte–macrophage colony-stimulating factor (GM-CSF) receptor on normal committed bone marrow progenitor cells and GM-CSF-dependent tumor cells. *Blood* 1995; **86**: 2732–2740.
175. McGraw KJ, Rosenblum MG, Cheung L and Scheinberg DA. Characterization of murine and humanized anti-CD33 gelonin immunotoxins reactive against myeloid leukemias. *Cancer Immunol Immunother* 1994; **39**: 367–374.
176. Strong RC, Uckun FM and Youle RJ. Use of multiple T cell directed ricin immunotoxins for autologous transplantation. *Blood* 1985; **66**: 627–635.
177. Uckun FM and Myers DE. Allografts and autograft purging using immunotoxins in clinical bone marrow transplantation for hematologic malignancies. *J Haematother* 1993; **2**: 155–163.
178. Vallera D and Uckun FM. Immunoconjugates. In: *Biological Response Modifiers and Cancer*. J Chiao (ed.), 1988: 17–21 (New York: Marcel Dekker).
179. Antin JH, Weinstein HJ, Bouloux C and Bierer BE. Immunotoxin-mediated depletion of CD5+ T cells from bone marrow for graft-versus-host disease prophylaxis. In: *Bone Marrow Processing and Purging: A Practical Guide*. AP Gee (ed.), 1991: 213–230 (Boca Raton FA: CRC Press).
180. Roy DC, Robertson MJ, Bélanger R et al. Engraftment following anti-MY9-BR depleted autologous marrow transplantation for patients with acute myeloid leukemia. *Blood* 1992; **80**: 376a.
181. Uckun FM, Kersey JH, Vallera DA et al. Autologous bone marrow transplantation in high-risk remission T lineage acute lymphoblastic leukemia using immunotoxins plus 4-hydroperoxycyclophosphamide for marrow purging. *Blood* 1990; **76**: 1723–1733.
182. Tondini C, Pap SA, Hayes DF et al. Evaluation of monoclonal antibody DF3 conjugated with ricin as a specific immunotoxin for in vitro purging of human bone marrow. *Cancer Res* 1990; **50**: 1170–1175.
183. Goldmacher VS, Bourett LA, Levine BA et al. Anti-CD38 blocked ricin: an imunotoxin for the treatment of mutiple myeloma. *Blood* 1994; **84**: 3017–3025.
184. Irvin JD and Uckun FM. Pokeweed antiviral protein: ribosome inactivation and therapeutic applications. *Pharmacol Ther* 1992; **55**: 279–302.
185. Uckun FM, Haissig S, Ledbetter JA et al. Developmental hierarchy during early human B cell ontogeny after autologous bone marrow transplantation using autografts depleted of CD19+ B cell precursors by an anti-CD19 pan B cell immunotoxin containing pokeweed antiviral protein. *Blood* 1992; **79**: 3369–3379.
186. Mykelbust AT, Godal A, Juell S et al. Comparison of two antibody-based methods for elimination of breast cancer cells from human bone marrow. *Cancer Res* 1994; **54**: 209–214.

187. Ghetie MA and Vitteta ES. Recent developments in immunotoxin therapy. *Curr Opin Immunol* 1994; **6**: 707–714.
188. Youle RJ. Mutations in diphtheria toxin to improve immunotoxin selectivity and understand toxin entry into cells. *Semin Cell Biol* 1991; **2**: 39–45.
189. Pastan IH, Pai LH, Brinkmann U and Fitzgerald DJ. Recombinant toxins: new therapeutic agents for cancer. *Ann NY Acad Sci* 1995; **758**: 345–354.
190. Lansdorp PM, Thomas TE, Schmidt CR *et al*. Marrow contamination: positive selection. In: *High-Dose Cancer Therapy*. JO Armitage and KH Antmann (eds), 1992: 276–288 (Baltimore, MD: Williams and Wilkins).
191. Collins NH, Gee AP and Henslee-Downey PJ. T-cell depletion of allogeneic bone marrow transplants by immunologic and physical techniques. In: *Stem Cell and Marrow Processing for Transplantation*. L Lasky and P Warkentin (eds), 1994: 149–168 (Bethesda, MD: American Association of Blood Banks).
192. Collins NH, Carabasi MY, Bleau S *et al*. New technology for the depletion of T cells from soybean lectin agglutinated, HLA-matched bone marrow grafts for leukemia, initial laboratory and clinical results. *Prog Clin Biol Res* 1992; **377**: 427–439.
193. Lebkowski J, Schain L, Harvey M *et al*. Isolation and culture of human CD34+ hematopoietic stem cells using AIS CELLectors™. In: *Hematopoietic Stem Cells: The Mulhouse Manual*. E Wunder, H Sovalat, PR Hénon and S Serke (eds), 1994: 215–230 (Dayton, OH: Alpha Med Press).
194. Lebkowski JS, Schain LR, Okrongly D *et al*. Rapid isolation of human CD34 hematopoietic stem cells – purging of human tumor cells. *Transplantation* 1992; **53**: 1011–1019.
195. Schain LR, Okrongly D, Okrama TB and Lebkowski JS. Separation of lectin-binding cells using polystyrene culture devices with covalently immobilised soybean agglutinin. *J Haematother* 1994; **3**: 37–46.
196. Heimfeld S and Berenson RJ. Clinical transplantation of CD34+ hematopoietic progenitor cells: positive selection using a closed automated avidin–biotin immunoadsorption system. In: *Hematopoietic Stem Cells: The Mulhouse Manual*. E Wunder, H Sovalat, PR Hénon and S Serke (eds), 1994: 231–239 (Dayton, OH: Alpha Med Press).
197. Shpall EJ, Jones RB, Franklin W *et al*. Transplantation of enriched autologous CD34 positive hematopoietic progenitor cells into breast cancer patients following high-dose chemotherapy. *J Clin Oncol* 1994; **12**: 28–36.
198. Shpall EJ, Gee AP, Cagnoni PJ *et al*. Stem cell isolation. *Curr Opinion Haematol* 1995; **2**: 452–459.
199. Gee AP. Immunomagnetic cell separation using antibodies and superparamagnetic microspheres. In: *Cell Separation Methods and Applications*. D Recktenwald (ed.), 1996. (New York: Marcel Dekker). In press.
200. Bieva C, Martiat P, Ferster E *et al*. Autologous bone marrow transplantation for acute leukemia using ferromagnetic microparticles and monoclonal antibody-purged marrows: demonstration of effectiveness by polymerase chain reaction. *Prog Clin Biol Res* 1991; **377**: 197–204.
201. Kemshead JT, Hancock J and Liberti P. Immunomagnetic colloids for the enrichment of tumor cells from peripheral blood and bone marrow: a model system. *J Haematother* 1994; **3**: 51–57.
202. Gee AP, Lee C, Sleasman JW *et al*. T lymphocyte depletion of human peripheral blood and bone marrow using monoclonal antibodies and magnetic microspheres. *Bone Marrow Transplant* 1987; **2**: 155–163.
203. Gee AP, Moss T, Mansour V *et al*. Large scale immunomagnetic separation system for the removal of tumor cells from bone marrow. *Prog Clin Biol Res* 1992; **377**: 181–188.
204. Kvalheim G, Sorensen O, Fodstad O *et al*. Immunomagnetic removal of B lymphoma cells from human bone marrow: a procedure for clinical use. *Bone Marrow Transplant* 1988; **3**: 31–41.
205. Hardwick RA, Kulcinski D, Mansour V *et al*. Design of large-scale separation systems for positive and negative immunomagnetic selection of cells using superparamagnetic microspheres. *J Haematother* 1992; **1**: 379–386.
206. Mansour V, Weiler M and Gee AP. Factors limiting the efficiency of immunomagnetic cell separation. *Prog Clin Biol Res* 1991; **377**: 169–180.
207. Moss TJ, Xu ZJ, Mansour VH, Hardwick A, Kulcinski D, Ishizawa L, Law P and Gee AP. Quantitation of tumor cell removal from bone marrow: a preclinical model. *J Haematother* 1992; **1**: 65–74.
208. Myklebust AT, Godal A, Juell S *et al*. Comparison of two antibody-based methods for elimination of breast cancer cells from human bone marrow. *Cancer Res* 1994; **54**: 209–214.
209. Gribben JG, Saporito L, Barber M *et al*. Bone marrows of non-Hodgkin's lymphoma patients with a *bcl-2* translocation can be purged of polymerase chain reaction-detectable lymphoma cells using monoclonal antibodies and immunomagnetic bead depletion. *Blood* 1992; **80**: 1083–1089.
210. Gee AP, Mansour V and Weiler M. T-cell depletion of human bone marrow. *J Immunogen* 1989; **16**: 103–115.
211. Gee AP, Mansour VH and Weiler MB. Effects of target antigen density on the efficacy of immunomagnetic cell separation. *J Immunol Methods* 1991; **142**: 127–133.
212. Wang MY, Kvalheim G, Kvaloy S *et al*. An effective immunomagnetic method for bone marrow purging in T cell malignancies. *Bone Marrow Transplant* 1992; **9**: 319–323.
213. Ishizawa L, Burgess J, Hardwick A *et al*. Selection of human CD34+ cells using indirect immunomagnetic procedures and a magnetic cell separation system. In: *Hematopoietic Stem Cells: The Mulhouse Manual*. E Wunder, H Sovalat, PR Hénon and S Serke (eds), 1994: 171–182 (Dayton, OH: Alpha Med Press).
214. Miltenyi S, Guth S, Radbruch A *et al*. Isolation of CD34+ hematopoietic progenitor cells by high-gradient magnetic cells sorting (MACS). In: *Hematopoietic Stem Cells: The Mulhouse Manual*. E Wunder, H Sovalat, PR Hénon and S Serke (eds), 1994: 201–213 (Dayton, OH: Alpha Med Press).
215. Yuan J, Phi-Wilson J, Kim K and Harding FA. Tumor purging by CD34+ selection in a model system using the AmCell/Amgen clinical grade immunomagnetic cell selector device. *Proceedings of the Fourth International Symposium on Blood Cell Transplant, Adelaide, SA*, 1996 (abstract).
216. Bender J. CD34+ cell selection using the Isolex™ device. *Proceedings of the Fourth International Symposium on Blood Cell Transplant, Adelaide, SA*, 1996 (abstract).
217. Guth S, Köster M, Thiel A *et al*. Multiparameter magnetic cell sorting using releasable super-paramagnetic microbeads

(MACS MultiSort) for rapid isolation of subsets of CD34+ human hematopoietic cells, *9th International Congress of Immunology, San Francisco, CA (abstract no. 2912)*, 1995.
218. *StemSep Magnetic Cell Separation System* (Vancouver, BC: StemCell Technologies).
219. de Wynter EA, Coutinho LH, Pei JC *et al*. Comparison of purity and enrichment of CD34+ cells from bone marrow, umbilical cord and peripheral blood (primed for apheresis) using five separation systems. *Stem Cells* 1995; **13**: 524–532.
220. Fruehauf S, Haberkorn M, Hoeft R *et al*. Isolation of CD34+ cells from leukapheresis products: evaluation of lymphoma purging. In: *Hematopoietic Stem Cells: The Mulhouse Manual*. E Wunder, H Sovalat, PR Hénon and S Serke (eds), 1994: 247–253 (Dayton, OH: Alpha Med Press).
221. Ross AA, Loudovaris M, Hazleton B *et al*. Immunocytochemical analysis of tumor cells in pre- and post-culture peripheral blood progenitor cell collections from breast cancer patients. *Exp Hematol* 1995; **23**: 1478–1483.

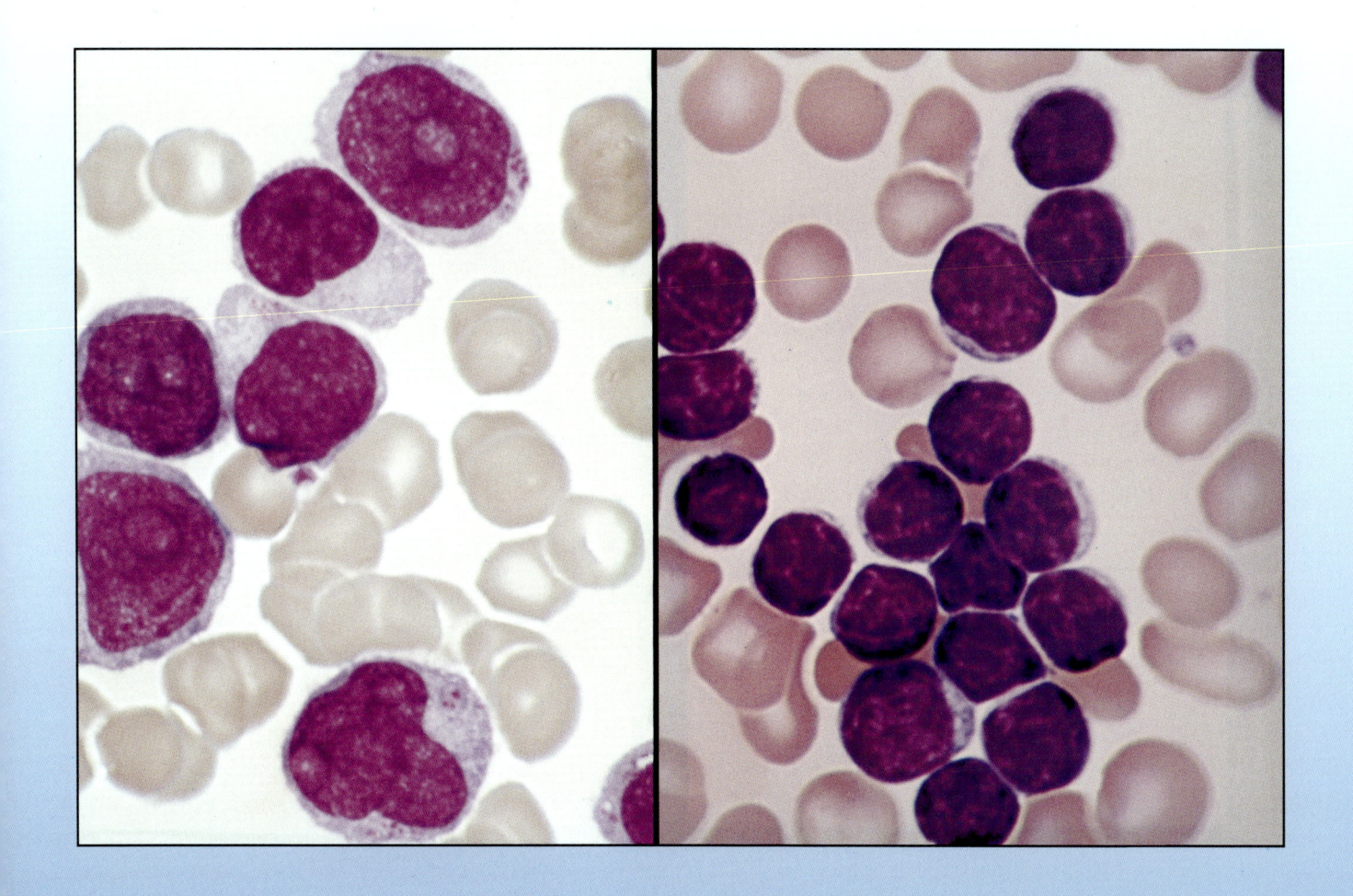

Chapter 34

Total body irradiation for bone-marrow transplant recipients

Chris Parker and Diana Tait

Historical background

Experiments in animals on the effects of total body irradiation (TBI) began soon after the discovery of radioactivity in 1898. As early as 1905, Heineke administered TBI to patients with leukaemia and round-cell sarcoma, and recorded brief responses [1]. One of the first dedicated TBI units was described by Hueblein in 1932 [2]. At the Memorial Hospital, New York, he carried out TBI in a lead-lined room with four beds. Each patient was between 5 and 7 metres away from a Coolidge 'deep therapy' X-ray tube, and simultaneous irradiation was possible. Although results were disappointing, and his methods were greeted with scepticism, his work was continued after his death. The total body dose given to patients was gradually increased until it reached 50% of the skin erythema dose (at that time the unit of dose was that which would produce just noticeable erythema in human skin, roughly equivalent to 7 Gy).

In 1942, Medinger and Craver published the Memorial Hospital results [3]. A total of 270 patients with leukaemia and lymphoma were treated at a distance of 3 metres from the X-ray tube. They found that doses up to 300 Roentgen (about 2.85 Gy), given as one continuous course over 10 days, were generally the upper limit for a fit patient, causing only mild upset. Using these methods they reported short-term remissions. Nevertheless, overall the results were disappointing, leading the authors to conclude that TBI could be dismissed as a treatment for acute leukaemia.

Interest, however, was revived after experiments by Lorenz et al. in 1951 showed that lethally irradiated animals could be rescued if fresh bone-marrow cells were infused following TBI [4]. Thomas demonstrated that dogs could completely recover from an otherwise lethal dose of 1200 Roentgen (11.5 Gy) if autologous bone marrow were given immediately afterwards [5]. With these promising results, Thomas then began treating leukaemic patients with end-stage disease. By 1966, over a time span of just four years, 417 allogeneic bone-marrow transplants (BMT) had been carried out, but with only three prolonged engraftments resulting. Later, it became clear that better results could be obtained if patients were in remission at the time of engraftment, and in a landmark paper in 1979, Thomas et al. reported a 60% three-year actuarial survival for patients with acute myeloid leukaemia (AML) in first remission [6]. This was at least comparable, if not superior, to results achieved by conventional chemotherapy alone. Since then, TBI has been widely used as part of the conditioning regime for BMT in the treatment of haematological malignancies. Less commonly, it has been used in the treatment of solid tumours [7], and of a variety of non-malignant conditions such as aplastic anaemia and certain inborn errors of metabolism. It has also been used, without marked success, as an immunosuppressive agent in the treatment of myasthenia gravis [8,9] and polymyositis [10].

Functions of total body irradiation

The two major functions of TBI, when used as part of the conditioning regime for BMT, are to provide adequate immunosuppression for marrow engraftment and to contribute to leukaemic cell kill. The issue of cell kill is obviously irrelevant when TBI is used in BMT for non-malignant disorders, and the rest of this chapter will be confined to the use of TBI in the treatment of leukaemia. The relative importance of immunosuppression and cell kill is a matter of dispute, and an important one, because it has major implications for the choice of TBI regimen. For example, if radiation-induced cell kill is important in the prevention of leukaemic relapse, then more intensive TBI schedules might improve the outcome of BMT. If, on the other hand, cell kill from TBI is relatively unimportant compared to that resulting from chemotherapy and graft-versus-leukaemia (GvL), and the major role of TBI is to provide immunosuppression, then one would not expect any advantage from intensifying TBI beyond the amount needed to allow engraftment.

Immunosuppression

The immunosuppression provided by TBI contributes to the prevention of allograft rejection (not a problem in the autograft setting). Animal data show a steep TBI dose–response for successful engraftment [11]. However, engraftment depends not just on TBI but also on other factors such as drug treatment with cyclophosphamide and cyclosporin, the degree of human leukocyte antigen (HLA) matching between host and donor, and whether or not the graft is T-cell depleted. In fact, it has not been possible in clinical practice to demonstrate any clear relationship between TBI parameters and the incidence of graft rejection. Furthermore, at least in the case of T-cell undepleted transplants from matched sibling donors, sustained engraftment is achieved in more than 98% of recipients [12]. It would therefore seem possible to modify commonly used TBI schedules to reduce toxicity without necessarily compromising marrow engraftment.

Cell kill

In practice, disease relapse is a much greater problem than failure to engraft. Most leukaemic cell lines are radiosensitive, so that TBI should add significantly to the cell kill achieved by cytotoxic drugs and by the GvL effect. Additionally, radiation may be particularly important for the eradication of disease from 'sanctuary' sites such as the testes and central nervous system. One approach has therefore been to intensify the TBI regimen, accepting major toxicity, in the hope of reducing the rate of relapse.

Two randomized trials from Seattle have investigated the effect of TBI dose escalation [13,14]. In both trials, fractionated TBI given as 12 Gy in six fractions was compared with 15.75 Gy in seven fractions prior to allogeneic BMT. The first trial comprised patients with AML, and the second, those with chronic myeloid leukaemia (CML). In both, there were significantly fewer relapses with the higher dose, suggesting that leukaemic cell kill by radiation was important. Unfortunately, however, the higher dose of TBI was associated with increased treatment-related mortality, so that there was no overall survival benefit with dose escalation (see Table 34.1). The lack of a survival benefit is obviously disappointing, but there may still be a place for intensifying radiotherapy. First, it may be that dose escalation would be of benefit in those patients at particularly high risk of relapse. Therefore, it would be interesting to repeat the Seattle studies in patients receiving autografts or T-cell depleted allografts. Second, the use of targeted radiotherapy (see later), which should spare important normal tissues relative to leukaemic cells, might allow dose escalation without unacceptable morbidity.

However, there are still those who argue that TBI cell kill is of little importance [15]. One argument is that the relapse rate following syngeneic BMT (that is, from an identical twin), in which there is no GvL, is much higher than after allografts. This observation suggests that, for allografts, GvL eradicates residual disease left after both chemotherapy and TBI. Furthermore, the relapse rate after autografting is similar to that after syngeneic BMT. It can be inferred that most relapses after autografts arise from persistent leukaemic cells in the recipient rather than the infused marrow, thus reflecting failure of the TBI to eradicate disease. However, these observations do not preclude the possibility that less intensive TBI would lead to even higher relapse rates.

Technical aspects of total body irradiation

Equipment

The technique used to deliver TBI varies considerably between centres. The ideal method should be comfortable for the patient, convenient for the department to administer alongside its routine workload, and deliver an accurate dose to the entire body in a specified distribution, at the desired dose-

Table 34.1 Results from the only two randomised trials of TBI dose escalation by Clift et al from Seattle

Study	AML [14]		CML [13]	
TBI protocol (Gy)	12	15.75	12	15.75
Number of cases	34	37	57	59
Treatment-related deaths	4	12	12	20
Median disease-free survival (months)	20	22	35	39

rate. Most radiotherapy centres do not have dedicated TBI units, and the techniques used in practice tend to reflect the facilities available, sometimes at the expense of some, or all, of these ideals. For example, difficulties in achieving a sufficiently large field size to irradiate the whole body has required, in some cases, the patient to assume the foetal position, often for long periods of time (Figure 34.1). Furthermore, these long treatment times, on general-purpose radiotherapy machines, can seriously disrupt the overall workload of a department. However, even with the most sophisticated of equipment, the actual dose distribution delivered may depend as much on the shape of the particular patient as on any technical factors.

The Royal Marsden Hospital has a purpose-built TBI unit consisting of two parallel opposed cobalt-60 sources, positioned 7 metres apart, with the treatment couch between them. The maximum field size, at the level of the couch, is 200 cm × 65 cm so that even the tallest of patients may lie full-length. The large source-to-patient distance helps to produce a relatively homogeneous dose distribution, and the dose rate may be varied by the use of attenuators placed in the beams. Because of the low energy of the cobalt sources compared with that of a linear accelerator, a light blanket placed over the patient provides sufficient build-up to avoid unwanted skin sparing. A dedicated unit, such as this, provides the luxury of treating patients independent of the general work of the department.

Dose distribution

As with most radiotherapy, it is usually considered desirable to deliver TBI with a homogeneous dose distribution. However, thinner parts of the body, such as the head and feet, tend to receive a higher dose than wider parts such as the trunk. These differences may be minimized by altering the proportion of time spent in the supine and lateral positions. In this way, it is usually possible to achieve less than 10% variation in dose across the body.

Some centres aim to restrict the dose to certain organs, such as lung, liver or kidneys, by the use of appropriate shielding, hoping to thus reduce treatment-related toxicity. Shielding organs smaller than the lungs is not really feasible because of the radiation scatter behind the blocks, and the difficulty in verifying block position for organs of typical soft-tissue density. Lung shielding (Figure 34.2), however, is practicable, at least in cooperative patients, and is used in many centres, although there is very little evidence to indicate whether or not it is beneficial. Rates of interstitial pneumonitis do seem to have fallen along with the introduction of shielding, but this has coincided with a move from single fraction towards fractionated TBI, so the reasons are unclear. The only randomized trial of shielding versus none failed to show a benefit for shielding [16], and Girinsky *et al.* have raised the concern that lung shielding could lead to an increased rate of leukaemic relapse [17]. The question of lung shielding should be addressed in future trials.

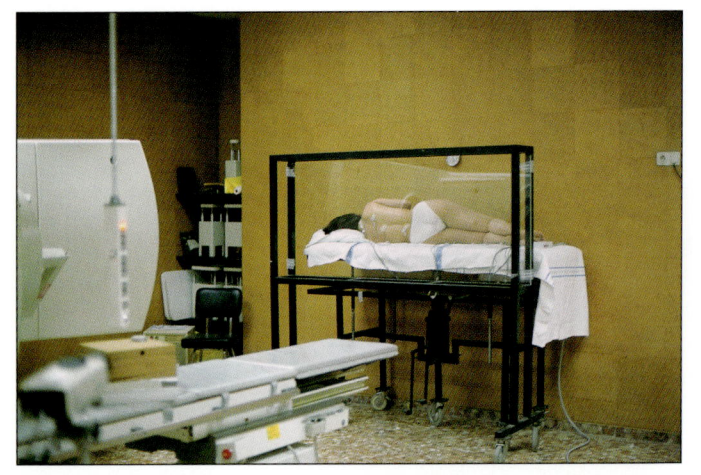

Figure 34.1 TBI using a conventional linear accelerator. The focus-to-skin distance is as long as possible to provide a sufficiently large field size.

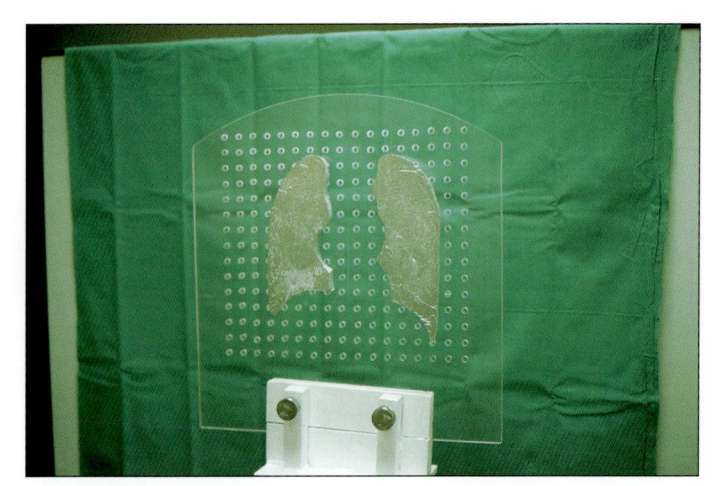

Figure 34.2 Lung shielding blocks.

Dosimetry

For the treatment itself the patient lies on the couch, either supine or in the lateral position, the proportion of time spent in each position depending upon the dose distribution. In the supine position, the hands are placed across the chest in order to provide some degree of lung sparing (Figure 34.3). Dosimetry may be based either on a pretreatment calculation method using patient dimensions, or on *in vivo* measurements, with either thermoluminescent dosimeters (TLD) or semiconductor diodes, taken during part of the treatment itself. TLDs have been widely used for many years, but they are time-consuming, both to prepare and to read, and semiconductor diodes, which provide an immediate readout, are becoming more popular. The TLDs or diodes are attached to the skin in specified positions, in order to measure the dose received at individual sites and to establish the dose distribution throughout the body (Figure 34.4).

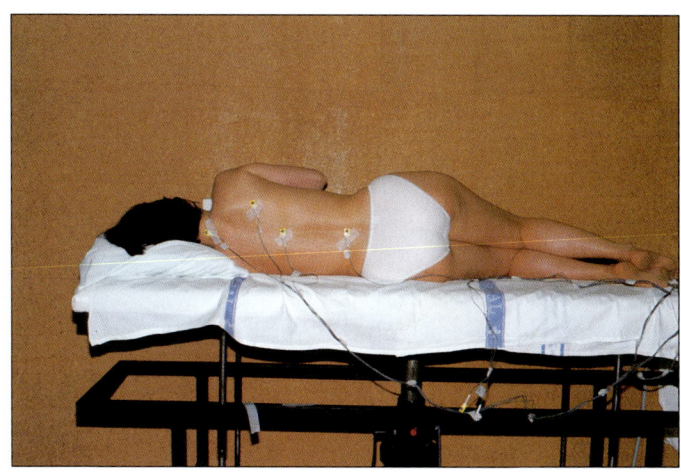

Figure 34.4 Semiconductor diodes in position for in vivo *dosimetry.*

Dose

Probably the most commonly used dose schedule is 12 Gy given in six fractions over three days. However, there are a number of variations on this. An alternative approach is to use a single-fraction treatment, usually of the order of 10 Gy, with the exact dose depending on the dose rate employed. At the Royal Marsden, the prescription is specified at the maximum lung dose, on the premise that it is lung toxicity which is dose-limiting. Other centres use a different prescription point, such as in the pelvis, where, if the separation is smaller than in the lungs, the dose absorbed may be higher. In other words, 10 Gy specified at the pelvis is likely to result in a lower overall dose than 10 Gy specified to the lungs. This variation in prescribing practice is one of several factors which makes it hard to compare results from different centres.

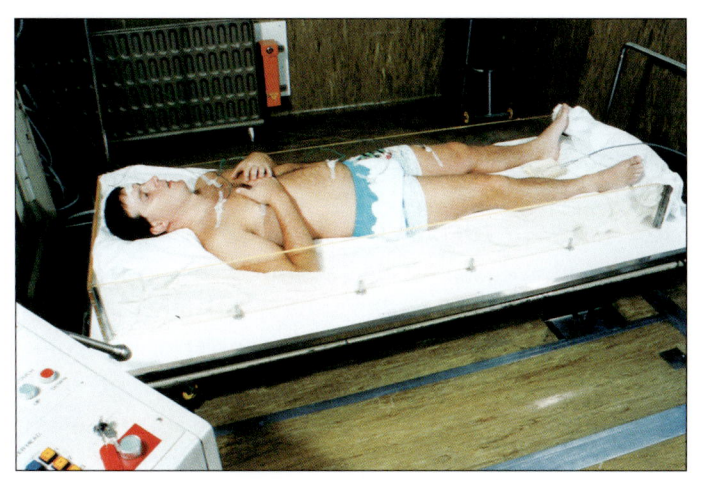

Figure 34.3 The field size on this dedicated TBI unit is large enough to allow the patient to lie full-length. Note the hands across the chest to provide some lung sparing.

Fractionation

The question of whether or not to fractionate TBI is controversial, and remains unresolved. Radiobiological theory predicts that for a given leukaemic cell kill, fractionation of TBI should spare late normal tissue effects, such as lung damage and growth impairment. Results from animal work [18], and some retrospective clinical series, are consistent with this theory [19,20]. However, it is hard to draw any conclusions from such series, as results are drawn from many centres, with different patient selection criteria, and TBI techniques which are likely to vary in ways other than fractionation. Unfortunately, there are no good randomized data addressing the question of fractionation. The one published, randomized trial included only 53 patients and was too small to provide any definitive answers [21]. In practice, most centres are now using fractionated TBI, a choice which is probably based as much on convenience as it is on theoretical considerations or clinical data. Fractionated TBI is commonly given at a dose rate of about 15 cGy/min so that each fraction takes about 20 minutes, allowing for time to change positions and to replace TLDs or diodes. On the other hand, single-fraction treatments are given at a lower dose rate of about 4 cGy/min, so the overall treatment time is 4–5 hours. With time added on for stoppages, single fractions usually take between 5 and 6 hours. Consequently, fractionation tends to cause less disruption to the routine workload of a department.

Clinical aspects of TBI

Patient selection and counselling

Before giving TBI, it must be established that the patient is fit for the procedure. Possible contraindications to TBI include previous irradiation, impaired lung function and advanced age. Abnormalities of lung function have been shown to be significant risk factors for death following BMT conditioned with TBI [22]. Patients are sometimes extremely wary of TBI, possibly associating it with unfavourable aspects of radiation, such as nuclear accidents. Proper counselling, therefore, takes considerable time, and should include a description of the procedure and the associated risks (see later) before obtaining patient consent.

Conditioning and preparation

The commonest conditioning regimen for BMT involves the use of TBI together with cyclophosphamide, TBI being given the day after the chemotherapy. A few hours prior to TBI the patient is premedicated with an anti-emetic, usually a 5-HT_3 antagonist such as ondansetron. Immediately before TBI, phenobarbitone 80 mg/kg is given, and repeated at three-hourly intervals during single-fraction treatments. The aim is to achieve sedation sufficient to help the patient keep still without compromising his cooperation. The use of phenobarbitone, rather than any other sedative, is historical, but it may prevent radiation-induced hyperpyrexia. If additional sedation is required a short-acting benzodiazepine, such as diazepam (5–10 mg), may be given.

Toxicity

BMT is a toxic treatment with the potential to cause numerous adverse effects. Undoubtedly, TBI contributes to this toxicity but transplantation is a complex process, involving many potentially toxic components, to which it is difficult to attribute specific toxicity. However, careful analysis of toxicity is important, not least because it is now possible to condition patients for BMT with drugs alone, thus avoiding TBI. It remains to be seen whether this approach will lead to a significant reduction in treatment-related toxicity.

Acute toxicity

Acute side-effects occurring during TBI include nausea and vomiting, headache and hyperthermia. Nausea and vomiting have been associated with anxiety [23], movement during irradiation [23], single-fraction treatment [24] and dose rates greater than 6 cGy/min [25]. However, since the introduction of 5-HT_3 antagonists, nausea and vomiting are seldom severe. For example, Schwella et al. report 'sufficient emesis control' in 22 out of 25 patients given ondansetron prior to fractionated TBI [26]. 5-HT_3 antagonists have been shown, in randomized controlled trials, to prevent TBI-induced nausea and vomiting more effectively than both placebo [27], and a combination of dexamethasone, metoclopramide and lorazepam [28]. Headache is seldom a problem but is associated with the use of 5-HT_3 antagonists [28]. Hyperthermia commonly occurs [29] but rarely causes symptoms and does not persist longer than 24 hours.

Other side-effects occurring within the first few days following TBI include xerostomia, jaw pain due to parotitis, diarrhoea, skin erythema and eye problems including photophobia, dry eye syndrome and conjunctival oedema. Parotid swelling and pain usually settle within 2–3 days, but xerostomia may persist for months. Diarrhoea is seen in about one-third of patients, and is more common in those who receive methotrexate as graft-versus-host disease prophylaxis. Skin erythema is inevitable except when very high-energy photons (18–20 MV) are used. Ocular problems have been reviewed by Spires [30].

Intermediate toxicity

Adverse effects occurring within weeks, or a few months, of TBI include interstitial pneumonitis, hepatic veno-occlusive disease, somnolence syndrome and alopecia. The hair loss is usually of little significance because almost all patients already have complete alopecia from their chemotherapy, and regrowth normally occurs within months. However, permanent alopecia after BMT has been reported and is associated with chronic graft-versus-host disease and prior cranial irradiation [31]. The somnolence syndrome is characterized by drowsiness, headache and anorexia occurring about 6 weeks after irradiation, and lasting for 1–2 weeks. Pneumonitis and hepatic veno-occlusive disease are two of the most important toxicities following BMT and will be discussed at more length.

Pneumonitis

Pneumonitis is common after BMT, and is frequently fatal. Data from the International Bone Marrow Transplant Registry [32] based on 932 patients show that pneumonitis occurred in 29%, and was fatal in 84% of these cases. The importance of radiation in the pathogenesis of pneumonitis remains unclear. Theory predicts that radiation pneumonitis will occur more commonly with higher radiation dose and dose rate, and will be less likely to occur with fractionation. Some retrospective series have indeed shown these associations [19,32]) but others have found no relationship between the incidence of pneumonitis and fractionation [33–35]. Furthermore, the only randomized trials of TBI dose escalation [13,14], of different dose rates [36], of fractionation [21], and of lung shielding [16], have failed to show any significant relationship between these variables and pneumonitis.

Factors other than radiation are certainly associated with pneumonitis. Evidence suggests that cytomegalovirus (CMV) infection [37], graft-versus-host disease [32], ganciclovir prophylaxis [38], type of transplant (allogeneic or autologous) [39], cyclophosphamide dose [40] and use of methotrexate [32] are all related to the incidence of pneumonitis. It would therefore appear that radiation is one of many contributory causes of pneumonitis, and possibly, a relatively unimportant one.

Hepatic veno-occlusive disease

Hepatic veno-occlusive disease (VOD) is another important cause of morbidity and mortality after TBI. In severe cases it presents with jaundice, hepatomegaly and ascites, and is thought to account for up to 10% of treatment-related deaths following BMT [41]. Reports of its incidence vary from 6–52%, the difference reflecting, at least in part, differences in diagnostic criteria. Elevated transaminases, female gender and the use of cytosine arabinoside all predispose to VOD, but TBI has also been implicated [41,42]. Once again, as for pneumonitis, there are conflicting data regarding the relationship of the different TBI parameters to the incidence of the disease. These have been recently summarized by Ozsahin *et al.* [43].

Late toxicity

The late effects of BMT have attracted a great deal of interest in recent years, partly because it is only now that information concerning them is becoming available, and partly because of the hope of avoiding them by the use of conditioning regimes excluding TBI.

Late effects of BMT in general are discussed fully in Chapters 55–57, and attention here will therefore be focussed on those late effects attributed to radiation, and the evidence concerning the extent to which TBI is, in fact, responsible. Such late effects include endocrine failure, growth impairment, cataract formation, renal dysfunction and second malignancies. For a more complete list see Table 34.2.

The endocrine late effects of note are hypothyroidism and gonadal failure. Hypothyroidism is common after BMT and is probably caused by TBI [44]. It is, of course, easily treatable. BMT is almost always followed by primary ovarian failure in women [45], and azoospermia in men [46]. Radiation to 10 Gy is certainly sufficient to cause permanent azoospermia, but is probably only one of several factors contributing to ovarian suppression, since doses as high as 16 Gy are needed to ensure ovarian ablation in other contexts. Indeed it is possible, especially for younger women, to retain ovarian function, and there are at least six reported cases of women who have borne children after TBI [47–50]. While paternity may be harder to establish with certainty, there is at least one case, proven by genetic testing, of a man who had previously received TBI, fathering a child [51].

Avoiding TBI may not, however, have a significant effect in terms of preserving gonadal function. The only published data which address this issue come from Chattergee *et al.* who measured pituitary-gonadal function in 15 women, both before, and 3–4 months after, BMT. As expected, the post-treatment results were abnormal, but no significant differences were found between those who had received radiation and those who had been conditioned with high-dose chemotherapy alone [52]. While these are interesting

Table 34.2 Toxicity of bone-marrow transplantation	
Early and intermediate	Late
Nausea and vomiting	Endocrine
Hyperthermia	infertility
Xerostomia	premature menopause
Skin erythema	hypothyroidism
Parotitis	growth impairment
Alopecia	
Interstitial pneumonitis	Ocular
Veno-occlusive disease	cataracts
	dry eyes
	Second malignancies
	Neurological
	necrotizing -
	leukoencephalopathy
	polyneuropathy
	intellectual impairment
	Renal
	impaired renal function
	haemolytic uraemic
	syndrome
	Skeletal
	exostoses
	osteoporosis
	aseptic necrosis
	Pulmonary
	bronchiolitis obliterans

Cataracts occur in 15–50% of those who survive five years after BMT, and may be inevitable with sufficiently long follow-up. The use of steroids for the treatment of graft-versus-host disease, high TBI dose rates, and single fraction treatments are associated with early cataract formation [58–61].

Renal impairment after BMT is common, which is not surprising in view of the number of nephrotoxic drugs to which these patients are exposed. Renal tolerance for radiotherapy has usually been regarded as 20 Gy in 2 Gy fractions. However, there is now some evidence that even the lower doses used in TBI impair renal function to some extent. In a retrospective study of 84 patients receiving allogeneic BMT after TBI, Miralbell *et al.* found that renal dysfunction was strongly related to TBI dose [62]. In this study, renal impairment did not lead to clinical problems, so the association with TBI is probably more of academic interest to radiobiologists, who may need to revise their estimates of renal tolerance, rather than of practical importance to bone-marrow transplanters.

There is much concern, although rather less data, about the risk of second malignancies following BMT [63]. There does appear to be a heightened risk of both lymphoproliferative disorders and solid tumours after BMT, although the magnitude of this risk is not known. One estimate, based on the follow-up of 700 patients who received BMT for aplastic anaemia, indicates an actuarial rate of malignancy of 14% at 20 years. In this study, TBI was an important prognostic factor for subsequent malignancy on multivariate analysis [64]. The hope of avoiding second malignancies has been a major impetus towards the development of conditioning regimes that do not include radiation.

data, longer follow-up is clearly required before reaching any firm conclusion.

BMT in children leads to significant growth impairment which is associated with growth hormone deficiency, and is more marked with single, rather than fractionated, TBI [53]. It occurs sooner, and is more likely, in those who have previously received prophylactic cranial irradiation [54,55], and is less severe in those whose transplant regimen does not include TBI [56,57]. This growth impairment responds to therapeutic growth hormone [54].

The future of TBI

Is TBI still necessary for BMT?

The role of TBI has been called into question by the advent of conditioning regimes for BMT that comprise drugs alone, usually a combination of busulphan and cyclophosphamide (BuCy). It was hoped that the omission of radiation would significantly reduce the morbidity and mortality associated with transplantation, and that the addition of busulphan would provide sufficient antileukaemic effect to offset the loss of TBI cell kill.

Five randomized trials (see Table 34.3) have been published comparing BuCy with cyclophosphamide and TBI (CyTBI) [65–69]. Perhaps surprisingly, no consistent differences have been found in short-term toxicity, including pneumonitis. In fact, hepatic veno-occlusive disease is more common with busulphan than with TBI, and in two of the five trials, conditioning with BuCy was associated with a significantly greater risk of treatment-related mortality. These two studies also showed an overall survival benefit for TBI [65,66].

However, it would be premature to conclude that CyTBI is superior to BuCy. Firstly, follow-up is short and it may be that BuCy will have an advantage in terms of late toxicity. Secondly, it may be possible to identify certain groups of patients for whom BuCy is at least an acceptable alternative, if not preferable, to CyTBI. This could certainly apply to those patients who have previously received near-tolerance doses of radiation. In addition, subgroup analysis appears to suggest that the survival advantage of TBI is confined to those with advanced, poor-risk disease. It may be that such patients, who have often been heavily pretreated, tolerate BuCy poorly. Further trials are ongoing and it will be interesting to see if this hypothesis is borne out. At present, therefore, TBI remains an established part of conditioning for BMT, and use of regimes such as BuCy is largely confined to clinical trials.

Targeted radiotherapy

Progress may come from attempts to modify the dose distribution of radiation in order to target sites of disease, with sparing of normal tissues. Two methods are being investigated. The first relies on conjugating I^{131} to antibodies directed against antigens expressed by haematopoietic cells. The second uses bone-seeking radionuclides emitting radiation of the appropriate energy, such as Sm^{153} or Ho^{166}, which are taken up by bone, and act on disease in the marrow by virtue of its proximity. Dosimetric studies using radiolabelled anti-CD45 antibodies have demonstrated that at least twice as much radiation can be delivered to bone as to lungs or liver [70]. This technique is now being tried in combination with conventional TBI and cyclophosphamide. If this approach proves successful, dose escalation of the radiolabelled antibodies may allow a dose reduction of conventional TBI, and, therefore, the hope of a less toxic treatment with an increased antileukaemic effect.

Table 34.3 Randomized studies comparing conditioning with BuCy and CyTBI

Study	Patients (n)	Randomization	Treatment-related mortality (%)	Overall survival (%)
Blaise et al. (1992) [66]	101	BuCy CyTBI	27 8*	51 (2 years) 75*
Ringden et al. (1994) [65]	167	BuCy CyTBI	28 9*	62 (3 years) 76*
Clift et al. (1994) [68]	142	BuCy CyTBI	18 24	80 (3 years) 80
Devergie et al. (1995) [67]	120	BuCy CyTBI	38 29	61 (5 years) 63
Dusenbury et al. (1995) [69]	35	BuCy CyTBI	16 16	24 (2 years) 50

*$P < 0.05$.

Conclusions

There remains considerable uncertainty concerning what constitutes the ideal TBI regimen. As discussed, this stems partly from the fact that the outcome of BMT depends on many factors other than the TBI parameters, making comparison between centres, and with historical controls, difficult to interpret. This difficulty is compounded by the paucity of good, randomized trials of different TBI protocols. Significant improvements over conventional TBI regimes are not likely to be made in the absence of large, randomized trials which would require the cooperation of many centres.

Acknowledgement

We would like to thank Dr B. Sanchez-Nieto for permission to use Figures 34.1, 34.2 and 34.4.

References

1. Heineke H. Experimentelle Untersuchungen über die Einwirkund der Röntgenstrahlen auf das Knochenmark, nebst einige Bemerkungen über die Röntgentherapie der Leukämie und Pseudoleukämie und des Sarcoms. *Deutsche Zeitschr fur Chirurg* 1905; **78**: 196–231.
2. Hueblein AC. A preliminary report on continuous irradiation of the entire body. *Radiology* 1932; **18**: 1051–1062.
3. Medinger FG and Craver LF. Total body irradiation. *Am J Roentgenol* 1942; **48**: 651–671.
4. Lorenz E, Uphoff D, Reid TR et al. Modification of irradiation injury in mice and guinea pigs by bone marrow injections. *J Nat Cancer Inst* 1951; **12**: 197–201.
5. Thomas ED and Ferrebee JW. Transplantation of marrow and whole organs: experiences and comments. *Canadian Med Ass J* 1962; **86**: 435–444.
6. Thomas ED, Buckner CD, Clift RA et al. Marrow transplantation for acute nonlymphoblastic leukaemia in first remission. *New Engl J Med* 1979; **301**: 597–599.
7. Horovitz ME, Kinsella TJ, Wexler LH et al. TBI and autologous bone marrow transplant in the treatment of high-risk Ewing's sarcoma and rhabdomyosarcoma. *J Clin Oncol* 1993; **11**(10): 1911–1918.
8. Durelli L, Ferrio MF, Urgesi A et al. TBI for myasthenia gravis: a long-term follow-up. *Neurology* 1993; **43**(11): 2215–2221.
9. Chassard JL, Martinent L, Bady B et al. Role of irradiation as a treatment for myasthenia gravis. A review of about 30 cases. *Bull Cancer Radiother* 1992; **79**(2): 137–148.
10. Cherin P, Herson S, Coutellier A et al. Failure of TBI in polymyositis: report of three cases. *Br J Rheumatol* 1992; **31**(4): 282–283.
11. Vriesendorp HM. Engraftment of haemopoietic cells. In: *Bone Marrow Transplantation, Biological Mechanisms and Clinical Practice*. DW Van Bekkum and B Lowenberg (eds), 1985: 73–145 (New York: Dekker).
12. Barrett AJ, Horovitz MM, Gale RP et al. Marrow transplantation for ALL: factors affecting relapse and survival. *Blood* 1989; **74**: 862–871.
13. Clift RA, Buckner CD, Appelbaum FR et al. Allogeneic marrow transplantation in patients with chronic myeloid leukaemia in the chronic phase: a randomised trial of two irradiation regimens. *Blood* 1991; **77**(8): 1660–1665.
14. Clift RA, Buckner CD, Appelbaum FR et al. Allogeneic marrow transplantation in patients with AML in first remission: a randomised trial of two irradiation regimens. *Blood* 1990; **76**(9): 1867–1871.
15. Gale RP, Butturini A and Bortin MM. What does TBI do in bone marrow transplants for leukemia? *Int J Radiat Oncol Biol Phys* 1991; **20**: 631–634.
16. Labar B, Bogdanic V, Nemet D et al. TBI with or without lung shielding for allogeneic BMT. *Bone Marrow Transplant* 1992; **9**: 343–347.
17. Girinsky T, Socie G, Ammarguellat H et al. Consequences of two different doses to the lungs during a single dose of TBI: results of a randomised study on 85 patients. *Int J Radiat Oncol Biol Phys* 1994; **30**(4): 821–824.
18. Appelbaum FR. The influence of total dose, fractionation, dose rate, and distribution of TBI on bone marrow transplantation. *Semin Oncol* 1993; **20**(4) (Suppl 4): 3–10.
19. Socié G, Devergie A, Girinsky T et al. Influence of the fractionation of TBI on complications and relapse rate for CML. *Int J Radiat Oncol Biol Phys* 1991; **20**: 397–404.
20. Deeg HJ, for the Seattle Marrow Transplant Team. Acute and delayed toxicities of TBI. *Int J Radiat Oncol Biol Phys* 1983; **9**: 1933–1939.
21. Deeg HJ, Sullivan KM, Buckner CD et al. Marrow transplantation for ANLL in first remission: toxicity and long-term follow-up of patients conditioned with single dose or fractionated TBI. *Bone Marrow Transplant* 1986; **1**: 151–157.
22. Crawford SW and Fisher L. Predictive value of pulmonary function tests before marrow transplantation. *Chest* 1992; **101**(5): 1257–1264.
23. Westbrook C, Glaholm J and Barrett A. Vomiting associated with whole body irradiation. *Clin Radiol* 1987; **38**: 263–266.
24. Barrett A. Total body irradiation before bone marrow transplantation in leukaemia: a cooperative study from the European Group for Bone Marrow Transplantation. *Br J Radiol* 1982; **55**: 562–567.
25. Cosset JM, Baume D, Pico JL et al. Single dose versus hyperfractionated total body irradiation before allogeneic bone marrow transplantation: a non-randomised comparative study of 54 patients at the Institut Gustave-Roussy. *Radiother Oncol* 1989; **15**: 151–160.
26. Schwella N, Konig V, Schwerdtfeger R et al. Ondansetron for efficient emesis control during TBI. *Bone Marrow Transplant* 1994; **13**(2): 169–171.
27. Tiley C, Powles R, Catalano J et al. Result of a double blind placebo controlled study of ondansetron as an antiemetic during total body irradiation in patients undergoing bone marrow transplantation. *Leukaemia Lymphoma* 1992; **7**: 317–321.
28. Prentice HG. Efficacy and safety of granisetron in the treatment of emesis caused by TBI: a comparison with standard anti-emetic therapy. *Proc Ann Meet Am Soc Clin Oncol* 1993; **12**: A1574.

29. Chaillet MP, Cosset J, Socie G et al. Prospective study of the clinical symptoms of therapeutic whole body irradiation. *Health Phys* 1993; **64**: 370–374.
30. Spires R. Ocular manifestations in bone marrow transplantation. *J Ophthalmic Nurs Technol* 1993; **12**(5): 208–210.
31. Vowels M, Chan LL, Giri N et al. Factors affecting hair regrowth after BMT. *Bone Marrow Transplant* 1993; **12**(4): 347–350.
32. Weiner RS, Bortin MM, Gale RP et al. Interstitial pneumonia after bone marrow transplantation. Assessment of risk factors. *Ann Intern Med* 1986; **104**: 168–175.
33. Kim TH, McGlave PB, Ramsay N et al. Comparison of two TBI regimens in allogeneic bone marrow transplantation for ANLL in first remission. *Int J Radiat Oncol Biol Phys* 1990; **19**: 889–897.
34. Frassoni F, Scarpati D, Bacigalupo A et al. The effect of total body irradiation dose and chronic GvHD on leukaemic relapse after allogeneic BMT. *Br J Haematol* 1989; **73**: 211–216.
35. Ozsahin M, Belkacemi Y, Pene F et al. Interstitial pneumonitis following autologous bone marrow transplantation conditioned with cyclophosphamide and TBI. *Int J Radiat Oncol Biol Phys* 1995; **34**(1): 71–77.
36. Ozsahin M, Pene F, Touboul E et al. Total body irradiation before bone marrow transplantation: results of two randomised instantaneous dose rates in 157 patients. *Cancer* 1992; **69**: 2853–2865.
37. Winston DJ, Ho WG, Champlin RE. CMV infections after allogeneic BMT. *Rev Infect Dis* 1990; **12**(Suppl): 776–792.
38. Schmidt GM, Horak DA, Niland JC et al. A randomised controlled trial of prophylactic ganciclovir for CMV pulmonary infection in recipients of allogeneic bone marrow transplants. *New Engl J Med* 1991; **324**: 1005–1011.
39. Deeg HJ. Interstitial pneumonitis. In: *A Guide to Bone Marrow Transplantation*. HJ Deeg, HG Klingemann and GL Phillips (eds), 1988: 114–122 (Berlin: Springer-Verlag).
40. Ozsahin M, Schwartz LH, Pene F et al. Is body weight a risk factor of interstitial pneumonitis after BMT? *Bone Marrow Transplant* 1992; **10**: 97.
41. Ganem G, Girardin MFSM, Kuentz M et al. Veno-occlusive disease of the liver after allogeneic BMT in man. *Int J Radiat Oncol Biol Phys* 1988; **14**: 879–884.
42. McDonald GB, Sharma P, Matthews DE et al. VOD after BMT: diagnosis, incidence and predisposing factors. *Hepatology* 1984; **4**: 116–122.
43. Ozsahin M, Pene F, Cosset JM and Laugier A. Morbidity after TBI. *Semin Radiat Oncol* 1994; **4**(2): 95–102.
44. Borgstrom B and Bolme P. Thyroid function in children after allogeneic BMT. *Bone Marrow Transplant* 1994; **13**(1): 59–64.
45. Sanders JE, Buckner CD, Amos D et al. Ovarian function following marrow transplantation for acute leukaemia. *J Clin Oncol* 1988; **6**: 813–818.
46. Sanders JE, Buckner CD, Leonard JM et al. Late effects on gonadal function of cyclophosphamide, TBI and marrow transplantation. *Transplantation* 1983; **36**: 252–255.
47. Giri N, Vowels MR and Barr AL. Successful pregnancy after TBI and BMT for acute leukemia. *Bone Marrow Transplant* 1992; **10**: 93–95.
48. Samuelsson A, Fuchs T, Simonsson B and Bjorkholm M. Successful pregnancy in a 28-year-old patient autografted for ALL following myeloablative treatment including TBI. *Bone Marrow Transplant* 1993; **12**(6): 659–660.
49. Russell JA and Hanley DA. Full term pregnancy after allogeneic transplantation for leukemia in a patient with oligomenorhoea. *Bone Marrow Transplant* 1989; **4**: 579–580.
50. Buskard N, Ballem P, Hill R et al. Normal fertility after total body irradiation and chemotherapy in conjunction with a bone marrow transplant for acute leukaemia. *Clin Invest* 1988; **2**(Suppl): C57.
51. Pakkala S, Lukka M and Helminen P. Paternity after BMT following conditioning with TBI. *Bone Marrow Transplant* 1994; **13**(4): 489–490.
52. Chattergee R, Mills W, Katz M et al. Prospective study of pituitary–gonadal function to evaluate short-term effects of ablative chemotherapy or TBI with autologous or allogeneic marrow transplantation in post-menarcheal female patients. *Bone Marrow Transplant* 1994; **13**(5): 511–517.
53. Thomas BC, Stanhope R, Plowman PN and Leiper AD. Growth following single fraction and fractionated TBI for BMT. *Eur J Paediatr* 1993; **152**(11): 888–892.
54. Bozzola M, Gorgiani G, Locatelli F et al. Growth in children after BMT. *Horm Res* 1993; **39**(3–4): 122–126.
55. Huma Z, Boulad F, Black P et al. Growth in children after bone marrow transplantation for acute leukaemia. *Blood* 1995; **86**(2): 819–824.
56. Brauner R, Fontoura M, Zucker JM et al. Growth and growth hormone secretion after BMT. *Arch Dis Child* 1993; **68**(4): 458–463.
57. Giri N, Davis EA and Vowels MR. Long-term complications following BMT in children. *J Paediatr Child Health* 1993; **29**(3): 201–205.
58. Hamon MD, Gale RF, MacDonald RM et al. Incidence of cataracts after single fraction total body irradiation: the role of steroids and GvHD. *Bone Marrow Transplant* 1993; **12**(3): 233–236.
59. Dunn JP, Jabs DA, Wingard J et al. Bone marrow transplantation and cataract development. *Arch Ophthalmol* 1993; **111**(10): 1367–1373.
60. Ozsahin M, Belkacemi Y, Pene F et al. TBI and cataract incidence: a randomised comparison of two instantaneous dose rates. *Int J Radiat Oncol Biol Phys* 1994; **28**(2): 343–347.
61. Fife K, Milan S, Westbrook K et al. Risk factors for requiring cataract surgery following TBI. *Radiother Oncol* 1994; **33**(7): 93–98.
62. Miralbell R, Bieri S, Mermillod B et al. Renal toxicity after allogeneic bone marrow transplantation: the combined effects of TBI and GvHD. *Blood* 1996; **14**(2): 579–585.
63. Deeg HJ and Witherspoon RP. Risk factors for the development of secondary malignancies after marrow transplantation. *Hem Oncol Clin North Am* 1993; **7**(2): 417–429.
64. Deeg HJ, Socie G, Schoch G et al. Malignancies after marrow transplantation for aplastic anemia and Fanconi anemia: a joint Seattle and Paris analysis of results in 700 patients. *Blood* 1996; **87**(1): 386–392.
65. Ringden O, Ruutu T, Remberger R et al. A randomised trial comparing busulphan with TBI as conditioning in allogeneic marrow transplant recipients with leukaemia: A report from the Nordic Bone Marrow Transplantation Group. *Blood* 1994; **83**(9): 2723–2730.

66. Blaise D, Maraninchi D, Archimbaud E *et al*. Allogeneic BMT for AML in first remission: a randomised trial of busulfan–cytoxan versus cytoxan–TBI as preparative regimen. A report from the Group d'Etudes de la Greffe de Moelle Osseuse. *Blood* 1992; **79**: 2578–2582.
67. Devergie A, Blaise D, Attal M *et al*. Allogeneic bone marrow transplantation for chronic myeloid leukaemia in first chronic phase: a randomised trial of busulphan–cytoxan versus cytoxan–TBI as preparative regimen. A report from the French Society of Bone Marrow Graft (SFGM). *Blood* 1995; **85(8)**: 2263–2268.
68. Clift RA, Buckner ED, Thomas WI *et al*. Marrow transplantation for chronic myeloid leukaemia: a randomised study comparing cyclophosphamide and TBI with busulfan and cyclophosphamide. *Blood* 1994; **84(6)**: 2036–2043.
69. Dusenbery KE, Daniels KA, McClure JS *et al*. Randomised comparison of cyclophosphamide–TBI versus busulfan–cyclophosphamide conditioning in autologous bone marrow transplantation for acute myeloid leukaemia. *Int J Radiat Oncol Biol Phys* 1995; **31(1)**: 119–128.
70. Matthews DC, Appelbaum FR, Eary JF *et al*. Use of radioiodinated anti-CD45 monoclonal antibody to augment marrow irradiation prior to marrow transplantation for acute leukemia. *Blood* 1992; **80**: 335a (Suppl 1) (Abstr).

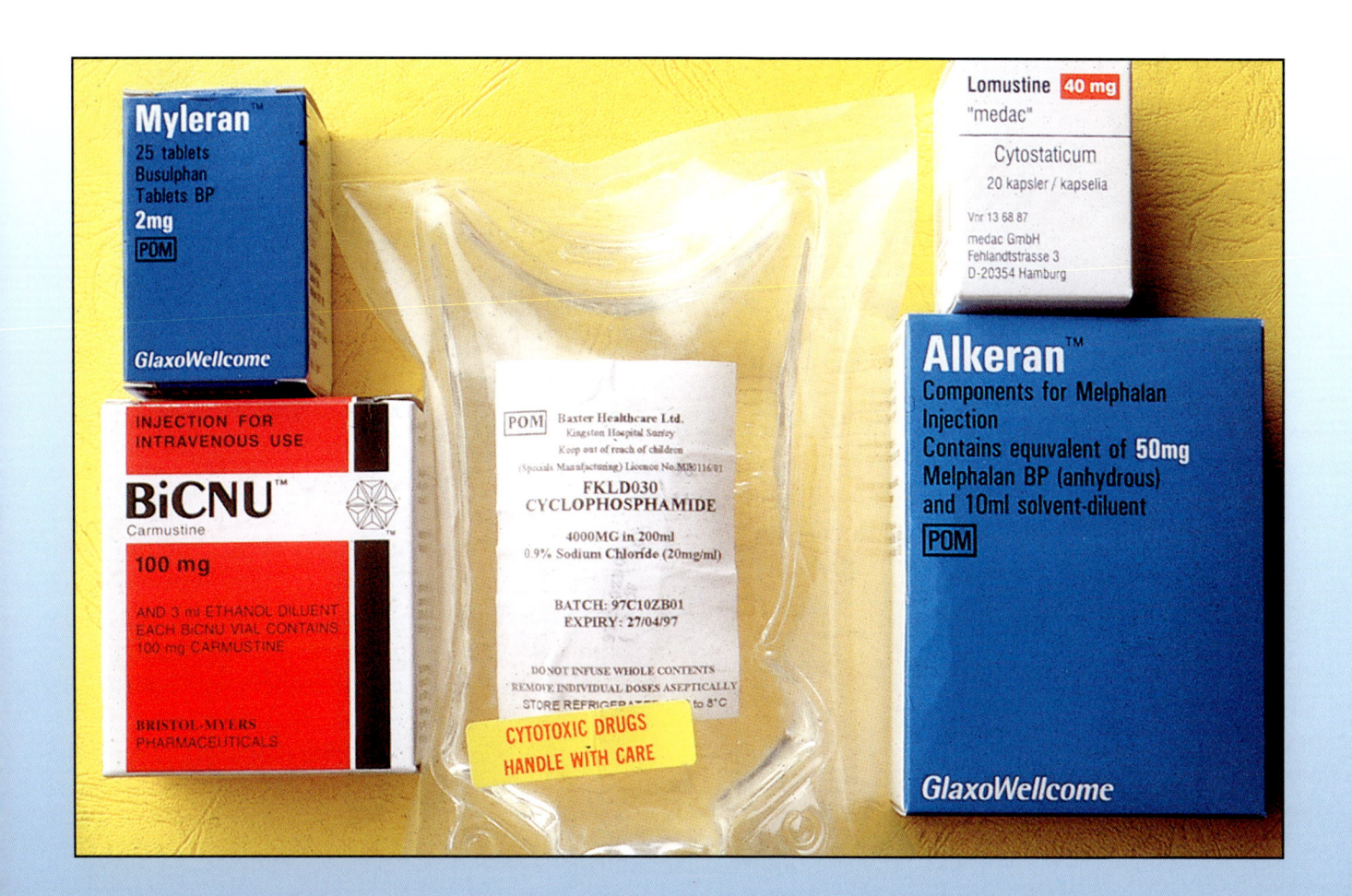

Chapter 35

Preparative regimens for allogeneic bone-marrow transplantation

John Barrett

Introduction

The preparative regimen given before bone-marrow transplantation (BMT) has three functions:
1. to immunosuppress the recipient to prevent graft rejection;
2. to provide myeloablation to allow reconstitution of 100% donor haematopoiesis;
3. to confer an antitumour effect.

The choice of preparative regimen depends upon the type of transplant. For example, transplants for severe aplastic anaemia require only immunosuppression to obtain engraftment, transplants for hereditary disorders with normal marrow cellularity require immunosuppression and myeloablation to permit establishment of 100% donor haematopoiesis, and transplants for malignant diseases demand an antitumour and an immunosuppressive preparative regimen. While these three functions are distinct, the agents used have overlapping properties. Thus, total body irradiation (TBI), used primarily as antileukaemia treatment is immunosuppressive and myeloablative (Figure 35.1).

Historically, preparative regimens were first used in the context of autologous BMT for malignant disorders, with the idea that dose escalation of antitumour therapy beyond that causing permanent bone-marrow failure can be safely applied if a marrow transplant 'rescue' is performed. Dose intensification is then only limited by non-haematopoietic side-effects. With the advent of allogeneic BMT in the 1970s, a combination of TBI with cyclophosphamide was used for leukaemia transplants. Non-radiation immunosuppressive regimens were developed for marrow grafts in non-malignant disorders. Cyclophosphamide was found to be a satisfactory transplant preparation in severe aplastic anaemia (SAA).

In transplants for non-malignant disorders with a normally cellular marrow, it was presumed that it would be necessary to make space for the incoming marrow by use of a myeloablative regimen. This led to the introduction of regimens combining cyclophosphamide with busulphan. Subsequently, much effort has been devoted to improving the immunosuppressive and antileukaemic qualities of the preparative regimens using variations of total body irradiation, and different chemotherapeutic agents. To reduce unwanted side-effects, radiation-free regimens have been developed and combinations of agents with different non-haematopoietic target susceptibilities are used to maximize antitumour activity, while diminishing specific organ damage. Maximum tolerated doses of radiation are now well characterized and radiation dose and fractionation can be selected to achieve the optimum therapeutic effect. Nevertheless, no preparative regimen is without some toxicity and treatment always involves a compromise between the desired and the unwanted effects. This chapter outlines the transplantation biology of engraftment and antileukaemia treatment, summarizes the properties and function of the agents used and describes preparative regimens in common use for specific diseases and transplant circumstances.

Marrow engraftment

Profound immunosuppression to the point of immune ablation is required to overcome the recipient's strong allogeneic response to donor bone-marrow cells and prevent prompt rejection of the transplant. Graft rejection manifests either as transient haematological recovery followed by aplasia, or by a complete absence of recovery (graft failure). Sometimes autologous recovery of haematopoiesis occurs. Haematopoietic progenitor cells express human leukocyte antigen (HLA) class I and II and minor histocompatibility

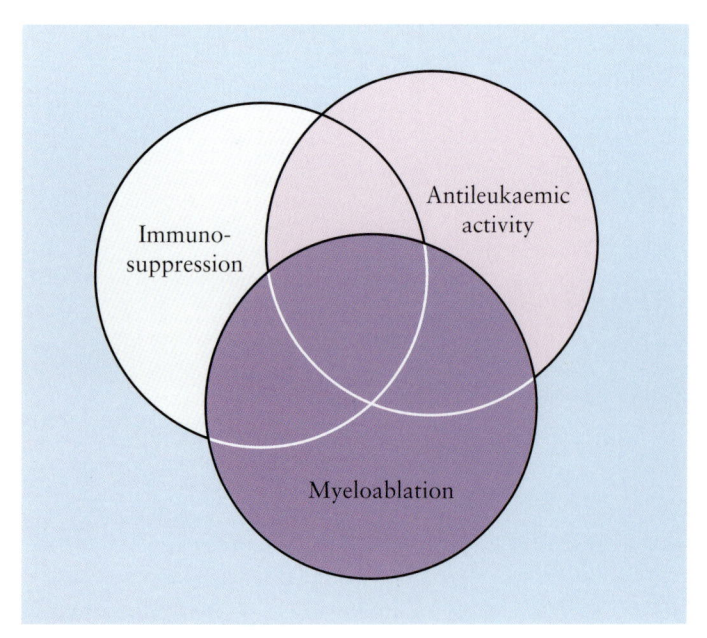

Figure 35.1 Effects of agents used in preparative regimens overlap.

antigens and are susceptible targets for allo-reacting cytotoxic T-cells. Between HLA-identical sibling pairs, rejection is mediated by minor histocompatibility antigen differences. In HLA-mismatched BMT, differences at major histocompatibility complex (MHC) class I and II loci further increase the risk of graft rejection [1–3], a risk which grows with increasing donor–recipient disparity. Natural killer (NK) cells can also reject allogeneic marrow: mice and humans with severe combined immunodeficiency disease (SCID) have no functioning T-cells, but can reject allogeneic marrow through NK activity [4,5].

In addition to the impact of the preparative regimen and the degree of histocompatibility, marrow engraftment is also determined by other factors associated with either the recipient or the donor (see Table 35.1).

Recipient factors determining engraftment

With the exception of identical twin donors and BMT for SCID, the infusion of donor bone marrow into a recipient not immunosuppressed by a preparative regimen results in prompt graft rejection by recipient T-cells. Transfusion-dependent patients with SAA or haemoglobinopathies readily become sensitized to minor histocompatibility antigens, which, if also present on transplanted cells, lead to graft rejection. The potential for rejection increases in proportion to the number of random transfusions received. However, because of the likelihood of sensitization to the donor's own antigens, transfusions from family members or the bone-marrow donor are especially hazardous [6,7]. Graft rejection rates vary according to the disorder being transplanted, due to the pre-BMT treatment as well as the type of preparative regimen used. For example, prior chemotherapy and the intensive preparative regimens used in leukaemia transplants reduce the potential for rejection, while prior transfusion in haemoglobinopathies and aplastic anaemia and the avoidance of irradiation in the preparative regimen increase the risk.

Donor factors determining engraftment

Animal studies demonstrate that the marrow-cell dose determines the rate and probability of engraftment [8]. Although it is not clear what stem-cell dose represents the lower limit for engraftment in man, recent data indicate that while CD34+ cell doses of $0.5–1 \times 10^6$/kg

Table 35.1 Factors determining marrow engraftment

	Probability of engraftment		
	High	Intermediate	Low
Histocompatibility	Identical twin	HLA identical sibling or family member	HLA mismatched or matched unrelated
Recipient	No transfusions No sensitization to HLA Intensified TBI preparative regimen Immune deficiency diseases	Less than 40 donor units HLA-sensitized CyTBI, BuCy Leukaemias, haemoglobinopathies	Greater than 40 donor units Sensitized to family donors Cy alone Aplastic anaemia
Donor	Donor buffy-coat transfusions after BMT High CD34+ cell dose	Undepleted donor marrow $1–2 \times 10^6$ CD34+ cells/kg	T-cell depletion $< 10^6$ CD34+ cells/kg
	Peripheral blood progenitor transplants	Bone-marrow transplants	Cord blood transplants in adults

Cy = cyclophosphamide, Bu = busulphan, TBI = total body irradiation.

permit engraftment in HLA-identical sibling BMT, they are associated with a significantly higher early transplant-related mortality [9]. A CD34 cell dose of $>1 \times 10^6$/kg for matched BMT, and larger doses in mismatched transplants, thus appears necessary.

The importance of T-lymphocytes in facilitating marrow engraftment is highlighted by the increased risk of graft failure observed in T-cell-depleted BMT [10–13]. Donor T-lymphocytes are responsible for an immune antihost response, acting in synergy with the preparative regimen, to deplete the recipient of lymphocytes and other cells responsible for rejection. Using molecular probes to identify minor residual recipient cell populations following BMT, a correlation can be found between graft rejection and clonable host lymphocytes persisting after T-depleted BMT [14–17]. This mixed chimaeric state is associated with a low incidence of graft-versus-host disease (GvHD) but an increased risk of graft failure. The type of T-depletion technique has an effect on rejection risk: experimental transplants in animals indicate that donor NK cells promote marrow engraftment. In clinical practice, physical methods of T-cell depletion (which spare NK cells) are less likely to cause graft failure [18–21]. Recently, the work of Ilstadt has drawn attention to a 'facilitator cell' with the novel phenotype CD3+ CD8+ but which is negative for the $\alpha\beta$ T-cell receptor [22]. This cell, present in bone marrow and peripheral blood in very small numbers, can confer engraftment with allogeneic or even xenogeneic stem cells.

Immunosuppressive agents

Chemotherapy
Cyclophosphamide is the most widely used immunosuppressive agent in BMT. It is used in conjunction with other agents to further increase marrow graft take. Thiotepa [23], busulphan [24], melphalan [25] and cytosine arabinoside [26] have all been used with or without cyclophosphamide and TBI to confer additional immunosuppressive activity.

Antibodies
Antilymphocyte globulin, antithymocyte globulin and monoclonal antilymphocyte antibodies are frequently used to achieve additional immunosuppression because of their low toxicity. A schedule using cyclophosphamide + antithymocyte globulin for HLA-matched sibling donor BMT for SAA reduced the rate of graft failure from 19% to <5% [27]. A monoclonal antibody to the leukocyte fixation antigen LFA-1 (CD11a) was extremely effective in achieving engraftment in haplo-identical BMT in children [28,29]. Similar results were achieved with an anti CD-5 monoclonal [30]. Increasingly, Campath-1 monoclonal antibody (anti-CD52) has been used in preparative regimens for unrelated BMT with apparent benefit on engraftment [31].

Radiation
Radiation has a profound effect on the lymphoid system and powerfully inhibits the ability of the recipient to reject grafted marrow. TBI, or radiation localized to the lymphoid system (either total lymph-node irradiation (TLI) or thoraco-abdominal irradiation (TAI), combined with cyclophosphamide have a strong immunosuppressive action. Enhanced irradiation schedules improve engraftment in T-depleted marrow transplant recipients and recipients of less than fully matched or unrelated BMT [32–34]. Manipulation of the dose, dose rate and schedule has a major effect on engraftment [35–36].

Single-fraction TBI is more effective than the same dose delivered in fractions. For single-fraction TBI, high-dose rates (>5 cGy/min) have a greater effect than lower rates. These factors are interdependent – the same radiobiological effect is achieved, for example, with 750 cGy at 30 cGy/min as with 1000 cGy at <5 cGy/min. Addition of extra fractions or limited field irradiation to the lymphatics and spleen is used to boost the immunosuppression while minimizing damage to other tissues [37].

Strategies for achieving marrow engraftment in transplants with a high risk of rejection

From the above considerations it is clear that the degree and quality of the immunosuppression used before BMT is critical for obtaining stable engraftment of bone-marrow cells. The problem is that the more intensive radiation-based preparative regimens needed to achieve engraftment in non-HLA identical sibling transplants carry a higher risk of regimen-related mortality. Compared with radiation and chemotherapy, monoclonal antilymphocyte antibodies, anti-T-cell sera, cyclosporin and methylprednisolone add only modestly to the toxicity of the regimen and are often used as immunosuppressants.

An adequate stem-cell dose and the presence of donor lymphocytes are also critical factors for engraftment. In designing immunosuppressive schedules for mismatched BMT, the investigator therefore has the choice of using an unmanipulated transplant to increase the chance of engraftment after a standard preparative regimen which risks GvHD, or an increased intensity regimen with a T-cell-depleted transplant, which risks increased regimen-related toxicity. In SAA, standard preparative schedules use T-cell unmanipulated transplants and an irradiation-free preparative regimen. Matched but unrelated or mismatched BMTs for SAA have a high risk of graft failure. To achieve graft take, these transplants require radiation-based preparation and an unmanipulated BMT. In unrelated transplants for haematological malignancies, practice is divided, with some investigators using T-cell depletion and enhanced immunosuppression and others using standard preparative regimens with undepleted BMT. In mismatched related donor BMT, most investigators have used intensified immunosuppression and T-cell depletion of the donor marrow.

The ability to provide 5–10-fold more $CD34^+$ cells from the donor by using granulocyte colony-stimulating factor (G-CSF)-mobilized peripheral blood progenitor cell (PBPC) transplants represents a new way of increasing the chance of engraftment following lower intensity preparative regimens, thus reducing regimen-related mortality [38]. The ability to give large stem-cell donations from single or multiple apheresis collections of PBPC makes their application in mismatched transplants particularly attractive. The main disadvantgae of PBPC transplants is the risk of GvHD from the large numbers of lymphocytes given in the unmanipulated donation. New techniques are being developed to perform T-cell depletion of the $CD34^+$-rich PBPC to allow engraftment without GvHD.

Use of the preparative regimen for myeloablation

The need to make 'space' for the incoming marrow has long been considered an important function of the preparative regimen. Patients with hemoglobinopathies, other inherited bone-marrow disorders, storage diseases and other congenital metabolic disorders have cellular marrows producing non-functioning abnormal or enzyme-deficient cells. The aim of the BMT is to replace the defective marrow with 100% donor hematopoiesis. However, the majority of recipients are infants and young children with a prolonged life expectancy, albeit with a compromised quality of life. Particular attention has been given to designing preparative regimens that avoid the long-term complications of growth arrest, gonadal failure and late malignancies. The standard approach is a combination of busulphan and cyclophosphamide (BuCy). The rationale for giving myeloablative treatment is that incoming donor stem cells must find a vacant niche in the bone marrow in order to establish haematopoiesis. It is, however, likely that the alloimmune response of the donor may be sufficient to deplete the recipient of residual stem cells. It has never been possible in man to determine whether myeloablation is an essential prerequisite to sustained engraftment, because the conditions necessary to immunosuppress inevitably create space by myeloablation. However, the question has recently been addressed in a congeneic mouse transplant model where the donor is distinguished from the female recipient by a male sex chromosome marker. Such experiments show that engraftment of donor stem cells occurs, albeit inefficiently, without prior myeloablation. The greater the stem-cell dose, the greater the degree of repopulation by donor cells [39]. These results challenge the assumption that creating empty stem-cell niches is a requirement for marrow engraftment. However, the preparative regimen may improve stem-cell 'homing' [40]. Pathological states which affect stem-cell homing such as splenomegaly and marrow fibrosis, also impair marrow engraftment [41].

The antileukaemic effect of the preparative regimen

In clinical practice, the therapeutic benefit of increasing the antileukaemic effect by intensifying treatment is eventually offset by increased mortality from regimen-related toxicity. Consequently, very high-intensity preparative regimens have not typically resulted in improved disease-free survivals [42,43]. The mechanism whereby increased treatment intensity improves the antileukaemic effect is complex: our perception of the function of the myeloablative preparative regimen has changed with the recognition of the contribution made by donor immune function in the eradication of malignant disease (the graft-versus-leukaemia or GvL effect) [44,45]. GvL reactivity makes a major contribution to the curative effect of allogeneic BMT for myeloid leukaemias, but plays a smaller role in BMT for acute lymphoblastic leukaemia. In addition to a direct action on the malignant cells, the increased intensity of the regimen improves immune ablation of the recipient, resulting in complete donor chimaerism. This, in turn, increases the incidence and severity of GvHD, which confers a correspondingly greater GvL effect [45]. It has been recently appreciated that TBI preparative regimens are responsible for stimulating recipient tissues to produce cytokines such as interleukin-1 (IL-1) and tumour necrosis factor (TNF). Increased preparative regimen intensity may further stimulate cytokine release which can activate donor immune cells and increase the potential for causing GvHD [46].

Regimens used for their antitumour effect

The pursuit of the ideal antileukaemic preparative regimen has resulted in a wide variety of schedules employing irradiation with additional chemotherapy.

TBI-based regimens

Total dose of TBI, dose rate and fraction number all impact on relapse [47–53]. These variables are interrelated, so that the same antileukaemic effect can be achieved with a relatively low single dose at a high-dose rate as with a larger total dose given at a low-dose rate in multiple fractions. The principle of fractionation is to allow time for normal tissues to repair between fractions, while tissues with lower repair capacity, such as leukaemia cells, fail to recover between fractions. Fractionation has been used in clinical BMT to decrease unwanted side-effects of TBI, while increasing the antileukaemic effect and also the immunosuppressive effect. Fractionation or hyper-fractionation (delivery of more than one fraction per day) permits total doses as high as 1500 cGy [54]. If the individual fraction is kept below 200 cGy, the acute dose rate of each fraction can be high without increasing the radiobiological effect. The dose–effect curve is steepest in the range 1200–1500 cGy, and within this range small increases in the dose received impact on both desired and and undesired effects of TBI [54].

Radiotherapy treatment units are primarily designed for cancer treatment where the aim is to deliver an accurate dose of radiation at a high-dose rate to a small area of tissue close to the machine source. TBI requires the opposite, namely, the delivery of a wide, evenly distributed beam of radiation to the whole body, at lower dose rates than used in conventional radiotherapy. Some ingenuity is therefore required to modify the physical set-up of the radiotherapy unit in order to deliver TBI. Dosimetry must take into account the variation in dose absorbed by different tissues. Since the most critical normal tissue affected by irradiation is the lungs, the total dose to the lungs should be particularly monitored. A distance of at least 3 metres is needed between the source and the patient in order to deliver a sufficiently wide and regular field to treat the whole body. Cobalt units tend to deliver low-dose rates and are best suited to single-fraction treatment. Linear accelerators deliver very high-dose rates and to achieve a satisfactory radiobiological effect requires fractionation. Such constraints determine the type of TBI schedule delivered in individual BMT units. Conventionally, TBI is preceded by a two-day treatment with cyclophosphamide 120 mg/kg to add further immuno-suppression (CyTBI). The schedule is described in detail in Appendix 1 at the end of this chapter. Radiation therapy is reviewed in Chapter 34.

Chemotherapy-based regimens

Over the last decade, chemotherapy-only preparative regimens have become more widely used. They have the advantage that the complicated technology and scheduling of TBI can be avoided and potentially, some of the long-term effects of radiotherapy. However, since there are few long-term survivors from these recently introduced regimens, the full spectrum of late effects has yet to be described. Another objective of using combinations of chemotherapeutic agents is to choose drug combinations at subliming doses with different non-haematopoietic toxicities, so as to increase the antileukaemic effect while diminishing damage to individual organ systems. Appendix 2 describes the characteristics of some of the more commonly used agents. Chemotherapy preparative regimens use alkylating agents such as busulphan [55] or melphalan [56], either alone or in combination with other agents. Melphalan is used at the myeloablative dose of 200–240 mg/m^2, busulphan at 12–16 mg/kg. The therapeutic range is limited by renal and gastrointestinal toxicity for melphalan and lung fibrosis and liver damage for busulphan. Attempts have been made to use high doses of drugs and combinations known to be effective at standard doses in particular malignant disorders.

Preparative regimen toxicity

The delivery of profound immunosuppression and myeloablation brings with it major side-effects. There is only at best a narrow therapeutic window between unacceptable toxicity and treatment intense enough to eradicate malignant disease. The unwanted effects of the preparative regimen can be separated into immediate side-effects during administration of chemotherapy and TBI, effects causing morbidity and mortality in the first weeks after the BMT, and delayed effects which may not be apparent for many years (Table 35.2). Nausea and vomiting are the commonest side-effects experienced during delivery of the intensive treatment. This complication is now much more readily controlled by the use of 5-hydroxytryptamine (5-HT) receptor and 5-HT$_3$ antagonists [57,58].

A rare but dangerous complication is cyclophosphamide-induced acute cardiac failure [59]. High-dose busulphan causes seizures, and phenobarbitone should be given in association with busulphan preparative regimens [60]. The most serious immediate post-transplant problem is hepatic veno-occlusive disease (VOD) [61,62] Factors predisposing to VOD are the use of chemotherapy and high-intensity preparative regimens, pre-existing liver dysfunction and extensive prior chemotherapy.

Interstitial pneumonitis occurring in the first few months after BMT is multifactorial but high-dose, single-fraction TBI contributes [63]. Delayed effects are beginning to be better characterized [64]. It is now clear that use of TBI but probably not cyclophosphamide is associated with a risk of developing solid tumours especially affecting, but not restricted to, skin and mucosa. Damage to the gonads, pituitary and thyroid

Table 35.2 Non-haematological effects of preparative regimens

During administration
  Nausea and vomiting
  Parotitis (TBI)
  Allergic reactions

Immediate: within weeks of administration
  Mucositis
  Haemorrhagic cystitis
  Veno-occlusive disease
  Cardiac failure
  Renal failure
  Interstitial pneumonitis
  Pigmentation, hair loss

Delayed
  Gonadal failure
  Delayed puberty
  Growth arrest
  Thyroid failure (TBI)
  Cataracts (TBI)
  Dental decay (TBI)
  Second malignancies

TBI = total body irradiation.

results in growth arrest and delayed or absent puberty in children [65,66], premature menopause in women, infertility and psychological disturbances [67]. In general, TBI regimens incur a greater frequency and severity of late effects than non-TBI multidrug regimens, or cyclophosphamide alone. However, regimens which include busulphan cause alopecia and infertility [68]. Several approaches to reducing regimen-related toxicity are being explored. In designing schedules, the use of multiple agents with different spectra of side-effects at subtoxic doses can achieve fewer unwanted effects while impacting more strongly on the recipient leukaemia and immune system. Various approaches are used to improve the delivery of increased doses of radiation to the bone marrow and the immune system. As mentioned previously, hyperfractionated or fractionated TBI is superior to single-fraction TBI, but satisfactory long-term results are also achievable with low-dose (500 cGy) single-fraction TBI [69.] Restricted field irradiation to the lymphatics (mantle and inverted Y) and boosting the rib cage by low energy beams can avoid lung toxicity [51].

In mismatched BMT, immunosuppression with antithymocyte globulin or antilymphocyte monoclonal antibodies can obviate the need for intensified chemotherapy and irradiation and reduce the risk of late effects. Recently, attention has focussed on the potential for tissue damage from cytokines (especially TNF-α and IL-1) released during the preparative regimen [46]. Irradiation, in particular, is a powerful initiator of cytokine release. This so-called 'cytokine storm' may enhance the severity of GvHD and increase the risk of hepatic veno-occlusive disease. Eliminating cytokines, for example by the use of anti-TNF antibodies, may in the future reduce some of these post-transplant problems.

Preparative regimens used in specific disorders

Immunodeficiency diseases

Immunodeficiency disorders represent a special situation where the very nature of the disorder favours engraftment. Almost without exception, children with severe combined immunodeficiency disease (SCID) receiving BMT from an HLA-matched donor engraft successfully without prior immunosuppression. However, a preparative regimen is essential for engraftment in transplants from HLA-mismatched or unrelated donors. Irrespective of the type of donor, transplants for immunodeficiency states other than SCID also require a fully immunosuppressive regimen [70,71]. Cyclophosphamide can be used as a single agent to prepare SCID recipients for mismatched BMT, and less severe immunodeficiency disorders, such as adenosine deaminase (ADA) deficiency, for HLA-matched BMT. The combination of BuCy is used for immunodeficiency disorders, states with significant residual T-cell function such as Wiskott–Aldrich disease and for mismatched BMT in immunodeficiency states other than SCID [72–74]. Although CyTBI regimens have also been used to achieve engraftment in disorders such as Wiskott–Aldrich disease, they carry a significantly higher transplant related mortality and should be avoided in these non-malignant conditions.

Inherited bone marrow disorders and inborn errors

Early attempts to transplant disorders such as thalassaemia with cyclophosphamide preparation alone, failed. Although patients with this group of disorders have abnomal marrow function, they have intact immune systems, unmodified by chemotherapy, and in the case of haemoglobinopathies they are often sensitized to HLA antigens by multiple transfusions. It has therefore proved necessary to use cyclophosphamide in combination with radiation or busulphan to achieve stable engraftment. Studies by Lucarelli et al. [75,76] in thalassaemic recipients made a major contribution to defining the best preparative regimen for children with inherited disorders in general. Dose-finding clinical trials and a multicentre survey showed that cyclophosphamide 200 mg/kg with busulphan 14 mg/kg achieved the best outcome – conferring a high rate of engraftment but avoiding some of the dose-limiting toxicities of busulphan [75,76]. This regimen is associated with spectacular results in non-malignant disorders of the marrow: greater than 95% disease-free survival in a series of thalassaemia and sickle-cell anaemia recipients [77–79]. (See also Chapters 18 and 19.) Mismatched or unrelated matched BMTs have a significant risk of rejection with this regimen. In these situations, additional treatment with antithymocyte globulin or monoclonal antilymphocyte antibodies can reduce rejection rate. The approaches for choosing a preparative regimen for immune deficiency diseases and congenital disorders are summarized in Table 35.3.

Fanconi anaemia

Gluckman et al. were the first to observe that Fanconi anaemia patients experience life-threatening problems of exfoliative dermatitis and enteritis associated with an increased susceptibility to the cyclophosphamide doses used in standard preparative regimens. It appears that the so-called DNA repair defect of Fanconi anaemia renders the proliferating tissues of the body especially susceptible to apoptosis caused by alkylating agents [80]. Gluckman and colleagues subsequently developed a safe preparative regimen of low-dose cyclophosphamide with irradiation to the lymph nodes (thoraco-abdominal irradiation, TAI), which greatly improved the outcome for Fanconi anaemia patients

Table 35.3 Preparative regimens for immune deficiencies and congenital disorders

Disorder	HLA-matched donor	HLA-mismatched related or matched unrelated donor
Severe combined immunodeficiency disease (SCID) – Swiss type, Bruton's	None	Cyclophosphamide 200 mg/kg
SCID – adenosine deaminase (ADA) deficiency; bare lymphocyte syndrome other combined immunodeficiencies	Cyclophosphamide 200 mg/kg	Busulphan 14 mg/kg Cyclophosphamide 200 mg/kg
Chediak–Higashi disease; Wiskott–Aldrich syndrome	Busulphan 14 mg/kg Cyclophosphamide 200 mg/kg	Busulphan 14 mg/kg, cyclophosphamide 200 mg/kg ± other immunosuppression
Congenital disorders without immunodeficiency; haemoglobinopathies; liposomal storage diseases; congenital cytopenias (pure red-cell aplasia, Kostmann's syndrome, Glanzman's disease)	Busulphan 14 mg/kg Cyclophosphamide 200 mg/kg	Busulphan 14 mg/kg, cyclophosphamide 200 mg/kg ± other immunosuppression

receiving BMT from HLA-identical siblings [81]. Whether the additional immunosuppression from TAI is essential for engraftment in every case is not definitively established. Arguing that the lymphocytes must share the same susceptibility to alkylating agents as other tissues, two Fanconi anaemia patients with short transfusion histories seen at the Hammersmith Hospital were conditioned with cyclophosphamide 20 mg/kg alone. Both had an uncomplicated course and showed 100% donor chimaerism (Dr Irene Roberts, personal communication). Patients with Fanconi anaemia receiving BMT from unrelated or mismatched donors are nevertheless at considerable risk of rejecting the transplant if given insufficient immunosuppression [82]. Fanconi anaemia patients who have developed a preleukaemic or leukaemic state present a therapeutic dilemma: the preparative regimen must be sufficiently intensive to reduce the leukaemic clone to a minimal residual disease state but must not cause mortality from major organ failure in the early transplant period. For Fanconi anaemia patients without a matched donor and those showing leukaemic progression, a regimen developed by the Cincinnati BMT Group achieves a satisfactory compromise using intermediate doses of TBI (450 cGy), 50 mg/kg cyclophosphamide, cytosine arabinoside (Ara-C) 200 mg/m^2 × 5 days and antithymocyte globulin (Dr Richard Harris, personal communication).

Severe aplastic anaemia

The aim of the preparative regimen in SAA is firstly to provide sufficient immunosuppression to allow engraftment, and secondly to treat the underlying immunological abnormality responsible for the aplasia in a proportion of patients. Evidence that cyclophosphamide plays a role in reversing a myelosuppressive mechanism in SAA comes from studies of BMT between identical twins. Despite full identity between donor and recipient, many transplants fail to engraft unless full transplant doses of cyclophosphamide are given [83]. For patients with SAA who are considered unsensitized to blood products (10–40 transfusions), cyclophosphamide alone is sufficient to permit engraftment in most cases. Once patients are sensitized by repeated transfusions, addition of antithymocyte globulin, Campath, total lymphoid irradiation, TAI or Ara-C are required to effect marrow engraftment

[6,7,23,24]. While effective, the CyTBI regimen is associated with high treatment-related mortality. Patients with SAA have been successfully grafted from matched unrelated donors with cyclophosphamide alone but the rate of graft rejection is high [82]. Improved results have been achieved with Ara-C, antithymocyte globulin, prednisolone, cyclophosphamide and TLI followed by T-cell-depleted BMT [84,85]. Mismatched transplants for SAA given cyclophosphamide alone universally fail to engraft. Engraftment can be achieved with CyTBI but there is a high mortality from GvHD [84]. Additional immunosuppression with TBI, Ara-C and monoclonal antilymphocyte antibodies followed by T-cell-depleted marrow grafts is achieving improved results [86]. Table 35.4 summarizes preparative regimens for SAA and Fanconi anaemia.

Haematological malignancies

When clinical BMT was in its infancy, patients with leukaemia were prepared with whole-body irradiation since it represented at the time the only available modality with sufficient antileukaemic activity to be effective in controlling disease in advanced leukaemia. Cyclophosphamide was added to the TBI because it was observed that some patients with end-stage leukaemia failed to achieve engraftment. Subsequently, much effort has gone into developing optimum dosimetry and scheduling. TBI schedules have become highly individualized in attempts to achieve minimal side-effects and maximum antileukaemic activity within the physical constraints of the available radiation equipment (see Chapter 34). While the CyTBI regimen is still the most widely used throughout the world, many teams have used other chemotherapeutic drugs with TBI to increase the antileukaemic potential of the treatment. Ara-C [26], melphalan [55,87], thiotepa [88], VP16 [89], vincristine [90] and piperazinedione [91] have been used singly or in combination with TBI, with or without standard doses of cyclophosphamide. These regimens have, in some instances, reduced relapse probability in high-risk malignancies. However, they are associated with their own individual patterns of toxicity which often contribute to increased transplant-related mortality. Since most of these preparative regimen variants have never been compared with CyTBI in prospective controlled trials, it is impossible in most instances to know whether these combinations differ significantly from standard CyTBI regimens in the disease-free survival they achieve. Table 35.5 summarizes common TBI and non-TBI-based preparative regimens [92–104].

Chemotherapy-only preparative regimens for haematological malignancies

In recent years, the variety of radiation-free regimens has increased considerably (see Table 35.5). Most experience, however, has been accumulated with the busulphan–cytoxan regimen developed by Santos *et al.*

Table 35.4 Preparative regimens for severe aplastic anaemia (SAA) and Fanconi anaemia (FA)

Condition	HLA-matched family donor*	HLA-matched unrelated donor
SAA good risk: <40 donor units, <6 months from diagnosis, uninfected	Cy200	Cy200; ATG; TAI/TBI
SAA poor risk: >40 donor units, >6 months from diagnosis, infected at BMT	Cy200; ATG	Cy200;ATG;TAI/TBI
FA unsensitized/sensitized	Cy20; TAI	Cy50; ATG; TAI
FA progressed to myelodysplastic syndrome (MDS)	Cy20; TBI450	Cy50; TBI450

Cy = cyclophosphamide, TAI = thoraco-abdominal irradiation, TBI = total body irradiation, ATG = antithymocyte globulin. Radiation doses in cGy, chemotherapy doses in mg/kg * = HLA-identical sibling or phenotypic family match.

Table 35.5 Preparative regimens used in allogeneic BMT for malignant disorders	
TBI-based	
CY120; TBI	
VP16; TBI [89,93,94]	*TBI variations:*
VP16; Cy; TBI [92,95,96,97]	Single fraction: from 500 cGy/30 cGy/min (high-dose rate, low total dose) to 1000 cGy <5 cGy/min (low-dose rate, high total dose)
VP16; BCNU; Cy; TBI [104]	
Ara-C; TBI [101,102,103]	Fractionated: 1200 – 1500 cGy in 6–8 fractions
Ara-C; Cy; TBI [98]	
Melphalan; TBI [56,87]	Hyperfractionated: up to 1500 cGy in 10–12 fractions
BuCy; TBI [99;100]	
Vincristine; TBI [90]	
Piperazinedione; TBI [91]	
Chemotherapy-based	
Busulphan/cyclophosphamide [105,107]	
'Small BuCy': Busulphan 1 mg/kg, Cy 120 mg/kg	
'Big BuCy': Busulphan 1 mg/kg, Cy 200 mg/kg	
BuCy; melphalan [109]	
Bu; Cy; Ara-C [111]	
Bu; Cy; VP16 [110,113]	
Bu; Cy; thiotepa [88]	
Cy; BCNU; VP16 [112]	
Thiotepa; Ara-C; melphalan [114]	
Bu = busulphan, Cy = cyclophosphamide, VP16 = etoposide, Ara-C = cytosine arabinoside. TBI = total body irradiation.	

[105]. Combinations of alkylating agents, nitrosoureas and etoposide have been widely explored. Table 35.5 lists the most commonly used combinations [106–114].

Comparison of chemotherapy and radiation-based regimens

The advantages and disadvantages of chemotherapy-only regimens are summarized in Table 35.6 and have been reviewed [115,116]. As a general rule, chemotherapy-only regimens and radiation-based treatments perform equally well in the disease-free survival they achieve. However, there is a tendency for higher relapse rates following chemotherapy and higher regimen-related mortality following TBI. The pattern of side-effects seen also differs: chemotherapy regimens using combinations of alkylating agents carry an increased risk of veno-occlusive disease. However, BuCy regimens have a minimal impact on growth and development. Furthermore, the incidence of second malignancies may be lower. For these reasons, chemotherapy-based regimens are particularly appropriate for BMT in infants and children [117].

In recent years several randomized studies comparing radiation with chemotherapy regimens have been carried out. These studies highlight specific transplant situations where chemotherapy-based regimens are at least as effective as TBI regimens. BuCy appears to be a satisfactory regimen for preparation of patients with

Table 35.6 Comparison of total body irradiation (TBI) versus chemotherapy-based preparative regimens

TBI	Chemotherapy
Dosimetry can be varied to avoid specific organ toxicities (e.g. lung shielding)	Combinations of agents with different target organ toxicities can be chosen to reduce damage to specific organs while maintaining intensity
Well tolerated – few immediate side-effects	Often poorly tolerated – nausea and vomiting and mucositis can be severe
Dose rate and fractionation can be tailored to achieve optimal engraftment and antileukaemia activity or lower non-haematological toxicity	Chemotherapy dose can be chosen to balance therapeutic effect against unwanted toxicity but the most commonly used drug, busulphan, has irregular absorption and individual doses received vary considerably
Requires motivated, sophisticated and experienced radiotherapy service with the capability of delivering TBI and monitoring received dose	Easily applied in centres without access to radiation therapy departments
Scheduling is limited by standard working hours of radiotherapy department and conflicting demands from patients receiving standard radiotherapy procedures	Easy to schedule. Chemotherapy can be given at weekends and some schedules applicable in an out-patient setting
Late effects can be severe (e.g. cataracts, growth arrest)	Late effects less frequent and severe (e.g. cataracts, growth arrest, delayed puberty)
Significant risk of second malignancies	Risk of second malignancies probably lower than for TBI regimens

chronic myeloid leukaemia [118,119], and some patients with acute myeloid leukaemia [120] but not acute lymphocytic leukaemia or advanced leukaemias, where the risk of relapse is higher with BuCy [121].

Preparative regimens for mismatched and unrelated BMT for leukaemia

Preparative regimens and BMT approaches for unrelated BMT have been developed from those already widely established for matched-sibling BMT. Because of the increased risk of severe GvHD, many protocols involve T-depletion of the donor marrow, further increasing the need for immunosuppression of the recipient to prevent graft rejection [122–127]. To offset the increased risk of graft rejection, additional immunosuppression is given. Much ingenuity has gone into designing novel preparative regimens. The increased risk of graft failure in mismatched BMT can be reduced by increasing the dose and number of TBI fractions or by adding additional chemotherapy. Several agents have been used successfully in combination with cyclophosphamide and TBI including high-dose Ara-C [122] and thiotepa [33]. Additional immunosuppression with antilymphocyte antibodies such as Campath during the preparative phase is also effective [121]. Gratifyingly, regimen-related toxicity is the same as for related HLA-matched BMT [128].

As mentioned above, chemotherapy-only regimens have been successfully used to achieve engraftment in transplants from donors other than HLA-identical siblings. It is also possible to achieve marrow engraftment in matched unrelated donor BMT without recourse to TBI by using busulphan and cyclophosphamide or other multi-agent chemotherapy preparative regimens. Although the graft failure rate may be somewhat higher, this disadvantage is offset by a lower regimen-related toxicity [129,130]. While it may be possible with the design of new preparative regimens to reduce early regimen-related mortality, the problems in mismatched and unrelated BMT of increased susceptibility to viral infections and complications from GvHD or its preventive treatment continue to pose a challenge.

Future developments

The lack of an ideal preparative regimen is a continuing challenge, and safer, more effective schedules require development. One promising area is to use the purine analogues fludarabine or 2-CDA as immunosuppressants [131]. These agents are relatively lymphocyte-specific, producing powerful and long-lasting suppression of T- and B-cell immune function. So powerful is the immune suppression produced, that patients receiving purine analogues as treatment for B-cell malignancies are at risk of developing transfusion-induced GvHD from random blood products. In pilot studies at the MD Anderson Hospital, purine analogues have been used as the sole immuno-suppressant to achieve marrow engraftment in older patients undergoing HLA-matched or mismatched BMT for leukaemia. Patients receiving fludarabine-containing preparative regimens had prompt engraftment and low regimen-related toxicity (Sergio Giralt, personal communication). Purine analogues might be ideally suited as a preparative therapy for Fanconi anaemia patients thus circumventing the need for cyclophosphamide immunosuppression.

To increase the antitumour effect without increasing unwanted side-effects, the Seattle Group are evaluating the use of short-acting radionuclides coupled to antibodies which target the bone marrow so as to increase local antileukaemic action [132,133]. Preliminary results suggest that it is possible to deliver higher doses of irradiation to the bone marrow, but many technical challenges remain to be solved before this approach can be fully evaluated.

References

1. Ferrara J, Lipton J, Hellman S et al. Engraftment following T-cell depleted marrow transplantation. I. The role of major and minor histocompatibility barriers. *Transplantation* 1987; **43**: 461–467.
2. Anasetti C, Amos D, Beatty P et al. Effect of HLA compatibility on engraftment of bone marrow in patients with leukemia or lymphoma. *New Engl J Med* 1989; **320**: 197–204.
3. Martin PJ. Determinants of engraftment after allogeneic marrow transplantation. *Blood* 1992; **79**: 1647–1650.
4. Lenarsky C and Parkman R. Bone marrow transplantation for the treatment of immune deficiency states. *Bone Marrow Transplant* 1990; **4**: 361–369.
5. Murphy WJ, Kumar V and Bennett M. Rejection of bone marrow allograft by mice with severe combined immunodeficiency disease. *J Exp Med* 1987; **165**: 1212–1217.
6. Champlin RE, Horowitz MM, van Bekkum DW et al. Graft failure following bone marrow transplantation for severe aplastic anemia: risk factors and treatment results. *Blood* 1991; **73**: 606–613.
7. Storb R and Champlin RE. Bone marrow transplantation for severe aplastic anemia. *Bone Marrow Transplant* 1991; **8**: 69–72.
8. Uharek L, Gassman W, Glass B et al. Influence of cell dose on graft-versus-host disease and rejection rates after allogeneic bone marrow transplantation. *Blood* 1992; **79**: 1612–1621.
9. Mavroudis D, Read E, Cottler-Fox M et al. CD34+ Cell dose predicts survival, post transplant morbidity and rate of hematologic recovery following allogeneic marrow transplants for hematologic malignancies. *Blood* 1996; **88**: 3223–3229.
10. Patterson J, Prentice HG, Brenner MK et al. Graft rejection following HLA-matched T-lymphocyte depleted bone marrow transplantation. *Br J Haematol* 1986; **63**: 221–230.
11. Martin PJ, Hansen JA, Torok-Storb B et al. Graft failure in patients receiving T-cell depleted HLA-identical allogeneic marrow transplants. *Bone Marrow Transplant* 1988; **3**: 445–456.
12. Marmont AM, Horowitz MM, Gale RP et al. T-cell depletion of HLA-identical transplants in leukemia. *Blood* 1991; **78**: 2120–2130.
13. Bunjes D, Wisneth M, Hertenstein B et al. Graft failure after T-cell depleted bone marrow transplantation: clinical and immunological characteristics and response to immuno-suppressive therapy. *Bone Marrow Transplant* 1990; **4**: 309–314
14. Terenzi A, Aversa F, Albi N et al. Residual clonable host cell detection for predicting engraftment of T-cell depleted BMTs. *Bone Marrow Transplant* 1993; **11**: 349–357.
15. Bunjes D, Theobald M, Wiesneth M et al. Graft rejection by a population of primed CDw52⁻ host T cells after *in vivo/ex vivo* T-depleted bone marrow transplantation. *Bone Marrow Transplant* 1993; **12**: 209–217.
16. McCann SR and Lawler M. Mixed chimerism: detection and significance following BMT. *Bone Marrow Transplant* 1993; **11**: 91–94.
17. Schouten HC, Sizoo W, Van't Veer MB et al. Incomplete chimerism in erythroid myeloid and B lymphocyte lineage after T-cell depleted allogeneic bone marrow transplantation. *Bone Marrow Transplant* 1988; **3**: 407–412.

18. Butturini A and Gale RP. New strategies for T-cell depletion. *Bone Marrow Transplant* 1990; **4**: 225–228.
19. Poynton CH. T-cell depletion in bone-marrow transplantation. *Bone Marrow Transplant* 1988; **3**: 265–279.
20. Martin PJ. The role of donor lymphoid cells in allogeneic marrow engraftment. *Bone Marrow Transplant* 1990; **4**: 283–290.
21. Martin PJ, Hansen JA, Duckner CD et al. Effects of *in vitro* depletions of T-cells in HLA identical allogeneic marrow grafts. *Blood* 1985; **66**: 664–672.
22. Kaufman CL, Colson Y, Wren SM, Watkins S, Simmons RL and Ilstadt ST. Phenotypic characterization of a novel bone marrow-derived cell that facilitates engraftment of allogeneic bone marrow stem cells. *Blood* 1994; **84**: 2436–2446.
23. Aversa F, Tabilo A, Terenzi A et al. Successful engraftment of T-cell depleted haploidentical 'three loci' incompatible transplantation in leukaemia patients by addition of recombinant human G-CSF mobilized peripheral blood precursor cells in bone marrow inoculum. *Blood* 1994; **84**: 3948–3955.
24. Buggia I, Locatelli F, Regazzi MB and Zecca M. Busulfan. *Ann Pharmacother* 1994; **28**: 1055–1062.
25. Van Besien K, Demuynck H, Lemaistre CF et al. High dose melphalan allows durable engraftment of allogeneic bone marrow. *Bone Marrow Transplant* 1995; **15**: 321–323.
26. Coccia PF, Strandjord SE, Warkentin PI et al High dose cytosine arabinoside and total body irradiation: an improved preparative regimen for bone marrow transplantation of children with acute lymphoblastic leukemia. *Blood* 1988; **71**: 888–893.
27. Bunin N, Leahey A, Kamani N and August C. Bone marrow transplantation in pediatric patients with severe aplastic anemia: cyclophosphamide and antithymocyte globulin conditioning followed by recombinant human granulocyte–macrophage colony stimulating factor. *J Paediatr Oncol* 1996; **18**: 68–71.
28. Storb R, Etzioni R, Anasetti C et al. Cyclophosphamide combined with antithymocyte globulin in preparation for allogeneic marrow transplants in patients with aplastic anemia. *Blood* 1994; **84**: 941–949.
29. Fischer A, Griscelli C, Blanche S et al. Prevention of graft failure by anti-LFA-1 monoclonal antibody in HLA mismatched bone marrow transplantation. *Lancet* 1986; **ii**: 1058–1061.
30. Van Dijken P, Ghagyur T, Mauch P et al. Evidence that anti-LFA-1 *in vivo* improves engraftment and survival after allogeneic bone marrow transplantation. *Transplantation* 1990; **49**: 882–886.
31. Koehler M, Hurwitz CA, Krance RA et al. XomaZyme-CD5 immunotoxin in conjunction with partial T cell depletion for prevention of graft rejection and graft versus-host disease after bone marrow transplantation from unrelated donors. *Bone Marrow Transplant* 1994; **13**: 571–577.
32. Hale G and Waldmann H. Control of graft-versus-host disease and graft rejection by T-cell depletion of donor and recipient with Campath-1 antibodies. Results of matched sibling transplants for malignant disease. *Bone Marrow Transplant* 1994; **13**: 597–613.
33. Soiffer RL, Mauch P, Tarbell NJ et al Total lymphoid irradiation to prevent graft rejection in recipients of of HLA non-identical T cell-depleted allogeneic marrow. *Bone Marrow Transplant* 1991; **7**: 23–34.
34. Ferrara J, Michelson J, Burakoff S and Mauch P. Engraftment following T-cell depleted marrow transplantation. III. Differential effects of increased total body irradiation on semiallogenic and allogenic recipients. *Transplantation* 1988; **45**: 948–952.
35. Slavin S, Or R, Weshler Z et al. The use of total lymphoid irradiation for abrogation of host resistance to T-cell depleted marrow allografts. *Bone Marrow Transplant* 1986; Vol 1 (Supp 1): 98.
36. O'Reilly RJ, Shank B, Collins N et al. Increased total body irradiation (TBI) abrogates resistance to HLA-matched marrow grafts depleted of T cells by lectin agglutination and E-rosette depletion (SBA-E-BMT). *Exp Haematol* 1985; **13**: 406–412.
37. Down J, Tarbell N, Thames H and Mauch P. Syngeneic and allogeneic bone marrow engraftment after total body irradiation. Dependence on dose, dose rate and fractionation. *Blood* 1991; **77**: 661–669.
38. Goldman JG. Peripheral blood stem cells for allografts. *Blood* 1995; **85**: 1413–1415.
39. Stewart PM, Crittenden RB, Lowry PA et al. Long-term engraftment of normal and post-5-fluorouracil murine marrow into normal nonmyeloablated mice. *Blood* 1993; **81**: 2566–2571.
40. Tavassoli M. The role of conditioning regimens in homing of transplanted hemopoietic cells. *Bone Marrow Transplant* 1992; **10**: 15–18.
41. Helenglass G, Treleaven JG, Parikh P, Aboud H, Smith C and Powles RL. Delayed engraftment associated with splenomegaly in patients undergoing bone marrow transplantation for chronic myelogenous leukemia. *Bone Marrow Transplant* 1990; **5**: 247–252.
42. Bearman SI, Applebaum FR, Buckner CD et al. Regimen related toxicity in patients undergoing bone marrow transplantation. *J Clin Oncol* 1988; **6**: 1562–1568.
43. Aurer I and Gale RP. Are new conditioning regimens for transplantation in acute myelogenous leukemia better? *Bone Marrow Transplant* 1991; **4**: 255–262.
44. Truitt RL and Atasoylu AA. Impact of pretransplant conditioning and donor T cells on chimerism, graft-versus-host disease, graft-versus-leukemia reactivity, and tolerance after bone marrow transplantation. *Blood* 1991; **77**: 2515–2523.
45. Horowitz MM, Gale RP, Sondel PM et al. Graft-versus-leukemia reactions after bone marrow transplantation. *Blood* 1990; **75**: 555–562.
46. Antin J and Ferrara JLM. Cytokine dysregulation and acute graft versus host disease. *Blood* 1992; **80**: 2964–2968.
47. Hagenbeek A and Martens ACM. The effect of fractionated versus unfractionated total body irradiation on the growth of the BN acute myelocytic leukemia. *Int J Rad Oncol Biol Phys* 1981; **7**: 80–85.
48. Vitale V, Scarpati D, Frassoni F and Corvo R. Total body irradiation: single dose, fractions, dose rate. *Bone Marrow Transplant* 1989; **4**(Suppl 1): 233–235.
49. Deeg HJ, Sullivan KM, Buckner CD et al. Marrow transplantation for acute non-lymphoblastic leukemia in first remission: toxicity and long-term follow up of patients conditioned with single dose or fractionated total body irradiation. *Bone Marrow Transplant* 1986; **1**: 151–157.
50. Thomas ED, Clift RA, Hersman J et al. Marrow transplantation for acute non-lymphoblastic leukemia in first

remission using fractionated or single dose irradiation. *Int J Radiat Oncol Biol Phys* 1982; **8**: 817–821.
51. Brockstein JA, Kernan NA, Groshen S *et al*. Allogeneic bone marrow transplantation after hyperfractionated total body irradiation and cyclophosphamide in children with acute leukemia. *New Engl J Med* 1987; **317**: 1618–1624.
52. Clift RA, Buckner CD, Applebaum FA *et al*. Allogeneic marrow transplants for patients with chronic myelogenous leukemia in the chronic phase: a randomized trial of two irradiation regimens. *Blood* 1991; **77**: 1660–1665.
53. Clift RA, Buckner CD, Applebaum FA *et al*. Allogeneic marrow transplants for patients with acute myelogenous leukemia in first remission: a randomized trial of two irradiation regimens. *Blood* 1988; **76**: 1867–1871.
54. Kim TH, Khan FM, Galvin JM. A report of the working party: Comparison of total body irradiation techniques for bone marrow transplantation. *Int J Radiat Oncol Biol Phys* 1980; **6**: 779.
55. Tutschka PJ, Copelan EA and Kapoor N. Replacing total body irradiation with busulfan as conditioning of patients with leukemia for allogeneic marrow transplantation. *Transplant Proc* 1989; **21**: 2952–2954.
56. Powles RL, Milliken S and Helenglass G. The use of melphalan in conjunction with total body irradiation as treatment for leukemia. *Transplant Proc* 1989; **21**: 2955–2957.
57. Hewitt M, Cornish J, Pamphillon D and Oakhill A. Effective emetic control during conditioning of children for bone marrow transplantation using ondansetron, a 5-HT$_3$ antagonist. *Bone Marrow Transplant* 1991; **7**: 431–434.
58. Hunter AE, Prentice HG, Pothecary K *et al*. Granisetron, a selective 5-HT$_3$ receptor antagonist for the prevention of radiation-induced emesis during total body irradiation. *Bone Marrow Transplant* 1991; **7**: 439–442.
59. Gardner SF, Lazarus HM, Bednaczyk EM *et al*. High dose cyclophosphamide-induced myocardial damage during BMT: assessment by positron emission tomography. *Bone Marrow Transplant* 1993; **12**: 139–144.
60. De la Camara R, Tomas JF and Figuera-Randa JM. High dose busulphan and seizures. *Bone Marrow Transplant* 1991; **5**: 363–364.
61. Baglin TP. Veno-occlusive disease of the liver complicating bone marrow transplantation. *Bone Marrow Transplant* 1994; **13**: 1–4.
62. Ozkaynak M, Weinberg K, Kohn D *et al*. Hepatic veno-occlusive disease post-bone marrow transplantation in children conditioned with busulfan and cyclophosphamide: incidence, risk factors, and clinical outcome. *Bone Marrow Transplant* 1991; **7**: 467–474.
63. Weiner RS, Bortin MM, Gale RP *et al*. Risk factors associated with interstitial pneumonia following allogeneic bone marrow transplantation for leukemia. *Transplant Proc* 1985; **17**: 470–474.
64. Kolb HJ and Bender-Gotze Ch. Late complications after allogeneic bone marrow transplantation. *Bone Marrow Transplant* 1990; **4**: 61–72.
65. Sanders JE, Pritchard S, Mahoney P *et al*. Growth and development following marrow transplantation for leukemia. *Blood* 1986; **68**: 1129–1135.
66. Leiper AD, Stanhope R, Lou T *et al*. The effect of total body irradiation and bone marrow transplantation during childhood and adolescence on growth and endocrine function. *Br J Haematol* 1987; **67**: 419–426.
67. Hinterberger-Fischer M, Kier P, Kahls P *et al*. Fertility, pregnancy and offspring complications after bone marrow transplantation. *Bone Marrow Transplant* 1991; **7**: 5–10.
68. Giorgiano G, Bozzola M, Locatelli F *et al*. Role of busulfan and total body irradiation on growth of prepubertal children receiving bone marrow transplantation and results of treatment with recombinant human growth hormone. *Blood* 1995; **86**: 825–831.
69. Fyles GM, Messner HA, Lockwood G *et al*. Long term results of bone marrow transplantation for patients with AML, ALL and CML prepared with single dose total body irradiation of 500 cGy delivered with a high dose rate. *Bone Marrow Transplant* 1991; **8**: 453–464.
70. Barrett AJ. Bone marrow transplantation, thymus transplantation and thymic factors in the treatment of congenital immune deficiency states. In: *Immunotherapy of Disease. Immunology and Medicine Series*. TJ Hamblin (ed.), 1989: 1–21 (Kluwer: Kluwer Academia, USA).
71. Fischer A, Landais P, Friedrich FW *et al*. Bone marrow transplantation (BMT) in Europe for primary immunodeficiency other than severe combined immunodeficiency disease: a report from the European Group for Immunodeficiency Disease. *Blood* 1994; **83**: 1149–1154.
72. Filipovitch AH, Shapiro RS, Ramsay NKC *et al*. Unrelated donor bone marrow transplantation for correction of lethal congenital immunodeficiencies. *Blood* 1992; **80**: 270–276.
73. Lenarsky C, Weinberg K, Kohn DB and Parkman R. Unrelated donor BMT for Wiskott–Aldrich syndrome. *Bone Marrow Transplant* 1993; **12**: 145–148.
74. Barrett AJ and McCarthy DM. Bone marrow transplantation for genetic disorders. *Blood Rev* 1990; **4**: 116–131.
75. Lucarelli G, Galimberti M, Polchi P *et al*. Bone marrow transplantation in patients with thalassemia. *New Engl J Med* 1990; **322**: 417–422.
76. Barrett AJ, Lucarelli G, Gale RP *et al*. Bone marrow transplantation for thalassaemia – a preliminary report from the International Bone Marrow Transplant Registry. In: *Advances and Controversies in Thalassaemia Therapy: Bone Marrow Transplantation and Other Approaches*. CD Buckner, RP Gale and G Lucarelli G (eds), 1989; 309: 173–186 (New York: Alan R Liss).
77. Lucarelli G, Polchi P, Izzi T *et al*. Marrow transplantation for thalassemia following treatment with busulfan and cyclophosphamide. *Lancet* 1985; **i**: 1355–1357.
78. Blazar DR, Ramsay NKC and Kersey JH. Pretransplant conditioning with busulfan and cyclophosphamide for non-malignant diseases. *Transplantation* 1985; **39**: 597–602.
79. Walters MC, Patience M, Leisenring W *et al*. Bone marrow transplantation for sickle cell disease. *New Engl J Med* 1996; **335**: 369–376.
80. Gluckman E, Devergie A and Dutreix J. Bone marrow transplantation for Fanconi's anaemia. In: *Fanconi Anemia. Clinical, Cytogenetic and Experimental Aspects*. TM Schroeder-Kurth, AD Auerbach and G Obe (eds), 1989: 60–68 (Berlin: Springer Verlag).
81. Socié G, Gluckman E, Raynal B *et al*. Bone marrow transplantation for Fanconi anemia using low dose thoraco-abdominal irradiation as conditioning regimen: chimersim study by PCR. *Blood* 1993; **82**: 2249–2256.
82. Bacigalupo A, Hows J, Gordon-Smith EC *et al*. Bone marrow transplantation for severe aplastic anemia from donors other

than HLA-identical siblings: a report from the BMT working party. *Bone Marrow Transplant* 1988; **3**: 531–535.

83. Champlin R, Feig SA, Sparkles RS *et al*. Bone marrow transplantation for identical twins in the treatment of aplastic anaemia: implications for the pathogenesis of the disease. *Br J Haematol* 1984; **56**: 455–463.

84. Castro-Malaspina H, Childs B, Laver J *et al*. Hyperfractionated total lymphoid irradiation and cyclophos-phamide for preparation of previously transfused patients undergoing HLA-identical marrow transplantation for severe aplastic anemia. *Int J Radiat Oncol Biol Phys* 1994; **29**: 847–854.

85. Gajewski JL, Ho WG, Feig ASA *et al*. Bone marrow transplantation using unrelated donors for patients with advanced leukemia and bone marrow failure. *Transplantation* 1990; **50**: 244–249.

86. Casper JT, Pietryga D, Camitta B *et al*. Bone marrow transplantation (BMT) for aplastic anemia using unrelated donors (UD). *J Cell Biochem* 1994; Suppl 18B: 69.

87. Helenglass G, Powles RL, McElwain TJ *et al*. Melphalan and total body irradiation (TBI) versus cyclophosphamide and TBI as conditioning for acute myeloblastic leukaemia. *Bone Marrow Transplant* 1988; **3**: 21–29.

88. Przepiorka D, Ippoliti C, Giralt S *et al*. A phase I–II study of high dose thiotepa, busulfan and cyclophosphamide as a preparative regimen for allogeneic bone marrow transplantation. *Bone Marrow Transplant* 1994; **14**: 449–453.

89. Blume KG, Long GD, Negrin RS *et al*. Role of etoposide (VP-16) in preparatory regimens for patients with leukaemia or lymphoma undergoing allogeneic bone marrow transplantation. *Bone Marrow Transplant* 1994; **14**(Suppl 4): S9–10.

90. Uderzo C, Rondelli R, Dini G *et al*. High dose vincristine, fractionated total body irradiation and cyclophosphamide as conditioning regimen in allogeneic and autologous bone marrow transplantation for childhood acute lymphoblastic leukaemia. *Br J Haematol* 1995; **89**: 790–797.

91. Dimitropoulos MA, Yau JC, Huan SD *et al*. Allogeneic bone marrow transplantation for leukaemia following piperazinedione and fractionated total body irradiation. *Am J Hematol* 1994; **46**: 82–86.

92. Spitzer TR, Peters C, Ortleib M *et al*. Etoposide in combination with cyclophosphamide and total body irradiation or busulfan as conditioning for marrow transplantation in adults and children. *Int J Radiat Oncol Biol Phys* 1994; **29**: 39–44.

93. Snyder DS, Negrin RS and O'Donnell MR. Fractionated total body irradiation and high dose etoposide as a preparatory regimen for allogeneic bone marrow transplantation for 94 patients with chronic myelogenous leukaemia in first clinical chronic phase. *Blood* 1994; **84**: 1672–1679.

94. Snyder DS, Chao NS, Amylon MD *et al*. Fractionated total body irradiation and high dose etoposide as a preparatory regimen for bone marrow transplantation for 99 patients with acute leukaemia in first complete remission. *Blood* 1993; **82**: 2920–2928.

95. Bostrom B, Weisdorf D, Kim T, Kersey JH and Ramsay NKC. Bone marrow transplantation for advanced stage acute leukemia: a pilot study of high energy total body irradiation, cyclophosphamide and continuous infusion etoposide. *Bone Marrow Transplant* 1990; **5**: 83–90.

96. Brown RA, Wolff SN, Fay JW *et al*. High dose etoposide, cyclophosphamide and total body irradiation with allogeneic bone marrow transplantation for patients with acute myeloid leukemia in untreated first relapse: a study by the North American Marrow Transplant Group. *Blood* 1995; **85**: 1391–1395.

97. Petersen FB, Buckner CD, Applebaum FR *et al*. Etoposide, cyclophosphamide and fractionated total body irradiation as a preparative regimen for marrow transplantation in patients with advanced hematological malignancy: a phase I study. *Bone Marrow Transplant* 1992; **10**: 83–88.

98. Petersen FB, Applebaum FR, Buckner CD *et al*. Simultaneous infusion of high dose cytosine arabinoside with cyclophosphamide followed by total body irradiation for the treatment of patients with advanced hematological malignancy. *Bone Marrow Transplant* 1988; **3**: 619–624.

99. Anderson JE, Appelbaum FR, Schoch G *et al*. Allogeneic marrow transplantation for myelodysplastic syndrome with advanced disease morphology: a phase II study of busulfan cyclophosphamide and total body irradiation and analysis of prognostic factors. *J Clin Oncol* 1996; **14**: 220–226.

100. Lynch MH, Petersen FB, Applebaum FR *et al*. A phase II study of busulfan, cyclophosphamide and fractionated total body irradiation as a preparatory regimen for allogeneic bone marrow transplantation in patients with advanced myeloid malignancies. *Bone Marrow Transplant* 1995; **15**: 59–64.

101. Woods WG, Ramsay NKC, Weisdorf D *et al*. Bone marrow transplantation for acute lymphoblastic leukemia utilizing total body irradiation followed by high doses of cytosine arabinoside: lack of superiority over cyclophosphamide containing conditioning regimens. *Bone Marrow Transplant* 1990; **4**: 9–16.

102. Riddell S, Applebaum FR, Buckner CD, *et al*. High dose cytarabine and total body irradiation with or without cyclophosphamide as a preparative regimen for marrow transplantation for acute leukemia. *J Clin Oncol* 1988; **6**: 576–582.

103. Weyman C, Graham-Pole J, Emerson S *et al*. Use of cytosine arabinoside and total body irradiation as conditioning for allogeneic marrow transplantation in patients with acute lymphoblastic leukemia: a multicenter survey. *Bone Marrow Transplant* 1993; **11**: 43–50

104. Wu DP, Milpied N, Moreau P *et al*. Total body irradiation, high dose cyclophosphamide, BCNU and VP-16 (CBV) as a new preparatory regimen for allogeneic bone marrow transplantation in patients with advanced hematologic malignancies. *Bone Marrow Transplant* 1994; **14**: 751–757.

105. Santos GW, Tutschka PJ, Brookmeyer R *et al*. Marrow transplantation for acute non-lymphocytic leukemia after treatment with busulfan and cyclophosphamide. *New Engl J Med* 1983; **309**: 1347–1353.

106. Copelan EA and Deeg HJ. Conditioning for allogeneic marrow transplantation in patients with lymphohemopoietic malignancies without the use of total body irradiation. *Blood* 1992; **80**: 1648–1658.

107. O'Donnell MR, Long GD, Parker PM *et al*. Busulphan/cyclophosphamide as conditioning regimen for allogeneic bone marrow transplantation for myelodysplasia. *J Clin Oncol* 1995; **13**: 2973–2979.

108. Anderson JE, Appelbaum FR, Scoch G *et al*. Allogeneic marrow transplantation for refractory anemia: a comparison of two preparative regimens and analysis of prognostic factors. *Blood* 1996; **87**: 51–58.

109. Locatelli F, Pession A, Bonetti F et al. Busulfan, cyclophosphamide and melphalan as conditioning regimen for bone marrow transplantation in children with myelodysplastic syndrome. *Leukaemia* 1994; **8**: 844–849.
110. Emminger W, Emminger-Schmidmeier W, Haas OA et al. Treatment of infant leukemia with busulfan cyclophosphamide + etoposide and bone marrow transplantation. *Bone Marrow Transplant* 1992; **10**: 313–318.
111. Ratanatharathorn V, Karanes C, Lum LG et al. Allogeneic bone marrow transplantation in high risk myeloid disorders using busulfan, cytosine arabinoside and cyclophosphamide (BAC). *Bone Marrow Transplant* 1992; **9**: 49–57.
112. Zander AR, Culbert S, Jaggenath S et al. High dose cyclophosphamide BCNU, and VP-1 (CBV) as a conditioning regimen for allogeneic bone marrow transplantation for patients with acute leukemia. *Cancer* 1987; **59**: 1083–1086.
113. Vaughan WP, Dennison JD, Reed EC et al. Improved results of allogeneic bone marrow transplantation for advanced hematologic malignancy using busulfan, cyclophosphamide and etoposide as cytoreductive and immunosuppressive therapy. *Bone Marrow Transplant* 1991; **8**: 489–495.
114. Cahn JY, Bordigoni P, Souillet G et al. The TAM regimen prior to allogeneic and autologous bone marrow transplantation for high risk acute lymphoblastic leukaemia: a cooperative study of 62 patients. *Bone Marrow Transplant* 1991; **7**: 1–4.
115. Kanfer EJ and McCarthy D. Cytoreductive preparation for bone marrow transplantation in leukaemia: to irradiate or not? *Br J Haematol* **71**: 447–450.
116. Copelan EA, Biggs JC, Avalos BR et al. Radiation-free preparation for allogeneic bone marrow transplantation in adults with acute lymphoblastic leukemia. *J Clin Oncol* 1992; **10**: 237–242.
117. Michel G, Gluckman E, Esperou-Bordeau H et al. Allogeneic bone marrow transplantation for children with acute myeloblastic leukemia in first complete remission: impact of conditioning regimen without total body irradiation: a report from the Société Française de Greffe de Moelle. *J Clin Oncol* 1994; **12**: 1217–1222.
118. Devergie A, Blaise D, Attal M et al. Allogeneic bone marrow transplantation for chronic myeloid leukemia in first chronic phase: a randomized trial of busulfan–cytoxan versus cytoxan–total body irradiation as preparative regimen: a report from the French Society of Bone Marrow Graft. *Blood* 1995; **85**: 2263–2268.
119. Clift RA, Buckner CD and Thomas D. Marrow transplantation for chronic myeloid leukaemia: a randomized study comparing cyclophosphamide and total body irradiation with busulfan–cyclophosphamide. *Blood* 1994; **84**: 2036–2043.
120. Ringden O, Ruutu T, Remberger M et al. A randomized trial comparing busulfan with total body irradiation as conditioning in allogeneic transplant recipients with leukaemia: a report from the Nordic Bone Marrow Transplant Group. *Blood* 1994; **83**: 2723–2730.
121. Blume KG, Kopecky KJ, Henslee-Downey JP et al. A prospective randomized comparison of total body irradiation–etoposide versus busulfan cyclophosphamide as preparatory regimens for bone marrow transplantation in patients with leukemia who were not in first remission: a Southwest Oncology Group Study. *Blood* 1993; **81**: 2187–2193.
122. Marks DA, Cullis JO, Ward KN et al. Allogeneic bone marrow transplantation for chronic myeloid leukemia using sibling and volunteer unrelated donors: a comparison of complications in the first two years. *Ann Intern Med* 1993; **119**: 207–214.
123. Gingrich RD, Ginder GD, Goekken NE et al. Allogeneic marrow grafting with partially mismatched unrelated marrow donors. *Blood* 1988; **71**: 1375–1381.
124. Gajewski JL, Ho WG, Feig SA, Hunt L, Kaufman N and Champlin RE. Bone marrow transplantation using unrelated donors for patients with advanced leukemia or bone marrow failure. *Transplantation* 1990; **50**: 244–249.
125. Lanino E, Lamparelli T, Dini G et al. BMT from unrelated donors: the Italian experience. *Bone Marrow Transplant* 1993; **11**(Supp 1): 88–89.
126. Beatty PG, Hansen JA, Longton GM et al. Marrow transplantation from HLA-matched unrelated marrow donors for treatment of hematological malignancies. *Transplantation* 1991; **51**: 443–447.
127. Casper J, Camitta B, Truitt R et al. Unrelated donor bone marrow transplants for children with leukaemia or myelodysplasia. *Blood* 1995; **85**: 2354–2363.
128. Davies SM, Ramsay NKC and Haake RJ. Comparison of engraftment in recipients of matched sibling or unrelated donor marrow allografts. *Bone Marrow Transplant* 1994; **13**: 51–58.
129. Mehta J, Powles RA, Mitchell P, Rege K, De Lord C and Treleaven J. Graft failure after bone marrow transplantation from unrelated donors using busulphan and cyclophosphamide for conditioning. *Bone Marrow Transplant* 1994; **13**: 583–588.
130. Kanfer EJ, MacDonald I, Hall G et al. Poor prognosis acute myeloid leukaemia treated by matched unrelated donor marrow transplant without preceding total body irradiation. *Bone Marrow Transplant* 1992; **9**: 67–69.
131. Cheson B. Infectious and immunosuppressive complications of purine analog therapy. Review article. *J Clin Oncol* 1995; **13**: 2431–2448.
132. Buckner CD. New chemotherapy/chemoradiotherapy preparative treatment regimens. In: *Clinical Bone Marrow Transplantation: A Reference Textbook*. K Atkinson (ed.), 1994 (New York: Cambridge University Press).
133. Storb R. Preparative regimens for patients with leukemia and severe aplastic anemia (overview): biological basis, experimental animal studies and clinical trials at the Fred Hutchinson Cancer Research Center. *Bone Marrow Transplant* 1994; **14**(Suppl 4): S1–3.

Appendix 1: A cyclophosphamide TBI preparative regimen for haematological malignancies

Total body irradiation 1360 cGy in eight fractions

Day −7	TBI	170 cGy a.m.	170 cGy p.m.
Day −6	TBI	170 cGy a.m.	170 cGy p.m.
Day −5	TBI	170 cGy a.m.	170 cGy p.m.
Day −4	TBI	170 cGy a.m.	170 cGy p.m.

Give dexamethasone 10 mg/m^2 every 12 h before first TBI fraction as anti-emesis.

Cyclophosphamide

Day −3	60 mg/kg as detailed below
Day −2	60 mg/kg as detailed below

Day −3

Hour	Treatment
0	Hydrate: normal saline 2.6 ml/kg/h 10 mEq/litre KCl (starting 12 hours pre-cyclophosphamide and continue hydration until 24 hours after last cyclophosphamide infusion)
11	Dexamethasone 10 mg/m^2 + granisetron 10 mg/kg i.v. Mesna 45 mg/kg i.v. in 100 ml D$_5$ or normal saline i.v. over 1 h Furosemide 20 mg i.v.
12	Cyclophosphamide 60 mg/kg i.v. in 250 ml dextrose over 1 h.
13	Mesna 45 mg/kg in 100 ml D$_5$ or normal saline i.v. over 8 h
21	Mesna 30 mg/kg in 100 ml D$_5$ or normal saline i.v. over 8 h
23	Dexamethasone 10 mg/m^2 + granisetron 10 mg/kg i.v.

Day −2
Repeat at midnight

Day −1
Stop i.v. hydration (24 hours after last cyclophosphamide dose). Monitor potassium level every 12 hours. If >4.5 mEq/litre stop KCl in hydration; if <3.0 mEq/litre increase to 25 mEq/litre. If urine output <1.5 ml/kg/h give additional 20 mg furosemide i.v. If body weight >2 kg over pre-cyclophosphamide value give additional furosemide 20 mg i.v.

Appendix 2: Common agents used in preparative regimens

Cyclophosphamide (Endoxan, Cytoxan)
Manufacturer: Asta Medica, Meade Johnson, Bristol Meyers Squibb, Orion Pharma International.

Action: Alkylating agent. Prevents cell division by binding DNA and preventing DNA replication. At a dose of 120–200 mg/kg this alkylating agent produces lymphopenia and pancytopenia. While the effect on immune function is profound and possibly permanent, total doses of 8–10 grams do not cause permanent marrow failure. Cyclophosphamide therefore appears to spare non-cycling stem cells. It is both immunosuppressive and myelosuppressive.

Metabolism: Converted in the liver by microsomal enzymes to active nitrogen mustard-like compounds. Excreted by the kidney as metabolites and unconverted cyclophosphamide.

Availability: 100, 200 and 500 mg vials.

Storage: Stable at room temperature. After reconstitution use within 24 hours.

Administration: Dissolved in 500 ml 5% dextrose and administered over 1 hour.

Precautions: To prevent haemorrhagic cystitis: give mesna as a bolus dose i.v. to 50% of the total dose of cyclophosphamide. Continue with 50% of total cyclophosphamide dose over the next 8 hours, then 25% of dose over the following 12 hours. Also ensure a urine output of over 100 ml/h by administering an i.v. fluid load of 1 litre normal saline + 20 mEq KCl in the 12 h preceding cyclophosphamide administration with furosemide 20–40 mg up to 12 hourly if necessary. Monitor potassium daily. Correct hypokalaemia with KCl 10–20 mEq/h.

Side-effects: Immediate – tingling and metallic taste, nausea and vomiting ADH syndrome, cardiotoxic at high doses (>70 mg/kg). Rare – pulmonary toxicity, cardiac damage, urticaria and flushing. Delayed – mucositis, alopecia, infertility.

Cyclophosphamide is the most widely used drug in BMT preparative regimens. It is generally well tolerated. Major side-effects are haemorrhagic cystitis – best prevented by administration of mesna which inactivates the active products of cyclophosphamide metabolism. High doses of cyclophosphamide carry a small risk of cardiac damage which limit the safe dose to 200 mg/kg.

Busulphan: (Myleran)
Manufacturer: Wellcome.

Action: Alkylating agent. Binds to DNA and inhibits DNA replication. Non cell-cycle specific. Myeloablative and immunosuppressive.

Metabolism: Up to 90% absorbed from upper gastrointestinal tract. Absorption is variable. Excreted in the urine as the inactive metabolite metasulphonic acid.

Availability: Manufacturer 2 mg tablets. More conveniently can be prepared in 25 mg and 50 mg tablets by pharmacy on site.

Administration: In four divided oral doses 4 mg/kg. Re-administer same dose if patient vomits within 3 hours of administration. Because the absorption varies between individuals, the optimal approach is to carry out a preliminary pharmacokinetic study monitoring plasma levels and adjusting total dose according to the efficiency of absorption.

Storage: Conserve below 25°C.

Side-effects: Pulmonary: restrictive lung disease and pulmonary fibrosis – uncommon due to busulphan in BMT schedules unless the patient has received prior long-term therapy with busulphan. Other: alopecia, gonadal damage, second malignancies.

The alkylating agent most widely used for its myeloablative action. Busulphan damages both cycling and non-cycling stem cells and depending on the total dose administered produces a profound and prolonged or irreversible marrow failure. The main dose-limiting side-effect is a restrictive lung disease and hepatic veno-occlusive disease. A disadvantage of busulphan is the lack of any approved intravenous preparation. The orally administered preparation shows extreme variability in its absorption. This variability can be partly overcome by adjusting the dose according to the busulphan level achieved in a pharmacokinetic study.

Melphalan: (Alkeran, L-Pan, L-Phenyalanine Mustard)
Manufacturer: Wellcome.

Action: Alkylating agent. Mustine derivative, binds to DNA and interferes with DNA replication. Non cell-cycle specific.

Metabolism: Administration i.v. results in rapid renal elimination of metabolites. Plasma half-life 6 hours.

Availability: 50 mg powder in vials.

Administration: Insoluble in water – reconstitute in 3 ml alcohol and administer into a fast-flowing i.v. infusion; 100–200 mg/m^2.

Storage: Conserve at 4°C; use immediately.

Precautions: Necrotizing! Avoid extravasation and contact with skin.

Side-effects: Gastrointestinal: nausea, vomiting, diarrhoea, weight loss and anorexia.

This alkylating agent was one of the first to be developed for treatment of malignant disease in the 1940s. Its properties are well known and its availability for intravenous administration make it preferred over busulphan by some investigators. Melphalan has profound immunosuppressive and myeloablative properties. It also causes a severe prolonged mucositis which makes intravenous feeding frequently necessary for patients receiving doses > 100 mg/m^2. Its dose-limiting side-effects are gastrointestinal damage, renal toxicity and an increased risk of veno-occlusive disease.

Thiotepa (triethylenethiophosphoramide)
Manufacturer: Lederle.

Action: Alkylating agent. Binds to DNA and inhibits DNA replication. Non cell-cycle specific. Myeloablative and immunosuppressive.

Metabolism: Rapid distribution after i.v. administration. Active form is rapidly metabolized by the liver.

Availability: 15 mg ampoules – powder with sterile water diluent.

Administration: i.v. 60 mg/m^2; i.v. by bolus or in 500 ml 5% dextrose.

Storage: Refrigerate.

Side-effects: Nausea and vomiting, mucositis. Veno-occlusive disease.

Thiotepa is principally used as an additional immunosuppressant to increase the probability of engraftment in mismatched T-cell-depleted transplants. It adds significant toxicity to the preparative regimen.

BCNU (carmustine)
Manufacturer: Bristol-Meyers

Action: Nitrosourea. An alkylating agent which crosses the blood–brain barrier. It binds to DNA and RNA interfering with DNA replication. Also inactivates a number of cytoplasmic proteins. It is active equally on cycling and non-cycling cells but has a major effect on cells in S phase. Myeloablative and immunosuppressive.

Metabolism: Administration i.v., the drug is distributed widely throughout the body reaching comparable levels in cerebrospinal fluid and plasma. Plasma half-life is approximately 36 hours. 70% excreted in the urine in 96 hours.

Availability: 100 mg powder ampoules.

Administration: Insoluble in water – reconstitute in 3 ml alcohol and administer into a fast-flowing i.v. infusion of 5% dextrose.

Storage: Refrigerate; protect from light. Use immediately when reconstituted.

Precautions: Necrotizing – avoid extravasation and contact with skin.

Side-effects: Causes tissue necrosis when extravasated. Gastrointestinal: nausea and vomiting, mucositis. Pulmonary: restrictive lung disease. Central nervous system: causes somnolence.

BCNU is used in combination chemotherapy preparative regimens to enhance the antileukaemia effect.

Etoposide (VP16, Epipodophylotoxin, Vepesid)
Manufacturer: Bristol Meyers Squibb.

Action: Alkaloid. One of the podophyllins. Blocks cells in G2 of the cell cycle by binding to the mitotic spindle. Myelosuppressive and immunosuppressive.

Metabolism: Administration i.v., binds rapidly to albumin. Half-life in plasma 18 hours.

Availability: Ampoules 100 mg with solvent.

Administration: For high doses used in BMT, it is necessary to dissolve first in alcohol and then reconstitute in 5% dextrose. Infuse in 500 ml 5% dextrose over 3–6 hours depending on dose.

Storage: Stable at room temperature after reconstitution for 96 hours.

Precautions: Necrotizing! Avoid extravasation and contact with skin.

Side-effects: Cardiovascular: high-dose administration can cause cardiac arrhythmias – use of a monitor is desirable. Gastrointestinal: nausea and vomiting – related to dose and rate of administration.

Etoposide has been used as an additional or alternative agent to cyclophosphamide in preparative regimens for high relapse risk leukaemias and especially acute lymphocytic leukaemia. It is usually well tolerated in high doses but regimens containing etoposide have an increased risk of veno-occlusive disease.

Cytosine arabinoside (Cytosar, Ara-C, Alexan, Cytarabine)
Manufacturer: Upjohn, Delta West.

Action: Antimetabolite. Phosphorylated intracellularly to active form Ara-C triphosphate. Blocks DNA polymerase and inhibits the conversion of cytidine to deoxycytidine. Blocks cells in S phase of the cycle. Myelosuppressive and immunosuppressive.

Metabolism: i.v. and s.c. administration. Metabolized in 2–3 hours in the liver by cytosine deaminase. The inactive metabolite uracil arabinoside is excreted in the urine.

Availability: 40, 100, 500 and 1000 mg vials of powder. Dilute in distilled water.

Administration: i.v. bolus up to 1 g/m^2. Higher doses (up to 3 g/m^2) should be diluted in saline to avoid toxicity from the diluent, depending on protocol.

Storage: 4°C; use within 24 hours once reconstituted.

Precautions: None.

Side-effects: Gastrointestinal: anorexia, nausea, vomiting, diarrhoea, stomatitis. Elevated liver-function tests. Central nervous system: somnolence and cerebellar damage from high doses more frequent in older (>60 years) individuals.

Cytosine arabinoside has been used as an additional or alternative immunosuppressive agent to cyclophosphamide in preparative regimens for mismatched transplants or high relapse risk acute lymphocytic leukaemia.

Fludarabine (Fludarabine Phosphate)
Manufacturer: Ben Verne Lab, Richmond CA.

Action: Purine analogue. Fludarabine is transformed intracellularly into the active form 2-fluoro-arabinofuranosiladenine triphosphate which inhibits DNA polymerase, ribonucleotide reductase and DNA primase. DNA synthesis is consequently inhibited.

Metabolism: A single intravenous injection maintains plasma levels for about 10 hours. Most of the drug is eliminated by the kidneys (23% in active form). Dose reductions are appropriate for renal dysfunction.

Availability and storage: 50 mg ampoules lyophilized powder stored at room temperature. Reconstituted in water it can be stored for up to 8 hours at 4°C.

Administration: i.v. 25 mg/m^2 in 200 ml 5% glucose over 30 minutes.

Campath-1 (Anti-CD52)
Manufacturer: Wellcome.

Action: Monoclonal antibody. Immunosuppressive. Binds to CD52 expressed on thymocytes, T-cells, B cells and some monocytes. Complement fixing.

Administration: i.v. over 4–6 hours. Control allergic side-effects with antihistamine and hydrocortisone.

Side-effects: The major side-effects are related to cytokine release, worse during the first dose. Allergic side-effects can also occur.

Campath-1 is a widely used immunosuppressant, effective both for increasing engraftment and also for reducing acute graft-versus-host disease.

Antilymphocyte globulin (ATG, Lymphoglobulin)
Manufacturer: Upjohn, Merieux.

Action: Antisera to human lymphocytes raised in horses or rabbits. Immunosuppressive. ATG has a potent but short-lived immunosuppressive action which falls short of immunoablation. ATG/ALG is therefore used as an adjunct to other immunosuppressive treatments.

Administration: i.v. over 4–6 hours. Control allergic side-effects with antihistamine and hydrocortisone.

Side-effects: The major side-effect is allergy to the animal protein.

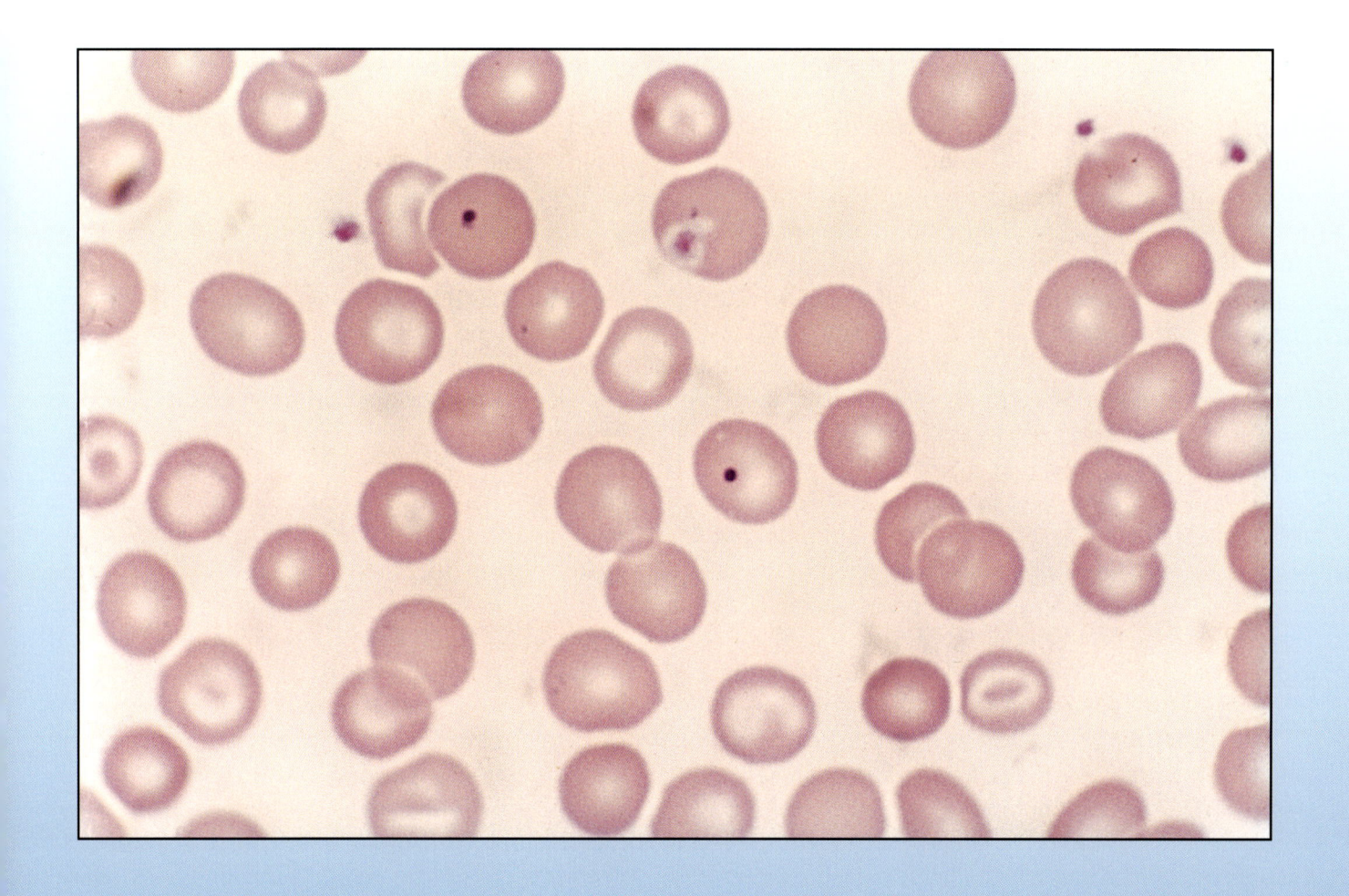

Chapter 36

High-dose regimens for autologous stem-cell transplantation

N. Claude Gorin

Introduction and general principles

High-dose regimens used for intensification before autografting are in principle defined as those capable of providing the highest antitumour effect achievable without taking into account the risks of myeloablation, since haematopoiesis is rescued by re-infusion of autologous haemopoietic stem cells (ASC). This statement emphasizes several important concepts. First, in contrast to allogeneic stem-cell transplantation, immunosuppression is generally not needed and, in fact, should be avoided. This may change in the near future if high-dose therapy with ASC transplant (ASCT) develops for the treatment of autoimmune diseases which will constitute an exception to the rule. Second, since a maximum antitumour effect is sought, it is obvious that each malignant disease treated will have its own peculiarities, and drugs and their combinations are chosen in relation to the known sensitivity of the tumour to the drugs.

The situation has, however, been somewhat different historically for haematological malignancies and for solid tumours. For haematological malignancies, experience of allogeneic transplants has provided regimens which have been directly transposed for ASCT. This has been the case in particular for the combination of cyclophosphamide (Cy) and total body irradiation (TBI) or for the combination of busulfan and Cy or etoposide or high-dose melphalan (HDM) which are used for both allogeneic and autologous transplants in leukaemias. For solid tumours, ASCT has brought a new concept which has generated its own tools, and the reference has mainly been past experience with conventional chemotherapy.

Identification of effective drugs for a given tumour has resulted chiefly from the considerable experience gained in phase I and II trials leading to the definition of maximum tolerated dose (MTD) in end-stage patients, and later to the observation of results achieved earlier in the course of the disease. High-dose regimens have been built by combining several effective drugs with the hope of increasing efficacy by cumulating their effects and/or by taking advantage of synergistic effects. However, MTD for single drugs is generally higher than those which can be given safely within combinations. Therefore, most high-dose regimens used for autografting today have resulted from phase I and II trials with escalating schedules, or from past empirical experience which has proven their tolerance and efficacy.

Drug combinations and use have been designed in keeping with several principles of chemotherapy which have been established over the past thirty years. These include:
- dose effect (the higher the dose, the higher the tumoricidal result); this is essentially the case for alkylating agents;
- absence of cross-resistance in the drugs selected to be combined;
- better likelihood of overcoming resistance by combining non-cross-resistant agents at the highest possible doses (MTD within the combination);
- higher chance of eradicating disease when using high-dose therapy early in the course of the disease, before it has been subjected to several chemotherapy approaches which may have generated resistance. This should occur ideally in a situation of minimal residual disease (MRD) where vascularization is good (for both optimal delivery and oxygenation) and in the absence of previous radiotherapy which may have caused sclerosis and made access to the tumor difficult The classical image is 'the hammer to kill a fly'.

Next, thorough knowledge of the drug pharmacology is necessary, in particular to ensure that the haemopoietic stem cells infused will not be exposed to direct or indirect (metabolites) toxicity. For example, a stem-cell transplant can be safely carried out 24 hours after administration of melphalan but not until 72 hours after etoposide. Finally, since haemopoietic toxicity is not the limiting factor, other organ toxicities must be taken into account and usually set dose limits. Examples of this include the cardiac toxicity seen after cyclophosphamide or anthracyclines, renal toxicity after platinum derivatives, liver toxicity (mostly veno-occlusive disease) after busulfan and lung toxicity after nitrosoureas.

After several years of therapeutic trials, it is accepted today that the best strategy for eradicating tumour is to use one aimed at firstly reaching the status of MRD with conventional chemotherapy, at which point high-dose intensification is given with ASCT. Most teams consider that the autograft should be purged of residual tumour cells as much as is feasible.

However, although there have been numerous observations supporting purging in particular for acute leukaemias, chronic myelocytic leukaemias, non-Hodgkin's lymphomas and neuroblastomas, including gene marking of the graft with the neomycin-resistance gene, some teams still consider that definitive proof for the beneficial effect of purging on patient outcome is lacking.

The concept of high-dose intensification has changed over years. From 1977, when the first successful autograft [1] was carried out in a patient with an acute myelocytic leukaemia (AML) until 1992, the autograft came from marrow-derived stem cells, and only a minority of patients underwent double intensification with a double ABMT. Peripheral blood stem-cell (PBSC) transplantation, which started in 1985, represented over 80% of all ASCT in 1996. It has introduced two important modifications:

- PBSC are mobilized by chemotherapy and haemopoietic growth factors, mainly granulocyte colony-stimulating factor (G-CSF), granulocyte–monocyte colony-stimulating factor (GM-CSF) and stem-cell factor (SCF). In some treatment strategies, the mobilizing chemotherapy is also chosen for its antitumour effect, so that strictly speaking, the concept of intensification should include this step of mobilization and its effect should be added to that of the high-dose regimen used immediately before transplant when the therapeutic evaluation is carried out.
- ASCT with peripheral blood is associated with faster kinetics of recovery of haemopoiesis, and in some institutions programmes of ambulatory ASCT exist. In addition, because the yields of peripheral blood by leukapheresis are usually high, it has become easier to use several intensifications (sequential intensifications). Successive high-dose regimens are either reduced in strength with regard to the original ones to enable repetition, or progressively escalated, with the last being the most intensive and possibly including TBI if pertinent.

Thus, the definition and scope of high-dose therapy pre-ASCT has changed over the years and become more complex. Indeed, regimens can only be studied separately according to disease. This chapter will concentrate only on principles, and describe almost exclusively high-dose regimens originally designed to be given as a single intensification procedure.

High-dose regimens in acute leukaemias

Table 36.1 lists examples of high-dose pretransplant regimens used for acute leukaemia. Schedules can be divided into two categories: those with total body irradiation and those consisting of chemotherapy combinations.

Total body irradiation (TBI)
Principle

The use of TBI, as indicated above, has been copied from the experience gained from allogeneic marrow transplantation [2–6], with the general assumption that, in combination with chemotherapy, it brings the highest possible tumour load reduction. Indeed, the BNML rat model of acute myelocytic leukaemia indicates that the combination of Cy with TBI can produce a reduction in leukaemic burden of up to 9 logs. The considerable immunosuppression associated with TBI, which is mandatory for allo BMT, is thought to be of no interest for ABMT, if not harmful, and several protocols have studied immune reinforcement post-autografting in an effort to further control MRD. As an example, administration of interleukin-2 (IL-2), interleukin-12 (IL-12) or linomide are being tested in an effort to boost natural killer (NK) cells and increase their antileukaemic activity.

Dose and fractionation

Thirty years of experience in preclinical models mainly with mice and dogs in parallel with the clinical experience in transplant units have provided several guidelines. Since it is not the scope of this chapter to review TBI, these are briefly summarized here:

- The tolerance of marrow stem cells is around 4 Gy.
- Above 10 Gy, other organ damage appears which can be fatal: gastrointestinal toxicity is first.
- A dose of 10 Gy delivered in a single fraction was the first tested and used with efficacy by the Seattle team [2–6].
- This dose delivered in a single fraction is associated with several toxicities: the most important are growth retardation in children, sterility, interstitial pneumonitis, cataracts and secondary malignancies.
- In an effort to reduce toxicity and also to increase antileukaemic efficacy, dose fractionation was

Table 36.1 Examples of high-dose therapy followed by stem-cell transplantation in leukaemia

Drugs (total doses)[†]	Duration (days)	Minimum interval before s.c. infusion (days)	Major specific toxicity[***]	Comment	Reference
Schedules including total body irradiation					
Cyclophosphamide (120 mg/kg) + sTBI (10 Gy)[*]	5	1		Standard	[2–5]
Cyclophosphamide (120 mg/kg) + F-TBI (12 Gy)[*]	7	2		F-TBI less toxic than sTBI (example: lower cataract incidence)	[2–5]
TBI Aracytine (12 g/m² or 24 g/m²)		1	Mucositis Toxicity of Ara-C treated with steroids	Described for ALL TAM 12: adults TAM 24: children	[17]
HDM (140 mg/m²)			Mucositis		[93]
Cyclophosphamide (120 mg/kg) Etopside (1500 mg/m²) F-TBI (10.2 Gy)	7	1	Mucositis (increased by etopside)		[94]
HF-TBI (1.25 Gy × 3/day × 4) Etopside (500 mg/m²) Cyclophosphamide (120 mg/kg)	9	2			
Schedules excluding total body irradiation					
Busulphan (16 mg/kg)[**] + CY4 (200 mg/kg)	8	2	Prophylaxis needed for busulphan-induced seizures. Liver veno-occlusive disease (multi-organ failure)	Plasma level busulphan monitoring recommended, with dose adjustment	[19,95]
BAVC [BCNU (800 mg/m²) Amsa (450 mg/m²) VP-16 (450 mg/m²) Aracytine (900 mg/m²)[††]]	3	1		Useful in older patients; called BAVC (C for Ara-C)	[30–32]
Busulphan (16 mg/kg) HDM (140–200 mg/m²)	5	1	Prophylaxis needed for busulphan-induced seizures		[28]
Busulphan (16 mg/kg) Etoposide (60 mg/kg)	5	3	Mucositis		
Busulphan (10–12 mg/kg) Cyclophosphamide (120–150 mg/kg) Thiotepa (450–750 gm/m²)			Mucositis		[29]

[*]Cyclophosphamide can be given before or after TBI. Two days interval needed between TBI and cyclophosphamide.
Lung shielding: sTBI = 8 Gy; F-TBI = 9 Gy.
One dose cyclophosphamide can be replaced by HDM (140 mg/m²) which crosses the blood-brain barrier.
[**]An alternative less toxic, but possibly less tumoricidal, regimen busulphan–CY2 uses cyclophosphamide at 120 mg/kg only over two days.
[***]Myelosuppression aside.
[†]Abbreviations: F-TBI = fractionated TBI; HDM = high-dose melphalan; HF-TBI = hyperfractionated TBI; sTBI = single-dose TBI;
TAM = TBI + Aracytine + high dose melphalan; TBI = total body irradiation. For other abbreviations, see text.
[††]Aracytine is cytosine arabinoside or Ara-C (C) in the BAVC regimen.

introduced with two specific regimens used today in many institutions [7–14]:

Fractionated TBI (F-TBI) consisting of two fractions of 2 Gy per day (morning and evening) for three days (total 12 Gy).

Hyperfractionated TBI (HF-TBI) consisting of 1.25 Gy three times a day for four days (total 15 Gy).

The major point of fractionation is to increase sparing of normal tissues by allowing repair of sublethal damage. It was first hoped that fractionation would increase leukaemic cell kill. This, at present, is unclear. It appears that 12 Gy fractionated is equivalent to 10 Gy single dose in this respect, and in fact, more antileukaemic effect would neccessitate higher doses of over 12 Gy, which can be given only as fractionated TBI, not as a single dose.

In a randomized trial of patients with AML in first complete remission and patients with chronic myelocytic leukemia (CML) who underwent allogeneic bone-marrow transplants in Seattle [8], 12 Gy fractionated TBI was compared with 15.75 Gy of HF-TBI. In patients who received adequate prophylaxis for graft-versus-host disease (GvHD), the relapse rate was 37% in the 12 Gy group but 0% in the 15.75 Gy group. However, this antileukaemic advantage was lost due to heavy toxicity with an increase in transplant-related mortality.

Toxicity also depends upon the instantaneous dose rate delivered at source. Several historical studies have shown that the incidence of interstitial pneumonitis is reduced with low dose rates [7,14]. Lung shielding is nowadays part of the routine procedure of TBI and is given at 8 Gy for single-dose TBI and at 9 Gy for F-TBI. Fractionation and lung shielding have reduced the incidence of interstitial pneumonitis considerably, and in recent series this no longer appeared to be linked to instant dose rate.

Dose rate may still remain an important factor in single-dose TBI, however. A recent report from our institution has confirmed the historical observation of a higher incidence of interstitial pneumonitis in the group irradiated at 0.15 Gy/min as compared with 0.06 Gy/min. The incidence of cataracts is also reduced with F-TBI [8,13] (see also below).

In the context of autografting, administration of TBI allows persistence in the body of stem cells with chromosome abnormalities which are detectable in the marrow by routine karyotype analysis. In a series of 66 patients transplanted in our institution following TBI, we were able to detect cytogenetic abnormalities at some time post-transplant. These were complex and concerned a minority of cells. Some were transitory and others modified with time [15].

Since similar abnormalities were not observed in other patients at our institution autografted following chemotherapy only, and because similar observations have been made in allotransplant recipients receiving T-depleted marrow but not unmanipulated marrow, the most likely explanation is that these altered cells are survivors of TBI which persist at a low level. To date, these abnormalities occurring specifically after TBI have not been linked to the development of secondary malignancies.

Chemotherapy combined with TBI or F-TBI

Total body irradiation is never given alone, and in fact both antileukaemic activity and toxicity should be considered in relation to the combination. The gold standard for acute leukaemias and for most haematological malignancies has been the Cy–TBI combination, with Cy given at 60 mg/kg/day for two days (total 120 mg/kg) followed by TBI or F-TBI after a two-day rest period [2–4,6]. The two-day rest is considered indispensible and allows normal tissue repair while not being long enough to enable leukaemic cell repair and survival. There have been several modifications to this basic scheme which has remained the core for most regimens used in haematological malignancies. These are:

- Cy can be given after, rather than before TBI, and in the rat model this has been shown to increase tumour kill by a further log.
- Cy–F-TBI is also often given as a reversed modality for practical reasons. F-TBI is delivered first in the radiotherapy unit to a patient who is not yet neutropenic and Cy is then given more safely in the transplant unit.
- several regimens have been created in an effort to increase antileukaemic activity and/or deliver drugs which cross the blood–brain barrier. Such regimens are usually used in higher risk patients, and most incorporate:

  etoposide (VP-16) at 60 mg/kg as a substitute for Cy [16];

high-dose cytosine arabinoside (Ara-C) at 3 g/m^2 to a total of 12 or 24 g/m^2 [17];

high-dose melphalan at 140 mg/m^2.

It should not be overlooked that chemotherapy may cause additional specific toxicities. The preventative role of mesna on Cy-induced haemorrhagic cystitis has been questioned, since in a recent randomized study, hyperhydration was shown to be equally effective [18]. There is also an association between haemorrhagic cystitis and presence of the BK virus in the urine. High-dose Ara-C can induce severe cutaneous toxicity with erythema, oedema, conjunctivitis and fever, which requires concomitant administration of steroids.

Chemotherapy-only regimens
The busulfan-cyclophosphamide combination

In 1983, the Baltimore group described initial results in patients with AML who had received a combination of Busulfan (Bu) and cyclophosphamide (Cy), in preparation for allogeneic BMT [19]. For simplicity, it may be considered that in this regimen BU takes the place of TBI. The original schedule of drug administration (so-called Bu–Cy4) consisted of Bu 1 mg/kg four times a day (4 mg/kg/day) for four consecutive days (total dose 16 mg/kg), followed by Cy (50 mg/kg/day × 4) for four additional days.

Since 1983, several comparative studies of allogeneic BMT have indicated that similar results in terms of leukaemia survival are achieved with either the Bu–Cy4 regimen or with conventional Cy–TBI [20–22]. The principal interest of Bu–Cy4 is that BMT becomes feasible in centres where TBI cannot be given, and also that its use removes the necessity for booking a TBI slot, thereby facilitating planning. This regimen also avoids growth retardation in children and may not cause definitive sterility. However, concern about toxicity, especially liver veno-occlusive disease, has led to major modifications:

- pharmacological studies have indicated the necessity for monitoring plasma busulfan levels to adjust oral intake. Differences in absorption are responsible for large variations in the area under the curve. Clearance of busulphan is higher in children, possibly because of higher levels of glutathione or an increased activity of gluthatione-S transferase. Monitoring of plasma levels leads to decreased liver toxicity in adults and enables administration of even higher doses in children. However, it is unfortunately not available in the majority of centres [23–25];
- the Colombus team, in an attempt to decrease toxicity while retaining antileukaemic activity has modified the original Baltimore regimen by reducing the dose of Cy to two doses of 60 mg/kg, to a total of 120 mg/kg instead of 200 mg/kg. They originally reported similar efficacy but this was later challenged [26];
- the French SFGM (Societé Français de Greffe de Moélle) group first started a randomized study comparing Cy + TBI versus Bu–Cy2 for conditioning AML patients for allografting. This was interrupted because of an increased relapse rate in the Bu–Cy2 group, and led to the conclusion that the antileukaemic efficacy of the reduced Bu–Cy was insufficient [27]. Instead, use of Bu–Cy4 was recommended. Subsequently, the busulphan component of Bu–Cy4 was reduced to 12 mg/kg instead of the original 16 mg/kg (3 mg/kg/day × 4) because of the high incidence of liver veno-occlusive disease. This regimen is currently in use by the French group for lymphomas.

Today, Bu–Cy is globally perceived as an alternative to Cy–TBI and both regimens are usually accepted in protocols assessing allogeneic and autologous stem-cell transplants. There are, however, exceptions where Cy–TBI is preferable (see below).

Modifications of busulphan–cyclophosphamide

Just as Cy–TBI has been the core around which changes have been made, similarly, adjustments to the original Bu–Cy protocol have been made to answer specific problems. In chronic myelocytic leukaemia (CML), Bu alone or the combination of Bu and HDM at 140 mg/kg have been tested [28]. Other combinations tested in acute leukaemia are Bu at the original dose and etoposide at 60 mg/kg, and a three-drug regimen combining 10–12 mg/kg Bu, Cy at doses of 120–150 mg/kg and thiotepa at 450–750 mg/m^2 [29].

The BAVC regimen

The BAVC regimen was initially described by the Rome team [30–32], and the results reported were, for some reason, better in patients with AML in second remission. In the original series, the leukaemia-free survival (LFS) was only 31% in first complete-remission patients. These poor results were possibly linked to re-infusion of tumour cells with unpurged marrow, since the relapse rate was greater in patients receiving the higher cell doses. In second complete remission, the LFS was 48% and this good result was largely attributed to the low TRM. In our institution we now use BAVC in patients over 55 years of age, with good results.

Other regimens

Several other so-called 'myeloablative regimens' have been used in the context of autografting for acute leukaemias. A possible interesting exception is the (BEAM) protocol (BCNU, etoposide, cytosine arabinoside, HDM), widely used for non-Hodgkin's lymphomas, which has apparently given results in AML comparable to series using regimens described above.

EBMT evaluation of pre-autografting regimens for acute leukaemias

The acute leukaemia registry of the European Cooperative Group for Blood and Marrow transplantation (EBMT) contains information on 14 487 patients transplanted as of January 1997 and includes 11 378 transplants since January 1987; 5776 patients have been autografted and 8711 allografted.

In AML, chemotherapy-only regimens for autografting have been used more frequently than TBI (54% versus 46%), mainly Bu–Cy, while acute lymphoblastic leukaemia (ALL) patients have mainly received TBI (82% versus 18%).

Interestingly, there was a tendency in favour of F-TBI which was more pronounced for ALL (61% of the patients received F-TBI and 21% single-dose TBI) than for AML (29% F-TBI, 17% single-dose TBI). When comparing with allogeneic BMT, one important difference concerned AML: pretransplant, 80% of patients received TBI either as a single dose or fractionated and only 22% received chemotherapy (Table 36.2).

Retrospective EBMT analyses have shown similar results, whatever the pre-autografting regimen for AML. There have, however, been suggestions that single-dose TBI has greater antileukaemic activity than F-TBI. A recent comparison of TBI and Bu–Cy (Bu-Cy 4 and Bu-Cy 2 combined) for both allogeneic and autologous transplants has been carried out by the

Table 36.2 Distribution of high dose regimens used in Europe for acute leukaemias (source EBMT)

	AML (%)	ALL (%)
TBI (total)	46	82
sTBI	17	21
F-TBI	29	61
Chemotherapy only	54	18

Acute Leukaemia Working Party of EBMT [22]: similar results emerged for both pretransplant modalities except in the case of patients with ALL in second remission or beyond who fared much worse if autografted following Bu–Cy. In fact, several previous retrospective studies of EBMT have repeatedly pointed out the superiority of TBI for ALL.

Other retrospective EBMT analyses have focused on toxicity: 1063 patients with acute leukaemia were analyzed for incidence of cataracts following either autologous or allogeneic transplantation after TBI [33]. The distribution was as follows: 567 patients had ALL and 490 AML; 688 were allografted and 375 autografted; single-dose TBI was given in 495 cases at a median dose of 10 Gy and F-TBI in 568 cases at a median dose of 12 Gy. The analyses took into account administration of steroids for any reason (316 patients) and administration of heparin for veno-occlusive disease prevention (195 patients). The global incidence of cataracts in the 1063 patients was 27% at five years and 50% at ten years. By multivariate analyses, factors promoting cataract formation were:
- older age (over 23 years);
- use of single-dose TBI (and not F-TBI) (relative risk (RR): 2.71);
- long-term steroid therapy;
- absence of heparin administration; and
- allogeneic transplantation rather than autologous (RR: 1.65) (Table 36.3).

Within single-dose TBI an instant dose rate > 0.04 Gy/min and a total dose over 8 Gy also increased the incidence. When analysing the need for cataract surgery in the global population, the most unfavourable factor was single-dose TBI which was associated with a seven fold increased relative risk.

Table 36.3 Factors promoting cataract formation (EBMT analysis)

- Older age (over 23 years)
- Use of single-dose TBI (and not F-TBI) (relative risk: 2.71)
- Long-term steroid therapy
- Absence of heparin administration
- Allogeneic transplantation rather than autologous (relative risk: 1.65)

High-dose regimens in lymphomas

Three regimens are primarily used for intensification in lymphomas, although broadly speaking, regimens potentially useful for lymphomas should be very similar to those used for acute leukaemias. These are CBV (cyclophosphamide, BCNU, VP-16), BEAM (BCNU, etoposide, cytosine arabinoside (Ara-C), high-dose melphalan) and regimens containing TBI. Only chemotherapy regimens will be reviewed here, since review of TBI for acute leukaemias applies also to lymphomas (Table 36.4).

Regimens
CBV regimen
The CBV regimen combines three drugs which have been shown in several models to be additive or synergystic with an absence of cross-resistance. The original CBV regimen [34] comprises Cy $1.5\,g/m^2$ from day –6 to day –3 (total $6\,g/m^2$), carmustine $300\,mg/m^2$ on day –6, and etoposide $300\,mg/m^2$ in two divided daily doses from day –6 to day –3. Stem cells are infused on day 0, i.e. 72 hours after the last dose of etoposide and six days after carmustine. These intervals are important in avoiding toxicity from residual drugs and metabolites. The toxicity of this original CBV is reported as low: 10% in the early days (1983–1989) but virtually nil in a more recent series of 105 patients treated from 1990 to 1993 in Omaha. As a consequence, patients with Hodgkin's disease in Omaha are nowadays transplanted on an out-patient basis.

Increases in the doses of the original CBV regimen have been attempted by several teams [35–44]:
- Cy has been increased to $7.2\,g/m^2$.
- Carmustine has been increased to $600\,mg/m^2$, and even to $800\,mg/m^2$ in one series.
- Etoposide has been increased up to $2.4\,g/m^2$.

The conclusion is predictable. With the most intense regimen containing Cy $7.2\,g/m^2$, BCNU $600\,mg/m^2$ and etoposide $2.4\,g/m^2$, the Vancouver team has achieved the highest antitumour activity (79% complete remission rate) associated with the highest transplant-related mortality (21%). However, with recent improvements in patient care including haemopoietic growth factors, it is possible that the transplant-related mortality will be reduced.

In a randomized study, the French GELA group has shown that high-dose intensification is associated with a better disease-free survival than conventional chemotherapy in patients with aggressive lymphomas in the high-risk group by the international prognostic index, even using one of the lowest doses of CBV [34].

There has been some attempt at adding a fourth drug to CBV:
- the Vancouver team has recently updated a series of patients with progressive Hodgkin's disease intensified with CBV + cisplatin (CBV + P) [45,46]. Their original regimen was made less intensive to reduce toxicity and consisted of Cy $7.2\,g/m^2$ over four days, BCNU $500\,mg/m^2$ and etoposide $2.4\,g/m^2$ by continuous infusion over 34 hours. Cisplatin was added at the conventional dose of $150\,mg/m^2$. The most recent patients received haemopoietic growth factors. Progression-free survival of the whole group has been 61% at eight years, with a clear relationship between number of adverse prognostic factors and risk of disease progression post-transplant;
- the San Antonio team has tested the CBV augmented with dacarbazine (DTIC) ($5\,g/m^2$ for one day) (CBVD) in a few patients, with no conclusive evidence of its superior antitumour efficacy;
- another approach tested in lymphomas by the French SFGM group is CBV–mitoxantrone which adds mitoxantrone at $30\,mg/m^2$ to the original CBV.

BEAM regimen
The BEAM regimen has remained the gold standard for intensification of non-Hodgkin's lymphoma and

Table 36.4 Examples of high-dose therapy followed by stem-cell transplantation in lymphomas and myelomas

Drugs (total doses)†	Duration (days)	Minimum interval before s.c. infusion (days)	Major specific toxicity**	Comment	Reference
Cyclophosphamide (6 g/m^2); BCNU (300 mg/m^2); etoposide (1 g/m^2)	4	3		So-called 'original CBV'	[34]
Cyclophosphamide (7.2 g/m^2); BCNU (600 mg/m^2); etoposide (1.6 g/m^2)	4	3		Doses of each drug for 'increased CBV' have varied among teams	[35,40]
BCNU (300 mg/m^2); Etoposide (800 mg/m^2); Ara-C (800 mg/m^2); HDM (140 mg/m^2)*	6	1	Mucositis	Standard BEAM regimen can be given with cytokines instead of a transplant [52–62]	[48,49, 52–54]
Cyclophosphamide (120–200 mg/kg) + sTBI or F-TBI (10–14.4 Gy)	5–7	1–2		Follicular non-Hodgkin's lymphoma	[96–97]
F-TBI (12 Gy); etoposide (60 mg/kg; cyclophosphamide (100 mg/kg)	7	2	Mucositis Skin mucositis	BCNU 450 mg/m^2 instead of F-TBI in patients previously irradiated	[98]
Thiotepa (750 mg/m^2); busulphan (10 mg/kg); cyclophosphamide (120 mg/kg)		2		Multiple myeloma	[99]
HDM (200 mg/m^2)		1		Double intensification programme 'Total therapy' multiple myeloma	[100]
HDM (140 mg/m^2) + TBI (8.5–10 Gy)		1			
^{90}Y +CBV				Experimental study of ^{90}Y in Hodgkin's disease	[89]

*BEAM. HDM has been replaced by cyclophosphamide in the USA: BEAC. **Myelosuppression aside.
Abbreviations: HDM = high-dose melphalan; TBI = total body irradiation; sTBI = single-dose TBI; F-TBI = fractionated TBI.

Hodgkin's disease [47–49]. Some teams, however, have used it with apparent success in AML.

BEAM consists of BCNU (300 mg/m^2), etoposide (800 mg/m^2), Ara-C (800 mg/m^2) and high-dose melphalan (HDM) (140 mg/m^2). It is given over six days and stem cells are infused on day 7, exactly one week after its initiation. On practical grounds, this renders transplant planning simple. In the past when HDM was not available in the USA, it was replaced by Cy at a dose of 1.5 g/m^2/day for four days (total 6 g/m^2) and called the BEAC. BEAM and BEAC have been used in all histological types with similar results. In the absence of any randomized study supporting the choice, TBI is preferred by several teams for intensification of low grade (follicular) lymphomas.

The randomized Parma study [50] has shown that intensification with BEAC and stem-cell support is better than conventional consolidation with the DHAP regimen in aggressive non-Hodgkin's lymphoma in chemosensitive relapse. By intention to treat, event-free survival at six years is 46% versus 12% (P = 0.001). In our own institution [51], the event-free survival and transplant-related mortality at five years on a total of 120 non-Hodgkin's lymphoma patients (64 aggressive, 56 low grade) treated with BEAM are shown in Table 36.5. These results clearly confirm the importance of intensification for MRD and for patients in good clinical condition, that is, preferably in first or second complete remission or partial remission but not later. An important finding in our series was that of the role of additional radiotherapy post-transplant on sites of previous involvement. By multivariate analysis, patients transplanted in first complete remission or first partial remission who received additional boost radiotherapy had an improved event-free survival (81 ± 11% versus 60 ± 8%,) and overall survival (89 ± 10% versus 77 ± 6%) at five years (p = 0.02).

While there is no question that BEAM is profoundly myelosuppressive and occasional observations following BEAM have shown long-lasting aplasia, our team has initiated a phase I study of BEAM first followed by GM-CSF [52,53] alone and later followed by the combination of GM-CSF + G-CSF + erythropoietin [54–56] in the absence of re-infused

Table 36.5 BEAM regimen results

Status at transplant	All types of NHL*	Aggressive	Low grade
Event-free survival			
First complete remission	75 ± 12%	75 ± 7%	73 ± 9%
First partial remission	54 ± 12%	58 ± 19%	46 ± 18%
Second or more complete remission	41 ± 14%	29 ± 16%	57 ± 24%
Resistant/refractory	9 ± 9%	10 ± 9%	43 ± 2%
P =	<0.0001	<0.0001	0.5
Transplant-related mortality at five years			
First complete remission	6 ± 4%	6 ± 6%	5 ± 5%
Second or more complete remission	6 ± 6%	11 ± 10%	0%
Partial remission	23 ± 13%	32 ± 21%	10 ± 7%
Resistant/refractory	59 ± 20%	71 ± 22%	–
P =	<0.0001	<0.0001	0.5

NHL = non-Hodgkin's lymphoma.

stem cells for patients with blood and/or marrow involvement precluding an autograft. Laboratory investigations in our institution have revealed a synergistic relationship between these three cytokines in *in vitro* long-term cultures, supporting the use of this combination. To date, a total of 23 patients have received BEAM plus three cytokines: 5 have died, (3 from progressive tumour, 1 from non-documented viral infection with liver involvement and encephalitis after haemopoietic recovery and 1 after haemopoietic recovery from liver haemorrhage following a biopsy for undefined severe aberration of liver function). In the 18 patients alive, the median times to recovery to 500 polymorphonuclear cells/mm^3 and 50 000 platelets/mm^3 were respectively, 18 and 25 days, not significantly different from 15 days and 23 days, respectively, in a parallel cohort of patients autografted in our institution with CD34$^+$ purified marrow stem cells [57]. This experience is unique, and indicates that the BEAM regimen, although very myelosuppressive, is not ablative and spares sufficient stem cells to allow amplification with cytokines *in vivo*.

Other chemotherapy regimens

The Toronto team [58] has used etoposide (60 mg/kg) over 5 or 32 hours and melphalan (160 or 180 mg/m^2) in a series of patients with chemotherapy-sensitive advanced aggressive or follicular transformed lymphomas which were first treated with salvage therapy to maximum response before transplant. In addition, patients with transformed, or any patient with T-cell phenotype received fractionated TBI (12 Gy). The total transplant-related mortality was 10% and the event-free survival at four years 45%, with status at transplant being the most important significant prognostic factor, as in many other series. Indeed, patients transplanted in complete remission had an event-free survival of 62%. A variant of this regimen is the combination of cyclophosphamide + etoposide + TBI used at the Sloan Kettering Hospital in New York [59].

The ICE (ifosfamide, carboplatin, etosposide) regimen, usually used for solid tumours, has been tested in non-Hodgkin's lymphoma. The GELA group is testing the feasibility of a double autografting programme in high-risk patients in a pilot study. Following a first intensification with BEAM, the second involves ICE (ifosfamide 3 g/m^2/day × 4; carboplatin 500 mg/m^2/day × 3; etoposide 500 mg/m^2/day × 4). Preliminary results in a limited number of patients indicate that this approach is feasible in the majority.

EBMT evaluation of pre-autografting regimens for lymphomas

In a recent EBMT survey covering 15 years on a total of 3750 patients treated in 141 institutions, distribution of high-dose regimens used is outlined in Table 36.6.

In agreement with the general principle of high-dose intensification, disease-free survival at ten years was better in patients intensified in first complete remission (70%), over very good partial remission (55%), over second remission (40%), over chemosensitive relapses (30%), with chemoresistant relapses doing the worst (15%).

In a 1995 retrospective study of progression-free survival of 872 patients with Hodgkin's disease and 645 patients with non-Hodgkin's disease, BEAM appeared superior to CBV for the former but inferior for the latter. Chemotherapy and TBI were superior to chemotherapy alone for lymphoblastic lymphomas, but equivalent to chemotherapy alone for other types of disease.

Table 36.6 Distribution of high dose regimens used in Europe for lymphomas

Regimen	Non-Hodgkin's lymphoma	Hodgkin's disease
BEAM	29%	44%
CBV	7%	26%
Chemotherapy + TBI	32%	5%
Other chemotherapy	32%	25%

High-dose regimens in solid tumours

As indicated in the introduction of this chapter, choice of the best pretransplant combination for high-dose intensification of solid tumours derives from knowledge of drug pharmacology, mechanisms of drug resistance, preclinical experience, results of therapy with conventional doses at various stages of the disease, and phase I and II trials of high-dose intensification with escalating schedules. This cannot be summarized here for so many different tumors, but we will review the general principles and give some pertinent information on the drugs most commonly included in the high-dose regimens.

Dose effect

Skipper and Schabel [60] first showed that alkylating agents demonstrate a steep and linear dose–antitumour relationship over a wide dose range in preclinical models. Since alkylating agents are predominantly toxic to bone marrow, considerable dose escalation is possible, limited only by extrahaematopoietic toxicity.

The commonest alkylating agents used for autografting are:
- cyclophosphamide (Cy)
- ifosfamide
- melphalan at high dose (PAM)
- busulfan used almost exclusively for haematological malignancies (see above)
- carmustine (BCNU)
- cisplatin (CDDP) and carboplatin
- thiotepa

Other drugs used include:
- etoposide
- mitoxantrone
- cytosine arabinoside (Ara-C) essentially for haematological malignancies
- paclitaxel used more recently for breast cancer.

Most alkylating agents can be used in the context of autografting at doses far above the doses used conventionally, the so-called 'standard doses'. The ratio of pretransplant dose to standard dose is between four and ten, with a maximum of 30-fold for thiotepa.

In the absence of resistance, there should be a linear increase of tumour log cell kill to dose. This is almost the case with alkylating agents which have a curvilinear relationship of dose to all kill-higher doses producing lower rates of cell kill, probably reflecting heterogeneity of the tumour cells for drug resistance. This is illustrated in Figure 36.1 where the MCF7 breast cancer cell line was incubated *in vitro* with various drugs (notably 4-hydroperoxy-Cy (4HC), the active catabolite of CY, L-PAM and thiotepa).

Another important interest of most alkylating agents is that induced resistance can be overcome by increasing the dose, which is not the case with other agents including anthracyclines. Therefore, almost all combinations used are centered around an alkylating agent which for practical purposes can be considered as the core.

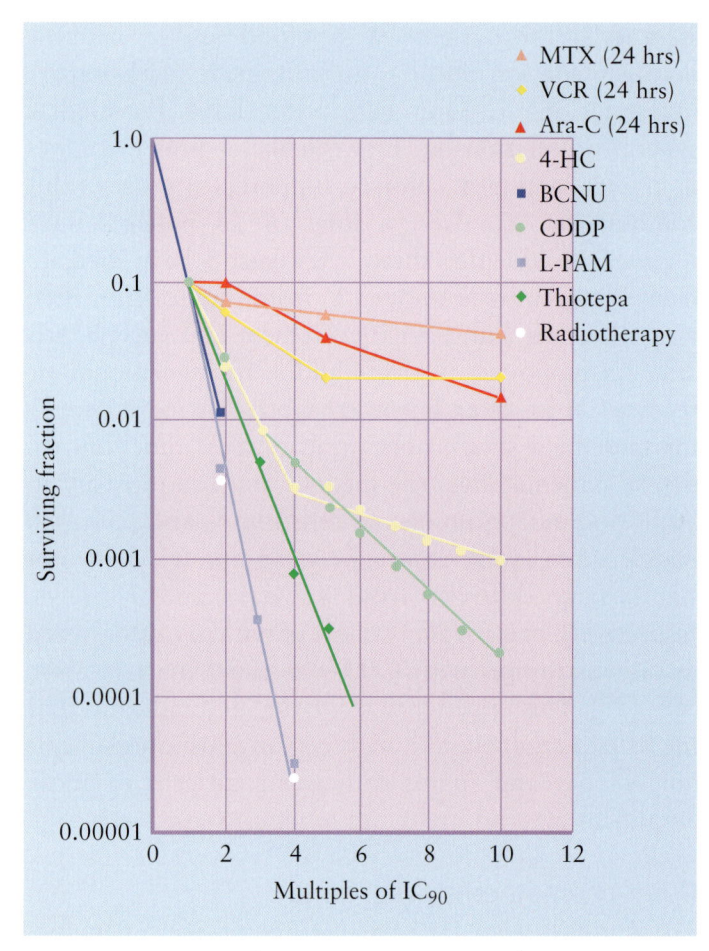

Figure 36.1 MCF7 (breast cancer) in vitro dose–response curves [78]. (Source: Frei E: Pharmacologic strategies for high dose chemotherapy. In: High dose cancer therapy. J Armitage, K Antman eds; Williams & Wilkins, Baltimore, 1995, 1–16).

Pharmacology of agents commonly used in relation to autografting for solid tumours

Cyclophosphamide

Cyclophosphamide, like alkylating agents in general, enters the cells by an active transport mechanism. It can be inactivated within the cytoplasm by conjugation with sulphydryl (SH)-delivering molecules such as glutathione. This explains present trials which are in progress with amifostine (WR 2721). This agent exerts protective effects against alkylators and radiation by combining several mechanisms including acting as an increased concentration of glutathione-SH [61].

Cyclophosphamide is a prodrug which is hydroxylated in the liver into 4-hydroperoxy-cyclophosphamide (4-HC), currently used for *in vitro* treatment in addition to its analogue mafosfamide which also generates directly *in vitro* 4-HC.

Amifostine is also a prodrug which is dephosphorylated by alkaline phosphatase to produce the free SH radical. Normal tissues in contrast to tumour have a higher absorption rate for amifostine, a higher content in alkaline phosphatase and improved activity of the enzyme because of a neutral pH (the pH in tumour cells is more acidic). As a consequence, when normal cells and tumour cells are combined, amifostine is more protective for normal cells. This has been applied to marrow purging in breast cancer [62] as well as in acute leukaemias [63]. In a randomized double-blind study, patients with breast cancer receiving high-dose intensification and autologous marrow purged by 4-HC have been shown to experience faster engraftment if the marrow has been protected before purging by amifostine. We are currently conducting a similar study in patients with acute leukaemia autografted with marrow purged with mafosfamide. Preclinical studies have confirmed the protective effect of amifostine on colony-forming cells of the granulocyte–macrophage lineage (CFU-GM) and the most immature progenitor cells, the long-term culture-initiating cells (LTCIC), and have also somewhat unexpectedly shown sensitization of the leukaemic cells to killing by mafosfamide, so that the differential log cell kill with the combination of amifostine followed by mafosfamide is of a six-order magnitude [63].

Phosphoramide mustard formed intracellularly after penetration by Cy is the predominant antitumour agent. Acrolein excreted in the urine is the toxic agent reponsible for haemorrhagic cystitis [64]. Doses of Cy used in the context of autografting for solid tumours range from 4 to 8 g/m^2. Of interest is the fact that the clearance of Cy increases over the days of administration. Ifosfamide has similar pharmacology to Cy.

Carmustine (BCNU)

BCNU is usually given at doses of 400–800 mg/m^2 as a two-hour infusion. It is prepared in a 10% ethanol solution which may produce hypotension. Its toxicity includes hepatic, lung and cardiac injury. There is a considerable variability in the area under the curve from patient to patient and the area may also be increased by previous drug exposure, specifically Cy. Because BCNU crosses the blood–brain barrier, it is usually used for brain tumours [65].

Thiotepa

Thiotepa has been used widely in the USA, but is less popular in Europe [65–68]. Its principal importance is that it is an alkylating agent which can be given to the patient at 10–50 times the conventional dose because of the autologous rescue. The limiting toxicities in this context are gastrointestinal, hepatic (veno-occlusive disease) and CNS. It is most frequently used in combinations for breast cancer [67–69] and ovarian carcinomas [70,71]. Interestingly, preclinical studies have shown that the antitumour activity of high-dose thiotepa can be increased by prior repeated administration of pentoxyfylline (see also below). This decreases haemopoietic toxicity for the same amount of tumour killing.

Etoposide

Etoposide is second only to alkylating agents in frequency of use. It blocks DNA topoisomerase type II which is important for DNA repair. It shows additive tumour killing with Cy and probably melphalan [72], has a dose-modifying effect for BCNU and is synergistic with platinum compounds. These drugs are therefore usually combined with etoposide. One very good example is the BEAM protocol used for lymphomas (see p. 584). Other examples are the high-dose regimens used for testicular cancers, ovarian cancers and some regimens for breast cancers.

Mitoxantrone

Mitoxantrone is an anthracycline which has a steep dose–response curve for haematopoietic toxicity. It has been given at up to fivefold the conventional dose (60–75 mg/m^2), over several days. It has a long half-life of 8–45 hours and, in addition, binds extensively to tissue. This may explain reports about impairment of marrow engraftment when the marrow has been infused less than seven days after its administration. It has largely been incorporated into regimens used for the treatment of breast cancer and ovarian carcinomas [73–75].

Paclitaxel

Paclitaxel is eliminated by hepatic metabolism and biliary excretion. Its half-life can reach 30 hours. Its toxicity includes peripheral neuropathy, mucositis, renal and lung injuries. The dose should be reduced in case of liver insufficiency. Marrow infusion is recommended after a minimum delay of five days. Paclitaxel so far has been incorporated into regimens for breast and ovarian cancers at total doses not exceeding 400 mg/m^2 [76,77].

Combinations

Combining drugs for better antitumour activity is a basic concept in oncology. It should be remembered that, while a tumour is clonal in origin, modifications occur in its evolution and include mutations and acquisition of drug resistance under the selective pressure of antitumour agents. As indicated above under general principles, combinations are built to overcome resistance by the choice of drugs with no cross-resistance, to take advantage of additive antitumour effects and possible synergistic effects without escalation of toxicity.

An example of an effective combination is cisplatin + bleomycin + vincristine for testicular cancers. Each drug has a different toxicity and all can be combined at full dosage. This has been modified into high-dose regimens using carboplatin instead of cisplatin, etoposide instead of vincristine and an alkylating agent such as cyclophosphamide or ifosfamide.

A quantitative estimate of the antitumour value of combinations has been proposed and referred to as the summation dose intensity SDI [78]: For a three-agent combination, A, B and C, the SDI is 3 if all three can be given at full dose with no reduction because of cumulative toxicity. As an example of this concept for high-dose intensification, the Dana Farber Cancer Center Group in Boston has calculated a SDI of 2.4 for the ICE regimen. Physicians in charge of patients undergoing high-dose regimens should be aware of the pattern of toxicity of each drug, of the increased toxicity potentially due to the combination and of potentially lethal manifestations: multi-organ failure – for example renal failure, veno-occlusive disease, and capillary leak syndrome. In this context, supportive care of the patient is of great importance. This includes, aside from haematological support, antibiotics, antiviral and antifungal agents, prevention of veno-occlusive disease with prostaglandin E$_2$ and/or low-molecular-weight heparins, and possibly other agents such as pentoxyfylline [79,80] which has been tested for its ability to reduce tumour necrosis factor excretion in the post-transplant period. Pentoxyfylline, also inhibits DNA repair and, if given with alkylating agents, can increase antitumour activity by up to tenfold *in vitro* at concentrations not achievable *in vivo*. Tables 36.7 and 36.8 give examples of high dose intensification regimens given for breast cancer and other solid tumours.

Pretransplant regimens and secondary malignancies

The observation that secondary malignancies occurred after allogeneic transplantation suggested that secondary malignancies would be observed following autografting. However, the first observations were only reported in 1993, after sufficient follow-up time had elapsed following the first autologous bone-marrow transplants.

A recent report from the IBMTR on a total of 9732 patients has indicated 109 secondary malignancies with an incidence of 0.6/100 person-years following allogeneic transplantation. A recent update from Seattle [81] has indicated a probability of secondary malignancies of 6% in patients prepared for transplant with chemotherapy-only regimens, but 20% in patients receiving TBI. This is consistent with the observation from the Hôpital Saint-Louis in Paris [82] of a projected incidence of secondary malignancy of 25% at 10 years in patients with aplastic anaemia conditioned with thoraco-abdominal irradiation.

Acquaintance with these data is important since a similar situation can be expected in autografting, namely a higher incidence of secondary malignancies following TBI.

One of the very first observations concerning myelodysplastic syndrome (MDS) made in our institution in 1986 was in a patient who had been autografted a year before for AML in remission. However, because of the initial diagnosis of AML, this complication was at the time confused with disease recurrence and its significance was missed. Numerous observations of MDS post-autografting were made later, in particular in patients autografted for lymphomas, and the incidence rates reported have varied from 9% at

Table 36.7 Examples of high-dose therapy followed by stem-cell transplantation for breast cancer

Drug combination (total dose)*	Duration (days)	Comment	Reference
Cyclophosphamide (6 g/m²); thiotepa (500 mg/m²); carboplatin (800–1600 mg/m²)		STAMP V 'standard'. Two courses possible for lower dose carboplatin	[67–69,101,102]
Thiotepa (900 mg/m²); CDDP* (200 mg/m²); cyclophosphamide (120 mg/kg)	10	Maximum tolerated dose. Renal and gastrointestinal toxicities	[103]
Cyclophosphamide (6 g/m²); carboplatin (2 g/m²); etoposide (625 mg/m²)	4	Mucositis. Reversible neuropathy. Two cycles well tolerated	[104]
Ifosfamide (20 g/m²); carboplatin (1.8 g/m²); etoposide (3 g/m²)		Maximum tolerated dose for ICE	[105]
Mitoxantrone (90 mg/m²); thiotepa (1200 mg/m²)		Maximum tolerated dose	[105]
Paclitaxel (360 mg/m²); mitoxantrone (75 mg/m²); thiotepa (900 mg/m²)		Maximum tolerated dose	[105]
Cyclophosphamide (6 g/m²); mitoxantrone (70 mg/m²); paclitaxel (250–400 mg/m²)	4	Excalation phase I/II study Ethylic alcohol infused with paclitaxel Bradycardia	[76]
Doxorubicin (165 mg/m²); etoposide (60 mg/m²); cyclophosphamide (100 mg/m²)	7	Mucositis Etoposide-related neuropathy	[106]
Mitoxantrone (60–90 mg/m²); HDM (140–180 mg/m²); carboplatin (1.5 g/m²); etoposide (1.5 g/m²)	4 3	Double ASCT programme Mucositis	[107]
Cyclophosphamide (5.6 g/m²); CDDP* (165 mg/m²); BCNU (600 mg/m²)	4	Outpatient care Pulmonary toxicity	[108.109]
Ifosfamide (12 g/m²); epirubicin (180 mg/m²); carboplatin (900 mg/m²)	5		[110]
HDM (180 mg/m²); etoposide (3000 mg/m²)	3	Mucositis Etoposide related neuropathy	[72]

*CDDP = cisplatin. For other abbreviations see text and Tables 36.1 and 36.4.

Table 36.8 Examples of high-dose therapy followed by stem-cell transplantation in solid tumours (other than breast cancer)

Disease	Drug combination (total dose)	Duration (days)	Comment	Reference
Testicular germ cell	Carboplatin (1500 mg/m²); etoposide (2400 mg/m²); ifosfamide (10 g/m²)	4	ICE regimen. Maximum tolerated dose in an escalating phase I/II study	[111]
	Carboplatin (≤ 2200 mg/m²); etoposide (1800 mg/m²); Cyclophosphamide (6.4 g/m²)	4	Carbopec regimen. Carboplatin dose dependent on creatinine clearance	[112,113]
	Carboplatin (875–1225 mg/m²); etoposide (1000–1250 mg/m²); ifosfamide (7.5–12.5 g/m²)	4	2 course programme	[114]
Ovarian cancer	Cyclophosphamide (120 mg/kg); carboplatin (1.5 g/m²); mitoxantrone (75 mg/m²)	6	Maximum tolerated dose renal toxicity: gastrointestinal tract, ears, renal	[74]
	Carboplatin (1.6 g/m²); mitoxantrone (36–60 mg/m²); thiotepa (500-600 mg/m²); etoposide (800 mg/m²)		Second course following a first course of HDM	[71]
	Carboplatin (1200 mg/m²); etoposide (1 g/m²); HDM (140 mg/m²)	5		[71]
Small-cell lung cancer	Carboplatin (750 mg/m²); ifosfamide (12 g/m²); etoposide (1500 mg/m²); epirubicin (150 mg/m²)		Chest + cranial irradiation post-transplant. Toxicity: mucositis	[115]
	Ifosfamide (10 g/m²); Carboplatin (1200 mg/m²); etoposide (1200 mg/m²)		Three cycles of intensification	[116]
Brain tumours	BCNU (800 mg/m²) or totemustine (800 mg/m²)	1 2	Wait 72 hours before ASCT. Radiotherapy after ASCT	[65]
Medulloblastoma	Carboplatin (1500 mg/m²); thiotepa (900 mg/m²); etoposide (750 mg/m²)			[117]
Neuroblastoma	Vincristine (5 mg); HDM (180 mg/m²); F-TBI (12 Gy)	5	French co-operative group regimen. Double intensification tested with this regimen as second	[118,119]
Melanoma	BCNU (600 mg/m²) or thiotepa (900 mg/m²); HDM (90 mg/m²)			[120]

Abbreviations: see Tables 36.1 and 36.4.

three years to 14.5% at five years. In the early observation period there was some indication that the incidence rate would be higher following peripheral blood stem-cell infusion than following marrow infusion, but this has not been confirmed [83–85].

Secondary malignancies are not only the consequence of the autograft *per se*, but result from the cumulative effects of the primary malignancy (the incidence of secondary malignancies is higher in patients with a primary malignancy), the number of courses of chemotherapy delivered and the pretransplant regimen, particularly if it includes TBI. It is likely that the incidence is higher in patients heavily pretreated before reaching intensification, and it can be argued that if high-dose intensification is given early in the course of the disease, it would be associated with a much lower incidence of secondary malignancy.

New approaches

The future for autografting will be directed towards defining new regimens which combine high antitumour activity and low toxicity. In this respect, higher selectivity for tumour cells would be a major achievement. Many teams are preparing and testing radiolabelled immunoglobulin therapy in both preclinical models and in man [86,87]. This can be included either in the pretransplant regimen or used after the autograft in an effort to eradicate persistent minimal residual disease.

Antibodies used are mainly monoclonal murine antibodies. Unfortunately, most patients develop human antimurine antibodies. Human monoclonal antibodies have been manufactured to bypass this obstacle. Currently, human IgM. Fab or $f(ab')_2$ fragments are preferred since they penetrate tumours better. These antibodies are chelated either to ^{111}In (indium) or ^{90}Y (yttrium), better antitumour activity being achieved with the latter.

Interesting results have been achieved in Hodgkin's disease with radiolabelled immunoglobulin therapy coupled or not coupled to ASCT with ^{111}In- or ^{90}Y-labelled antiferritin [88,89]. Results have also been reported in patients with AML (more specifically, AML3) with ^{131}I-labelled anti-CD33 monoclonal antibody (IM-195) [90,91], and in patients with breast cancer with ^{90}Y-labelled antibodies against the human milk fat globulin and human mammary epithelial antigens (the epitope named BrE-3) [92].

Conclusion

The notion of a pretransplant regimen, especially in the field of autografting, has changed over the past twenty years. Today, it cannot only be regarded as a high-dose regimen given in the few days preceding the infusion of stem cells. It must be approached as a strategy rather than a regimen which begins with the first step of conventional tumour load reduction, continuing to the mobilization of stem cells to be cryopreserved and then infused, and including high-dose intensification which may be sequential. It finishes with whatever additional therapy may be offered to the patient post-transplant such as cytokines, radiotherapy, immunotherapy and, in the future, radiolabelled immunoglobulin therapy.

The future may well lie in the direction of what we, in our institution, refer to as the 'smart combination'. First, an autologous stem-cell transplant to utilize the best antitumour regimen without the potential toxicity of an allograft, followed by infusion of allogeneic stem cells to take advantage of an antitumour immune reaction.

References

1. Gorin NC, Najman A and Duhamel G. Autologous bone marrow transplantation in acute myelocytic leukemia. *Lancet* 1997; **14**: 1050.
2. Thomas ED, Ashley CA and Lochte HE. Homograft of bone marrow in dogs after lethal total body irradiation. *Blood* 1959; **14**: 720–736.
3. Thomas ED, Buchner T, Clift RA *et al*. Marrow transplantation for acute non-lymphoblastic leukemia in first remission. *New Engl J Med* 1979; **301**: 597–599.
4. Thomas ED, Buchner CD, Banaji M *et al*. One hundred patients with acute leukemia with chemotherapy, total body irradiation and allogeneic marrow transplantation. *Blood* 1977; **49**: 511–533.
5. Thomas ED, Clift RA, Herman J *et al*. Marrow transplantation for acute non-lymphoblastic leukemia in first remission using fractionated or single dose irradiation. *Int J Radiat Oncol Biol Phys* 1982; **8**: 817–821.
6. Thomas ED. Total body irradiation regimens for marrow grafting. *Int J Radiat Oncol Biol Phys* 1990; **19**: 1285–1288.
7. Barrett A, Depledge MH and Powles RL. Interstitial pneumonitis following bone marrow transplantation after low dose rate TBI. *Int J Radiat Oncol Biol Phys* 1983; **9**: 1029–1033.
8. Deeg HJ, Flournoy N, Sullivan K *et al*. Cataracts after total body irradiation and marrow transplantation. Effect of dose fractionation. *Int J Radiat Oncol Biol Phys* 1984; **10**: 957–964.
9. Clift RA, Buckner D, Appelbaum R *et al*. Allogeneic marrow transplantation in patients with acute myeloid leukemia in

first remission: a randomized trial of 2 irradiation regimens. *Blood* 1990; **76**: 1867–1871.

10. Socie G, Devergies A, Gerinsky T *et al*. Influence of fractionation of total body irradiation on complications and relapse rate for chronic myelogenous leukemia. *Int J Radiat Oncol Biol Phys* 1991; **20**: 397–404.

11. Oszahin M, Pene F, Touboul E *et al*. Total body irradiation before bone marrow transplantation. Results of two randomized instantaneous dose rate in 157 patients. *Cancer* 1992; **69**: 2853–2865.

12. Gorin NC. High-dose therapy for acute myelocytic leukemia. In: *High-Dose Cancer Therapy*, 2nd edn. JO Armitage and KH Antman (eds), 1995: 635–678 (Baltimore, MD: Williams & Wilkins).

13. Belkacemi Y, Oszahin M, Pene F *et al*. Cataractogenesis after total body irradiation. *Int J Radiat Oncol Biol Phys* 1996; **35**: 53–60.

14. Ozsahin M, Belkacemi Y, Pene F *et al*. Interstitial pneumonitis following autologous bone marrow transplantation conditioned with cyclophosphamide and total-body irradiation. *Int J Radiat Oncol Biol Phys* 1996; **34**: 71–77.

15. Perot C, Van Den Akker J, Laporte JPh *et al*. Multiple chromosome abnormalities in patients with acute leukemia after autologous bone marrow transplantation using total body irradiation and marrow purged with mafosfamide. *Leukaemia* 1993; **7**: 509–515.

16. Blume KG, Forman SEJ, O'Donnell MR *et al*. Total body irradiation and high-dose etoposide: a new preparatory regimen for bone marrow transplantation in patients with advanced hematological malignancies. *Blood* 1987; **69**: 1015–1020.

17. Cahn JY, Bordigoni P, Souillet G *et al*. The TAM regimen prior to allogeneic and autologous bone marrow transplantation for high-risk acute lymphoblastic leukemias: a cooperative study of 62 patients. *Bone Marrow Transplant* 1991; **7**: 1–4.

18. Vose JM, Reed ED, Pippert GC *et al*. Mesna compared with continuous bladder irrigation as uroprotection during high-dose chemotherapy and transplantation: a randomized trial. *J Clin Oncol* 1993; **11**: 1306–1310.

19. Santos GW, Tutschka PJ, Brookmeyer R *et al*. Marrow transplantation for acute non-lymphocytic leukemia after treatment with busulfan and cyclophosphamide. *New Engl J Med* 1983; **309**: 1347–1353.

20. Blume KG, Kopecky KJ, Henslee-Downey JP *et al*. A prospective randomized comparison of total body irradiation–etoposide versus busulfan–cyclophosphamide as preparatory regimens for bone marrow transplantation in patients with leukemia who were not in first remission: a South-West Oncology Group Study. *Blood* 1993; **81**: 2187–2193.

21. Ringden O, Ruutu T, Remberger M *et al*. A randomized trial comparing busulfan with total body irradiation as conditioning in allogeneic marrow transplant recipients with leukemia. A report from the Nordic Bone Marrow Transplantation Group. *Blood* 1994; **83**: 2723–2730.

22. Ringden O, Labopin M, Tura S *et al*. A comparison of busulfan versus total body irradiation combined with cyclophosphamide as conditioning for autograft or allograft bone marrow transplantation in patients with acute leukaemia. *Br J Haematol* 1996; **93**: 637–645.

23. Grochow LB, Jones RJ, Brundrett RB *et al*. Pharmacokinetics of busulfan: correlation with veno-occlusive disease in patients undergoing bone marrow transplantation. *Cancer Chemother Pharmacol* 1989; **25**: 55–61.

24. Vassal G, Deroussent A, Hartmann O *et al*. Dose dependent neurotoxicity of high dose busulfan in children: a clinical and pharmacological study. *Cancer Res* 1990; **50**: 6203–6207.

25. Grochow LB. Busulfan disposition: the role of therapeutic monitoring in bone marrow transplantation induction regimens. *Semin Oncol* 1993; **20**: 18–25.

26. Tutschka PJ, Copelan EA, Klein JP *et al*. Bone marrow transplantation for leukemia following a new busulfan and cyclophosphamide regimen. *Blood* 1987; **70**: 1382–1388.

27. Blaise D, Maraninchi D, Archimbaud E *et al*. Allogeneic bone marrow transplantation for acute myeloid leukemia in first remission: a randomized trial or a busulfan/cytoxan versus citoxan/total body irradiation as preparative regimen: a report from the Groupe d'Etudes de la Greffe de Moelle Osseuse. *Blood* 1992; **79**: 2578–2582.

28. Mittchel PL, Shepherd VD, Proctor HM *et al*. Peripheral blood stem cells used to augment autologous bone marrow transplantation. *Arch Dis Child* 1994; **70**: 237–240.

29. Przepiorka D, Dimopoulos M, Smith T *et al*. Thiotepa, busulfan and cyclophosphamide as a preparative regimen for marrow transplantation: risk factors for early regimen-related toxicity. *Ann Haematol* 1994; **68**: 183–188.

30. Meloni G, De Fabritiis P, Carella AM *et al*. Autologous bone marrow transplantation in patients with AML in first complete remission: results of two different conditioning regimens after the same induction and consolidation therapy. *Bone Marrow Transplant* 1990; **5**: 29–32.

31. Meloni G, De Fabritiis P, Petti MC *et al*. BAVC regimen and autologous bone marrow transplantation in patients with acute myelogenous leukemia in second remission. *Blood* 1990; **12**: 2282–2285.

32. Meloni G, Vignetti M, Andrizzi C *et al*. Autologous BMT in AML: the nine-year experience at Hematology University 'La Sapienza' of Rome. 21st Annual Meeting of the European Group for Bone Marrow Transplantation, Harrogate, UK, March 13–17 1994. *Bone Marrow Transplant*, 529a.

33. Belkacami Y, Labopin M, Vernant JP *et al*. Cataract incidence after total body irradiation (TBI) and marrow transplantation (BMT) for acute leukemia (AL) in complete remission (CR). An EBMT study. *Int J Radiat Oncol* 1998, in press.

34. Haioun C, Lepage E, Gisselbrecht Ch *et al*. A GELA study: autologous bone marrow transplantation versus sequential chemotherapy for aggressive non-Hodgkin's lymphoma in first complete remission: a study of 542 patients (LNH 87-2 protocol). *Bone Marrow Transplant* 1996; **17**(Suppl 1): S144.

35. Ratanatharathorn V, Uberti J, Karanes C *et al*. Prospective comparative trial of autologous versus allogeneic bone marrow transplantation in patients with non-Hodgkin's lymphoma. *Blood* 1994; **84**: 1050–1055.

36. Carella AM, Congiu AM, Gaozza E *et al*. High-dose chemotherapy with autologous bone marrow transplantation in 50 advanced resistant Hodgkin's disease patients: an Italian Study Group report. *J Clin Oncol* 1988; **6**: 1411–1416.

37. Ahmed T, Ciavarella D, Feldman E *et al*. High-dose potentially myeloablative chemotherapy and autologous bone marrow transplantation for patients with advanced Hodgkin's disease. *Leukaemia* 1989; **3**: 19–22.

38. Wheeler C, Antin JH, Churchill WH et al. Cyclophosphamide, carmustine and etoposide with autologous bone marrow transplantation in refractory Hodgkin's disease and non-Hodgkin's lymphoma: a dose finding study. J Clin Oncol 1990; 8: 648–656.

39. Armitage JO, Bierman PJ, Vose JM et al. Autologous bone marrow transplantation for patients for relapsed Hodgkin's disease. Am J Med 1991; 91: 605–611.

40. Reece DE, Barnett MJ, Connors JM et al. Intensive chemotherapy with cyclophosphamide, carmustine and etoposide followed by autologous bone marrow transplantation for relapsed Hodgkin's disease. J Clin Oncol 1991; 9: 1871–1879.

41. Weaver CH, Appelbaum FR, Petersen FB et al. High-dose cyclophosphamide, carmustine and etoposide followed by autologous bone marrow transplantation in patients with lymphoid malignancies who have received dose limiting radiation therapy. J Clin Oncol 1993; 11: 1329–1335.

42. Bierman PJ, Bagin RG, Jagannath S et al. High-dose chemotherapy followed by autologous hematopoietic rescue in Hodgkin's disease: long-term follow up in 128 patients. Ann Oncol 1993; 4: 767–773.

43. Vose JM, Andersson JR, Kessinger A et al. High-dose chemotherapy and autologous hematopoietic stem cell transplantation for aggressive non-Hodgkin's lymphoma. J Clin Oncol 1993; 11: 1846–1851.

44. Martin-Algarra S, Bierman PJ, Anderson J et al. Cyclophosphamide, BCNU and VP-16 followed by autologous bone marrow or peripheral blood stem cell transplantation in Hodgkin's disease. Retrospective analysis of 10 year experience at the University of Nebraska Medical Center. Blood 1994; 84: 536a.

45. Reece DE, Connors JM, Spinelli JJ et al. Intensive therapy with cyclophosphamide, carmustine, etoposide + cisplatin and autologous bone marrow transplantation for Hodgkin's disease in first relapse after combination chemotherapy. Blood 1994; 83: 1193–1199.

46. Reece DE, Barnett MJ, Sheperd JD et al. High-dose cyclosphosphamide, carmustin (BCNU) and etoposide (VP16-213) with or without cisplatin (CBV + P) and autologous transplantation for patients with Hodgkin's disease who fail to enter a complete remission after combination chemotherapy. Blood 1995; 86: 451–456.

47. Philip T, Biron P, Maraninchi D et al. Massive chemotherapy with autologous bone marrow transplantation in 50 cases of bad prognosis non-Hodgkin's lymphoma. Br J Haematol 1985; 60: 599–609.

48. Philip T, Armitage JO, Spitzer ERG et al. High-dose therapy and ABMT after failure of conventional therapy in adults with intermediate grade or high-grade non-Hodgkin's lymphoma. New Engl J Med 1987; 316: 1493–1498.

49. Mills W, Chopra R, McMillan A et al. BEAM chemotherapy and autologous bone marrow transplantation for patients with relapsed or refractory non-Hodgkin's lymphoma. J Clin Oncol 1995; 13: 588–595.

50. Philip T, Guglielmi C, Hagenbeck A et al. Autologous bone marrow transplantation as compared with salvage chemotherapy in relapses of chemotherapy-sensitive non-Hodgkin's lymphoma. New Engl J Med 1995; 333: 1540–1545.

51. Fouillard L, Labopin M, Laporte JPh et al. Autologous stem cell transplantation for non Hodgkin's lymphomas. The role of graft purging and radiotherapy post transplantation. Results of a retrospective analysis on 120 patients autografted in a single institution. 1997. Submitted.

52. Fouillard L, Gorin NC and Laporte JPh. Recombinant human granulocyte–macrophage colony-stimulating factor + the BEAM regimen instead of ABMT. Lancet 1989; i: 1460.

53. Laporte JPh, Fouillard L and Douay L. GM-CSF instead of autologous bone marrow transplantation after the BEAM regimen. Lancet 1991; 338: 601–602.

54. Laporte JPh, Lesage S and Woler M. Administration of three cytokines instead of bone marrow transplantation in an HIV-positive patient with high-grade lymphoma. [Letters to the Editor.] Eur J Haematol 1994; 53: 123–125.

55. Laporte JPh, Karrakassis D, Lesage S et al. Can hemopoietic growth factors replace autologous bone marrow transplantation (ABMT) in lymphoma patients when tumoral marrow infiltration precludes it? Blood 1995; 86(Suppl 1): 439a.

56. Laporte JPH, Karakassis D, Lesage S et al. How can cytokines help? Bone Marrow Transplant 1997; 19(Suppl 1): S20.

57. Gorin NC, Lopez M, Laporte JPh et al. Preparation and successful engraftment of purified CD34+ bone marrow progenitor cells in patients with non-Hodgkin's lymphoma. Blood 1995; 85: 1647–1654.

58. Prince HN and Keating A. Autologous bone marrow and blood cell transplantation with etoposide and melphalan for poor prognosis non-Hodgkin's lymphoma: the importance of disease status at transplant. In: Autologous Marrow and Blood Transplantation. Proceedings of the 7th International Symposium, Arlington, Texas. KA Dicke and A Keating (eds), 1995: 339–356 (Arlington TX: Cancer Center and Educational Institute Arlington).

59. Gulati S, Yahalom J, Acaba L et al. Treatment of patients with relapsed and resistant non-Hodgkin's lymphoma using total body irradiation, etoposide and cyclophosphamide and autologous bone marrow transplantation. J Clin Oncol 1992; 10: 936–941.

60. Schabel FM, Griswold DP, Corbett TH et al. Testing therapeutic hypotheses in mice and men: observation of therapeutic activity against advanced solid tumors in man treated with anticancer drugs that have demonstrated potential clinical utility for treatment of advanced solid tumors in mice. In: Methods in Cancer Research. VT DeVita and H Bush (eds), 1979: 3–51 (Orlando FL: Academic Press).

61. Capizzi RL. Amifostine: the preclinical basis for broad-spectrum selective cytoprotection of normal tissues from cytotoxic therapies. Semin Oncol 1996; 23(Suppl 8): 2–17.

62. Shpall EJ, Stemmer SM, Hami L et al. Amifostine (WR 2721) shortens the engraftment period of 4-hydroperoxycyclophosphamide purged bone marrow in breast cancer patients receiving high-dose chemotherapy with autologous bone marrow support. Blood 1994; 83: 3132–3137.

63. Douay L, Chen Hu, Giarratana MC et al. Amifostine improves the antileukemic therapeutic index of mafosfamide: implications for bone marrow purging. Blood 1995; 86: 2849–2855.

64. Cox PJ. Cyclophosphamide cystitis. Identification of acrolein as the causative agent. Biochem Pharmacol 1979; 28: 2045–2049.

65. Hildebrand J, Sahmoud T, Mignolet F, Brucher JM and Afra D. Adjuvant therapy with dibromodulcitol and BCNU

increases survival of adults with malignant gliomas. EORTC Brain Tumor Group. *Neurology* 1994; **44**(8): 1479–1483.

66. Herzig G (ed.). *High-dose Thiotepa and Autologous Bone Marrow Transplantation in Advances in Cancer Chemotherapy*, 1987. (New York: John Wiley).

67. Antman K, Ayash L, Elias A *et al*. A phase II study of high dose cyclophosphamide, thiotepa and carboplatin with autologous marrow support in women with measurable advanced breast cancer responding to standard dose therapy. *J Clin Oncol* 1992; **10**: 102–110.

68. Antman K, Ayash L, Elias A *et al*. High dose cyclophosphamide thiotepa and carboplatin with autologous marrow support in women with measurable advanced breast cancer responding to standard dose therapy: analysis by age. *J Nat Cancer Inst* 1994; **16**: 91–94.

69. Perry J, Cruz J, Hopkins J *et al*. High-dose cyclophosphamide, thiotepa and carboplatin (CTCb) with autologous stem cell transplantation (ASCT) for poor prognosis breast cancer. *Proc Am Soc Clin Oncol* 1994; **13**: 93.

70. Shpall E, Jones RB, Bearman SI and Purdy MP. Future strategies for the treatment of advanced epithelial ovarian cancer using high-dose chemotherapy and autologous bone marrow support. *Gynaecol Oncol* 1994; **54**: 357–361.

71. Viens P and Maraninchi D. High-dose chemotherapy and autologous marrow transplantation for common epithelial ovarian carcinoma. In: *High-Dose Cancer Therapy*, 2nd edn. J Armitage and K Antman (eds), 1995; 847–854 (Baltimore MD: Williams and Wilkins).

72. Razis ED, Samonis G, Cook P *et al*. Phase one trial of high-dose melphalan, high-dose etoposide and autologous bone marrow reinfusion in solid tumors: an Eastern Cooperative Oncology Group (ECOG) study. *Bone Marrow Transplant* 1994; **14**: 443–448.

73. Smyth JF, MacPherson JS, Warrington PS *et al*. The clinical pharmacology of mitoxantrone. *Cancer Chemother Pharmacol* 1986; **17**: 149–152.

74. Stiff PJ, McKenzie RS, Alberts DS *et al*. Phase I clinical and pharmacokinetic study of high-dose mitoxantrone combined with carboplatin, cyclophosphamide and autologous bone marrow rescue: high response rate for refractory ovarian carcinoma. *J Clin Oncol* 1994; **12**: 176–183.

75. Stiff PJ, Bayer R, Camarda M *et al*. A phase II trial of high-dose mitoxantrone, carboplatin and cyclophosphamide with autologous bone marrow rescue for recurrent epithelial ovarian carcinoma: analysis of risk factors for clinical outcome. *Gynaecol Oncol* 1995; **57**: 278–285.

76. Glück S, Cano P, Dorreen M *et al*. High-dose cyclophosphamide (CTX), mitoxanthrone (MXT) and paclitaxel (Taxol, TXL) for the treatment of metastatic breast cancer with stem cell support. *8th International Symposium on Autologous Marrow and Blood Transplantation*, Arlington, Texas, August 18–21 1994.

77. Sonnichsen DS, Hurwitz CA, Pratt CB *et al*. Saturable pharmacokinetics and paclitaxel pharmacodynamics in children with solid tumors. *J Clin Oncol* 1994; **12**: 532–538.

78. Frei E. Pharmacologic strategies for high-doses chemotherapy. In: *High-Dose Cancer Therapy*. J Armitage and K Antman (eds), 1995: 1–16 (Baltimore MD: Williams & Wilkins).

79. Dezube BJ, Fridovich-Keil JL, Bouvard I *et al*. Pentoxifylline and well-being in patients with cancer. *Lancet* 1990; **335**: 662.

80. Teicher BA, Holden SA, Herman TS *et al*. Effect of pentoxifylline as a modulator of alkylating agent activity *in vitro* and *in vivo*. *Anticancer Res* 1991; **11**: 153–158.

81. Witherspoon RP, Storb R, Pepe M *et al*. Cumulative incidence of secondary solid malignant tumors in aplastic anemia patients given marrow graft after conditioning with chemotherapy alone. *Blood* 1992; **79**: 289–290.

82. Socié G, Henry-Amar M, Cosset JM *et al*. Increased incidence of solid malignant tumors after bone marrow transplant for severe aplastic anemia. *Blood* 1991; **78**: 277–279.

83. Miller JS, Arthur DC, Litz CE *et al*. Myelodysplastic syndrome after autologous bone marrow transplantation: an additional late complication of curative cancer therapy. *Blood* 1994; **83**: 3780–3786.

84. Traweek T, Slovak M, Nadermanee A *et al*. Clonal karyotypic hematopoietic cell abnormalities occurring after autologous bone marrow transplantation for Hodgkin's disease and non-Hodgkin's lymphoma. *Blood* 1994; **84**: 957–963.

85. Stone RM. Myelodysplastic syndrome after autologous transplantation for lymphoma: the price of progress? *Blood* 1994; **83**: 3437–3440.

86. Goldenberg DM. New developments in monoclonal antibodies for cancer detection and therapy. *CA Cancer J Clin* 1994; **44**: 43–63.

87. Vriesendorp HM, Quadri SM, Stinson RL *et al*. Selection of reagents for human radioimmunotherapy. *Int J Radiat Oncol Biol Phys* 1992; **22**: 37–45.

88. Quadri SM, Lai J, Mohammadpour H *et al*. Assessment of radiolabeled stabilized f(ab')$_2$ fragments of monoclonal antiferritin in NUD mouse model. *J Nucl Med* 1993; **34**: 2152–2159.

89. Vriesendorp HM and Quadri SM. Hodgkin's disease: a perpetual paradigm for new therapeutic approaches. In: *Autologous Marrow and Blood Transplantation*. Proceedings of the 7th International Symposium, Arlington, Texas. KA Dicke and A Keating (eds), 1995: 709–719. (Arlington TX: Cancer Treatment Research and Educational Institute Arlington).

90. Scheinberg DA, Lovett D, Divgi CR *et al*. A phase I trial of monoclonal antibody M-195 in acute myelogenous leukemia: specific bone marrow targeting and internalization of radionuclide. *J Clin Oncol* 1991; **9**: 478–479.

91. Caron PC, Jurcic JG, Scott AM *et al*. A phase Ib trial of humanized monoclonal antibody M-195 (anti-CD 33) in myeloid leukemia: specific targeting without immunogenicity. *Blood* 1994; **83**: 1760–1768.

92. Jones RB, Stemmer SM, Kasliwal R *et al*. Intensive radiolabeled antibreast monoclonal antibody ^{90}Y-BrE-3 with autologous hematopoietic cell support preliminary results. In: *Autologous Marrow and Blood Transplantation*. *Proceeding of the 7th International Symposium*, Arlington, Texas. KA Dicke and A Keating (eds), 1995: 727–734 (Arlington TX: Cancer Center and Educational Institute Arlington).

93. Kantarjian AM, Talpaz M, Andersson D *et al*. High-doses of cyclophosphamide, etoposide and total body irradiation followed by autologous stem cell transplantation in the management of patients with chronic myelogenous leukemia. *Bone Marrow Transplant* 1994; **14**: 57–61.

94. Gulati S, Acaba L, Hahalom J *et al*. Autologous bone marrow transplantation for acute myelogenous leukemia using 4-hydroperoxycyclophosphamide and VP-16 purged bone marrow. *Bone Marrow Transplant* 1992; **10**: 1–6.

95. Vassal G. Pharmacological-guided dose adjustment of busulfan in high-dose chemotherapy regimens: rationale and pitfalls [Review]. *Anticancer Res* 1994; **14**(6a): 2363–2370.
96. Gribben JG, Freedman AS, Neuberg D *et al*. Immunologic purging of marrow assessed by PCR before autologous bone marrow transplantation for B-cell lymphoma. *New Engl J Med* 1991; **325**: 1525–1533.
97. Haas R, Murea S and Moss M. Myeloablative high-dose therapy with peripheral blood stem cell (PBSC) transplantation in low grade non-Hodgkin's lymphomas (NHL). *8th International Symposium on Autologous Marrow and Blood Transplantation, Arlington, Texas, August 18–21* 1994.
98. Horning SJ, Negrin RS, Chao JC *et al*. Fractionated total body irradiation, etoposide and cyclophosphamide + autografting in Hodgkin's disease and non-Hodgkin's lymphoma. *J Clin Oncol* 1994; **12**: 2552–2558.
99. Dimipoulos MA, Ester J, Huh Y *et al*. Intensive chemotherapy with blood progenitor transplantation for primary resistant multiple myeloma. *Br J Haematol* 1994; **87**: 730–734.
100. Vesole DH, Barlogie B and Jagannath S. High-dose therapy for refractory multiple myeloma: improved prognosis with better supportive care and double transplants. *Blood* 1994; **84**: 950–956.
101. Ayash L, Elias E, Wheeler C *et al*. Double dose intensive chemotherapy with autologous marrow and peripheral blood progenitor cell support for metastatic breast cancer: a feasibility study. *J Clin Oncol* 1994; **12**: 37–44.
102. Ayash L, Wheeler C, Fairclough D *et al*. Prognostic factors for prolonged progression free survival with high-dose chemotherapy with autologous stem cell support for advanced breast cancer. *J Clin Oncol* 1995; **13**: 2043–2049.
103. Ghalie R, Richman CM and Adler SS. Treatment of metastatic breast cancer with a split course high-dose chemotherapy regimen and autologous bone marrow transplantation. *J Clin Oncol* 1994; **12**: 342–346.
104. Brown ER, Sridhara R, Sledge GW *et al*. Tandem autotransplantation for the treatment of metastatic breast cancer. *J Clin Oncol* 1995; **13**: 2050–2055.
105. Perkins J, Elfenbein G, Fields K *et al*. Novel high-dose regimens for the treatment of breast cancer. *8th International Symposium, Arlington, Texas, August 18–21* 1994.
106. Somio G, Dorochow JH, Forman SJ *et al*. High-dose doxorubicin, etoposide and cyclophosphamide with stem cell reinfusion in patients with metastatic or high-risk primary breast cancer. City of Hope Bone Marrow Oncology Team. *Cancer* 1994; **73**: 1678–1685.
107. Patrone F, Ballestrero A, Ferrando F *et al*. Four step high-dose sequential chemotherapy with double hematopoietic progenitor cell rescue for metastatic breast cancer. *J Clin Oncol* 1995; **13**: 840–846.
108. Peters WP, Ross M, Vredenburgh JJ *et al*. High-dose chemotherapy and autologous bone marrow support as consolidation after standard dose adjuvant therapy for high-risk primary breast cancer. *J Clin Oncol* 1993; **11**: 1132–1143.
109. Peters WP, Ross M, Vredenburgh JJ *et al*. The use of intensive clinic support to permit out patient autologous bone marrow transplantation for breast cancer. *Semin Oncol* 1994; **21**: 25–31.
110. Hochaus S, Pförsich M, Murea S *et al*. Immunomagnetic selection of CD34$^+$ peripheral blood stem cells for autografting in patients with breast cancer. Submitted.
111. Siegert W, Beyer J, Strohsheer I *et al*. High-dose treatment with carboplatin, etoposide and ifosfamide followed by autologous stem cell transplantation in relapsed or refractory germ cell cancer: a phase I–II study. The German Testicular Cancer Cooperative Study Group. *J Clin Oncol* 1994; **12**: 1223–1231.
112. Droz JP *et al*. Prediction of long-term response after high-dose chemotherapy with autologous bone marrow transplantation in the salvage treatment of non-seminomatous germ cell tumors. *Eur J Cancer* 1993; **29a**: 818–821.
113. Pico JL, Fadel E, Ibrahim A *et al*. High-dose chemotherapy followed by hematological support: experience in the treatment of germ cell tumors. *Bull Cancer (Paris)* 1995; **82**(Suppl 1): 56S–60S.
114. Lotz JP, Andre T, Donsimoni R *et al*. High dose chemotherapy with ifosfamide, carboplatin and etoposide combined with autologous bone marrow transplantation for the treatment of poor prognosis germ cell tumors and metastatic trophoblastic disease in adults. *Cancer* 1995; **75**: 874–885.
115. Brugger W, Frommhold H, Pressler K *et al*. Use of high-dose etoposide–ifosfamide–carboplatin–epirubicin and peripheral blood progenitor cell transplantation in limited disease small cell lung cancer. *Semin Oncol* 1995; **22**(Suppl 2): 3–8.
116. Leyvraz S, Rosti G, Lange A *et al*. Multiple cycles of high-dose ICE chemotherapy with peripheral blood stem cells (PBSC) in small cell lung cancer (SCLC). EBMT study. *8th International Symposium of Autologous Marrow and Blood Transplantation, Arlington, Texas, August 18–21* 1994.
117. Dunkel IJ and Finlay JL. High-dose chemotherapy with autologous stem cell rescue for medulloblastoma and supratentorial PNET. *8th International Symposium of Autologous Marrow and Blood Transplantation, Arlington, Texas, August 18–21* 1994.
118. Philip T, Zucker JM, Bernard JL *et al*. Improved survival at 2 and 5 years in the LMCE1 on selected group of 72 children with a stage IV neuroblastoma older than 1 year of age at diagnosis: is cure possible in a small subgroup? *J Clin Oncol* 1991; **9**: 1037–1044.
119. Philip T, Ladenstein R, Zucher JM *et al*. Double megatherapy and autologous bone marrow transplantation for advanced neuroblastoma: the LMCE-2 study. *Br J Cancer* 1993; **67**: 119–127.
120. Herzig RH. Dose intensive therapy for advanced melanoma. In: *High-Dose Cancer Therapy*, 2nd edn. J Armitage and K Antman (eds), 1995; 873–878 (Baltimore MD: Williams & Wilkins).

Problems after transplantation

Part 3

Graft-versus-host disease
Acute graft-versus-host disease
Chronic graft-versus-host disease
The histopathology of graft-versus-host disease

Take, rejection and relapse
Graft failure: diagnosis and management
Minimal residual disease in acute leukaemia
Relapse and its management

Infection
Bacterial infections
Cytomegalovirus
Other viral infections
Fungal infections
Other infections
Reimmunisation after transplantation
General infection prophylaxis

Other considerations
Complications in the early post-transplant period
Neurological aspects of stem-cell transplantation
Blood transfusion support
Nutritional support
Re-adaptation to normal life

Late effects of transplantation
Paediatric problems
Endocrine and reproductive dysfunction in adults
Fertility

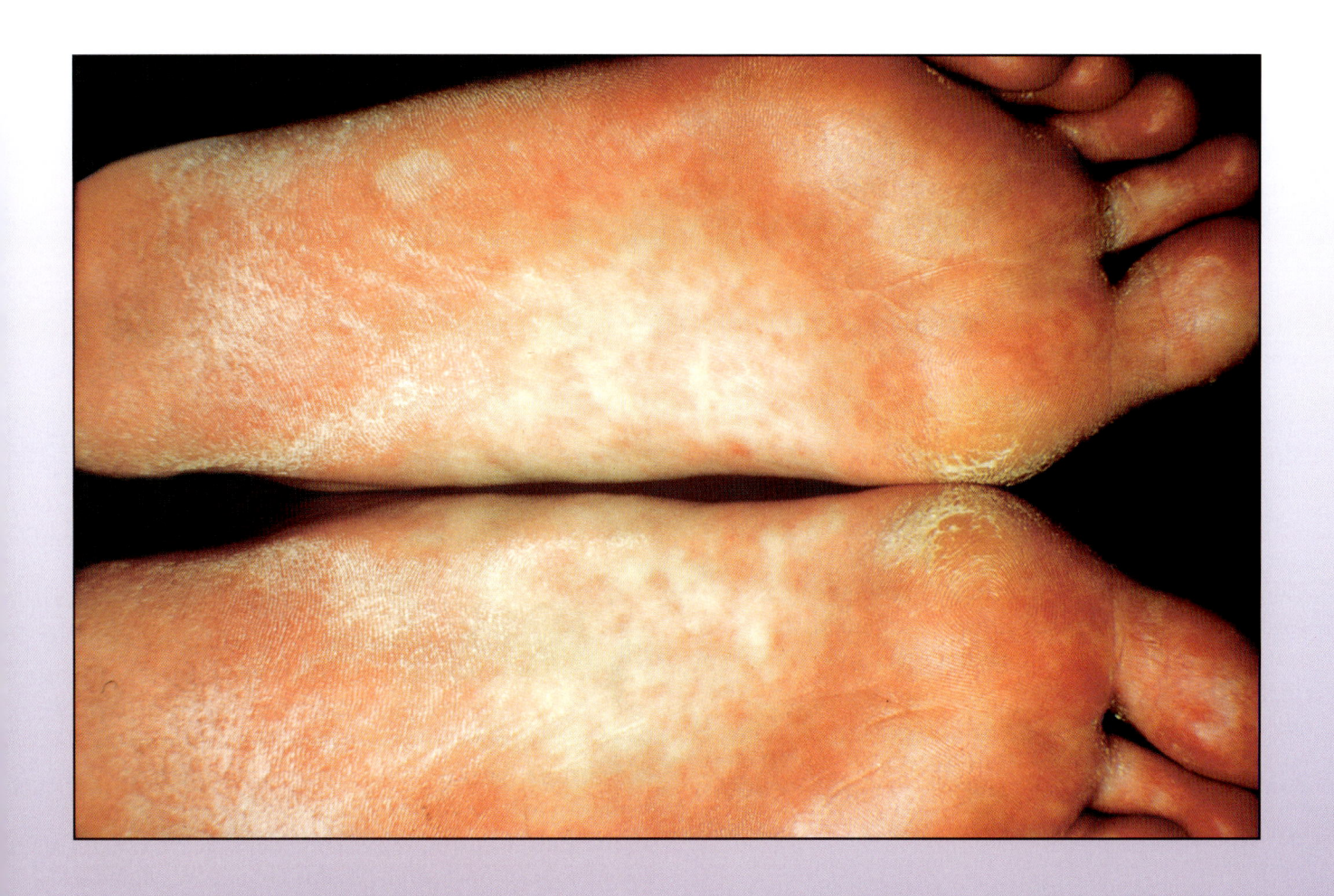

Chapter 37
Acute graft-versus-host disease

Gérard Socié and Jean-Yves Cahn

Introduction

Acute graft-versus-host disease (GvHD) remains a major cause of morbidity and mortality following allogeneic bone-marrow transplantation (BMT). A recent, comprehensive, survey of the European Group for Blood and Bone Marrow Transplantation summarized activity of haematopoietic cell transplants in Europe in 1994: 3502 allogeneic transplants were performed, most (2677; 76%) from a human leukaemia antigen (HLA) -identical sibling donor [1]. Since more than one-third of these patients will develop significant acute GvHD, this leads to an approximate conservative estimate of 1200 patients per year in Europe at risk of developing this life-threatening complication.

A similar estimate can be drawn from the number of transplants performed in 1994 in the United States and reported to the International Bone Marrow Transplant Registry (IBMTR): 1569 allogeneic transplants (908 from an HLA-identical sibling donor), with 28% of patients developing moderate to severe acute GvHD (MM Horowitz and PA Rowlings, personal communication). This huge number of patients illustrates well the extent of the problem. Here, the current thoughts about the pathophysiology of this disease are briefly summarized, and the incidence, risk factors, prophylaxis and treatment of acute GvHD are described. Finally, future prospects in the management of acute GvHD are examined. Since the main aim of this book is to review the current situation, we have not made any attempt to be exhaustive, but have instead focused on the literature which includes sufficient patients and/or seems to provide major insights into the management of this disease.

Current thoughts about the pathophysiology of acute GvHD

In this section we summarize the current thoughts about the pathophysiology of this disease, and in particular provide the reader with some of the basic premises which have led, or will lead to the use of various therapeutic modalities. It is over thirty years since Billingham (1966) defined the essential elements of acute GvHD [2]:

1. The graft must contain immunologically competent cells.
2. The recipient must express tissue antigens that are not present in the transplant donor.
3. The recipient must be unable to mount an effective response to destroy the transplanted cells.

We now know that these immunocompetent cells are T-lymphocytes [3,4]. However, despite numerous studies in patients with acute GvHD, there is no clear evidence that a specific subset is involved in the initiation of acute GvHD. Recent studies have attempted to characterize the lymphocyte infiltrate within acute GvHD lesions. A study by Gaschet et al., [5] in two recipients of mismatched transplant, allowed *in situ* isolation of cytotoxic T-cells against four graft mismatches (CD8$^+$ T-lymphocytes against class I HLA antigens and of CD4$^+$ T-lymphocytes against HLA class II antigens).

Two papers by Dietrich et al. aimed to analyze T-cell receptor variability in patients with acute GvHD [6,7]. The T-cell repertoire was analyzed in peripheral blood as well as in skin samples. Analysis of the α- and β-amplified products showed substantial differences between peripheral blood mononuclear cells and skin lymphocyte RNA, and a detailed analysis in one patient allowed identification of several recurrent transcripts in the skin (with only some present in the patient's blood).

While in humans the role of these CD3/αβ-positive T-cells seems predominant in acute GvHD lesions, the role, if any, of γδ T-cells in human GvHD is poorly understood (although the latter cells seem to play a significant role in acute GvHD in the murine system). Finally, recent knowledge concerning the biology of T-cells may assume importance in the future in understanding the pathophysiology of acute GvHD, and may therefore possibly influence treatment. This is especially true where the discovery of a second activation pathway for T-lymphocytes through the interaction between the CD28/CTLA4 and the CD80 (B7-1)/CD86 (B7-2) molecules [8–11] is concerned.

The second stated by Billingham requirement is that the recipient must express tissue antigens not present in the donor. While in HLA-mismatched transplants either CD4 cells recognize major histocompatibility complex (MHC) class II mismatched antigen, or CD8 cells recognize class I mismatched antigen, the molecules that are recognized in HLA-identical sibling transplants (the most frequent clinical situation) have been characterized only very recently [12–17]. These are the so-called 'minor histocompatibility antigens' (mi-HAg).

Finally, Billigham's third requirement stipulates that the recipient of T-cells must be immuno-compromised, a requirement that is obviously met in recipients of allogeneic BMT, following conditioning therapy.

GvHD is currently understood as a multistep process and has been reviewed [18–23]. In step one, recipient tissue is damaged either directly by the conditioning therapy, or indirectly by infection-induced cytokines, including: interleukins IL-1, IL-6; tumour necrosis factor-α, (TNFα). The target organs, skin, gut, and liver ducts, then exhibit an increased expression of HLA molecules, adhesion molecules (such as VCAM1 or ELAM1) or other products with procoagulant activities. Together with this increase in HLA molecule expression on epithelial cells, a number of antigens are processed and presented by antigen-presenting cells to T-lymphocytes. These lymphocytes recognize recipient peptide–HLA complexes (allo-antigens) in which either the HLA molecules (mismatched transplants), the bound peptides, or non-shared mi-HAg are recognized as foreign by the donor T-lymphocytes. These phenomena then lead to activation of individual T-cells, autocrine production of IL-2 and γ-interferon (IFNγ), and expression by activated T-cells of the IL2-receptor.

These activated T-lymphocytes then expand and differentiate (clonal proliferation and differentiation). They secrete IL-2 which activates newly engrafted mononuclear cells to secrete more inflammatory cytokines such as IL-1, TNFα or IFNγ. The resulting inflammatory response causes an additional release of cytokines and amplifies local organ injury, leading to a 'cytokine storm' [23]. In addition to these indirect, cytokine-mediated pathological changes, a direct cytolytic action of the activated T-cell also occurs.

The role, if any, of other cell subsets in human acute GvHD, such as macrophages and natural killer (NK) cells, is the subject of ongoing controversy.

Acute GvHD: incidence and risk factors

Data concerning the incidence and analysis of risk factors for the development of acute GvHD largely come from international registry data or from large institutions. However, even if they are of major importance for the analysis of clinical results, such studies cannot accurately define the degree of GvHD that will occur in an individual patient. HLA disparity between donor and recipient is a powerful factor, and the use of T-depleted versus T-replete grafts strongly influences the incidence of acute GvHD. In this section, the incidence and risk factors for acute GvHD in recipients from sibling donors is described, and in the second part, recent data on this problem in patients grafted from mismatched related or unrelated donors is analyzed.

Incidence and risk factors after transplants from sibling donors

A number of parameters have been recognized as being risk factors for developing acute GvHD. These can be divided into those which are inherent features of the patient or the donor (such as age or gender); treatment-related factors (such as lymphocyte number) which can be modified to reduce the risk of severe GvHD, and post-transplant events (such as cytomegalovirus (CMV) infection) that appear to precipitate GvHD (trigger or amplify) (Figure 37.1).

The largest group of patients analyzed to date, comes from data reported to the IBMTR [24] from 1978 to 1985. This study involved 2036 recipients of HLA-identical sibling non-T-cell-depleted marrow, grafted for leukaemia or aplastic anaemia. The two-year probability of developing acute GvHD was 54% for absent or mild and 46% for moderate-to-severe GvHD. During this time, most (1235) patients received methotrexate or cyclosporine (710) alone as prophylaxis, and occasional patients received both drugs (29). Factors predictive for developing moderate-to-severe acute GvHD include donor–recipient sex match (female-to-male the greatest, relative risk = 2.0). This was markedly increased if female donors for male recipients were previously pregnant or transfused (relative risk = 2.9). Older patients were at increased risk of GvHD (relative risk = 1.6).

A recent analysis from the IBMTR aimed to study acute GvHD severity (see discussion on severity/grading systems below) and updated the registry data on the incidence of acute GvHD in adult patients transplanted for leukaemia between 1986 and 1992 [25]. In this study, two cohorts of patients were analysed: the first included 2129 patients who received methotrexate plus cyclosporin as prophylaxis, and the other included 752 patients who received a T-cell-depleted graft. The incidence of none-to-mild (grades 0

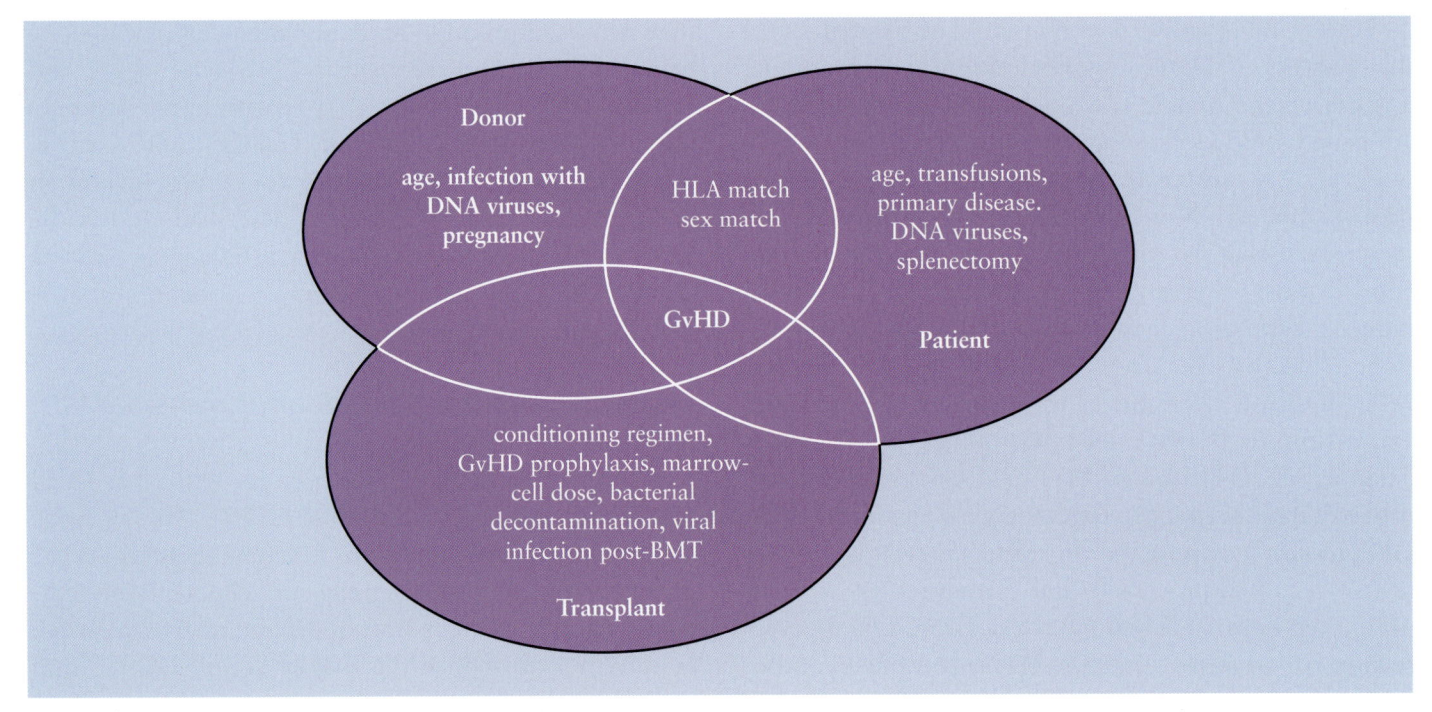

Figure 37.1 Factors associated with acute GvHD.

to I) acute GvHD was 66% and 73% in the T-repleted and T-depleted group, respectively, while moderate-to-severe (grades II to IV) were 35% and 28%, respectively. The data clearly shows a reduced incidence of the moderate-to-severe form of the disease during the most recent period. This may be partly due to the introduction of methotrexate plus cyclosporin as prophylaxis, or to newly introduced gnotobiotic measures. However, whatever the reasons, this highlights the need for a reassessment of risk factors for acute GvHD according to the treatment period and prophylaxis regimen.

The study by Nash *et al.* [26] who reported a retrospective analysis of risk factors for developing acute GvHD in a cohort of 446 patients transplanted in Seattle from 1981 to 1988 and who received cyclosporin plus methotrexate as prophylaxis, is of great interest. The incidence of grades II–IV and grades III–IV (severe) acute GvHD were 36% and 16%, respectively. In a multivariate Cox regression analysis, risk factors associated with the onset of moderate-to-severe GvHD were sex mismatch and donor parity, increased total body irradiation dose and reduction of methotrexate or cyclosporin to less than 80% of the scheduled dose. When only patients who developed grades II–IV acute GvHD were considered, the more severe (grades III–IV) acute GvHD was associated with increased patient age (40 years or older), and dose reductions of cyclosporin. Serological status for CMV, HLA-antigen subtypes at the A and B loci, and laminar air-flow isolation, all previously identified as affecting acute GvHD, were not confirmed as risk factors in this study population.

Other single-institution studies have suggested that some additional factors might be linked to the occurrence of moderate-to-severe acute GvHD. Some authors have particularly emphasized the role of herpes viruses [19]. In their most recent multivariate analysis (including 291 recipients of HLA-identical sibling transplants from 1975 to 1993), the Swedish group [27] showed that monotherapy (methotrexate or cyclosporin), donor seropositivity for several herpes viruses, recipient seropositivity for CMV and early engraftment were the principal risk factors for acute GvHD. Finally, the Essen group in Germany recently pointed out that sustained suppression of intestinal anaerobic bacteria reduces the risk of acute GvHD after sibling BMT [28].

Incidence and risk factors after transplants from alternative donors

Data concerning BMT from related donors other than HLA-identical siblings are scarce. The largest study comes from the IBMTR [29] and concerns 470 transplants from alternative related donors compared with 3648 transplants from HLA-identical siblings. This study clearly shows that the likelihood of adverse outcome correlates with increasing HLA disparity. The risk of acute GvHD increases with increasing donor–recipient HLA disparity. The risk of acute GvHD after HLA phenotypically matched and one-antigen mismatched transplants is not significantly higher than after HLA-identical sibling transplants. In contrast, the relative risk of acute GvHD after two- and three-antigen mismatched transplants was 3.1 and 4.4, respectively.

The role of HLA disparity in the incidence and severity of acute GvHD is even more striking in recipients of unrelated donors. In this situation the incidence of severe acute GvHD (grades III–IV) ranged between 20 and 50% but seems to be clearly linked with the degree of matching that is strictly related to the method used to assess it (serological versus molecular). The incidence of acute GvHD and the role of HLA allele disparity in influencing severity of the disease in large studies are summarized in Table 37.1. From these data it also seems that the incidence of acute GvHD in unrelated transplants is linked to the age of the patient and perhaps to disease stage.

Acute GvHD: *in vitro* predictive tests

Inability to predict GvHD in an individual patient has led to the development of a number of *in vitro* predictive tests. In HLA genotypically identical sibling transplants, a mixed leukocyte culture assay (MLC) is often performed in addition to HLA typing. A large study from the Fred Hutchinson Cancer Research Center, involving 783 patients, questioned the usefulness of the MLC, since there was no association between increased donor antirecipient MLC reactivity pretransplant and the incidence or severity of subsequent acute GvHD [30]. However, in a limited number of patients (40 cases), the Hadassah group used a modified MLC assay, with improved sensitivity, which appears to detect fine antigenic disparities between HLA-identical siblings [31].

More recently, limiting dilution analysis systems have been used to estimate the frequency of allo-reactive cytotoxic T-lymphocyte precursors (CTL-p) in the peripheral blood of donors. While it has proven useful in recipients from unrelated donors [32–34] it was not clear if this CTL-p assay was sensitive enough to detect allo-reactivity between HLA-identical sibling donor–recipient pairs. Two groups have developed an assay to quantify antirecipient helper (interleukin-2-producing) T-lymphocyte precursors (HTL-p) [35,36]. Both CD4+ and CD8+ T-cell subsets seem to contribute in comparable frequencies to host and donor HTL-p pre- and post-transplant [37,38]. Recognition of mi-HAg by CD8+ appeared to be class I HLA restricted, whereas CD4+ HTL-p operated in a class II-restricted fashion. However, it is our understanding that a clinically practical *in vitro* test for the prediction of GvHD must be simple, time-saving, sensitive and specific. Although sensitive and relatively specific, the above-mentioned tests do not seem to reach a sufficient level of simplicity and of time-saving. Prospective cooperative studies would be helpful in the search for the most clinically practical assay to predict GvHD in BMT between HLA-identical siblings [39].

Help may come in the near future from recent advances in the understanding of mi-HA [40]. After years of intensive research, some of the mi-HA have recently been characterized [13], and correlations between mi-HA mismatches and increased risk of severe acute GvHD suggested [16]. Up to now, however, these mismatches at mi-HA loci can only be detected by cytotoxic T-cell clones [16,41,42], but molecular typing may soon be feasible. Finally, DNA polymorphism within two genes (CD31-PECAM-1 and TNFα) has also been been recently linked to increased GvHD severity [43; and E. Holler, personal communication 1996). Of note, it is not known if these two latter gene polymorphisms act as true mi-HA. The real importance of mi-HA typing in predicting acute GvHD incidence and severity will, however, only be determined by multivariate analysis using factors which have already been defined as covariates.

Clinical features of acute GvHD

The classically recognized target organs of acute GvHD in man are skin, gastrointestinal tract and liver, although other tissues may also be involved.

Dermal features

The initial manifestation of acute GvHD is often a maculopapular rash (Figure 37.2). The median onset

Table 37.1 Acute GvHD, incidence in unrelated transplant and impact of HLA-matching

Study	Patients (n)	Patient population	Incidence (%)	Impact of HLA-matching
Spencer et al. [127]	115	CML (all TCD BMT)	Grade III–IV; 24	Impact of HLA class I identity (IEF)
Balduzzi et al. [128]	88	Children, various diagnosis	Grade III–IV; 49	GvHD grade II–IV; 83% vs. 98% in matched versus BMT
Petersdorf et al. [129]	364	Various ages and diagnosis	Overall incidence grade III–IV; not stated	Influence of DRB1 matching (grade III–IV risk 48 versus 70)
Davies et al. [130]	211	Various ages and diagnosis	Grade II–IV; 64	Influence of HLA A and B incompatibility in adults
Casper et al. [131]	50	Children, ALL and MDS	Grade II–IV; 33	No influence of one-antigen mismatch
Kernan et al. [132]	462	Various ages and diagnosis	Grade III–IV; 47	No influence of MM (serology) for grade III–IV
Schiller et al. [133]	55	Acute leukaemia advanced stage	Grade III–IV; 36	Not stated
Marks et al. [134]	46	CML	Grade II–IV; 66	Not stated
McGlave et al. [135]	196	CML	Grade III–IV; 54	Infuence of HLA matching on DFS

CML = chronic myeloid leukaemia; TCD = T-cell depletion; BMT = bone-marrow transplantation; ALL = acute lymphoblastic leukaemia; MDS = myelodysplastic syndrome; IEF = iso-electro focussing; DFS = disease free survival; MM = mismatched.

of skin rash is the third week post-transplant (median day 19, range 5–47) [44]. It initially involves the palms, soles and ears, although it can begin in other areas of the body, such as the back, shoulders or face. As the rash intensifies, confluent lesions occur, often associated with papule formation (Figure 37.3). Formation of bullae and generalized erythroderma occur in the more severe cases (Figures 37.4 and 37.5). The rash is usually pruritic and/or burning. These subjective symptoms may appear before a rash is visible. There may be an associated rise in body temperature. A hyperacute form of GvHD has been described by Sullivan and coworkers [45] which includes fever, generalized erythroderma and desquamation due to dermo-epidermal separation. This develops 7–14 days after transplantation and resembles toxic epidermal necrolysis or staphylococcal skin syndrome. The differential diagnosis of post-transplant skin rash classically includes toxic rash induced by the chemotherapy/radiotherapy conditioning regimen, drug allergy and viral infections. If associated with other GvHD features such as liver or gastrointestinal-tract involvement, diagnosis should be unequivocal. However, if only a maculopapular rash is present, the diagnosis may be in doubt. Although skin biopsies help to establish the diagnosis, histological changes, especially those due to chemoradiotherapy, can be indistinguishable from those seen with GvHD.

Hepatic and intestinal involvement usually appear several days after the rash, but may manifest

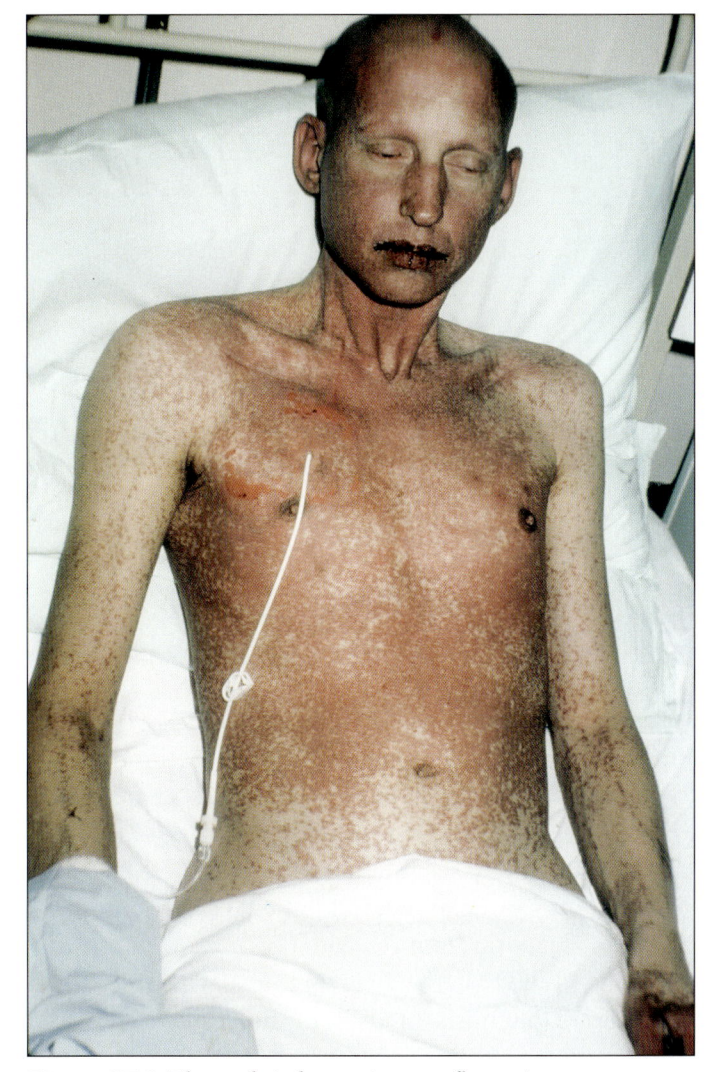

Figure 37.3 The rash is becoming confluent in some areas.

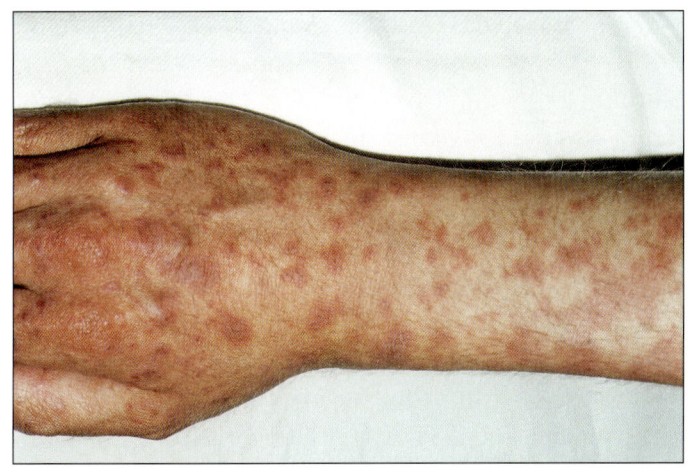

Figure 37.2 The typical maculopapular rash of early acute graft-versus-host disease.

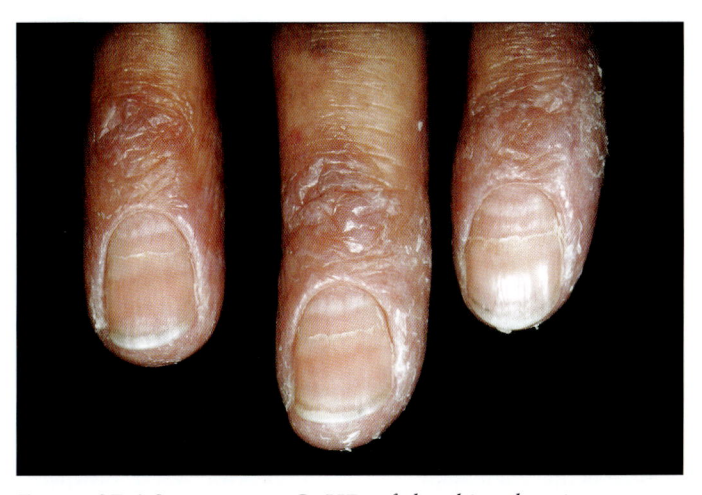

Figure 37.4 Severe acute GvHD of the skin, showing desquamation and blister formation. The finger-nails also show the horizontal ridges and cracks associated with earlier chemoradiotherapy, which temporarily halted growth.

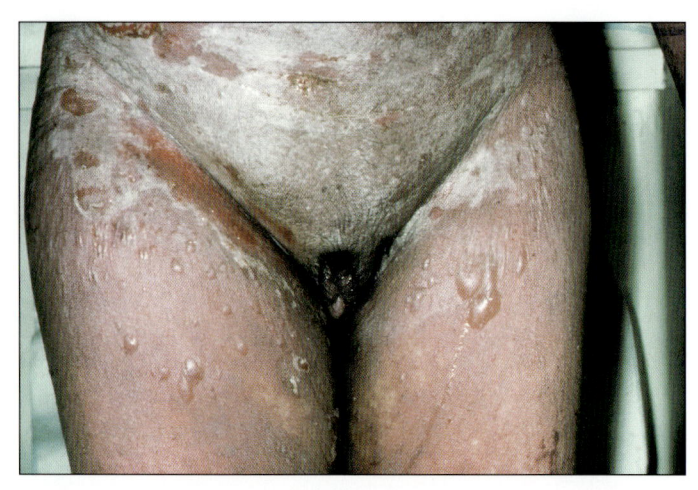

Figure 37.5 Severe acute GvHD of the skin (see Fig 37.4).

concurrently. However, it is rare to see liver or gut involvement before skin disease is apparent [44–47].

Hepatic features

Liver dysfunction commonly develops within two to four weeks of transplantation. There is generally a gradual rise in bilirubin. In parallel, there is a rise in alkaline phosphatase and transaminases (AST, ALT). The liver may be enlarged, but patients rarely complain of pain. Hepatic failure with encephalopathy due solely to GvHD of the liver is unusual [22,48]. The differential diagnosis of liver dysfunction early post-transplant is broad. Mild-to-moderate function abnormalities may be related to hepatic veno-occlusive disease (VOD), infection, drug toxicity (including that of cyclosporin) and parenteral nutrition. Although hepatic GvHD can be distinguished from hepatic VOD by the rare occurrence of weight gain or pain in the right upper quadrant in the former, pathological studies have shown the frequent association of both diseases in patients with chronic cholestasis [49].

Gastrointestinal features

Symptoms of acute GvHD of the distal small bowel and colon include diarrhoea, intestinal bleeding, crampy abdominal pain and ileus. The diarrhoea is often mucoid, due to a mixed watery exudate and exfoliated mucosae. Even with cessation of oral intake, voluminous secretion may persist and stool volumes represent an important parameter of the grading system for severity of the disease. The differential diagnosis of enteric GvHD is primarily chemoradiotherapy effects and intestinal infection (CMV in particular). Diarrhoea is frequently seen within a week of the transplant, secondary to preparative therapy. It usually resolves within a few weeks. Infection is a much more difficult differential diagnosis, since superinfection is common in patients with biopsy-proven gut GvHD, and CMV infection can trigger development of GvHD [48].

Endoscopic findings of enteric GVHD range from normal to extensive oedema and mucosal shedding [45,50]. Lesions may be most prominent in the caecum and ileum. Histology reveals crypt-cell necrosis. More recently, an upper gastrointestinal form of GvHD has been described [51]. This syndrome, presenting clinically as anorexia, dyspepsia, food intolerance and vomiting, was recognized and confirmed histologically in 62 of 469 patients undergoing allogeneic bone-marrow transplantation (13% by Kaplan–Meier estimates). Non-specific symptoms of upper gastrointestinal GvHD require histological and microbiological studies to confirm the diagnosis. Apparently more common in older patients, upper-tract disease responds well to immunosuppressive therapy.

Acute GvHD grading systems

While clinical manifestations of acute GvHD after allogeneic BMT were first described in the early 1960s by Mathé, the first detailed criteria for grading GvHD were published in 1974 by Glucksberg and coworkers [44], and slightly modified one year later by Thomas *et al.* [46]. Glucksberg's criteria [44] take into account different stages of skin, liver or gut disease based upon the extent and severity of the rash, serum level of AST, bilirubin and volume of diarrhoea. The combination of stages was used to assign an overall grade from I to III, and patients with 'extreme constitutional symptoms' were designated grade IV. It should be emphasized that Glucksberg's original report included only 61 patients and that methotrexate alone was given as GvHD prophylaxis. These criteria were modified by Thomas *et al.* in 1975 [46]. Grades II and IV then were distinguished on the severity of skin or gut involvement, and AST was no longer used for staging. Since then, these criteria have been widely used for grading GvHD and are summarized in Tables 37.2 and 37.3. Recently, a consensus evaluated the validity of this grading system with the use of cyclosporin and modern supportive care [52]. Standard GvHD grading criteria were found to distinguish different mortality risks. Analysis of new data suggested that persistent nausea with histological evidence of GvHD but no diarrhoea should be included as stage 1 gastrointestinal GvHD. Additional studies were recommended to evaluate heterogeneity of outcome within GvHD grades prior to making further revisions.

Such a study has been recently completed by the IBMTR [25]. Data on 2881 adult patients receiving HLA-identical sibling T-cell depleted (n = 752) or non-T-cell-depleted (n = 2129) transplants for leukaemia between 1986 and 1992 were analyzed. Relative risk of relapse, treatment-related mortality and treatment failure were calculated for patients with Glucksberg grades I, II or III/IV versus those without GvHD, and for patients with distinct patterns of organ involvement, regardless of Glucksberg grade. Using data for non-T-cell-depleted transplants, a Severity Index was developed, grouping patients with patterns of organ involvement associated with similar risk of treatment-related mortality and treatment failure. Higher Glucksberg grade predicted poorer outcome. However, patients with the same grade but different patterns of skin, liver or gut involvement often had significantly different outcomes. Patients were thus classified into four categories (A–D) with increased relative risk of treatment failure and treatment-related mortality. Compared to patients without GvHD, relative risks of treatment failure were 0.85 for Severity Index A, 1.21 with B, 2.19 with C and 5.69 with D. Prognostic utility of these categories was then tested in patients receiving T-depleted transplants, and similar relative risks were found. Such an index could be of outstanding practical importance in enhancing design and interpretation of clinical trials in the current era of allogeneic BMT, but must be prospectively validated to compare with the classical Glucksberg grading system.

Table 37.2 Clinical grading of acute graft-versus-host disease

Grade	Degree of organ involvement
I	+ to ++ skin rash; no gut or liver involvement; no decrease in clinical performance
II	+ to +++ skin rash; + gut or liver involvement (or both); mild decrease in clinical performance
III	++ to +++ skin rash; ++ to +++ gut or liver involvement (or both); marked decrease in clinical performance
IV	similar to grade III and profound decrease in clinical performance

Table 37.3 Acute GvHD grading Thomas et al. [47]

Stage	Skin: maculopapular rash	Liver: bilirubin	Intestinal tract: diarrhoea
+	< 25% of body surface	2–3 mg/dl (34–50 µ/L)	>500 ml
++	25–50% body surface	3–6 mg/dl (51–102 µ/L)	>1000 ml
+++	Generalized erythroderma	6–15 mg:dl (103–255 µ/L)	>1500 ml
++++	Generalized erythroderma with bullae and desquamation	>15 mg:dl (>255 µ/L)	Severe abdominal pain with or without ileus

Acute GvHD prevention

Strategies for prevention of acute GvHD are aimed at interfering with the afferent phase of the GvH response, that is, they attempt to eliminate donor T-cells or block their activation [22]. Removal of T-cells results in a lower incidence of acute GvHD but a higher incidence of graft failure and relapse. T-cell depletion is discussed in full in Chapter 32. Another approach to the prophylaxis of acute GvHD is the use of immunosuppressive drugs such as methotrexate, cyclosporin and cyclophosphamide, either singly or combined with other agents including prednisone. Recently, the use of antibodies to the IL-2 receptor has been tested for GvHD prophylaxis. Finally, the use of intravenous immunoglobulin, protective isolation and gut decontamination (gnotobiotic measures) have also been shown to decrease the incidence of acute GvHD.

The following summarizes the data on immunosuppressive drugs and monoclonal antibodies with special emphasis on large randomized trials and long-term results.

Prevention via immunosuppressive drugs
Single-agent immunosuppression

On the basis of animal studies, post-transplant immunosuppression to prevent GvHD was incorporated into clinical practice. Procarbazine, cyclophosphamide and methotrexate (MTX) were found to be effective in murine and canine models [45,53,54].

Standard MTX prophylaxis was given at a dose of 15 mg/m^2 on day 1, 10 mg/m^2 on days 3, 6, 11, and weekly thereafter to day 102. While initial studies involving small numbers of patients gave contradictory results [55], a prospective randomized trial comparing standard 102-day MTX prophylaxis with an abbreviated 11-day course of MTX found a significant increase in the incidence of grades II to IV acute GvHD when immunosuppression was discontinued early (25 versus 59%, $P < 0.002$) [56].

In the early 1980s, pilot studies demonstrated effective prevention of GvHD with cyclosporin (CSP) prophylaxis [57–59]. Cyclosporin was given intravenously at a dose of 1.5 mg/kg every 12 hours starting on day –1 and continuing until oral dosing was tolerated. Starting at day 50, oral CSP was tapered 5% each week and discontinued by day 180. Subsequent controlled trials comparing standard MTX with a six-month course of CSP showed no difference in the rate of acute (and chronic) GvHD, leukaemic relapse, interstitial pneumonitis and event-free survival [60,61]. A large retrospective study by the IBMTR examined this issue in 2286 patients transplanted for acute leukaemia in first remission or for chronic myeloid leukaemia (CML) in first chronic phase [62]: 608 received MTX, 977 CSP and 669 combined MTX + CSP. In adults, CSP or MTX leads to comparable risks of acute and chronic GvHD. Compared with MTX, CSA was associated with less interstitial pneumonitis, less treatment-related mortality, more relapses (especially in acute lymphoblastic leukaemia) and less treatment failure (relapse or death from any cause). Finally, one randomized Italian study addressed the question of CSP dosage (1 mg/kg versus 5 mg/kg) from day –1 to day +20 in patients transplanted for acute leukaemia [63]. After stratification for age, grade II or more was significantly lower in the higher dose group, but the actuarial risk of relapse in patients in first remission was higher (43%) in this patient group, as compared to that of the lower dose group (9%, $P = 0.0001$).

Combined-agent immunosuppression

Subsequent studies indicated that combined therapy is more effective in preventing acute GvHD than either MTX or CSP used alone, although few were randomized [64–67]. The group from City of Hope has used steroids (prednisone) since the early 1980s in combination with MTX or CSP (see below). Finally, recent reports examined the two- versus three-drug regimen.

The Seattle group undertook two randomized trials of combined MTX + CSP. The first compared MTX and CSP versus CSP alone for prophylaxis of acute GvHD in patients given HLA-identical marrow grafts for leukaemia. Patients randomly assigned to receive MTX + CSP were given 15 mg/m^2 of MTX body surface on day 1, and 10 mg/m^2 on days +3, +6 and +11. Cyclosporin was delivered as described above. The results of this trial involving 93 patients were first reported in 1986, and two long-term follow-up reports updated the results at 3.0–4.5 and 6–8.5 years, respectively [64, 65]. Patients receiving CSP alone had a more than two-fold higher risk of developing acute GvHD than those receiving MTX + CSP (grade II–IV cumulative incidence 60% versus 30%). The incidence of chronic GvHD was identical in the two groups.

Patients who received CSP alone experienced a higher probability of non-relapse death compared to patients who received MTX + CSP. Among patients with acute myeloid leukaemia (AML) this disadvantage was offset by a higher leukaemic relapse rate. In patients with CML, relapse curves were identical for the two groups. No significant improvement in event-free survival was noted in the long term. The second randomized trial compared GvHD prevention with MTX alone to CSP + MTX in 46 patients given marrow grafts for severe aplastic anaemia [66–68]. Patients given MTX alone developed grades II–IV acute GvHD more often (53% incidence) than those given MTX + CSP (18% incidence). This increased risk for patients receiving MTX alone was confirmed in a Cox regression analysis which included age, lack of laminar air-flow isolation and prior transfusions as possible risk factors. Long-term follow-up reports updated the results at 3–6 and 9–12 years, respectively [66,67]. Long-term survival rates were slightly better for the MTX + CSP group (73%) as compared to the MTX alone group (58%) but did not reach statistical significance (but the number of patients in each treatment group was 22 only and 24).

Data from the IBMTR on 669 patients transplanted for early leukaemia and receiving MTX + CSP were compared with those of 977 patients with the same disease stage but receiving CSP alone [62]. In this study, adults receiving the combination had significantly less acute and chronic GvHD and less interstitial pneumonitis. Treatment failure was marginally reduced (relative risk 0.8, $P < 0.05$). Finally, the MTX + CSP regimen was recently evaluated in a series of 101 patients who underwent BMT for haematological malignancies after a busulfan-cyclophosphamide conditioning regimen [69]. The incidence (9.2%) of grades II–IV acute GvHD in this series was surprisingly low in 72 patients receiving optimal GvHD prophylaxis (that is, full MTX and achieving therapeutic CSP concentrations).

Between 1983 and 1985, the City of Hope group conducted a randomized study which compared MTX + prednisone and CSP + prednisone for acute GvHD prophylaxis [70]. This study involved 107 patients and the reported incidence of grades II–IV acute GvHD was 47% versus 28% ($P < 0.05$) in patients receiving MTX + prednisone and CSP + prednisone, respectively.

Since then, the role of prednisone in the prevention of acute GvHD has been re-evaluated by the Seattle group in a randomized study [71]. This study involved 147 patients with leukaemia or aplastic anaemia. Although a total accrual of 340 patients had been planned, the study was terminated early on the basis of results from an interim analysis. All patients were given MTX + CSP, as described above, and were randomized to receive, or not, prednisone from day 0 to day 35 (1 mg/kg day 0 to day 22, 0.5 mg/kg day 22 to day 35). The cumulative incidence of grades II–IV was 36% in the MTX + CSP arm and 45% in the MTX + CSP + prednisone arm ($P = 0.28$). Among HLA-identical patients, these figures were 25% versus 46% ($P = 0.02$). A subsequent analysis of this trial showed an increased risk of infection in patients who were receiving prednisone. The authors concluded that addition of prednisone to their standard MTX + CSP regimen is not beneficial in recipients of HLA-identical marrow grafts. The problem of early termination of this study should, however, be emphasized.

Finally, the triple immunosuppressive drug regimen (MTX + CSP + prednisone) has recently been compared with CSP + prednisone in a randomized fashion [72]. One hundred and fifty patients with early leukaemia were enrolled in this study. All patients received total body irradiation (13.20 Gy) and etoposide (60 mg/kg) in preparation for BMT from HLA-identical sibling donors. Patients receiving the triple-drug regimen had a significantly lower incidence of grade II–IV acute GvHD (9%) than those receiving CSP + prednisone (23%, $P = 0.02$). Multivariate analysis confirmed that a higher risk was associated with CSP + prednisone alone.

Results and unanswered questions in combined agent immunosuppression are outlined in Table 37.4.

All randomized studies summarized here involved patients who were grafted from sibling donors. All these patients were grafted from HLA-identical siblings with the exception of one randomized study [71] in which 25 patients received one-HLA locus mismatched sibling transplants. However, as described earlier in this chapter, acute GvHD is an even greater problem in marrow transplants from unrelated donors. Furthermore, in a significant number of recipients, moderate-to-severe acute GvHD still occurs despite

Table 37.4 Acute GvHD prophylaxis after HLA-identical sibling BMT: combined immunosuppression

Results of randomized studies	Unanswered questions
MTX + CSP > CSP in leukaemia	MTX + CSP > CSP in aplastic anaemia?
MTX + CSP > MTX in aplastic anaemia	MTX + CSP + pred < MTX + CSP in leukaemia
CSP + pred > MTX + pred in leukaemia	CSP + pred versus MTX + CSP in leukaemia?
CSP + MTX + pred > CSP + pred in leukaemia	Omission of day +11 MTX dose?
MTX = methotrexate; CSP = cyclosporin; pred = prednisone.	

optimum immunosuppressive prophylaxis. In both HLA-identical sibling and unrelated transplants, T-cell depletion is the most effective method of preventing GvHD but is associated with increased risks of both graft failure and relapse. There are few controlled comparative trials of T-cell depletion [73–75]. Only one of these trials compared T-depletion with the CSP + MTX combined immunosuppressive regimen [75]. Long-term follow-up of this latter trial comparing 48 adult leukaemic recipients of HLA-identical sibling marrow has recently been published. The median observation time was 5.5 years. While noticeable differences in the leukaemia-free survival of patients with CML (25% versus 51% in the CSP + MTX and T-cell-depleted group, respectively) exist, the difference did not reach statistical significance, probably due to the low number of patients enrolled in this trial (10 patients with CML in each group). Overall probability of leukaemia-free survival was similar in the two groups. Thus, data from these three randomized trials and from a large retrospective study from the IBMTR [76] permit the conclusion that T-cell depletion is clearly associated with a lower disease-free survival in patients with CML. It is not yet clear whether the same is true in patients with acute leukaemia, and especially in patients with ALL.

In the light of promising results using monoclonal antibodies for the treatment of steroid-resistant acute GvHD (see below) and of results of phase I and II studies that suggested monoclonal antibodies might be effective in GvHD prevention [77–79], it seems justified to test these new reagents for acute GvHD prophylaxis in phase III trials. Two such trials have recently been completed. The first involved 101 patients with early leukaemia who were randomly assigned to receive an IL-2-receptor antibody in addition to the MTX + CSP regimen [80]. All patients were grafted from an HLA-identical sibling donor. The antibody did not significantly affect the cumulative frequency of GvHD of grade II or worse (38% versus 46%). Furthermore, with a nearly five-year median follow-up, the antibody-treated patients had a significantly lower leukaemia-free survival, mainly because of a progressive increase in the rate of late relapses. A similar double-blind placebo-controlled multicentre trial has recently been completed in recipients from unrelated donors [81]. The first analysis of this study which used a humanized anti-IL2 receptor antibody showed no efficacy of this agent in preventing GvHD or improving outcome in recipients of unrelated donor marrow.

Acute GvHD treatment

While numerous studies have demonstrated the efficacy of a variety of approaches for prophylaxis, GvHD nonetheless remains a frequently encountered, life-threatening complication of marrow transplantation, particularly when the donor is not an HLA-identical sibling. In the past, studies have reported the efficacy of glucocorticoids, antithymocyte globulin and cyclosporin in the treatment of acute GvHD. More recently, monoclonal antibodies have been used in the treatment of steroid-resistant acute GvHD. However, in contrast to the number of studies assessing GvHD prophylaxis, there are surprisingly few controlled studies of GvHD treatment. This disparity most probably reflects the difficulty and complexity in evaluating the results of treatment. Only a few randomized trials have been reported [82], and the largest reported only 77 patients.

In addition to these trials, large retrospective analyses of GvHD treatment have been carried out by both the Seattle and the Minneapolis groups. Results of the randomized studies and of the two large retrospective studies will be summarized first, followed by those of phase I–II studies, and the one randomized study which used monoclonal antibodies.

One of the first studies of the treatment of acute GvHD reported the relative effectiveness of antithymocyte globulin (ATG) in reversing human GvHD [83]. In 1981, the first randomized study was published [84]. This trial compared 20 patients who received corticosteroids (2 mg/kg for 10 days) to 17 patients who received ATG (7 mg/kg every other day for six days). All patients received MTX alone as prophylaxis, and all had grade II or more acute GvHD. Both treatment modalities were associated with a mild decrease in severity of GvHD and there was no statistical difference between treatment groups, whether assessed by improvement in specific organs or in the overall grade of acute GvHD.

The second trial aimed to compare 14-days treatment with corticosteroids (2 mg/kg) and CSP (12–15 mg/kg orally or 3–5 mg/kg intravenously) [85]. This trial involved 77 patients with grade II–IV acute GvHD despite MTX prophylaxis. Sixty-one percent of the patients treated with CSP responded, as compared to 41% of the patients treated with steroids ($P = 0.039$), leading to the conclusion that CSP has at least a comparable efficacy to methylprednisolone.

The last trial compared ATG + CSP with or without methylprednisolone [86]. Forty-eight patients with grade II–IV acute GvHD despite MTX prophylaxis were enrolled. This trial involved 18 patients grafted from non-identical sibling donors. The addition of steroids did not appear to be beneficial and was even detrimental in this patient cohort because of the large number of infectious deaths in the group receiving steroids. It should be emphasized that all of these early trials involved patients who received MTX alone as GvHD prophylaxis. Furthermore, since now most, if not all, patients are given CSP (alone or in combination with MTX or prednisone), the results of the randomized study of CSP versus steroids for the treatment of acute GvHD cannot be used for therapeutic decision-making. Thus, in the cyclosporin era, steroids are considered the gold standard for acute GvHD first-line therapy. In this regard, the Minneapolis randomized study of short- versus long-term steroids treatment is of interest [87]. Thirty patients responding to 60 mg/m^2 steroids given from day 14 were randomized either to short treatment (2275 mg/m^2 over 12 weeks) or long taper (6300 mg/m^2 over 21 weeks). This study suggests that rapid administration of high-dose prednisone to a cumulative dose of 2000 mg/m^2 might lead to complete response of acute GvHD.

The Minneapolis group also performed two retrospective analyses on the impact of treatment of moderate-to-severe acute GvHD [88,89]. In the first they analyzed the long-term outcome of 197 patients who were treated for grade II–IV acute GvHD [88]. Among these 197 patients, 41% achieved complete and continuing resolution of acute GvHD after a median of 21 days of therapy (steroids in 160 patients). Analysis of clinical features associated with complete response identified more favourable responses in patients without liver involvement with ALL, and for donor–recipient pairs other than male patients with female donors.

In the second study [89] involving 272 patients with acute GvHD and transplanted more recently, the response to primary therapy (steroids for 209 patients) was the single most important factor predicting improved long-term survival. In multivariate analysis, transplantation from a mismatched or an unrelated donor was not of independent importance in predicting treatment response.

A similar analysis has been performed by the Seattle group. Late in 1990 and early in 1991, Martin *et al.* published two reports on initial and secondary treatment, respectively [90,91]. In the first study they analyzed data on 740 patients with grade II–IV acute GvHD [90]. Initial treatment was steroids in 531 patients, ATG in 156, and CSP and/or monoclonal antibody in 170 patients. Overall, complete or partial responses were seen in 44% of patients. Prophylaxis with MTX and CSP was associated with favourable treatment outcome, and treatment with glucocorticoids or cyclosporin was more successful than treatment with ATG.

A secondary treatment study analyzed data on 427 patients [91]. Secondary treatment was with glucocorticoids ($n = 249$), cyclosporin ($n = 80$), ATG ($n = 114$) or monoclonal antibody ($n = 19$), either singly ($n = 390$) or in combination ($n = 37$). Overall, complete or partial responses were seen in 40% of patients. The highest complete response rate with secondary treatment was seen when the GvHD recurred during tapering of primary glucocorticoids.

From the data summarized above, and from the experience of almost all centres, it thus appears that steroids are the treatment of choice as first-line treatment of acute GvHD. However, a number of issues remain unresolved concerning this first-line treatment:

1. **Optimum starting dose.** Although 2 mg/kg is generally the starting dose, use of steroids as prophylaxis leads some groups to begin at 5 mg/kg.
2. **Duration of administration.** The optimum duration of administration has not been defined. Many patients 'relapse' after withdrawal of steroids regardless of whether lower doses or relatively high doses have been given, and require re-instigation of therapy.
3. **Definition of so-called cortico-resistance and cortico-dependence.** While a number of studies have been published on the use of high-dose and 'mega-dose' steroids, there is no definitive proof of a dose–effect of steroids in the treatment of acute GvHD.

Beside the use of systemic therapy, topical steroids may be of help in the management of either skin or intestinal disease [92]. Also, somatostatin analogues might be of help in the management of acute gastrointestinal disease [93].

More recently, monoclonal antibodies (mAb) and IL-1 receptor antagonists have been used for the treatment of steroid-resistant acute GvHD. Data on phase I–II studies are summarized in Table 37.5. From these data, mAb appeared to be promising in the treatment of steroid-resistant acute GvHD. As in other studies of acute GvHD therapy, there was, however, the inherent problem of the definition of steroid resistance and of the definition of response criteria. Furthermore, as with other therapies, liver disease seemed to be less amenable to improvement with mAb and, whatever the target organ, the problem of acute GvHD relapse at the end of treatment still persists with mAb.

Thus, a phase-III double-blind placebo-controlled trial seemed timely. A multicentre European trial has

Table 37.5 Phase I–II studies of monoclonal antibodies for the treatment of acute GvHD

Authors	Patients (n)	Type of mAb	Response*
Hebart et al. [136]	14	Anti-CD3/TCRab	3/5 CR with anti-CD3
			5/7 PR with anti-TCR, no CR
Anasetti et al. [137]	11	Anti-CD25	1 CR
Byers et al. [138]	34	Anti-CD5-ricin A	2
Hervé et al. [139]	32	Anti-IL-2R	21 CR
Hervé et al. [140]	19	Anti-TNFα	8 very good PR, 6 PR
Anasetti et al. [141]	17	Anti-CD3	5 CR, 8 PR
Anasetti et al. [142]	20	Human anti-IL-2Ra	4 CR, 4 PR
Antin et al. [143]	17	IL-1-RA	2 CR, 8 PR
Racadot et al. [144]	15	Anti-CD2, anti-IL-2R, anti-TNFα	5 CR, 4 very good PR, 2 PR
Heslop et al. [145]	10	CBL1	5 CR, 4 PR

*CR = complete response; PR = partial response.

recently been completed by Cahn and coworkers [94]. Sixty-nine patients participated in this study, which excluded non-genotypically identical allogeneic marrow transplant recipients. The trial compared the efficacy of the combination of *in vivo* anti-CD25 mAb, CSP and steroids, versus placebo and CSP + steroids. However, despite promising preliminary results in the treatment of steroid-resistant acute GvHD, the role of first-line treatment of such a mAb remains to be determined since there was no difference in the response rate or in survival at one year in the two groups. Further understanding of allo-reactivity mechanisms (including cells, receptors and cytokines) associated with GvHD will, however, probably lead to new therapeutic approaches for this complication of BMT (see below).

Besides therapy with immunosuppressive drugs and mAb, supportive care is of obvious major importance in the practical management of patients with acute GvHD. Gut rest, hyperalimentation, pain control and antibiotic prophylaxis are routine aspects of supportive care of patients with acute GvHD [45].

As stated above, a somatostatin analogue appears to be of benefit in controlling secretory diarrhoea in some patients. Antiviral prophylaxis (and treatment if there is a CMV-associated infection) may be particularly important in preventing interstitial pneumonitis in patients with refractory acute GvHD. Finally, fungal infections are one of the main causes of increased morbidity and mortality in these patients. New antifungal agents such as thiazoles and liposomal amphotericin may be of benefit in preventing and treating serious mycotic infections.

Acute GvHD: recent developments and future prospects

From the data reviewed above, it seems clear that acute GvHD remains one of the most persistent problems of allogeneic BMT. It is still a major cause of both morbidity and mortality despite significant progress in prophylaxis although less progress in treatment. Over the past few years, advances have been made in both understanding and knowledge of human haematopoietic stem cells and the process of T-cell activation. Furthermore, the new sources of haematopoietic stem cells (cord blood and allogeneic peripheral blood stem cells) are currently being investigated worldwide as sources of transplantable cells in either HLA-identical sibling transplants or in mismatched situations. Finally, new drugs are currently under investigation for prophylaxis and/or treatment of acute GvHD. These recent developments are summarized in the last section of this chapter.

A point of major biological and clinical importance, that is, the close interrelationship between GvHD and the graft-versus-leukaemia (GvL) phenomenon should be emphasized. GvHD/GvL interrelationships are reviewed in Chapter 42. Although it is not currently clear if the GvL phenomenon can be separated from the GvHD process on a cellular level [95], it has been statistically apparent since the late 1980s that there is a correlation between the severity of acute and/or chronic GvHD and subsequent decrease in relative risk of relapse after allogeneic BMT for leukaemia [96,97]. This is supported by evidence from murine models [98]. However, proof for this principle has only recently arisen through the use of donor lymphocyte infusions, given as sole therapy to patients for relapse of their primary malignant disease [99].

Thus, one of the major goals of allogeneic stem-cell transplantation over the ensuing years will be to take advantage of the current knowledge in basic haematology and immunology and to move from transplantation of unseparated products to the use of stem cells for haematological reconstitution and of lymphocytes (and dendritic cells) to allow engraftment and GvL: in other words, to move from transplantation of unseparated cells to component allogeneic cell therapy.

New sources of transplantable allogeneic cells

Umbilical cord blood

The first umbilical cord blood transplant was performed at the Hopital Saint Louis (Paris) in 1987 in a patient with Fanconi anaemia. Since then, growing numbers of such transplants have been performed worldwide both from HLA-matched and mismatched siblings. More recently, the use of cryopreserved cord blood from unrelated donors has been investigated by several groups in Europe and in the United States. It is currently unclear if these cells lead to a decreased or similar incidence of acute GvHD, although it has been proven that a single human umbilical cord blood provides sufficient stem cells to allow long-term engraftment. Data from *in vitro* studies suggest that cord blood lymphocytes may be naive and less immunogenic, that they bear an immature phenotype, and that from a functional aspect they lack constitutional perforin expression, and cytotoxic cells seems to comprise mostly a NK cell subset [100,101] (Table 37.6).

Data from the International Cord Blood Transplant Registry [102] show a low incidence of grade II–IV (2%) acute GvHD for patients with HLA-identical or HLA-1 antigen disparate sibling donor grafts, and this occurs even in patients with two- or three-antigen disparate sibling donors or unrelated donors. Whether or not greater HLA disparities between donor and recipient can be tolerated by the use of umbilical cord blood is currently under investigation worldwide.

Since the incidence of GvHD strongly correlates with recipient age, and most cord blood transplants have been performed in children where donor and recipient herpes virus species infections are absent and where few T-lymphocytes have been infused, analysis of larger numbers of patients and comparisons with marrow transplant recipients with the same GvHD risk factors are required to define the true incidence and risk factors of acute GvHD following cord blood transplantation.

Allogeneic peripheral blood stem cells

Peripheral blood stem cells have been use as a source of support after high-dose chemotherapy in autologous transplants for about ten years. The first allogeneic PBSC transplants were reported in 1994, and since then this approach been increasingly used. By mid 1995, the first three series were published [103–106], all including less than 10 patients.

In October of the same year, the first International Symposium on Allogeneic PBSC was held in Geneva under the auspices of the EBMT [107], updating and extending data on the use of this approach in allogeneic transplantation. Data on large series of unmanipulated PBSC transplants presented at this symposium are summarized in Table 37.7. Large numbers of T-cells were infused, and grade II–IV acute GvHD incidence ranged from 13 to 52%. As reviewed in a recent Editorial [108], among the issues raised by the use of allogeneic PBSC was that of grafting with material containing a minimum of more than one order of magnitude of T-cells, as compared to the number in a marrow graft, thus potentially increasing the risk of acute GvHD. Although it was initially claimed that this incidence might even be less than in conventional bone-marrow grafting, one can assume today that the incidence of acute GvHD following allogeneic PBSC transplantation is approximately comparable to that after marrow transplantation.

A randomized study comparing these two sources of haematological stem cells, therefore, seems timely and warranted to address the question of the incidence and risk factors of acute and chronic GvHD. Such a study has been initiated by the EBMT and will hopefully bring some of the answers in the near future.

Transplantation of allogeneic CD34+ cells

Over the past few years, convincing *in vitro* data have shown that human haematopoietic stem cells are contained within the CD34+ cell population [109]. Furthermore, studies on allogeneic PBSC grafts have shown that they contain three- to four-fold more CD34+ than a bone-marrow graft. Immunoselection of the CD34+ cell population allows recovery of a high number of CD34+ cells and, in the same procedure, a 2–3 log T-cell depletion of the graft [110]. T-cells may be frozen and used for delayed add-back with a fixed number of T-cells to tentatively overcome the increased relapse rate associated with T-cell depletion.

The use of such CD34+-enriched grafts from peripheral blood, with or without bone marrow, has recently been reported in a limited number of patients (all series included approximately 10 patients). All transplants were performed from HLA-identical sibling donors. Somewhat surprisingly, despite a 2–3 log T-cell

Table 37.6 Features of cord blood cells

Cord blood lymphocytes may be naive and less immunogenic
They bear an immature phenotype
They lack constitutive perforin expression
Cytotoxic cells seems to comprise mostly a NK cell subset

Table 37.7 Peripheral blood stem cell transplantation. Data reviewed in [150]

Study	Patients (n)	CD34+ 10^6/kg	PMN engraftment	Platelet engraftment	CD3+ 10^6/kg	Acute GvHD Grade >2
EBMT [146]	60	6.7	15 days (9–27)	16 days (9–67)	360	48%
Seattle [147]	41	12	14	10	412	38%
Houston [148]	25		10	18		42%
Omaha [107]	14		11 days (9–16)		740	57%
Calgary [107]	26	5.1	16 days (11–28)	13.5 days (12–32)		37%
Dallas [149]	19	8.3	13	14	320	13%
São Paulo [107]	17		14 days (10–20)	14 days (9–88)		52%

depletion leading to the injection of $0.5–1.8 \times 10^6$ CD3+/kg, the reported incidence of moderate-to-severe acute GvHD was significant (more than 80% if patients were given CSP alone as prophylaxis) [107,111]. However, it should be noted that these transplants were performed in older patients with advanced disease. Data on more patients are thus required to obtain a true picture concerning acute GvHD incidence and risk factors following allogeneic CD34+ cell transplantation. Finally, although some CD34+ cell transplants have been performed in patients grafted from unrelated donors, no data are yet available.

Mega-dose T-cell-depleted PBSC and marrow for mismatched transplants

Most patients who might benefit from transplantation do not have an HLA-matched sibling donor. Since the mid 1980s, studies on the feasibility and safety of transplants from partially matched family members have been demonstrating that HLA-matching is the critical and limiting factor in marrow transplantation. Three major problems have emerged from these types of transplant [112]:
1. Poor graft function or graft rejection.
2. Increased incidence and severity of acute GvHD.
3. A profound (and long-lasting) immunodeficient state.

Based on data from a murine model [113], the Perugia group recently reported on the use of mega-doses of T-cell-depleted PBSC and marrow cells in haplo-identical (three-loci incompatible) transplants in patients with advanced haematological malignancies [114, 115]. These authors reported a high incidence of engraftment (34 out of 36 patients, with 4 patients being transplanted twice), and a relatively low incidence of acute GvHD (17%). Nevertheless, the immunodeficient state seems to persist as a major problem in these transplants, since 10 patients died of infectious complications. These promising results should be confirmed in patients with less advanced disease, and such trials are in progress.

New drugs or reagents to prevent or treat acute GvHD

New immunosuppressants

A number of molecules with potent immunosuppressive activity are currently being studied in animal models, in organ transplantation, or as phase I studies in allogeneic BMT. These include, among others: brequinar sodium, deoxypergualin and its derivatives, mizoribine, rapamycin, trimetrexate, mycophenolic acid, tepoxalin, FK506 and RS-61443 [116]. Until now, sufficient clinical data have only been published on the use of FK506 in allogeneic BMT. While the mechanism of action of this compound is similar to CSP, its immunosuppressive activity has been claimed to be superior in liver transplantation. In allogeneic BMT it has been used in steroid-resistant acute or chronic GvHD [117–119] with noticeable activity in nearly 25% of the patients. Two studies enrolling 18 and 27 patients, respectively, aimed to study its efficacy, alone or in combination with methotrexate or steroids, as prophylaxis after HLA-matched sibling transplants [120,121]. The incidence of acute GvHD of grades II–IV was 44% and 41%, respectively, and the main toxicity was renal. Randomized studies comparing standard prophylaxis (CSP + methotrexate and/or prednisone) and FK506 (+ methotrexate and/or prednisone) therefore seem timely and warranted.

Blocking costimulatory signals as a tool to prevent or treat acute GvHD

Antigen-specific T-cell activation requires interaction of the T-cell specialized antigen-presenting cells (APC). In the peripheral blood, dendritic cells, activated B-cells and monocytes can present antigen. In skin, keratinocytes and Langerhans cells serve this function. Antigens coupled to class I MHC molecules are recognized by T-cell receptor (TCR)/CD3 in the context of an associated CD8 molecule, whereas recognition of antigens coupled to class II requires CD4. After crosslinking of TCR by antigen-MHC, T-cells are competent to recognize a number of potential second signals, termed 'costimulation'. Presentation of antigen to the T-cell receptor without costimulation results in a state of antigen-specific unresponsiveness on rechallenge, known as 'anergy' *in vitro* and 'tolerance' *in vivo*. Mounting evidence suggests that inhibition of the costimultatory pathway CD80 (B7-1) / CD86 (B7-2) (on APC) with CD28 / CTLA4 (on T-cells) is both necessary and sufficient to induce antigen-specific anergy [8–10] (Figure 37.6).

These recent advances may be of major importance in the biology of organ transplantation and in allogeneic BMT. Indeed, some murine models have demonstrated that *in vivo* treatment aiming at blocking this costimulatory pathway (through CTLA4-Ig) during the initial period of donor allo activation can completely abort the subsequent development of GvHD [122]. In this model, although T-cells are retained, treatment reduces endogenous cytokine production and arrests the subsequent expansion of donor T-cells.

A recent *in vitro* study has also demonstrated that complete blockade of B7 family-mediated costimulation is necessary to induce human alloantigen-specific anergy [123]. Complete blockade of B7 family-mediated costimulation, but not of MHC recognition or adhesion, induces host alloantigen-specific anergy by reducing cytokine production below the threshold necessary for common chain signalling. The associated reduction of allo-reactive HTL-p frequency below that thought to be predictive for GvHD, without depletion of either non-allospecific T-cells or haematopoietic progenitors seems a promising avenue to explore in the prophylaxis and the treatment of acute GvHD.

Suicide gene for specific in vivo T-cell depletion

Although effectively preventing GvHD, *ex vivo* T-cell depletion increases graft rejection and reduces the GvL effect. The *ex vivo* transfer of the herpes simplex virus thymidine kinase suicide gene (*HSV-tk*) into T-cells before their infusion could allow allo-selective *in vivo* depletion of these T-cells with ganciclovir if subsequent GvHD were to occur. Such *HSV-tk* transduced T-cells have recently been generated [124,125] and the use of such cells is currently being investigated in allogeneic BMT recipients.

Promiscuous binding to class II MHC molecule of synthetic copolymer as a tool to prevent GvHD

A recent study in a murine model of transplantation across minor histocompatibility barriers also presents new possibilities in the prophylaxis of acute GvHD. The Stamford group used a synthetic random basic copolymer with promiscuous binding to class II MHC molecules, and showed that it inhibits T-cell proliferative responses to major and minor histocompatibility antigens *in vitro* and confers the ability to prevent murine GvHD *in vivo* [126]. This new approach in prophylaxis of acute GvHD may well prove of significance in the future, and further studies are under way.

Acknowledgements

The clinical figures were kindly provided by Dr Peter Mortimer.

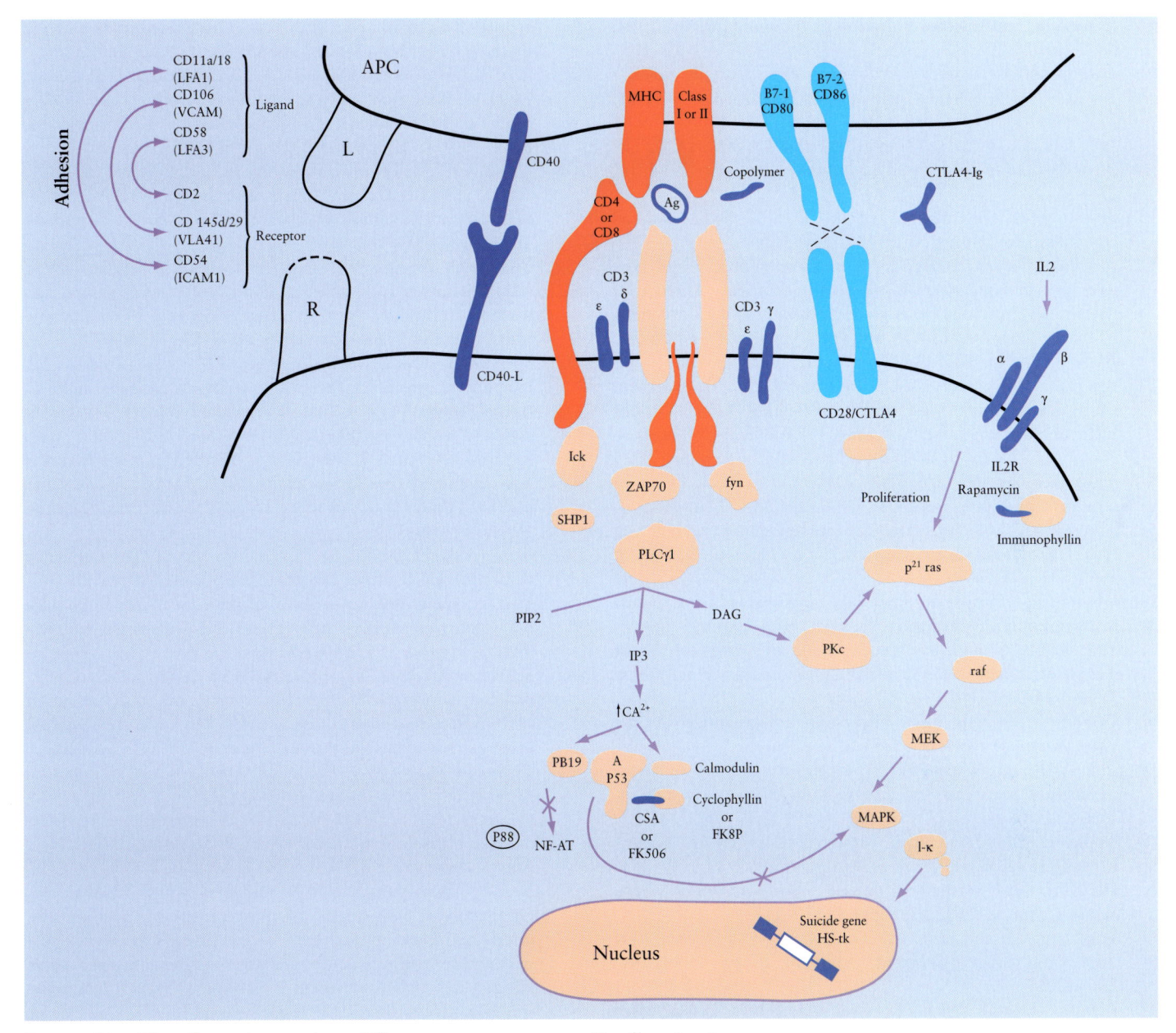

Figure 37.6 The allogenic reaction; different ways to prevent T-cell activation.

References

1. Gratwohl A, Hermans J and Baldomero H. Hematopoietic precursor cell transplants in Europe: activity in 1994. Report from the European Group for Blood and Marrow Transplantation (EBMT). *Bone Marrow Transplant* 1996; **17**: 137–148.
2. Billingham RE. The biology of graft-versus-host reactions. *Harvey Lectures* 1966; **62**: 21–78.
3. Masuko K, Kato S, Hagihara M *et al*. Stable clonal expansion of T cells induced by bone marrow transplantation. *Blood* 1996; **87**: 789–799.
4. Kasten–Sportes C, Masset M, Varrin F, Devergie A and Gluckman E. Phenotype and function of T lymphocytes infiltrating the skin during graft-versus-host disease following allogeneic bone marrow transplantation. *Transplantation* 1989; **47**: 621–624.
5. Gaschet J, Mahe B, Milpied N *et al*. Specificity of T-cells invading the skin during acute graft-vs-host disease after semiallogeneic bone marrow transplantation. *J Clin Invest* 1993; **91**: 12–20.
6. Dietrich PY, Caignard A, Diu A *et al*. Analysis of T-cell receptor variability in transplanted patients with acute graft-versus-host disease. *Blood* 1992; **80**: 2419–2424.
7. Dietrich PY, Caignard A *et al*. In vivo T-cell clonal amplification at time of acute graft versus host disease. *Blood* 1994; **84**: 2815–2820.
8. Guinan EC, Gribben JG, Boussiotis VA, Freeman GJ and Nadler LM. Pivotal role of the B7:CD28 pathway in

transplantation tolerance and tumor immunity. *Blood* 1994; **84**: 3261–3282.
9. Thompson CB. Distinct roles of the costimulatory ligands B7-1 and B7-2 in T helper cell differentiation. *Cell* 1995; **81**: 979–982.
10. June CH, Bluestone JA, Nadler LM and Thompson CB. The B7 and CD28 receptor families. *Immunology Today* 1994; **15**: 321–331.
11. Bluestone JA. New perspectives of CD28-B7-mediated T-cell costimulation. *Immunity* 1995; **2**: 555–559.
12. Brochu S, Baron C, Belanger R and Perreault C. Graft-host tolerance in bone marrow transplant chimeras. Absence of graft-versus-host disease is associated with unresponsiveness to minor histocompatibility antigens expressed by all tissues. *Blood* 1994; **84**: 3221–3228.
13. den Haan JMM, Sherman NE, Blokland E et al. Identification of a graft versus host disease-associated human minor histocompatibility antigen. *Science* 1995; **268**: 1476–1480.
14. Perreault C, Decary F, Brochu S et al. Minor histocompatibility antigens. *Blood* 1990; **76**: 1269–1280.
15. Goulmy E, Voogt P, van Els C, De Bueger M and van Rood J. The role of minor histocompatibility antigens in GvHD and rejection: a mini-review. [Review.] *Bone Marrow Transplant* 1991; **7**(Suppl 1): 49–51.
16. Goulmy E, Schipper R, Pool J et al. Mismatches of minor histocompatibility antigens between HLA-identical donors and recipients and the development of graft-versus-host disease after bone marrow transplantation. *New Engl J Med* 1996; **334**: 281–285.
17. Goulmy E. Human minor histocompatibility antigens. *Curr Opin Immunol* 1996; **8**: 75–81.
18. Jadus MR and Wepsic HT. The role of cytokines in graft-versus-host reactions and disease *Bone Marrow Transplant* 1993; **11**: 89.
19. Appleton AL and Sviland L. Pathogenesis of GvHD – role of herpes viruses. *Bone Marrow Transplant* 1993; **11**: 349–355.
20. Deeg HJ. Graft-versus-host disease – host and donor views. *Semin Hematol* 1993; 30 (Suppl 4) 110–118.
21. Vogelsang GB and Hess AD. Graft-versus-host disease: new directions for a persistent problem. *Blood* 1994; **84**: 2061–2067.
22. Ferrara JL and Deeg HJ. Graft-versus-host disease [see comments]. [Review.] *New Engl J Med* 1991; **324**: 667–674.
23. Antin JH and Ferrara JL. Cytokine dysregulation and acute graft-versus-host disease. [Review.] *Blood* 1992; **80**: 2964–2968.
24. Gale RP, Bortin MM, Van Bekkum DW et al. Risk factors for acute graft-versus-host disease. *Br J Haematol* 1987; **67**: 397–406.
25. Rowlings PA, Przepiorka D, Klein JP and Horowitz MM. A revised grading system for acute graft-vs-host disease. *Blood* 1994; **84**(Suppl 1): 539a.
26. Nash RA, Pepe MS, Storb R et al. Acute graft-versus-host disease: analysis of risk factors after allogeneic marrow transplantation and prophylaxis with cyclosporin and methotrexate [see comments]. *Blood* 1992; **80**: 1838–1845.
27. Hagglund H, Bostrom L, Remberger M et al. Risk factors for acute graft-versus-host disease in 291 consecutive HLA-identical bone marrow transplant recipients. *Bone Marrow Transplant* 1995; **16**: 747–753.
28. Beelen DW, Haralambie E, Brandt H et al. Evidence that sustained growth suppression of intestinal anaerobic bacteria reduces the risk of acute graft-versus-host disease after sibling marrow transplantation. *Blood* 1992; **80**: 2668–2676.
29. Ash RC, Horowitz MM, Gale RP, Van Bekkum DW, Casper JT et al. Bone marrow transplantation from related donors other than HLA-identical siblings: effect of T-cell depletion. *Bone Marrow Transplant* 1991; **7**: 443–452.
30. Degast GC, Mickelson EM, Beatty PG et al. Mixed leukocyte culture reactivity and graft-versus-host disease in HLA-identical marrow transplantation for leukemia. *Bone Marrow Transplant* 1992; **9**: 87–90.
31. Bishara A, Brautbar C, Nagler A et al. Prediction by a modified mixed leukocyte reaction assay of graft-versus-host disease and graft rejection after allogeneic bone marrow transplantation. *Transplantation* 1994; **57**: 1474–1479.
32. Spencer A, Brookes PA, Kaminski EM et al. Cytotoxic T lymphocyte precursor frequency analyses in bone marrow transplantation with volunteer unrelated donors – value in donor selection. *Transplantation* 1995; **59**: 1302–1308.
33. Kaminski E, Hows J, Man S et al. Prediction of graft versus host disease by frequency analysis of cytotoxic T-cells after unrelated donor bone marrow transplantation. *Transplantation* 1989; **48**: 608–613.
34. Roosnek E, Hogendijk S, Zawadynski S et al. The frequency of pretransplant donor cytotoxic T-cell precursors with anti-host specificity predicts survival of patients transplanted with bone marrow donors other than HLA-identical siblings. *Transplantation* 1993; **56**: 691–696.
35. Schwarer AP, Jiang YZ, Brookes PA et al. Frequency of anti-recipient alloreactive helper T-cell precursors in donor blood and graft-versus-host disease after HLA-identical sibling bone-marrow transplantation. *Lancet* 1993; **341**: 203–205.
36. Theobald M, Nierle T, Bunjes D, Arnold R and Heimpel H. Host-specific interleukin-2-secreting donor T-cell precursors as predictors of acute graft-versus-host disease in bone marrow transplantation between HLA-identical siblings. *New Engl J Med* 1992; **327**: 1613–1617.
37. Nierle T, Bunjes D, Arnold R, Heimpel H and Theobald M. Quantitative assessment of posttransplant host-specific interleukin-2-secreting T-helper cell precursors in patients with and without acute graft-versus-host disease after allogeneic HLA-identical sibling bone marrow transplantation. *Blood* 1993; **81**: 841–848.
38. Theobald M and Bunjes D. Pretransplant detection of human minor histocompatibility antigen-specific naive and memory interleukin-2 secreting T-cells within class-I major histocompatibility complex (MHC)-restricted CD8+ and class-II MHC-restricted CD4+ T-cell subsets. *Blood* 1993; **82**: 298–306.
39. Johnsen HE. Predictors of acute graft-versus-host disease in bone marrow transplantation between HLA-identical siblings. *New Engl J Med* 1993; **328**: 1497.
40. Kernan NA and Dupont B. Minor histocompatibility antigens and marrow transplantation. *New Engl J Med* 1996; **334**: 323–324.
41. Niederwieser D, Grassegger A, Aubock J et al. Correlation of minor histocompatibility antigen-specific cytotoxic T-lymphocytes with graft-versus-host disease status and analyses of tissue distribution of their target antigens. *Blood* 1993; **81**: 2200–2208.
42. De Bueger M, Bakker A, Bontkes H, Van Rood JJ and Goulmy E. High frequencies of cytotoxic T-cell precursors

against minor histocompatibility antigens after HLA-identical BMT – absence of correlation with GvHD. *Bone Marrow Transplant* 1993; **11**: 363–368.
43. Behar E, Chao NJ, Hiraki DD *et al*. Polymorphism of adhesion molecule CD31 and its role in acute graft-versus-host disease. *New Engl J Med* 1996; **334**: 286–291.
44. Glucksberg H, Storb R, Fefer A *et al*. Clinical manifestation of graft-vs-host disease in human recipients of marrow from HLA-matched sibling donors. *Transplantation* 1974; **18**: 295–304.
45. Sullivan KM. Graft-versus-host disease. In: *Bone Marrow Transplantation*. SJ Forman, KG Blume and ED Thomas (eds), 1994: 339–359 (Cambridge, MA: Blackwell Scientific).
46. Thomas ED, Storb R, Clift RA, Fefer A, Johnson FL *et al*. Bone marrow transplantation. *New Engl J Med* 1975; **292**: 895–902.
47. Thomas ED, Storb R, Clift RA *et al*. Bone marrow transplantation. *New Engl J Med* 1975; **292**: 832–843.
48. Vogelsang GB, Hess AD and Santos GW. Acute graft-vs-host disease: clinical characteristics in the cyclosporin era. *Medicine* 1988; **67**: 163–174.
49. Bertheau P, Hadengue A, Cazalshatem D, Devergie A, Schretzenmeyer C *et al*. Chronic cholestasis in patients after allogeneic bone marrow transplantation: several diseases are often associated. *Bone Marrow Transplant* 1995; **16**: 261–265.
50. Deeg HJ and Cottler-Fox M. Clinical spectrum and pathophysiology of acute graft-vs-host disease. In: *Graft-vs-Host Disease*. SJ Burakoff, HJ Deeg, J Ferrara and K Atkinson (eds), 1990: 311–335 (New York: Marcel Dekker).
51. Weisdorf DJ, Snover DC, Haake R, *et al*. Acute upper gastrointestinal graft-vs-host disease: clinical significance and response to immunosuppressive therapy. *Blood* 1990; **76**: 624–629.
52. Przepiorka D, Weisdorf D, Martin P *et al*. Consensus Conference on Acute GvHD Grading. *Bone Marrow Transplant* 1995; **15**: 825–828.
53. Ringden O. Management of graft-versus-host disease. *Eur J Haematol* 1993; **51**: 1–12.
54. Pietryga D. Prevention and treatment of acute graft-versus-host disease. *Am J Pediatr Hematol Oncol* 1993; **15**: 28–48.
55. Lazarus HM, Coccia PF and Herzig RH. Incidence of acute graft-versus-host disease with and without methotrexate prophylaxis in allogeneic bone marrow transplant patients. *Blood* 1984; **64**: 215–220.
56. Sullivan KM, Storb R, Buckner CD *et al*. Graft-versus-host disease as adoptive immunotherapy in patients with advanced hematologic neoplasms. *New Engl J Med* 1989; **320**: 828–834.
57. Powles RL, Clink H and Spence D. Cyclosporin-A to prevent graft-versus-host disease in man after allogeneic bone marrow transplantation. *Lancet* 1980; **i**: 327–329.
58. Tutschka PJ, Beschorner WE, Hess AD and Santos GW. Cyclosporin-A to prevent graft-versus-host disease: a pilot study in 22 patients receiving allogeneic marrow transplants. *Blood* 1983; **61**: 318–325.
59. Gluckman E, Lokiek F and Devergie A. Use of cyclosporin for prevention of acute graft-versus-host disease after allogeneic bone marrow transplantation. *Transplant Proc* 1988; **20**: 461–469.
60. Storb R, Deeg HJ, Fisher L *et al*. Cyclosporin vs methotrexate for graft-versus-host disease prevention in patients given marrow grafts for leukemia: long term follow-up of three controlled trials. *Blood* 1988; **71**: 293–298.
61. Storb R, Martin P, Deeg HJ *et al*. Long-term follow-up of three controlled trials comparing cyclosporin versus methotrexate for graft-versus-host disease prevention in patients given marrow grafts for leukemia. [Letter.] *Blood* 1992; **79**: 3091–3092.
62. Ringden O, Horowitz MM, Sondel P *et al*. Methotrexate, cyclosporin, or both to prevent graft-versus-host disease after HLA-identical sibling bone marrow transplants for early leukemia. *Blood* 1993; **81**: 1094–1101.
63. Bacigalupo A, Van Lint MT, Occhini D *et al*. Increased risk of leukemia relapse with high dose cyclosporin-A after allogeneic marrow transplantation for acute leukemia. *Blood* 1991; **77**: 1423–1428.
64. Storb R, Deeg HJ, Pepe M *et al*. Methotrexate and cyclosporin versus cyclosporin alone for prophylaxis of graft-versus-host disease in patients given HLA-identical marrow grafts for leukemia: long-term follow-up of a controlled trial. *Blood* 1989; **73**: 1729–1734.
65. Storb R, Pepe M, Deeg HJ *et al*. Long-term follow-up of a controlled trial comparing a combination of methotrexate plus cyclosporin with cyclosporin alone for prophylaxis of graft-versus-host disease in patients administered HLA-identical marrow grafts for leukemia. [Letter.] *Blood* 1992; **80**: 560–561.
66. Storb R, Deeg HJ, Pepe M *et al*. Graft-versus-host disease prevention by methotrexate combined with cyclosporin compared to methotrexate alone in patients given marrow grafts for severe aplastic anaemia: long-term follow-up of a controlled trial. *Br J Haematol* 1989; **72**: 567–572.
67. Storb R, Leisenring W, Deeg HJ *et al*. Long-term follow-up of a randomized trial of graft-versus-host disease prevention by methotrexate/cyclosporin versus methotrexate alone in patients given marrow grafts for severe aplastic anemia. *Blood* 1994; **83**: 2749–2750.
68. Storb R, Deeg HJ, Farewell V *et al*. Marrow transplantation for severe aplastic anemia: methotrexate alone compared with a combination of methotrexate and cyclosporin for prevention of acute graft-versus-host disease. *Blood* 1986; **68**: 119–125.
69. Vonbueltzingsloewen A, Belanger R, Perreault C *et al*. Acute graft-versus-host disease prophylaxis with methotrexate and cyclosporine after busulfan and cyclophosphamide in patients with hematologic malignancies. *Blood* 1993; **81**: 849–855.
70. Forman SJ, Blume KG, Krance RA, Miner PJ, Metter GE *et al*. A prospective randomized study of acute graft-versus-host disease in 107 patients with leukemia: methotrexate/prednisone v cyclosporin/prednisone. *Transplant Proc* 1987; **19**: 2605–2607.
71. Storb R, Pepe M, Anasetti C *et al*. What role for prednisone in prevention of acute graft-versus-host disease in patients undergoing marrow transplantation? *Blood* 1990; **76**: 1037–1045.
72. Chao NJ, Schmidt GM, Niland JC *et al*. Cyclosporin, methotrexate, and prednisone compared with cyclosporine and prednisone for prophylaxis of acute graft-versus-host disease. *New Engl J Med* 1993; **329**: 1225–1230.
73. Maraninchi D, Gluckman E, Blaise D *et al*. Impact of T-cell depletion on the results of allogeneic bone marrow transplantation for standard risk leukaemia: a randomized study of the GEGMO. *Lancet* 1987; **ii**: 175–178.

74. Mitsuyasu RT, Champlin RE, Gale RP et al. Treatment of donor bone marrow with monoclonal anti-T-cell antibody and complement for prevention of graft-versus-host disease: a prospective, randomized, double-blind trial. *Ann Intern Med* 1986; **105**: 20–26.
75. Ringden O, Remberger M, Aschan J et al. Long-term follow-up of a randomized trial comparing T-cell depletion with a combination of methotrexate and cyclosporin in adult leukemic marrow transplant recipients. *Transplantation* 1994; **58**: 887–891.
76. Marmont A, Horowitz MM, Gale RP et al. T-cell depletion of HLA-identical transplants in leukemia. *Blood* 1991; **78**: 2120–2130.
77. Blaise D, Maraninchi D, Mawas C et al. Prevention of acute graft-versus-host-disease by monoclonal antibody to interleukin-2 receptor. *Lancet* 1989; **ii**: 1333–1334.
78. Belanger C, Esperou-Bourdeau H, Bordigoni P et al. Use of an anti-interleukin-2 receptor monoclonal antibody for GvHD prophylaxis in unrelated donor BMT. *Bone Marrow Transplant* 1993; **11**: 293–297.
79. Anasetti C, Martin PJ, Storb R et al. Prophylaxis of graft-versus-host disease by administration of the murine anti-IL-2 receptor antibody 2A3. *Bone Marrow Transplant* 1991; **7**: 375–381.
80. Blaise D, Olive D, Michallet M et al. Impairment of leukaemia-free survival by addition of interleukin-2-receptor antibody to standard graft-versus-host prophylaxis. *Lancet* 1995; **345**: 1144–1146.
81. Anasetti C, Lin AY, Gluckman E et al. A phase II/III randomized, double blind, placebo-controlled multicenter trial of humanized anti-tac for prevention of acute graft-versus-host disease in recipients of marrow transplants from unrelated donors. *Blood* 1995; **86**(Suppl 1): 621a.
82. Deeg HJ and Henslee-Downey PJ. Management of acute graft-versus-host disease. *Bone Marrow Transplant* 1990; **6**: 1–8.
83. Storb R, Gluckman E, Thomas ED et al. Treatment of established human graft-versus-host disease by antithymocyte globulin. *Blood* 1974; **44**: 57–75.
84. Doney KC, Weiden PL, Storb R and Thomas ED. Treatment of graft-versus-host disease in human allogeneic marrow graft recipients: a randomized trial comparing antithymocyte globulin and corticosteroids. *Am J Hematol* 1981; **11**: 1–8.
85. Kennedy MS, Deeg HJ, Storb R, Doney K, Sullivan KM et al. Treatment of acute graft-versus-host disease after allogeneic bone marrow transplantation: randomized study comparing corticosteroids and cyclosporine. *Am J Med* 1985; **78**: 978–983.
86. Deeg HJ, Loughran TP, Storb R et al. Treatment of human acute graft-versus-host disease with antithymocyte globulin with or without methylprednisolone. *Transplantation* 1985; **40**: 162–166.
87. Hings IM, Filipovich AH, Miller WJ et al. Prednisone therapy for acute graft-versus-host disease – short-term versus long-term treatment. *Transplantation* 1993; **56**: 577–580.
88. Weisdorf D, Haake R, Blazar B et al. Treatment of moderate/severe acute graft-versus-host disease after allogeneic bone marrow transplantation: an analysis of clinical feature and outcome. *Blood* 1990; **75**: 1024–1030.
89. Hings IM, Severson R, Filipovich AH et al. Treatment of moderate and severe acute GvHD after allogeneic bone marrow transplantation. *Transplantation* 1994; **58**: 437–442.
90. Martin PJ, Schoch G, Fisher L et al. A retrospective analysis of therapy for acute graft-versus-host disease: initial treatment. *Blood* 1990; **76**: 1464–1472.
91. Martin PJ, Schoch G, Fisher L et al. A retrospective analysis of therapy for acute graft-versus-host disease: secondary treatment. *Blood* 1991; **77**: 1821–1828.
92. Baehr PH, Levine DS, Bouvier ME et al. Oral beclomethasone dipropionate for treatment of human intestinal graft-versus-host disease. *Transplantation* 1995; **60**: 1231–1238.
93. Ely P, Dunitz J, Rogosheske J and Weisdorf D. Use of a somatostatin analogue, octreotide acetate, in the management of acute gastrointestinal graft-versus-host disease. *Am J Med* 1991; **90**: 707–710.
94. Cahn JY, Bordigoni P, Tiberghien P et al. Treatment of acute graft-versus-host disease with methylprednisolone and cyclosporin with or without an anti-interleukin-2 receptor monoclonal antibody – a multicenter phase III study. *Transplantation* 1995; **60**: 939–942.
95. Antin JH. Graft-versus-leukemia – no longer an epiphenomenon. *Blood* 1993; **82**: 2273–2277.
96. Horowitz MM, Gale RP, Sondel PM et al. Graft-versus-leukemia reactions after bone marrow transplantation. *Blood* 1990; **75**: 555–562.
97. Sullivan KM, Weiden PL, Storb R et al. Influence of acute and chronic graft-vs-host disease on relapse and survival after bone marrow transplantation from HLA-identical siblings as treatment of acute and chronic leukemia. *Blood* 1989; **73**: 1720–1728.
98. Sosman JA and Sondel PM. The graft-versus-leukemia effect: implications for post marrow transplant antileukemia treatment. *Am J Pediatr Hematol Oncol* 1993; **15**: 185–195.
99. Kolb HJ, Schattenberg A, Goldman JM et al. Graft-versus-leukemia effect of donor lymphocyte transfusions in marrow grafted patients. *Blood* 1995; **86**: 2041–2050.
100. Berthou C, Legrosmaida S, Soulie A et al. Cord blood T lymphocytes lack constitutive perforin expression in contrast to adult peripheral blood T lymphocytes. *Blood* 1995; **85**: 1540–1546.
101. Bensussan A, Gluckman E, Elmarsafy S et al. BY55 monoclonal antibody delineates within human cord blood and bone marrow lymphocytes distinct cell subsets mediating cytotoxic activity. *Proc Natl Acad Sci USA* 1994; **91**: 9136–9140.
102. Wagner JE, Kernan NA, Steinbuch M, Broxmeyer HE and Gluckman E. Allogeneic sibling umbilical-cord-blood transplantation in children with malignant and non-malignant disease. *Lancet* 1995; **346**: 214–219.
103. Korbling M, Przepiorka D, Huh YO et al. Allogeneic blood stem cell transplantation for refractory leukemia and lymphoma: potential advantage of blood over marrow allografts. *Blood* 1995; **85**: 1659–1665.
104. Schmitz N, Dreger P, Suttorp M et al. Primary transplantation of allogeneic peripheral blood progenitor cells mobilized by filgrastim (granulocyte colony-stimulating factor). *Blood* 1995; **85**: 1666–1672.
105. Bensinger WI, Weaver CH, Appelbaum FR et al. Transplantation of allogeneic peripheral blood stem cells mobilized by recombinant human granulocyte colony-stimulating factor. *Blood* 1995; **85**: 1655–1658.
106. Korbling M, Huh YO, Durett A et al. Allogeneic blood stem cell transplantation: peripheralization and yield of donor-

derived primitive hematopoietic progenitor cells (CD34(+) Thy-1(dim)) and lymphoid subsets, and possible predictors of engraftment and graft-versus-host disease. *Blood* 1995; **86**: 2842–2848.
107. Proceedings of the First International Symposium on Allogeneic Peripheral Blood Progenitor Cell Transplantation: An EBMT Symposium. *Bone Marrow Transplant* 1996; **17**(Suppl 2): S1–S82.
108. Goldman J. Peripheral blood stem cells for allografting. *Blood* 1995; **85**: 1413–1415.
109. Krause DS, Fackler MJ, Civin CI and May WS. CD34: Structure, biology, and clinical utility. *Blood* 1996; **87**: 1–13.
110. Link H, Arseniev L, Bahre O et al. Combined transplantation of allogeneic bone marrow and CD34(+) blood cells. *Blood* 1995; **86**: 2500–2508.
111. Link H, Arseniev L, Bahre O et al. Transplantation of allogeneic CD34+ blood cells. *Blood* 1996; **87**: 4903–4909.
112. Hervé P, Cahn JY and Beatty P. Graft-vs-host disease after bone marrow transplantation from donors other than HLA-identical siblings. In: *Graft-vs-Host Disease*. SJ Burakoff, HJ Deeg, J Ferrara and K Atkinson (eds), 1990: 425–454 (New York: Marcel Dekker).
113. Bacharlustig E, Rachamim N, Li HW, Lan FS and Reisner Y. Megadose of T-cell-depleted bone marrow overcomes MHC barriers in sublethally irradiated mice. *Nature Medicine* 1995; **1**: 1268–1273.
114. Aversa F, Tabilio A, Terenzi A et al. Successful engraftment of T-cell-depleted haploidentical 'three-loci' incompatible transplants in leukemia patients by addition of recombinant human granulocyte colony-stimulating factor-mobilized peripheral blood progenitor cells to bone marrow inoculum. *Blood* 1994; **84**: 3948–3955.
115. Aversa F, Terenzi A, Tabilio A et al. Addition of PBPC to the marrow inoculum allows engraftment of mismatched T-cell depleted transplants for acute leukemia. *Bone Marrow Transplant* 1996; **17**(Suppl 2): S58–S61.
116. Sharma V, Li B, Khanna A, Sehajpal PK and Suthanthiran M. Which way for drug-mediated immunosuppression? *Curr Opin Immunol* 1994; **6**: 784–790.
117. Kanamaru A, Takemoto Y, Kakishita E et al. FK506 treatment of graft-versus-host disease developing or exacerbating during prophylaxis and therapy with cyclosporin and/or other immunosuppressants. *Bone Marrow Transplant* 1995; **15**: 885–889.
118. Koehler MT, Howrie D, Mirro J et al. FK506 (tacrolimus) in the treatment of steroid-resistant acute graft-versus-host disease in children undergoing bone marrow transplantation. *Bone Marrow Transplant* 1995; **15**: 895–899.
119. Hemenway C. FK506 in bone marrow transplantation. *Blood* 1995; **86**: 3611–3612.
120. Nash RA, Etzioni R, Storb R et al. Tacrolimus (FK506) alone or in combination with methotrexate or methylprednisolone for the prevention of acute graft-versus-host disease after marrow transplantation from HLA-matched siblings: A single-center study. *Blood* 1995; **85**: 3746–3753.
121. Caux C, Massacrier C, De Zutterdambuyant C et al. Human dendritic Langerhans cells generated *in vitro* from CD34(+) progenitors can prime naive CD4(+) T cells and process soluble antigen. *J Immunol* 1995; **155**: 5427–5435.
122. Hakim FT, Cepeda R, Gray GS, June CH and Abe R. Acute graft-vs-host reaction can be aborted by blockade of costimulatory molecules. *J Immunol* 1995; **155**: 1757–1766.
123. Gribben JG, Guinan E, Boussiotis VA et al. Complete blockade of B7 family-mediated costimulation is necessary to induce human alloantigen specific anergy: a method to ameliorate graft-vs-host disease and extend donor pool. *Blood* 1996; **87**: 4887–4893.
124. Tiberghien P, Reynolds CW, Keller J et al. Ganciclovir treatment of herpes simplex thymidine kinase-transduced primary T lymphocytes: An approach for specific *in vivo* donor T-cell depletion after bone marrow transplantation? *Blood* 1994; **84**: 1333–1341.
125. Tiberghien P. Use of suicide genes in gene therapy. *J Leukocyte Biol* 1994; **56**: 203–209.
126. Schlegel PG, Aharoni R, Chen Y et al. A synthetic random basic copolymer with promiscuous binding to class II major histocompatibility complex molecules inhibits T-cell proliferative responses to major and minor histocompatibility antigens *in vitro* and confers the capacity to prevent murine graft-versus-host disease *in vitro*. *Proc Natl Acad Sci USA* 1996; **93**: 5061–5066.
127. Spencer A, Szydlo RM, Brookes PA et al. Bone marrow transplantation for chronic myeloid leukemia with volunteer unrelated donors using *ex vivo* or *in vivo* T-cell depletion. Major prognostic impact of HLA class I identity between donor and recipient. *Blood* 1995; **86**: 3590–3597.
128. Balduzzi A, Gooley T, Anasetti C et al. Unrelated donor marrow transplantation in children. *Blood* 1995; **86**: 3247–3256.
129. Petersdorf EW, Longton GM, Anasetti C et al. The significance of HLA-DRB1 matching on clinical outcome after HLA-A, B, DR identical unrelated donor marrow transplantation. *Blood* 1995; **86**: 1606–1613.
130. Davies SM, Shu XO, Blazer BR et al. Unrelated donor bone marrow transplantation: Influence of HLA A and B incompatibility on outcome. *Blood* 1995; **86**: 1636–1642.
131. Casper J, Camitta B, Truitt R et al. Unrelated bone marrow donor transplants for children with leukemia or myelodysplasia. *Blood* 1995; **85**: 2354–2363.
132. Kernan NA, Bartsch G, Ash RC et al. Analysis of 462 transplantations from unrelated donors facilitated by the National Marrow Donor Program. *New Engl J Med* 1993; **328**: 593–602.
133. Schiller G, Feig SA, Territo M et al. Treatment of advanced acute leukaemia with allogeneic bone marrow transplantation from unrelated donors. *Br J Haematol* 1994; **88**: 72–78.
134. Marks DI, Cullis JO, Ward KN et al. Allogeneic bone marrow transplantation for chronic myeloid leukemia using sibling and volunteer unrelated donors – a comparison of complications in the first two years. *Ann Intern Med* 1993; **119**: 207–214.
135. McGlave P, Bartsch G, Anasetti C et al. Unrelated donor marrow transplantation therapy for chronic myelogenous leukemia – initial experience of the National Marrow Donor Program. *Blood* 1993; **81**: 543–550.
136. Hebart H, Ehninger G, Schmidt H et al. Treatment of steroid-resistant graft-versus-host disease after allogeneic bone marrow transplantation with anti-CD3/TCR monoclonal antibodies. *Bone Marrow Transplant* 1995; **15**: 891–894.
137. Anasetti C, Martin PJ, Hansen JA et al. A phase I-II study evaluating the murine anti-IL-2 receptor antibody 2A3 for treatment of acute graft-versus-host disease. *Transplantation* 1990; **50**: 49–54.

138. Byers V, Henslee PJ, Kernan NA *et al.* Use of an anti-pan-T lymphocyte ricin A chain immunotoxin in steroid-resistant acute graft-versus-host disease. *Blood* 1990; **75**: 1426–1432.
139. Hervé P, Wijdenes J, Bergerat JP *et al.* Treatment of corticosteroid resistant graft-versus-host disease by *in vivo* administration of anti-interleukin-2 receptor monoclonal antibody (B-B10). *Blood* 1990; **75**: 1017–1023.
140. Hervé P, Flesch M, Tiberghien P *et al.* Phase I–II trial of a monoclonal anti-tumor necrosis factor alpha antibody for the treatment of refractory severe acute graft-versus-host disease. *Blood* 1992; **79**: 3362–3368.
141. Anasetti C, Martin PJ, Storb R *et al.* Treatment of acute graft-versus-host disease with a nonmitogenic anti-CD3 monoclonal antibody. *Transplantation* 1992; **54**: 844–851.
142. Anasetti C, Hansen JA, Waldmann TA *et al.* Treatment of acute graft-versus-host disease with humanized anti-Tac: an antibody that binds to the interleukin-2 receptor. *Blood* 1994; **84**: 1320–1327.
143. Antin JH, Weinstein HJ, Guinan EC *et al.* Recombinant human interleukin-1 receptor antagonist in the treatment of steroid-resistant graft-versus-host disease. *Blood* 1994; **84**: 1342–1348.
144. Racadot E, Milpied N, Bordigoni P *et al.* Sequential use of three monoclonal antibodies in corticosteroid-resistant acute GvHD: a multicentric pilot study including 15 patients. *Bone Marrow Transplant* 1995; **15**: 669–677.
145. Heslop HE, Benaim E, Brenner MK *et al.* Response of steroid-resistant graft-versus-host disease to lymphoblast antibody CBL1. *Lancet* 1995; **346**: 805–806.
146. Schmitz N, Bacigalupo A, Labopin M *et al.* Transplantation of allogeneic peripheral blood progenitor cells – the EBMT experience. *Bone Marrow Transplant* 1996; **17**: S40–S46.
147. Gandhi V, Estey E, Keating MJ, Chucrallah A and Plunkett W. Chlorodeoxyadenosine and arabinosylcytosine in patients with acute myelogenous leukemia: pharmacokinetic, pharmacodynamic, and molecular interactions. *Blood* 1996; **87**: 256–264.
148. Korbling M and Fliedner T. The evolution of clinical peripheral blood stem cell transplantation. *Bone Marrow Transplant* 1996; **17**: S4–S11.
149. Rosenfeld C, Collins R, Pineiro L, Agura E and Nemunaitis J. Allogeneic blood cell transplantation without posttransplant colony-stimulating factors in patients with hematopoietic neoplasm: a phase II study. *J Clin Oncol* 1996; **14**: 1314–1319.
150. Russell N, Gratwohl A and Schmitz N. The place of blood stem cells in allogeneic transplantation. *Br J Haematol* 1996; **93**: 747–753.

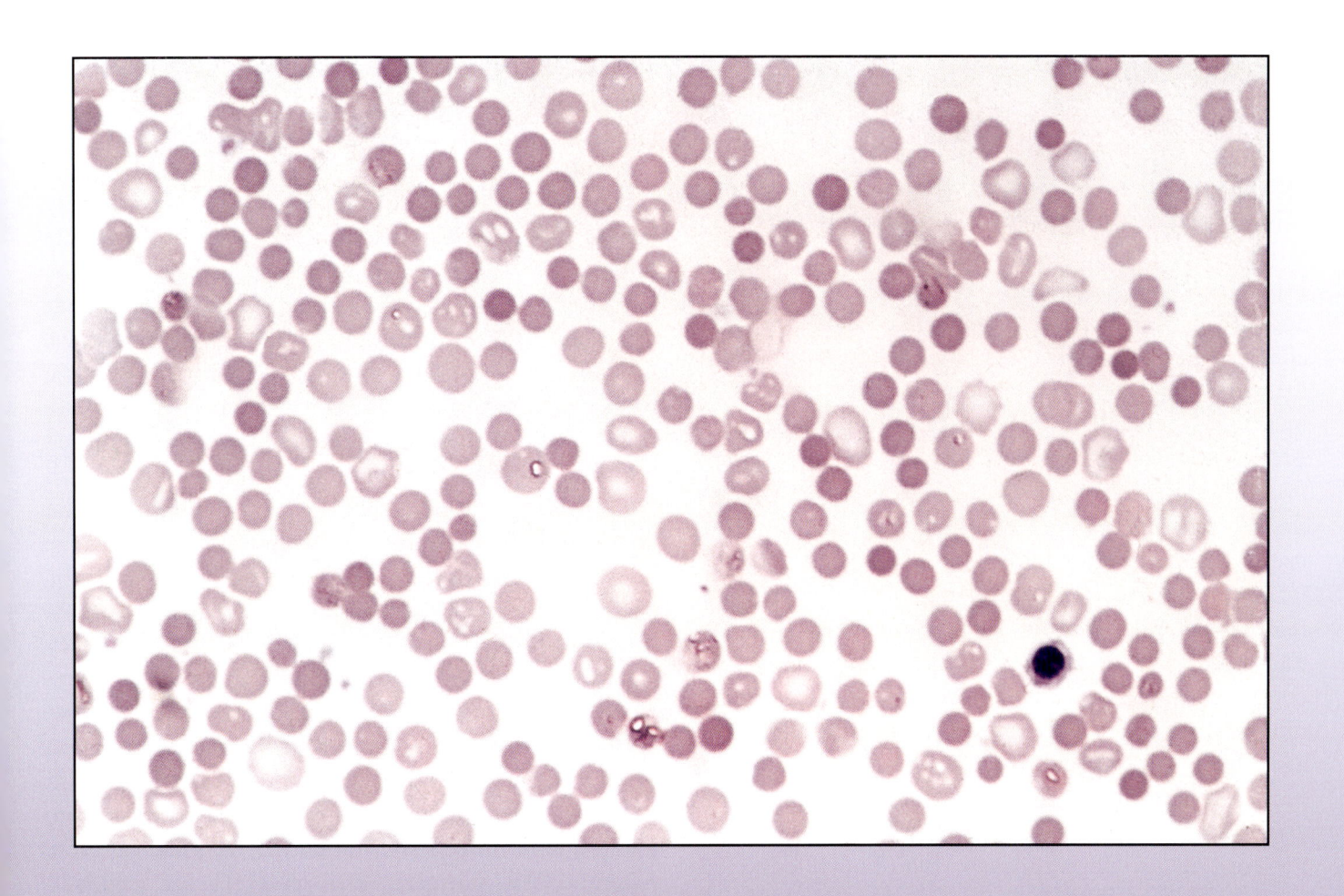

Chapter 38
Chronic graft-versus-host disease

Adriana Seber and Georgia B. Vogelsang

Introduction

Chronic graft-versus-host disease (cGvHD) is rapidly becoming one of the most significant problems faced by allogeneic bone-marrow transplant (BMT) patients. It is reported to occur in 25–60% of patients surviving more than four months after allogeneic transplantation. Significant advances in the treatment and prevention of acute GvHD (aGvHD) have been achieved but these advances have not translated into decreased rates of cGvHD. This persistently high incidence of cGvHD may be explained by the fact that BMT has been performed in patients with progressively higher risk of cGvHD. It is known that the incidence of cGvHD increases with age, with the use of mismatched or unrelated donors, and with the infusion of donor leukocytes to prevent or treat the relapse of underlying malignancies after BMT (Table 38.1). The age of patients receiving transplants has continued to increase, so that many transplant centres now offer allogeneic transplants to patients up to the age of 65 years. Increasing numbers of patients are receiving transplants from mismatched or unrelated donors, or are receiving donor leukocyte infusions. Patients receiving vigorously lymphocyte-depleted marrow grafts have a lower incidence of cGvHD. A history of acute GvHD or the finding of GvHD on a skin or oral biopsy by day 100 after transplant despite the lack of clinically evident GvHD, are strong predictors for subsequent development of cGvHD. Finally, there is a suggestion that patients receiving allogeneic peripheral blood stem-cell transplants may have a lower incidence of aGvHD, but a higher incidence of cGvHD than comparable patients receiving marrow grafts.

Understanding of cGvHD has lagged significantly behind our understanding of aGvHD. In most patients with cGvHD, autoreactive T-cells can be demonstrated, as would be expected in a disease that can resemble most of the known autoimmune diseases. In animal models, the investigation of the pathophysiology of cGvHD is very expensive and time-consuming. Patients have frequently already returned home by the time they develop cGvHD, a fact which compromises the ability to investigate the immunobiology and clinical features of cGvHD. The early manifestations of the disease can be missed if the patients are seen at long intervals. Assumptions regarding cGvHD are influenced by the frequency patients are seen at the transplant centres.

The first thorough review of cGvHD published by Sullivan *et al.* in 1981 [1], described the manifestation of severe end-stage cGvHD, the initial experience with its treatment and, perhaps the most important lesson, the frequent infectious complications seen in these patients. All patients with cGvHD are severely immunocompromised. Their death is usually not due to the manifestations of GvHD, but related to infections. All patients should be maintained on prophylactic antibiotics and given strict warnings about the potential for rapid development of significant infectious complications.

Table 38.1 Risk factors for the development of chronic GvHD

Older age
Donors with mismatched HLA
Unrelated donors
Use of donor leukocyte infusions
History of acute GvHD
Positive skin or oral biopsy at day 100 post BMT
Use of peripheral blood stem cells instead of bone marrow

Classification of chronic GvHD

There is no standardized classification of cGvHD, and this severely limits comparison of patients entered into different clinical trials. Chronic GvHD can be classified according to the type of onset, the clinical manifestations and the extent of the disease. Patients in whom cGvHD evolves directly from aGvHD have a progressive onset. These patients usually have the most severe cGvHD, with a very high mortality. In the quiescent onset, the aGvHD is followed by a period with no detectable GvHD before the development of cGvHD. Finally, a rare group of patients have *de novo* cGvHD. That is, there is no antecedent aGvHD. We have recently described a fourth type of onset – explosive GvHD – in which patients develop acute onset of multi-organ involvement of GvHD, which shifts within days of presentation from erythroderma (severe acute) to a diffuse lichenoid eruption (chronic). Patients have both acute organ GvHD involving the liver and/or gut, and chronic manifestations of GvHD in the mouth and eyes. As opposed to progressive cGvHD, many of these patients have not had prior aGvHD, and some have had known cGvHD. Explosive GvHD is usually associated with abrupt cessation of immunosuppressive agents or severe skin injury (sunburn, herpes infections, and drug eruptions). The survival of patients with explosive GvHD is extremely poor.

Chronic GvHD can also be classified as limited and extensive disease. Limited GvHD is defined as localized skin involvement with or without mild hepatic dysfunction. Extensive GvHD is defined as either generalized skin involvement, or localized skin involvement associated with severe hepatic (progressive hepatitis, bridging necrosis, or cirrhosis at the liver biopsy), ocular, oral or any other target organ involvement. In other words, patients with extensive disease have multi-organ involvement as defined by skin in addition to any organ other than the liver, unless the liver shows significant damage at liver biopsy. Although this classification of cGvHD is relatively easy, its utility has not yet been demonstrated.

Finally, cGvHD can be divided according to the cutaneous manifestations as lichenoid and sclerodermatous. The lichenoid form is the most common presentation. It usually occurs earlier after BMT, and sometimes evolves into a sclerodermatous form later in the course of poorly controlled cGvHD. A distinction between these two forms of GvHD is essential due to the different therapeutic approach adopted in the treatment of each of them, as discussed later in this chapter. Table 38.2 summarizes the classifications of GvHD.

Clinical manifestations

These are summarized in Table 38.3. The organ most commonly involved in cGvHD is the skin, although occasional patients have isolated oral, ocular, or hepatic disease.

Skin

Skin which is damaged by either aGvHD, sun, or herpetic infections seems to be more susceptible to developing cGvHD. Lichenoid GvHD presents as a papular pruriginous rash which resembles lichen planus (Figures 38.1A,B). As opposed to aGvHD, there is no typical distribution. Simultaneous involvement of the lacrimal and salivary glands is common,

Table 38.2 Classification of chronic GvHD

Criteria	Type of cGvHD	Characteristics
Onset	Progressive	Direct evolution from aGvHD
	Quiescent	Onset after complete resolution of aGvHD
	De novo	No antecedent aGvHD
	Explosive	Acute and chronic GvHD features are concomitant at the time of onset and very aggressive
Extension	Limited	Skin (localized) associated/not to mild liver involvement
	Extensive	Skin (generalized) and/or liver (severe), eye, mouth, or any other target organ involvement
Clinical presentation	Sclerodermatous	Thickening and tautness of the skin, usually patchy, occasional blisters and ulcers. Associated or isolated fascial involvement causes severe limitation in the range of motion
	Lichenoid	Maculo-papular rash. Skin is thick and rough. Common oral and ocular involvement. Can evole to scleroderma

Table 38.3 Clinical manifestations of chronic GvHD

Organ	Clinical manifestation	Evauluation	Intervention
Skin	Papular rash (lichenoid) or thick, taut, fragile skin, with poor healing (sclerodermatous)	Clinical and biopsy to confirm the diagnosis of GvHD	Moisture (ideally with petroleum jelly), treat local infection, protect from further trauma
Nails	Vertical ridging, fragile, cracked	Clinical	Nail polish or SuperGlue may help to decrease further damage
Sweat glands	Inflammation leading to risk of hyperthermia		Avoid excessively warm places
Hair	Scalp and body hair is thin and fragile, can be partially or completely lost	Clinical	
Eyes	Dryness, photophobia, and burning. Progression to corneal abrasion if appropriate care is not initiated	Regular ophthalmological evaulation including Schirmer's test	Preservative-free tears during the day and preservative-free ointment at night
Mouth	Dry, sensitivity to toothpaste, spicy food, tomato ketchup. Whitish non-detachable plaques in the cheeks and tongue identical to lichen planus. Erythema and painful ulcerations, mucosal scleroderma with decreased sensitivity to temperature can also happen	Regular dentist evaulation (with appropriate endocarditis prophylaxis. Viral and fungal cultures at diagnosis and at any worsening exam or symptoms	Avoid substances which are not tolerated, as well as extreme temperatures. Toothpastes without mint are better tolerated. Regular dental care preceded by appropriate endocarditis prophylaxis
Respiratory tract	Bronchiolitis obliterans can manifest as dyspnoea, wheezing, cough with normal computed tomography scan and marked obstruction at pulmonary function tests. Chronic sinopulmonary symptoms and/or infections are also common	Periodic pulmonary function tests including FEV_1, FVC, DLCO helium lung volumes. Computed tomography (CT) scan in symptomatic patients. With abnormal chest CT must rule out infections. Lung biopsy if clinically indicated. CT scan of the sinuses if clinically indicated	Replacement of IgG may decrease the incidence of brochiolitis

Table 38.3 Continued

Organ	Clinical manifestation	Evaluation	Intervention
Gastrointestinal tract	Abnormal motility and strictures can happen. Infrequently reflux, dysphagia, substernal pain, diarrhoea, malabsorption, weight loss	Swallowing studies, endoscopy if clinically indicated. Nutritional evaluation	Systemic treatment of GvHD; endoscopic/surgical treatment of strictures. Nutritional intervention as early and effective as possible is essential for overall improvement
Liver	Cholestasis (increased bilirubin, alkaline phosphatase). Isolated liver involvement must have histological confirmation of GvHD	Periodic liver-function test checks. Liver biopsy if clinically indicated	No specific therapy is proven efficacious. FK506 may have better liver concentration
Musculoskeletal system	Fasciitis manifests as limitation of the capacity to slide the skin over the muscle and decrease in the range of motion. Myositis is rare. Osteoporosis may happen due to hormonal deficits, use of steroids, decreased activity	Periodic physical therapy evaluation to document the range of motion. Bone density evaluation especially in patients using steroids	Aggressive physical therapy programme. Do *not* send patients for surgical release of joints
Immune system	Profound immunodeficiency. Functional asplenia. High risk of pneumococcal sepsis, PCP and invasive fungal infections. Variable IgG levels	Assume all patients as severely immunocompromised and asplenic	PCP prophylaxis (until 6 months after no GvHD) and pneumococcal prophylaxis (lifetime). Replace IgG to keep level >500 mg/dl. Delay vaccinations to 6 months after GvHD has resolved
Haematopoietic system	Variable cytopenias, involving any series. Occasional eosinophilia	Haemogram and whenever indicated bone-marrow aspirate and biopsy, antineutrophil and antiplatelet antibodies	No specific intervention besides systemic treatment of GvHD
Others	Virtually all autoimmune disease manifestations have already been described in association with chronic GvHD, including the presence of	As clinically indicated	

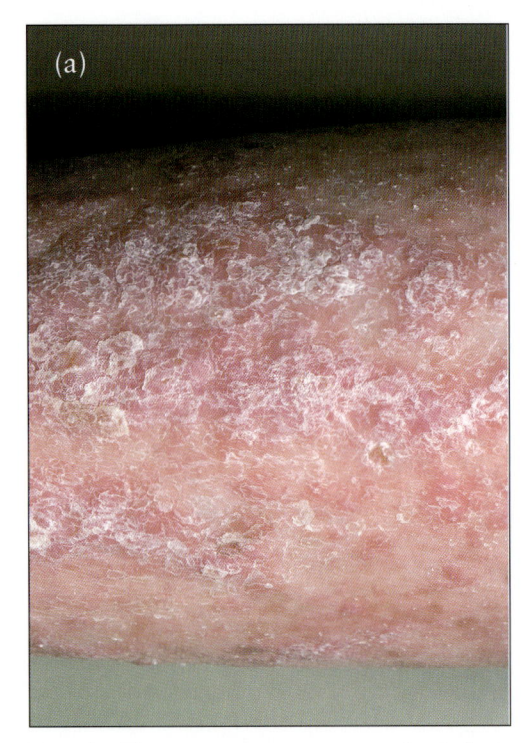

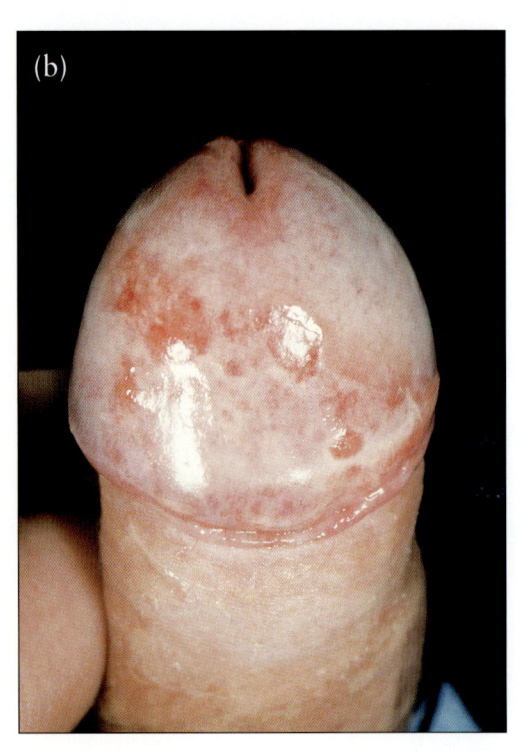

Figures 38.1(a,b) The appearances seen in the lichenoid form of chronic graft-versus-host disease of the skin. There is a papular, pruriginous rash with no typical distribution.

manifesting as dry eyes and dry mouth (sicca syndrome). Clinically, it resembles lichen planus.

The sclerodermatous form of the disease is clinically similar to systemic sclerosis. It can involve the dermis and/or the muscular fascia. The skin is very thick, fragile, and healing is extremely poor (Figures 38.2). Patients can develop blisters and/or skin ulcerations, which represent severe manifestation of sclerodermatous cGvHD. Pigmentation can be abnormally increased or decreased (Figures 38.3 and 38.4). Sclerosis histologically involves the dermis, causing hair loss and loss of sweat glands (Figure 38.5). Isolated sclerodermatous fascial GvHD is manifested as a normal skin with decreased mobility, firmly attached to the muscles. It can involve joint areas, dramatically decreasing the range of motion. Since the two manifestations, scleroderma and fasciitis, have different therapeutic approaches, it is important to make a precise diagnosis.

Eyes

Dry eyes (Sjögren's syndrome) are the most common manifestation due to lacrimal gland involvement by GvHD. Photophobia and burning are common symptoms. Patients can also be completely asymptomatic, with ocular GvHD being diagnosed only at the time of corneal damage. To avoid such complications, all patients with cGvHD should periodically be monitored by Schirmer's test to measure tear production. Conjunctival GvHD can be diagnosed by an ophthalmologist experienced in GvHD. There is conjunctival hyperaemia and formation of pseudomembranes. This is usually a manifestation of severe chronic GvHD and carries a very poor prognosis.

Mouth

Oral disease is commonly seen in association with ocular GvHD. In its earliest manifestations, patients may simply complain of xerostomia (dryness of the mouth) or increased sensitivity (typically to toothpaste and and spicy foods), and a mild erythema may be seen on examination. As the disease progresses, however, patients can have odynophagia (pain on swallowing) and lichenoid changes can be noted in the buccal mucosa, which are whitish plaques mimicking oral lichen planus or thrush (Figure 38.6). Erythema, ulcerative lesions and mucosal atrophy may develop. Atrophy of the gums can occur which predisposes to severe dental damage. Advanced dental caries can result from the decreased secretions and deficiencies in

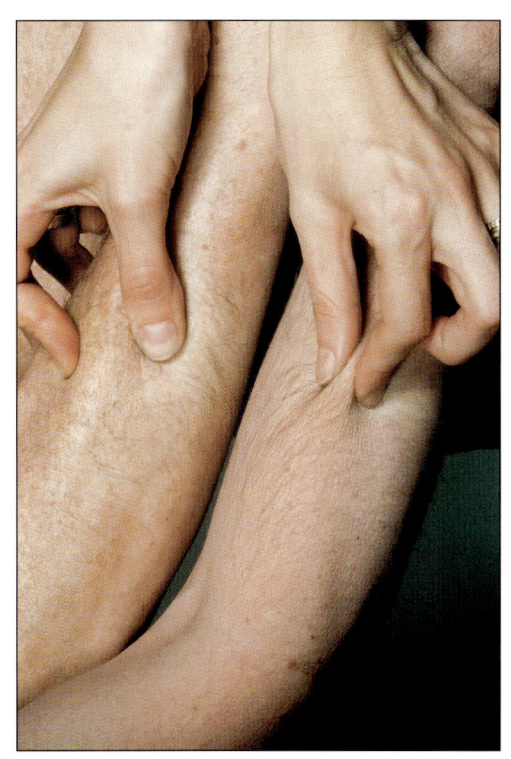

Figure 38.2 The sclerodermatous form of chronic graft-versus-host disease, showing reduced skin mobility and thickening, sometimes with tethering to underlying tissues.

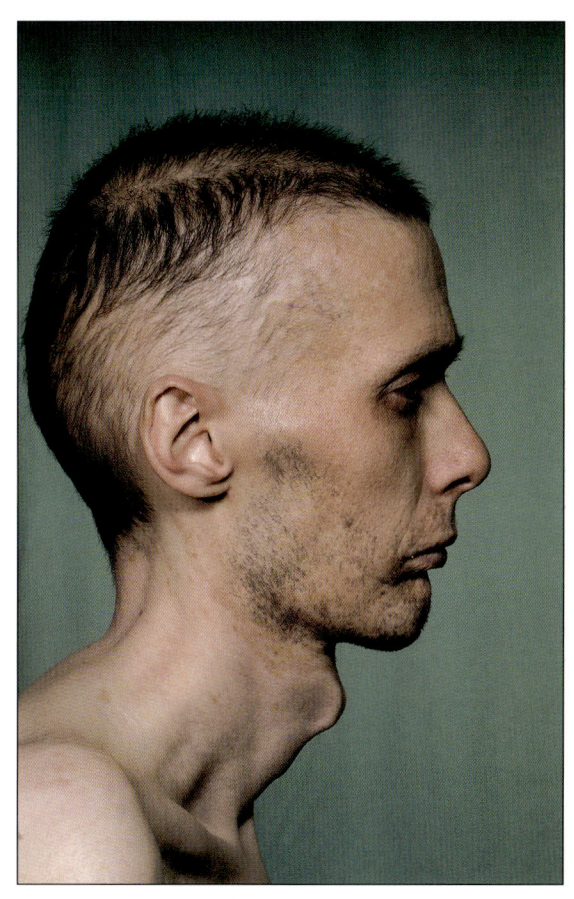

Figure 38.4 Chronic graft-versus-host disease of the skin as also described in Figure 38.3.

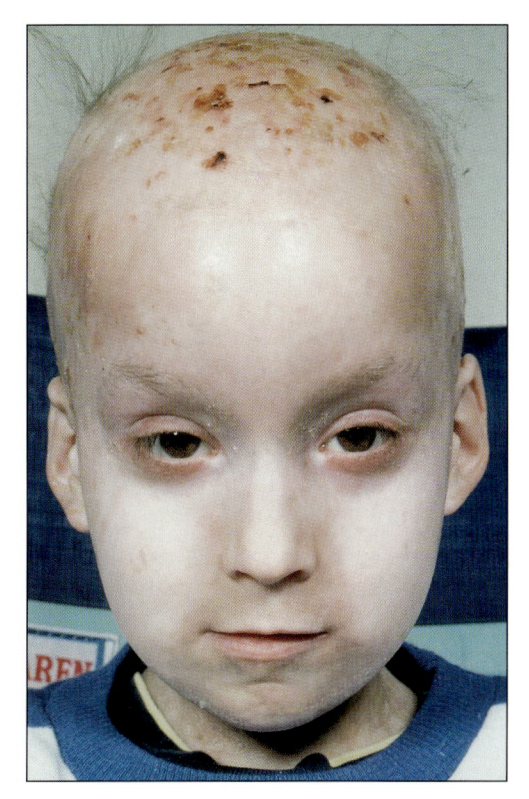

Figures 38.3 Chronic graft-versus-host disease of the skin showing increased fragility, poor healing and poor hair growth.

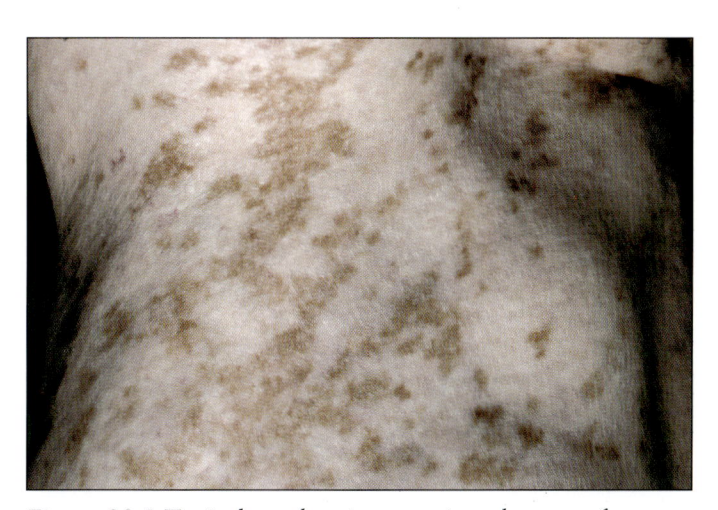

Figure 38.5 Typical patchy pigmentation changes of chronic graft-versus-host disease.

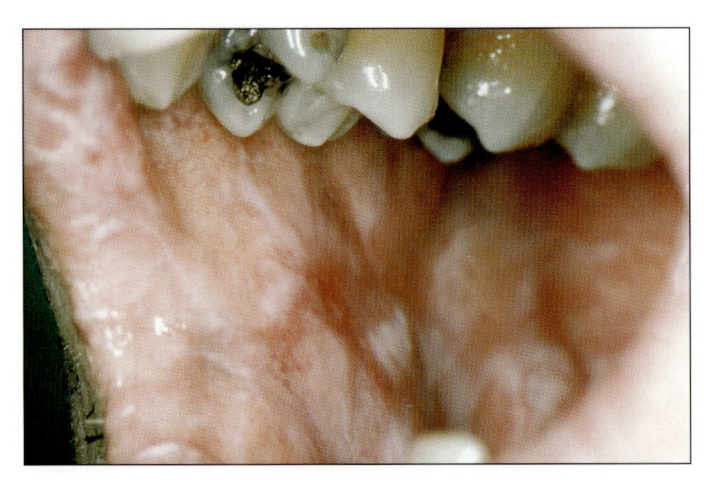

Figure 38.6 The lichenoid changes within the mouth seen with advanced chronic GvHD.

local immunity. All dental procedures should be preceded by a period of antibiotic therapy to prevent bacteraemia. Salivary gland and mucosal involvement can be demonstrated by simple mucosal biopsy. Secondary infections are common, especially with herpes simplex and yeasts (Figure 38.7), and may have atypical presentations. Changes in symptoms are frequently due to local infection. Cultures should be obtained at least at diagnosis and with any complaint of increased oral symptoms.

Respiratory tract
Chronic sinopulmonary infections, cough and bronchospasm are observed in some patients with cGvHD. Bronchiolitis obliterans is a severe manifestation of cGvHD involving the lungs. Unlike interstitial pneumonitis, which generally occurs early during the first 100 days after transplant, obliterative bronchiolitis occurs late. Symptoms include progressive dyspnoea, wheezing and cough. Chest radiographs may be completely normal or they may show signs of hyperinflation and hyperlucencies consistent with bleb formation, together with presence of interstitial pneumatosis, pneumothorax or pneumomediastinum. Pulmonary function tests reveal a marked reduction in expiratory flow when compared to the reduction in vital capacity and increase in the residual lung volume. These findings are all consistent with the presence of obstructive lung diseases. Obliterative bronchiolitis can have an acute or insidious onset and may progress rapidly. Lung biopsies are usually diagnostic. Patients with bronchiolitis obliterans have a very poor prognosis and no therapy has been shown to substantially improve their survival.

Gastrointestinal tract
Signs and symptoms of gastrointestinal tract involvement include oesophageal reflux, dysphagia, substernal pain and diarrhoea as a result of malabsorption. Abnormal motility, mucosal desquamation and formation of webs or strictures may also be seen, most commonly in the oesophagus. We frequently observe a wasting or 'failure to thrive' syndrome in patients with severe cGvHD, which usually improves with adequate GvHD treatment.

Liver
Hepatic disease is fairly common in cGvHD. Patients present mainly with cholestasis, with an elevated serum alkaline phosphatase and bilirubin. These findings are not specific and liver biopsy is necessary to make the diagnosis in patients with isolated liver involvement or, if indicated, for the differential diagnosis between GvHD and viral hepatitis, or drug toxicity. Patients have very few symptoms referable to the liver, unless the disease becomes severe.

Muscle
Fascial involvement is very common in sclerodermatous GvHD, although underrecognized. Many patients have fairly pliable skin but have severe restriction in the range of movement due to fasciitis. Patients developing cGvHD should be carefully

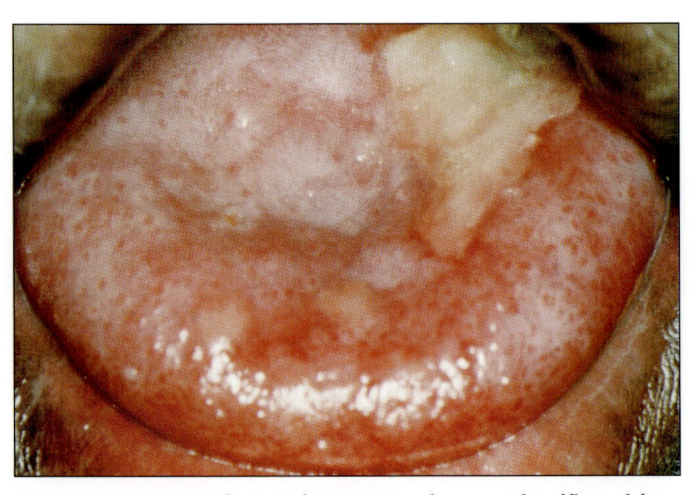

Figure 38.7 Secondary infections in the mouth afflicted by cGvHD are common and are likely to be fungal or herpetic in origin.

monitored by physical therapists regarding their range of movement. Muscular cramps are very frequent, although the physiopathology is poorly understood. Rarely, patients have myositis with tender muscles and elevated muscle enzymes. Myasthenia gravis can also be occasionally seen.

Immune system
Patients with cGvHD are profoundly immuno-incompetent, due to both the GvHD and its treatment. They may have functional asplenia, sometimes with circulating Howell–Jolly bodies. They must be treated similarly to splenectomized patients regarding precautions against sepsis by encapsulated bacteria. These patients are also at significant risk for *Pneumocystis carinii* pneumonia, and fungal infections are common. All GvHD patients should be very carefully monitored for bacterial, viral and fungal infections, since these are the main causes of death. Immunoglobulin levels may be elevated, normal, or depressed. Supplementation with intravenous IgG is frequently used in patients with low IgG levels (≤ 500 mg/dl).

Haematopoietic system
Many patients with cGvHD have suppression of marrow function. This may be either due to stromal damage or to a specific autoimmune manifestation. Leukopenia, anaemia and/or thrombocytopenia can be seen with cGvHD. Occasionally, patients may have eosinophilia. Thrombocytopenia has been described as a marker for severe cGvHD, although in our patients it reflected a progressive onset of cGvHD.

Gynaecological
Vaginal dryness and strictures can occur. Patients who have received mediastinal radiation are at increased risk of breast cancer and should be carefully monitored in this regard.

Other autoimmune disorders
Essentially, every known autoimmune disorder has been reported in patients suffering from cGvHD, including autoimmune cytopenias, myasthenia gravis, myositis, serositis, vasculitis, etc. Although autoantibodies can be demonstrated in many patients with cGvHD, there is neither a pathognomonic pattern, nor an established clinical significance of such antibodies. These manifestations are frequently fascinating, but they may simply be a reflection of the disordered immune system of these patients.

Histology
Skin
The histopathological findings in the lichenoid skin lesions of cGvHD resemble those of idiopathic lichen planus. Changes include hyperkeratosis, acanthosis, dyskeratosis and vacuolar alterations in the basal cell layer, together with monocytic and lymphocytic infiltrates in the papillary dermis. The intensity of inflammation in the lichenoid form of cGvHD is less pronounced than that seen in idiopathic lichen planus. These lesions heal without dermal fibrosis or loss of elastic tissue. In contrast, the sclerodermatous form of cGvHD is associated with sclerosis and thickening of the reticular dermis, loss of distinction between the papillary and reticular dermis, increased collagen deposition and a mild perivascular lymphocytic infiltrate. Characteristically, the sweat glands are infiltrated by lymphocytes and melanophages.

Eyes
Lymphocytic infiltration, fibrosis and destruction of the lacrimal glands result in decreased tear production and chemosis, corneal scarring and ulceration. These pathological changes in the lacrimal apparatus resemble those seen in the sicca syndrome of Sjögren.

Mouth
The histopathological features of the lichenoid oral lesions are similar to those seen in the lichenoid form of cutaneous cGvHD. Fibrosing sialoadenitis, as seen in the Sjögren sicca syndrome, may be demonstrated by biopsy of minor salivary glands.

Respiratory tract
Infiltration of submucosal glands with lymphocytes and plasma cells is common, but these cellular infiltrates are not seen in the bronchial and bronchiolar mucosa. Histopathological findings of bronchiolitis obliterans are best seen in the terminal bronchioles. In these areas, lymphocytic and mononuclear cell infiltrates and hyperplasia of bronchiolar smooth muscle may be noted. Focal or transmural necrosis of bronchioles and bronchi can be present. The most striking feature is the intraluminal accumulation of

inflammatory cells and granulation tissue, leading to partial of even complete occlusion of the bronchioles. Mucus plugging with atelectasis or emphysema of distal air spaces may be present. Hyperplasia of bronchial mucous glands and destruction of alveoli, as seen in chronic bronchitis and emphysema, is absent in cases of obliterative bronchiolitis. Although focal interstitial inflammatory reactions may occur in obliterative bronchiolitis, the intensity and extent of these changes are minimal, as opposed to the situation in interstitial pneumonitis.

Gastrointestinal tract
While mucosal or submucosal fibrosis is most commonly observed in the oesophagus and only very rarely in the large intestine, it may occur anywhere along the upper gastrointestinal tract. Mononuclear cell infiltrates as seen in the lamina propria may be observed anywhere in the gastrointestinal tract. The cellular infiltrates are associated with shortening of the villi and hyperplasia of the crypts of Lieberkuhn, which is most evident in the small intestine.

Liver
The portal triads show dense infiltration by lymphocytes, histiocytes, and often eosinophils and plasma cells. The infiltrate extends into the lobule with piecemeal hepatocellular involvement. The bile ducts usually show lymphocyte-associated necrosis of the epithelium, and periportal bile stasis is prominent. There can be increased portal fibrosis, occasionally leading to micronodular cirrhosis. After long-standing active disease, the ducts in the portal triads may be decreased in number, or absent.

Prognostic factors
Wingard *et al.* [2] evaluated factors which predicted for a poor outcome from cGvHD. In 85 patients with cGvHD, baseline characteristics before therapy were examined to determine if there were risk factors for death. In a multivariant proportional hazards analysis, three baseline factors emerged as independent predictors of death: progressive presentation of cGvHD, lichenoid changes on skin histology and elevated serum bilirubin (Table 38.4). Patients with one of these risk factors had a 70% survival at six years, where as patients with two or three of these risk factors had a survival of only 20%.

Thrombocytopenia, although found to be a prognostic factor by other authors, merely reflected the progressive onset of GvHD in our patients.

Table 38.4 Adverse prognostic factors

| Progressive presentation |
| Lichenoid skin histology |
| Bilirubin greater than twice normal |
| Thrombocytopenia |

Evaluation
It is highly recommended to histologically confirm the diagnosis of cGvHD. It is common to have patients referred for refractory GvHD who, in fact, have no active disease or who have other complications of BMT not related to GvHD. Biopsy of at least one affected organ such as the skin or oral mucosa to demonstrate the presence and activity of the disease can be very helpful in making a differential diagnosis. A comprehensive evaluation of all organs and systems most frequently affected by chronic GvHD, despite the presence or absence of symptoms, can help to access the extent of the disease and guide therapy.

Eyes
Schirmer's test is positive when tear production in five minutes is <5 ml). Evaluation of the cornea is especially important prior to the use of psoralen and ultraviolet A light (PUVA) or etretinate. Fundal examination may be helpful to rule out infections when indicated. Evaluation regarding development of cataracts secondary to total body irradiation (TBI) or steroids is also of importance.

Mouth
Dental evaluation should be carried out in order to permit treatment of pathologies that can increase trauma to the buccomucosa. Cultures for herpes simplex virus and yeast at the onset of oral GvHD and whenever the patient has any new or worsening oral signs or symptoms is advisable.

Respiratory tract
Pulmonary function tests should be carried out, including spirometry and diffusing capacity, to rule out obstruction compatible with bronchiolitis obliterans. If the FEV_1 or DLCO are significantly decreased, helium lung volumes should also be estimated to assess residual volume which is increased in air trapping, and thus compatible with an obstructive process.

Gastrointestinal tract
Nutritional evaluation is imporant to access absorption and to rule out infections and GvHD-related strictures if clinically pertinent. Many patients need dietary complements.

Liver
Periodic checks of liver function tests (liver enzymes alkaline phosphatase, bilirubin) should be run even in the absence of clinical symptoms.

Musculoskeletal system
Physical therapy can be extremely helpful in the evaluation of range of movement, strength and functional ability, all of which can be compromised by either GvHD or its treatment. Bone density should be assessed to guide early intervention should osteoporosis occur.

Immune system
IgG level should be checked at monthly intervals to guarantee levels >500 mg/dl.

Endocrine function
Thyroid function should be routinely checked every year after BMT. Children should have growth and development recorded and growth hormone levels checked if indicated. All patients should have their sex hormones checked and replaced as indicated. Oestrogens are especially important due to concomitant use of steroid therapy in patients with GvHD, potentially worsening osteoporosis.

Gynaecological
Gynaecological and breast examinations should be carried out as indicated by age and symptoms.

Treatment of chronic graft-versus-host disease

One of the first papers describing cGvHD also established the need for therapy in most patients [1]. Based on these findings, Sullivan et al. undertook a randomized double blinded study using prednisone plus placebo versus prednisone and azathioprine as treatment for extensive chronic GvHD [3]. A third group of patients was treated with prednisone alone due to thrombocytopenia. One hundred and seventy-nine patients were enrolled and 164 were evaluated. The median duration of therapy was two years. Infection and recurrence of malignancy were the most common causes of death. Non-relapse mortality differed markedly among the groups. Twenty-one percent of patients received prednisone alone and 40% of patients received prednisone and azathioprine. Survival was markedly different: 61% with prednisone alone and 47% with the combination therapy. For patients receiving combination therapy, the increased death rate was due to infections. Patients treated with prednisone alone due to thrombocytopenia did poorly due to both infections and progressive disease.

The same group treated high-risk (based on thrombocytopenia) or refractory chronic GvHD with prednisone alternating with cyclosporin (CsA) [4]. For the 40 patients receiving primary treatment for high-risk chronic GvHD, the actuarial survival was 51%, and for the 21 patients receiving salvage therapy, the actuarial survival was 67%. Causes of death, again, were primarily related to infections and relapse of the malignant disease.

Treatment of cGvHD depends upon the extent of the disease. Isolated oral involvement can be treated exclusively with topical steroids. Systemic disease should be treated with standard therapy, which in our institution is CsA and prednisone, daily for approximately two weeks (Table 38.5). After the disease is controlled, CsA and prednisone are tapered to an alternate-day schedule (see below). Patients not responding to standard doses can be enrolled in refractory GvHD protocols, involving the use of pulsed steroids, PUVA, etretinate, thalidomide and so on. Evaluation of cGvHD activity is difficult because many patients with severe GvHD have permanent sequelae, despite optimal treatment. The criterion adopted in our institution is to maintain therapy for at least three months after the patent has failed to

Table 38.5 Standard systemic treatment of chronic GvHD	
Agent	Treatment
Prednisone	1 mg/kg/day. After two weeks, taper by 25% per week to 1 mg/kg/day every other day
CsA	10 mg/kg/day (based on ideal or actual weight, whichever is lower). After the steroid taper is completed to every other day schedule start CsA taper by 25% per week on alternate days to a final dose of 10 mg/kg/day every other day, not coinciding with steroid day
Length of treatment: the same therapy must be continued for at least three months after the patient stopped having any improvement. Then the drugs can be tapered off over 30–60 days.	

show any improvement in the disease. Drugs are then slowly tapered, one at a time.

Immune suppressants

Standard treatment

Prednisone
1 mg/kg/day (based on actual weight), as a once-daily oral dose. Two weeks after starting therapy and with GvHD not active, prednisone can be tapered by 25% a week on alternate days, to a final dose of 1 mg/kg every other day.

Cyclosporin A (CsA)
10 mg/kg/day orally, divided into two doses daily (the only drug for the treatment of GvHD where the dose is based on ideal or actual weight, whichever is lower). The dose must be adjusted for serum creatinine, keeping trough levels between 200 and 500 ng/ml. After the steroids have been tapered and with GvHD under control, CsA is tapered by 25% per week on alternate days. Thus, within one month the 'maintenance' CsA dose is 10 mg/kg/day, divided into two doses, on alternate days. CsA and prednisone should not be given on the same day. They should not be discontinued abruptly or before the patient has experienced no further improvement in the GvHD for at least three months.

Alternative treatments

These are summarized in Table 38.6.

Tacrolimus (FK506)
FK506 is largely used for solid organ transplants. It can be used as an alternative to CsA in patients who cannot tolerate the latter due to malignant hypertension, seizures, haemolytic–uraemic syndrome or thrombocytopenic thrombotic purpura. Patients with refractory hepatic GvHD may also benefit from FK506 instead of CsA due to better concentrations of the drug in the liver. It should be started at 0.1 mg/kg (as with CsA, dosage is based upon ideal body weight and actual weight, whichever is lower). Within 3–4 weeks, trough levels 5–20 ng/ml should be reached.

Psoralen and ultraviolet A light (PUVA)
PUVA is routinely used for the treatment of psoriasis. It is only active against the cutaneous manifestations of GvHD. In our institution, 40 patients with either refractory cGvHD (35) or high-risk disease (5) were treated with PUVA [6]. Eleven patients were treated for isolated cutaneous disease. Five obtained a complete response. Twenty-two patients had systemic disease with lichenoid cutaneous histology. The skin responses were complete in 11 and partial in 6 patients. Unfortunately, no systemic effects were seen in the

Table 38.6 Alternative systemic treatment of chronic GvHD
Tacrolimus (FK506)
Psoralen–ultraviolet light A (PUVA) (lichenoid disease)
Etretinate (sclerodermatous disease)
Thalidomide
Total lymphoid irradiation (TLI)

patients with multi-organ disease. PUVA is *not* indicated for sclerodermatous skin disease, but it may benefit patients with cutaneous GvHD which has not responded to conventional therapy, patients with very extensive cutaneous disease, or with repeated flares of the GvHD when steroids are tapered.

The initial UV light dose is based on skin type. Treatments are given three to four times a week for no more than two consecutive days, for a total of 32 treatments (12 weeks). The light sensitizer used prior to PUVA is Methoxypsoralen Ultra, 0.3 mg/kg to the nearest 10 mg, one hour prior to each treatment. We recommend that patients eat two hours prior to taking the pills, take any anti-emetic medicine a half-hour prior to each dose, and that they then remain with no oral intake except for medicines for three hours prior to the PUVA therapy. 8-Methoxypsoralen (8-MOPP) 0.6 mg/kg two hours prior to each treatment can be used as an alternative if Methoxypsoralen Ultra is not available, although this may cause more nausea. Patients should avoid sun exposure for 24 hours after taking Methoxypsoralen Ultra or 8-MOPP and they should use protective spectacles distributed by the dermatologist (not regular sunglasses), which completely filter out UVA and UVB. If PUVA is being used for refractory or extensive GvHD in combination with steroids and CsA, tapering to alternate days should only be started six weeks after the start of PUVA therapy, instead of after two weeks as in the regular protocol. Oral PUVA can also be used for oral GvHD which is refractory to topical steroids.

Etretinate

Etretinate is a vitamin A derivative with established use in some dermatological conditions. It can have good results in the treatment of sclerodermatous and/or fascial cGvHD. Although the mechanism of action is unknown, it appears to play a role in breaking down scar tissue. The initial recommended dose is 0.6 mg/kg/day in two to four divided doses, rounded to 10 mg or 25 mg tablets. Most patients notice erythema with dryness and peeling of the palms, soles and lips. The dose can be increased to the maximum tolerated if desired. If severe toxicity occurs, the drug should be stopped for two weeks and then resumed at 50% of the original dose. The main concern is liver toxicity, which may necessitate interruption of treatment. Triglycerides, cholesterol and liver-function tests should be checked two and four weeks after starting the drug, and monthly thereafter. Etretinate should not be taken with milk because this increases absorption of the drug. Vitamin A supplementation should be discouraged because this can cause additive toxic effects. Severe birth defects are known to occur when etretinate is taken before or during pregnancy. The period during which pregnancy must be avoided has not been determined.

Thalidomide

A phase I–II trial of thalidomide for GvHD for high-risk patients and patients failing initial therapy has been reported [7]. Forty-four patients were treated on this study, with 23 being treated for refractory disease. Even including the refractory patients, the median platelet count of the entire group was 90 000, suggesting that this group of patients was very similar to the patients reported by Sullivan *et al.*, who had progressive and high-risk cGvHD treated with CsA and prednisone.

The overall survival was 64% (78% in patients with refractory cGvHD and 48% in high-risk patients). Again, infection was the major cause of death. This study suggested that thalidomide may be effective therapy for patients with high-risk or refractory disease. The drug is currently being evaluated in another phase II trial, combined with CsA and PUVA.

Total lymphoid irradiation (TLI)

Socié *et al.* reported the use of low-dose TLI. In 9 patients receiving 100 cGy thoraco-abdominal irradiation, 6 had significant improvement in their chronic GvHD. The irradiation was given as a single dose and side-effects were minimal [5].

Topical treatment of oral GvHD

If oral GvHD is isolated or does not respond to systemic treatment, topical therapy can be given after oral infections have been excluded. dexamethasone (Decadron) Elixir (0.5 mg/ 5 ml as a 2–3 minutes rinse and spit, four times daily), or oral PUVA may be tried. In cases of GvHD resistant to initial therapy, Dexamethasone solution 1 mg/cc or beclomethasone can be used. Topical antifungal prophylaxis must be used while patients are receiving topical GvHD therapy (Table 38.7).

> **Table 38.7 Topical therapy for oral GvHD (Decadron Elixir 0.1 mg/ml)**
>
> Swish for 2–3 minutes and spit at least four times a day. Can be used alone or in association with systemic therapy. Essential to associate with topical prophylactic antifungal therapy

Infectious diseases prophylaxis (See Table 38.8).

Infections are the main cause of death in patients with GvHD, and maximal effort should be made therefore to educate patients about the wisdom of taking prophylactic medications and calling their physician if they experience fever or malaise.

Pneumocystis carinii (PCP)

Prophylaxis is with sulfamethoxazole 800 mg and trimethoprim 160 mg orally twice daily, twice a week, or with alternative drugs and schedules currently used in AIDS and BMT centres.

Table 38.8 Infectious disease prophylaxis

Disease agent	Treatment
Pneumocystis carinii	Sulfamethoxazole 800 mg and trimethoprim 160 mg oral twice a day on two consecutive days of the week
Encapsulated bacteria	Penicillin V 250 mg oral twice a day
Fungus	Topical oral prophylaxis if oral GvHD is under treatment with topical steroids
Cytomegalovirus (CMV)	Frequent surveillance cultures and antigen detection in patients (or donors) who are CMV-positive
Herpes simplex virus	Culture mouth if new symptoms. Treat only acute episodes
Varicella zoster virus	Intravenous therapy immediately due to risk of dissemination. Treat only acute episodes

PCP prophylaxis should be maintained until GvHD is not active *and* any GvHD therapy has been stopped for more than six months.

Pneumococcal prophylaxis

Patients with chronic GvHD may develop fulminant sepsis due to encapsulated organisms, most frequently *Pneumococcus*. This is due to their functional asplenia. Life-long prophylaxis should be considered using penicillin V (250–500 mg, oral, twice daily) or erythromycin (Estolate 250 mg, oral, twice daily). Prior to all invasive procedures, including dental work, patients with cGvHD should receive antibiotic 'endocarditis' prophylaxis, as recommended by the American Heart Association, to avoid bacteraemia.

Fungus infections

Systemic antifungal therapy is not routinely used. Topical antifungal prophylaxis is necessary if oral GvHD is present and the patient is using topical steroids.

Viruses

Cytomegalovirus (CMV)

CMV surveillance blood cultures (antigen detection and cultures) in CMV-positive patients *or* donors should be taken at least twice a month while patients are receiving GvHD treatment. Patients with previous CMV disease may be maintained on ganciclovir while receiving steroids or when they have active GvHD.

Herpes simplex virus (HSV)

Long-term acyclovir therapy should be avoided due to possibility of developing resistant herpes viruses. Worsening oral GvHD should always raise a strong suspicion of secondary local infection by either virus or fungus. Other mucosal lesions may occur, affecting the nasal and perineal areas. Cultures should be obtained as clinically indicated. HSV infections should be treated if active.

Varicella zoster virus (VZV)

Chickenpox, shingles, or disseminated zoster frequently occur in patients with cGvHD. They should be treated promptly, usually with intravenous aciclovir.

Vaccinations

Vaccinations should be postponed until one year after stopping all GvHD treatment, when there are no signs of active GvHD. It is recommended to start with diphtheria, tetanus toxoid (dT), inactivated poliomyelitis (IPV) and influenza. Polyvalent pneumococcal, meningococcal and *Haemophilus influenzae B* (Hib) vaccines can be also be given at this time. Influenza vaccine can be given annually. Pneumococcal vaccine should be boosted every 5–10 years. Measles, or measles, mumps and rubella should be given two years after resolution of GvHD.

Hypogammaglobulinaemia
IgG levels should be checked monthly. If levels are <500 mg/dl, IgG 400–500 mg/kg should be administered.

Special recommendations (Table 38.9)
Protection from sun
The skin is usually very sensitive in the presence of GvHD, and extremely sensitive when PUVA or etretinate are being used. Sunburn can trigger GvHD even in previously unaffected areas. We recommend a factor #15 sunscreen to be used at all times to block both UVA and UVB.

Topical skin care
This can be carried out with any commercial perfume-free and alcohol-free moisturizing lotions.

Eyes
Patients with sicca syndrome should have careful ophthalmologic follow-up to prevent long-term damage to the eyes. Patients with a positive Schirmer's test (≤ 5 mm) or symptoms of dry eyes should use preservative-free tears at least every four hours, and preservative-free ointment at night. They may also benefit from temporary or permanent lacrimal duct occlusion.

Oral care
Decrease in the production of saliva can increase the incidence of caries. Regular dental evaluations should be carried out, with 'endocarditis prophylaxis' prior to any procedure. Artificial saliva may be used to control symptoms.

Nutrition
Poor appetite is common in these patients and malnutrition frequently results in a cycle of worsening wasting, poor healing, decreased strength, and decreased appetite. Nutritional monitoring is important to maintain the patient's well-being.

Physical therapy
Physical therapy or an oriented activity programme is essential to maintain mobility and strength while patients are receiving GvHD therapy, especially in those who are receiving steroids. Aggressive physical therapy programmes can maintain mobility even in critically compromised patients.

Muscle cramps
These are frequent among patients with chronic GvHD. Although the causes are unknown, general recommendations including electrolyte replacement (calcium, magnesium, potassium, sodium), dantrolene, calcium-channel blockers, sodium-channel blockers or quinine, can be helpful. Quinine is usually the first choice starting at 260 mg orally at dinner time. Dantrolene is started at 25 mg daily and gradually increased in increments of 25 mg at 4–7-day intervals, up to 100 mg twice to four times a day, with a maximum of 400 mg daily. The major side-effects of this drug are muscle weakness, drowsiness, severe diarrhoea and liver-function test abnormalities. It should be used with caution in patients with cardiac or pulmonary impairment. It can also cause photosensitivity and should not be used with PUVA.

Summary
Chronic GvHD is a complex disorder and requires careful multisystem management. Although progress has been made in caring for these patients, many

---

Table 38.9 Special recommendations

- Vaccinations should be postponed until resolution of GvHD
- Replace IgG to keep levels greater than 500 mg/dl
- Avoid sunburn. Always use sunscreen factor #15
- Moisturize skin with any perfume-free and alcohol-free product
- Special attention to nutritional status

patients are left with severe disabilities. Aggressive management can improve the quality of life for these patients many of whom are cured from their original condition.

Acknowledgements

The clinical figures were kindly provided by Dr Peter Mortimer.

References

1. Sullivan KM, Schulman HM, Storb R *et al*. Chronic graft-versus-host disease in 52 patients: adverse natural outcome and successful treatment with combination immunosuppression. *Blood* 1981; **52**: 267–276.
2. Wingard J, Piantadosi S, Vogelsang G *et al*. Predictors of death from chronic graft-versus-host disease after bone marrow transplantation. *Blood* 1989; **74**: 1428–1435.
3. Sullivan KM, Witherspoon R, Storb R *et al*. Azathioprine compared with prednisone and placebo for treatment of chronic graft-versus-host disease: prognostic influence of prolonged thrombocytopenia after allogeneic marrow transplantation. *Blood* 1988; **72**: 546–554.
4. Sullivan K, Witherspoon R, Storb A *et al*. Alternating day cyclosporine and prednisone for treatment of high risk chronic graft versus host disease. *Blood* 1988; 72: 555–561.
5. Socié G, Devergie A, Cosset J *et al*. Low dose total lymphoid irradiation for extensive, drug resistant chronic graft-versus-host disease. *Transplantation* 1990; **49**: 657–658.
6. Vogelsang GB, Wolff D, Altomonte V, Farmer E, Morison WL, Corio R and Horn T. Treatment of chronic graft-vs-host disease with PUVA. *Bone Marrow Transplant* 1996; **17**: 1061–1067.
7. Vogelsang GB, Farmer ER, Hess AD *et al*. Thalidomide for the treatment of chronic GvHD. *New Engl J Med* 1992; **325**(16): 1055–1058.

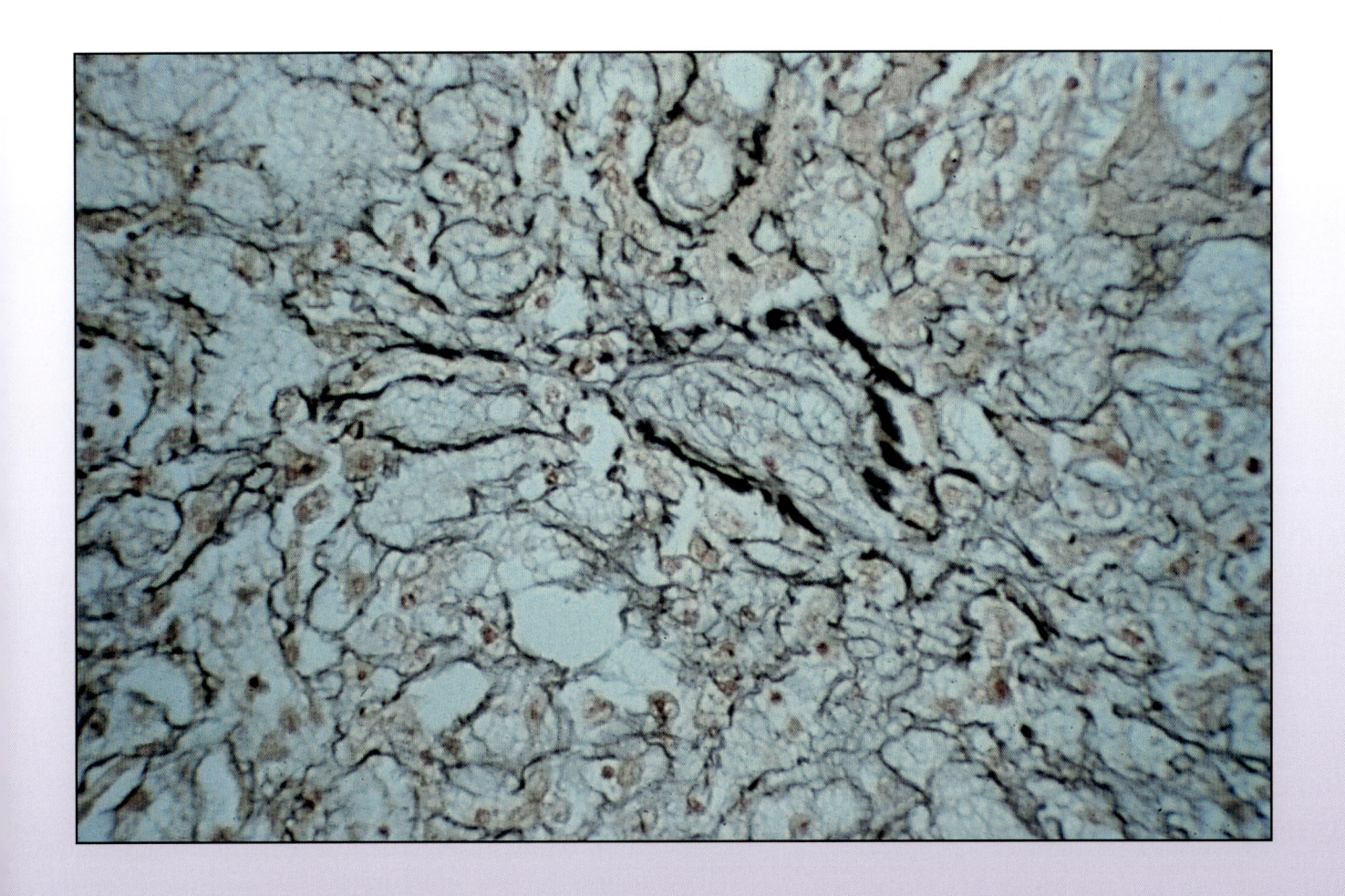

Chapter 39

The histopathology of graft-versus-host disease

Keith P. McCarthy

Introduction

Graft-versus-host disease (GvHD) is the result of the introduction of immune-competent cells into genetically different individuals. It occurs when the donor lymphocytes recognize class I or II or minor histocompatibility antigen differences in the host and, although it may be seen in a number of situations, it occurs most commonly following allogeneic bone-marrow transplantation when it is seen in approximately 50% of cases [1] and when it is thought to be at least contributory to 40% of deaths [2]. GvHD may also be seen followings stem-cell transplantation as a treatment for a variety of haematological disorders, although it is apparently less common following umbilical cord blood transplantation [3].

There has been much research into GvHD, and much is known about its clinical and pathological features and about its treatment, but the pathogenetic mechanisms which underlie it are still incompletely understood. Since T-cell depletion of the donor marrow results in reduced severity and incidence of GvHD, it is assumed that T-cells are of fundamental importance, but tissue factor have also been shown to be involved in the undoubtedly complex and multifactorial genesis of the disease [4].

Although there is a subdivision of GvHD into acute and chronic forms, to a certain extent this division is arbitrary, albeit with certain distinguishing features. Thus, chronic GvHD, which is defined as GvHD occurring 100 days or more after transplantation, may arise *de novo*, following prolonged or recurrent acute GvHD or following acute GvHD after a long remission. Acute GvHD usually commences 7–14 days post-transplant and classically affects mainly the skin, colon and liver. This predilection, currently unexplained, accounts for the symptoms of acute GvHD: skin rash, jaundice and gastrointestinal symptoms, principally diarrhoea. Chronic GvHD may affect a much wider range of organs, although the skin, colon and liver are again the three main sites affected. From these facts alone it can be seen that acute and chronic GvHD, although related, are very different diseases.

Skin

Acute GvHD

The clinical picture of acute GvHD is characterized by a rash which, in its less severe form, may be confined to the palms and soles and malar areas of the face; in its more severe form the rash may cover the entire body. The rash is classically said to be maculopapular and pruritic, although in mild cases it may be merely erythematous and non-specific in character. In severe cases, the rash may be exfoliative with blistering and marked erythroderma, resembling Stevens–Johnson syndrome.

The histological changes which occur in acute skin GvHD correlate fairly well with the clinical appearances but are not completely coincident. Essentially, acute skin GvHD is characterized by a lichenoid infiltrate of small lymphocytes; this term is used because it has a resemblance to the inflammatory skin condition lichen planus in which there is a band-like infiltrate of small lymphocytes within the upper dermis, extending into the lower levels of the epidermis and associated with degenerative changes within the basal keratinocytes of the epidermis. In the context of GvHD, the infiltrate of small lymphocytes, although important (see below) for the diagnosis, may be sparse and patchy. This is not surprising given the inevitable lymphodepletion which is seen immediately post-transplant. With increasing severity, the degenerative changes become more prominent: coalescence of the necrotic cells results in clefting at the epidermal–dermal junction which, in its severest form, may produce complete sloughing of the epidermis. The changes affect not only the epidermis but also the superficial parts of the skin appendages, especially the hair follicles and sweat ducts. Topographically, the changes are more likely to be seen in skin which is clinically affected, a phenomenon which it is important to bear in mind when skin is biopsied for histological diagnosis of GvHD.

This spectrum of changes seen in GvHD has given rise to the grading system which is most commonly used today (Table 39.1). This was first published by Lerner *et al.* in 1974 [5]. Whilst this has proved a durable and useful grading system, there are certain points which need to be emphasized. The changes are far from specific for GvHD for they may be seen in a variety of conditions including lichen planus, erythema multiforme and even in AIDS [6]. However, careful clinical evaluation will usually exclude such conditions. The most difficult aspect is grade I GvHD which is characterized by epidermal basal abnormalities. If a lichenoid infiltrate is present, it is

Table 39.1 Histopathological grading of acute GvHD of the skin [5]	
Grade 1:	Vacuolation seen within basal cells of the epidermis
Grade 2:	Individually necrotic keratinocytes within epidermis
Grade 3:	Bullae at epidermal–dermal junction
Grade 4:	Complete epidermal sloughing

possible to make a diagnosis of Grade I GvHD, but epidermal basal abnormalities, in the absence of a lichenoid lymphocytic infiltrate, may be seen in skin biopsies of patients with or without rashes and may even be found in biopsies taken before the transplant [7]. Moreover, a histologically normal biopsy may be found in the presence of clinical evidence of GvHD [1].

It is assumed that the epidermal basal abnormalities which are found in the absence of clinical GvHD are drug-induced [8], an effect of radiotherapy [9], or possibly both. It is interesting to speculate whether it is purely coincidental that the regimens which are used in bone-marrow transplantation produce such mimicry of GvHD or whether there is, in fact, an association. There is a small amount of evidence to support a causal link, at least in the case of chronic GvHD [10], and it has been shown that comparison with pretransplant biopsies shows a greater degree of epidermal basal damage in post-transplant, pre-GvHD biopsies [11]. It has been shown that the lymphocytic infiltrate in GvHD is not present at the clinical onset, suggesting that it is, in fact, not the primary event in the evolution of GvHD [7].

Whatever its relationship to true GvHD, the presence of epidermal basal abnormalities in the absence of clinical GvHD, together with the occurrence of histologically normal skin biopsies in the presence of GvHD, mean that there is considerable difficulty in the diagnosis of early skin GvHD. This problem can be alleviated by undertaking immunohistochemical analysis.

Immunohistochemistry shows the infiltrating lymphocytes to be T-cell in phenotype with an admix of natural killer cells and macrophages. The T-cells are a combination of CD4+ and CD8+ cells. Although the overall proportion of T-cells expressing the $\delta\gamma$ T-cell receptor does not appear to be increased, there is a significant concentration of these cells around blood vessels [12]; this is not a diagnostic feature, however [13].

There has been much interest in Langerhans cells in GvHD, since these cells have a role in the normal immunological processes of the skin. Although their numbers are considerably reduced by the conditioning regimen, some recipient Langerhans cells do remain and it has been suggested that these are the target of donor lymphocytes [14,15]. More recent research, however, indicates that preferential sites of attack in GvHD are the epithelial stem cell within the rete ridge of the epidermis and the parafollicular hair bulge stem cells of the hair follicle [16,17].

If the lymphocytic infiltrate is not a primary event in GvHD, what is? Examination of a range of cytokines has proved fruitful in the search for the both the pathogenetic mechanism of GvHD and a means of diagnosing early GvHD [18]. It has been known for some years that human leukocyte antigens (HLA)-DR antigens on epidermal keratinocytes are upregulated early in the course of the disease [14,19]; this is not specific for GvHD and may be seen in many inflammatory disorders of the skin. It should be noted, however, that normal keratinocytes do not express HLA-DR. There is upregulation of other cytokines as well, including γ-interferon (IFN-γ), interleukin-2 (IL-2), interleukin-4 (IL-4), tumour necrosis factor-α (TNF-α) and tumour necrosis factor-β (TNF-β) [18,20] (Table 39.2). Such observations are not merely of academic interest. Anti-TNF-α and anti-IFN-γ antibodies have been shown to be of use in the prevention [21,22] and treatment of GvHD [23].

The expression of other cytokines is altered in GvHD. Molecules involved in cell adhesion are either

Table 39.2 Cytokines upregulated during acute GvHD
γ-interferon (IFN-γ)
Interleukin-2 (IL-2)
Interleukin-4 (IL-4)
Tumour necrosis factor-α (TNF-α)
Tumour necrosis factor-β (TNF-β)

upregulated (ICAM-1 on keratinocytes [11], ELAM-1 on endothelium and VCAM-1 on dermal dendritic cells [24]) or downregulated (CD34 on endothelium [25]). The former three molecules all promote lymphocyte adhesion, the latter diminishes it (Table 39.3). These changes suggest a mechanism whereby cytokine production in the dermal blood vessel endothelium, dermal dendritic cells and keratinocytes facilitates the entry of donor T-lymphocytes into the skin. They also suggest a possible method for the early histological diagnosis of GvHD since immuno-histochemical positivity for VCAM-1 on perivascular dendritic cells and for HLA-DR on keratinocytes appears to be specific of GvHD and to occur before there is significant infiltration by donor T-lymphocytes [12]. Figures 39.1 and 39.2 show the histological features of acute GvHD of the skin.

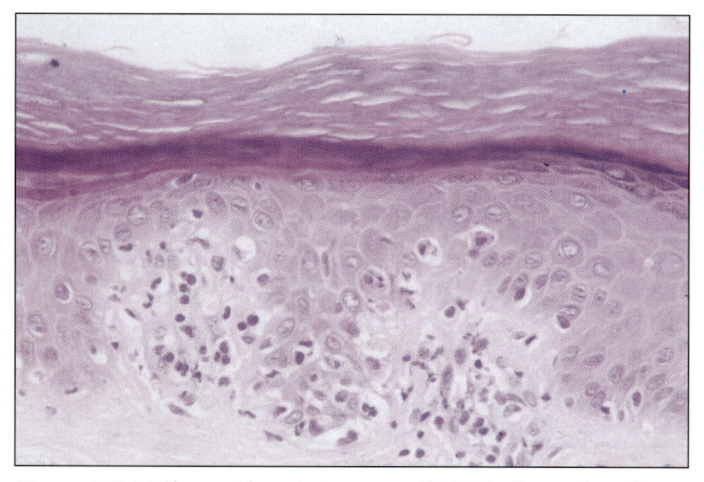

Figure 39.1 The epidermis in acute GvHD shows basal vacuolation and individual epithelial cell necrosis together with junctional mononuclear cell infiltrate.

Chronic GvHD

There are two histological forms of chronic GvHD – lichenoid and sclerodermatous.

- As its name suggests, lichenoid chronic GvHD resembles acute GvHD in that it is characterized by a dermal lymphoid infiltrate. This infiltrate is denser (possibly merely because, occurring at a later time after transplantation, there are more donor T-lymphocytes), and accompanied by epidermal hyperplasia and pigmentary incontinence (melanophages in the dermis) due to release of melanin from the chronic damage to the basal epidermis.
- Sclerodermatous chronic GvHD (Figure 39.3) may follow the lichenoid variant or it may occur *de novo*. It is so called because its histological appearance resembles scleroderma with marked fibrosis and elastosis of the dermis accompanied by atrophy of skin adnexal structures and possibly the epidermis. These changes are reflected in the clinical appearance of tight, shiny skin with alopecia. They may be generalized or focal. Immunohistochemical staining shows deposition of IgM in the region of the epidermal basement membrane.

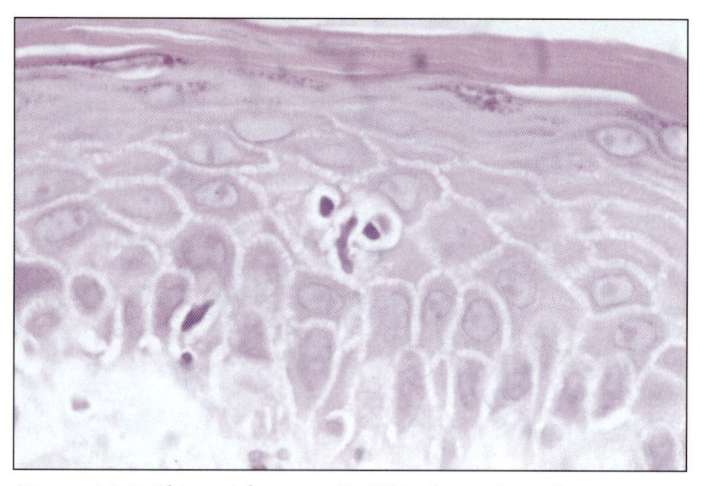

Figure 39.2 Skin with acute GvHD shows lymphocytes attached to surrounding individual necrotic epithelial cells, a process called 'satellitosis'.

Table 39.3 Adhesion molecules in GvHD
Upregulated molecules (all promote lymphocyte adhesion)
ICAM-1 on keratinocytes
ELAM-1 on endothelium
VCAM-1 on dermal dendritic cells
Downregulated molecules (diminish lymphocyte adhesion)
CD34 on endothelium
ICAM = intracellular adhesion molecule
ELAM = endothelial leucocyte adhesion molecule
VCAM = vascular cell adhesion molecule

Gastrointestinal tract

Although it is the ileum and large intestine which are most frequently affected by GvHD [26], the disease may occur at any point along the gastrointestinal tract. For obvious reasons of relative ease and high

Table 39.4 Histopathological grading of acute GvHD of the intestine [5]

Grade 1:	Individual cell necrosis in gland crypts
Grade 2:	Loss of individual gland crypts
Grade 3:	Loss of two or more adjacent crypts
Grade 4:	Mucosal sloughing

probability of obtaining positive results, it is the rectum which has been most frequently biopsied, but it should be remembered that the histological changes of GvHD may be focal, so that a negative biopsy does not exclude the diagnosis. Moreover, a negative rectal biopsy result may be obtained in the uncommon instances in which symptoms indicate involvement of predominantly the upper gastrointestinal tract.

The histological changes within the rectum and intestine are comparable to those found in the skin with the primary target appearing to be glandular epithelial cells. Thus, in mild cases there may be only loss of individual glandular epithelial cells, but with increasing severity of disease, more and more cells are lost so that whole crypts disappear ('exploding crypts'), epithelial ulceration occurs and eventually there is mucosal sloughing (Table 39.4); (Figures 39.4 and 39.5). Although these appearances can mimic chronic inflammatory bowel disease, there is relative sparing of enterochromaffin cells, a distinguishing feature [27].

The sigmoidoscopic findings range from mild mucosal reddening and swelling through frank ulceration to widespread loss of mucosa. It should be noted that although the agreement between sigmoidoscopic and histological findings is good [26], it is not complete and that microscopic changes of GvHD may be found in the presence of a normal sigmoidoscopic examination [28].

Another correlation with cutaneous GvHD is the relative lack of specificity of the changes which characterize the lower grades. Thus, individual necrosis of glandular epithelial cells may be produced by the conditioning regimen [29], although the microscopic appearances revert to normal with time [30]. Other conditions which may mimic low-grade GvHD include cytomegalovirus (CMV) infection, a

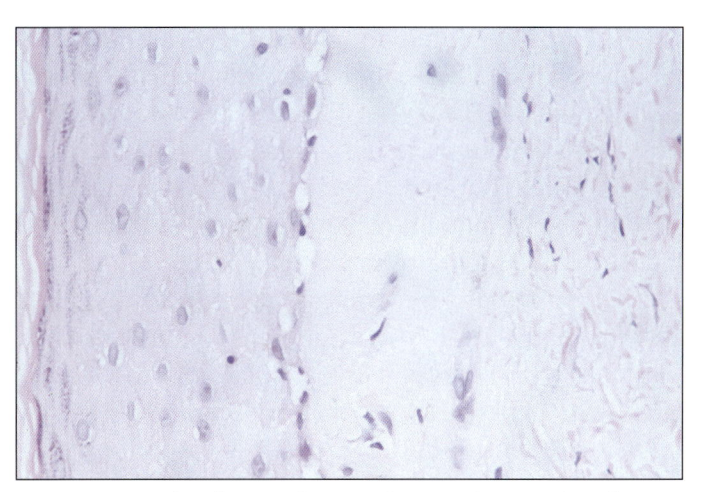

Figure 39.3 The skin in chronic GvHD shows scleroderma-like changes with fibrosis of the papillary dermis.

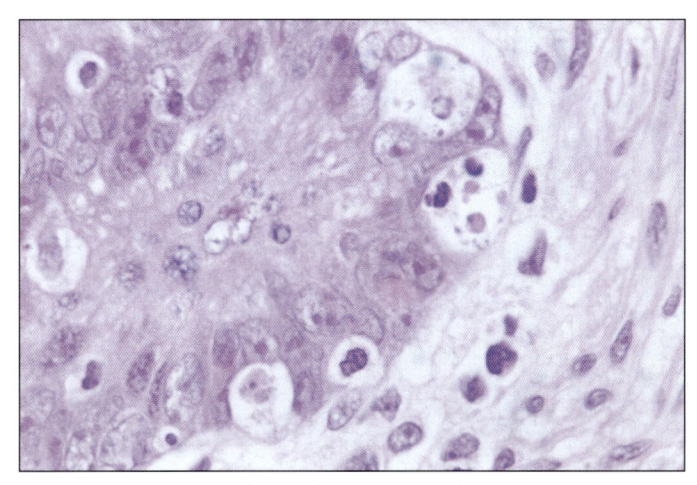

Figure 39.4 Crypt of rectal mucosa with acute GvHD shows the characteristic individual epithelial cell necrosis and abundant karyorrhexic debris.

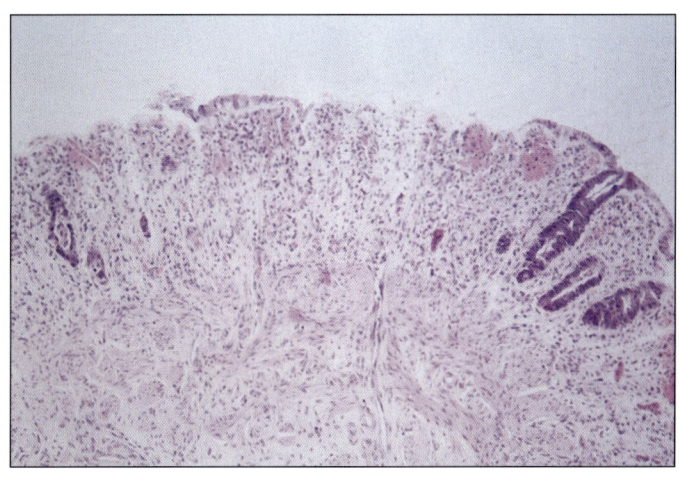

Figure 39.5 Rectal mucosa with grade III GvHD changes shows loss of three or more contiguous crypts.

disease which is common in the immunocompromised condition which follows bone-marrow transplantation [31]. It has been suggested that synchronous CMV infection might increase the severity of GvHD [32]. A careful search for the characteristic viral inclusions, backed up by immunohistochemistry if necessary, should exclude or confirm this possibility.

Another histological appearance which has been found to be of use in the diagnosis of acute GvHD is the finding of a 'focal periglandular infiltrate' [33]. This is the presence of a lymphocytic infiltrate in the lamina propria around crypts and is associated with individual cell apoptosis.

Immunohistochemical analysis of the infiltrate found in the intestine in GvHD shows differences with the skin [34]. Thus, although there is upregulation of HLA-DP and then HLA-DR early in the disease [35,36], there is decrease in the ratio of $CD4^+$ to $CD8^+$ cells due mainly to an absolute fall in numbers of $CD4^+$ cells [4]. Numbers of natural killer cells are also increased and there is upregulation of CD16 on macrophages, an Fc receptor for IgG. The precise significance of these findings is as yet unclear, as is the precise sequence of events.

Chronic GvHD does not affect the stomach and intestine so severely, but the changes correlate with those seen in the skin, with increased numbers of chronic inflammatory cells and fibrosis of the submucosal tissues being present.

Interestingly, the squamous mucosa of the oesophagus, if involved at all, is affected in a manner similar to the epidermis; this applies to both acute and chronic GvHD. A consequence of chronic GvHD affecting the oesophagus may be stricturing and dysphagia.

Liver

The liver is the third major site of GvHD and it is usually seen in association with GvHD in the skin and gastrointestinal tract. Biochemical evidence of hepatic dysfunction is extremely common following bone-marrow transplantation, but this is multifactorial in pathogenesis; the conditioning regimen, infection and veno-occlusive disease may all contribute. The characteristic lesion of hepatic GvHD is centred on small bile ducts, although hepatocytes themselves may be affected. As with the changes seen in the skin and gastrointestinal tract, the appearances seen may be mimicked by other disease processes, although the conditioning regimen does not appear to cause significant changes within small bile ducts [37].

Histologically, the small bile ducts show cytological atypia with nuclear enlargement and pleomorphism. Some cells may appear individually necrotic or have pyknotic nuclei; anucleate cells may even be seen. There is usually cell debris within bile duct lumina. Although it may be possible to identify an infiltrate of small lymphocytes within portal tracts, this may be minimal due to the lymphodepletion of bone-marrow transplantation; occasionally lymphocytes are seen within the bile duct epithelium. Cholestasis is also usually present (Table 39.5). Hepatocyte damage and necrosis are frequently seen but this is variable and non-specific for GvHD [37]. The large bile ducts may also show abnormalities similar to those seen in the small ducts.

It has been claimed that 'endothelialitis' or 'endotheliitis' (the attachment of small lymphocytes to the vascular wall with subsequent endothelial damage), although only found in 40% of cases, is a specific finding in hepatic GvHD [38] (Figure 39.6). This appearance, however, can also be seen in a variety of inflammatory liver diseases including viral infection, alcoholic hepatitis, primary biliary cirrhosis and non-specific reactive hepatitis [39].

Immunohistochemistry shows that the predominant lymphocyte within the affected portal tracts is T-cell in phenotype; as with GvHD in the gastrointestinal tract, these are predominantly $CD8^+$ cells. Macrophages and natural killer cells are also observed.

Table 39.5 Histological changes of acute hepatic GvHD

Nuclear enlargement and pleomorphism. Individual necrotic cells, cells with pyknotic nuclei or anucleate cells
Cell debris within bile duct lumina
Possibly small lymphocytes within portal tracts; occasionally lymphocytes are present within the bile duct epithelium
Cholestasis usually present

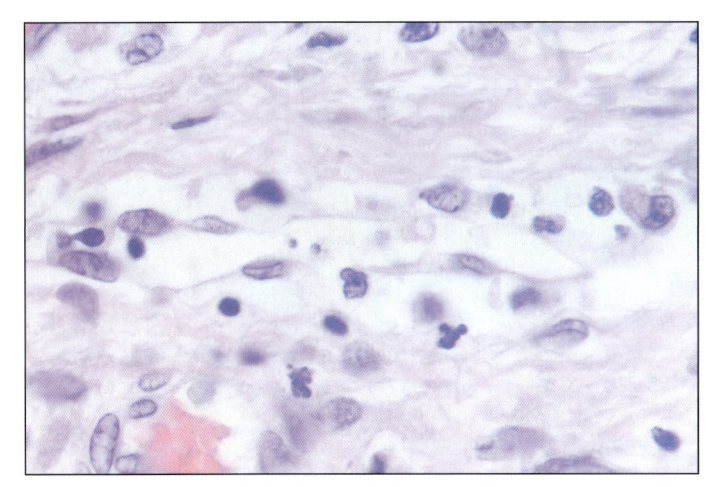

Figure 39.6 'Endothelialitis' of the portal vein is a specific feature of acute hepatic GvHD.

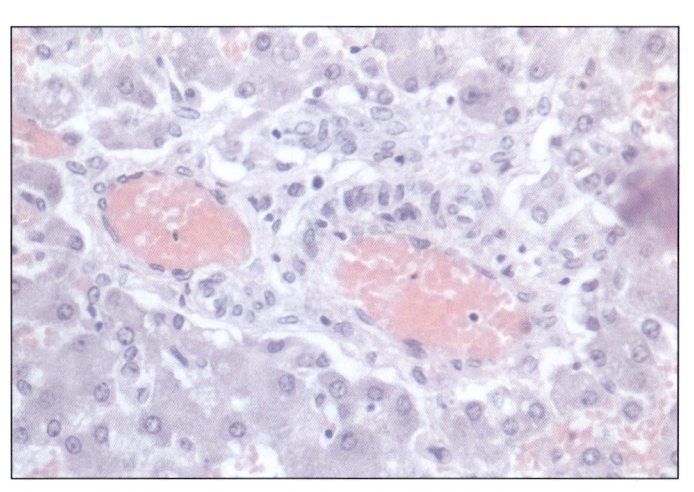

Figure 39.8 Portal tract in chronic GvHD shows absent interlobular bile duct with intact arteriole and a venule, and minimal inflammation. A phenomenon called 'vanishing bile duct syndrome'.

Although a grading system, analogous to those used in skin and gut GvHD, has been proposed, its usefulness is open to question since it relies on the percentage of small bile ducts which show the changes of GvHD [5] (Figure 39.7). Since the diagnosis has to be made on small liver biopsies, there is the possibility of sampling error introducing major inaccuracy. In addition, the prognostic value of the grading system is open to question [38].

Chronic liver GvHD can be seen as essentially indistinguishable from the acute form save in the severity of the changes which are seen. Thus, bile ducts appear more severely damaged and may disappear completely – 'vanishing bile duct syndrome' (Figure 39.8). With lymphoid reconstitution, the lymphocytic infiltrate becomes more severe and, as with chronic GvHD elsewhere, fibrosis becomes a significant feature. Cirrhosis has even been reported as a consequence of GvHD [40].

Lungs

There is considerable controversy about whether GvHD really does affect the lungs. Undoubtedly, patients who have undergone bone-marrow transplantation do have pathological changes within their lungs which correspond to the presence of GvHD at other sites. The characteristic lesion – bronchiolitis obliterans – affects small airways with narrowing of their lumina by oedema, fibrosis and smooth-muscle hyperplasia; this is accompanied by infiltration by both small lymphocytes and polymorphonuclear neutrophils [41].

It has been claimed that both interstitial pneumonitis and lymphocytic bronchitis are also part of the spectrum of changes seen in lung GvHD. The evidence for this assertion is not good, although there is some evidence from animal experiments [42].

Lymphoid organs

It seems counterintuitive that GvHD should not affect the lymphoreticular system yet the evidence is at best equivocal [30]. Undoubtedly, there is splenic

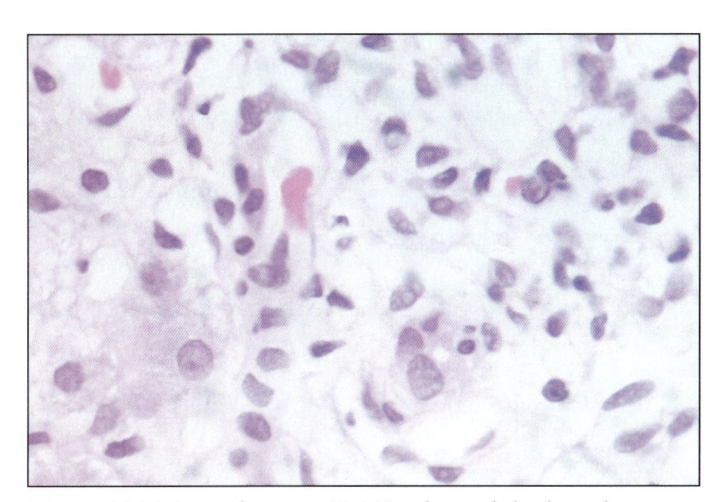

Figure 39.7 Acute hepatic GvHD shows bile duct damage. There is loss of some epithelial cells with interepithelial lymphocyte infiltration. Adjacent venule shows swollen endothelium.

enlargement in GvHD [43], although no specific histological abnormality has been identified. The polymerase chain reaction (PCR) has been used to detect cytokine expression within the spleen in GvHD: IL-4, TNF-α and TNF-β mRNAs have all been detected, albeit in post-mortem samples [20].

Cytokine expression within circulating blood mononuclear cells has been analyzed using PCR and a tendency to increased expression of the interleukin-2 receptor and interleukin-6 receptor has been reported [44]. The precise significance and usefulness of this finding is not clear.

Perhaps not surprisingly, the bone marrow is also affected by GvHD [45]. GvHD has been found in mice to decrease haematopoietic reserve within the marrow with a consequent increase in extramedullary haematopoiesis in the liver and spleen.

The lymph nodes are invariably lymphodepleted following bone-marrow transplantation but no specific histological features have been found. There are reports of individual cell necrosis, analogous to that seen in the skin, gastrointestinal tract and liver, within the thymic epithelium, although this is disputed [46,47].

Other organs

Although it less often and less severely affected by GvHD, the squamous epithelium of the oropharynx shows changes similar to those seen in the skin. The salivary glands are rarely affected but damage to the glandular epithelium has been reported in acute GvHD [48]. Chronic GvHD is more likely to affect them, producing atrophy of the glandular mucosa and duct ectasia. If these changes also occur in the lacrimal glands, there may be a sicca syndrome.

The pancreas may also be affected by GvHD in a manner similar to that seen in the bile ducts of the liver [49]. The endocrine pancreas is not affected.

Acknowledgement

All figures were kindly provided by Dr N. Al-Nasiri.

References

1. Sloane JP. Graft-versus-host disease – a histological perspective. *Blood Rev* 1990; **4**: 196–203.
2. Gale RP. Graft-versus-host disease. *Immunol Rev* 1985; **88**: 193–224.
3. Wagner JE. Umbilical cord blood transplantation. *Transplantation* 1995; **35**: 619–621.
4. Forbes GM, Erber WN, Herrmann RP, Davies JM and Collins BJ. Immunohistochemical changes in sigmoid colon after allogeneic bone marrow transplantation. *J Clin Pathol* 1995; **48**: 308–313.
5. Lerner KG, Kao GF, Storb R, Buckner CD, Clift RA and Thomas ED. Histopathology of graft-versus-host reaction (GvHR) in human recipients of marrow from HLA-matched sibling donors. *Transplant Proc* 1974; **6**: 367–371.
6. Rico MJ, Kory WP, Gould EW and Pennys NS. Interface dermatitis in patients with the acquired immune deficiency syndrome. *J Am Acad Dermatol* 1987; **16**: 1209–1281.
7. Elliott CJ, Sloane JP, Sanderson KV, Vincent M, Shepherd V and Powles R. The histological diagnosis of cutaneous graft versus host disease: relationship to marrow purging and other clinical variables. *Histopathology* 1987; **11**: 145–155.
8. Sale GE, Lerner KG, Barker EA, Shulman HM and Thomas ED. The skin biopsy in the diagnosis of acute graft-versus-host disease in man. *Am J Pathol* 1977; **89**: 621–636.
9. LeBoit P. Subacute radiation dermatitis: a histologic imitator of acute cutaneous graft-versus-host disease. *J Am Acad Dermatol* 1989; **20**: 236–241.
10. Socié G, Gluckman E, Cosset JM, Devergie A, Girinski T, Esperou H and Dutreix J. Unusual localization of cutaneous chronic graft-versus-host disease in the radiation fields in four cases. *Bone Marrow Transplant* 1989; **4**: 133–135.
11. Norton J and Sloane JP. Epidermal damage in skin of allogeneic marrow recipients: relative importance of chemotherapy, conditioning and graft v. host disease. *Histopathology* 1992; **21**: 529–524.
12. Norton J, Al-Saffar N and Sloane JP. An immunohistological study of gamma/delta lymphocytes in human cutaneous graft-versus-host disease. *Bone Marrow Transplant* 1991; **7**: 205–208.
13. Drijkoniger M, DeWolf-Peeters C, Tricot G, Degreef H and Desmet V. Drug-induced skin reactions and acute cutaneous graft-versus-host reaction: a comparative immunohistochemical study. *Blut* 1988; **56**: 69–73.
14. Lampert IA, Suitters AJ and Chisholm PM. Expression of Ia antigen on epidermal keratinocytes in graft-versus-host disease. *Nature* 1981; **293**: 149–150.
15. Suitters AJ and Lampert IA. The loss of Ia+ Langerhans' cells during graft-versus-host disease in rats. *Transplantation* 1983; **36**: 540–546.
16. Sale GE and Beauchamp M. Parafollicular hair bulge in human GvHD: a stem cell-rich primary target. *Bone Marrow Transplant* 1993; **11**: 223–225.
17. Sale GE, Beauchamp MD and Akiyama M. Parafollicular bulges, but not hair bulb keratinocytes, are attacked in graft-versus-host disease of human skin. *Bone Marrow Transplant* 1994; **14**: 411–413.
18. Cohen J. Cytokines as mediators of graft-versus-host disease. *Bone Marrow Transplant* 1988; **3**: 193–197.
19. Sloane JP, Elliott CJ and Powles RP. HLA-DR expression in epidermal keratinocytes after allogeneic bone marrow transplantation. *Transplantation* 1987; **46**: 840–844.
20. Rowbottom AW, Norton J, Riches PG, Hobbs JR, Powles RP and Sloane JP. Cytokine gene expression in skin and lymphoid organs in graft versus host disease. *J Clin Pathol* 1993; **46**: 341–345.

21. Mowat AM. Antibodies to IFN-gamma prevent immunologically mediated intestinal damage in murine graft-versus-host reaction. *Immunology* 1989; **68**: 18–23.
22. Shalaby MR, Fendly B, Sheehan KC, Schrieber RD and Ammann AJ. Prevention of the graft-versus host reaction in newborn mice by antibodies to tumour necrosis factor-alpha. *Transplantation* 1989; **47**: 1057–1061.
23. Hervé P, Bordigoni P, Cahn JY et al. Use of monoclonal antibodies in vivo as a therapeutic strategy for acute GvHD in matched and mismatched bone marrow transplantation. *Transplant Proc* 1991; **23**: 1692–1694.
24. Norton J, Sloane JP, Al-Saffar N and Haskard DO. Vessel-associated adhesion molecules in normal skin and acute graft-versus-host disease. *J Clin Pathol* 1991; **44**(7): 586–591.
25. Norton J, Sloane JP, Delia D and Greaves MF. Reciprocal expression of CD34 and cell adhesion molecule ELAM-1 on vascular endothelium in acute cutaneous graft-versus-host disease. *J Pathol* 1993; **170**: 173–177.
26. Sale GE, Shulman HM, McDonald GB and Thomas ED. Gastro-intestinal graft-versus-host disease in man: a clinicopathological study of the rectal biopsy. *Am J Surg Pathol* 1979; **3**: 291–299.
27. Bryan RL, Antonakapolous GN, Newman J and Milligan DW. Intestinal graft-versus-host disease. *J Clin Pathol* 1991; **44**: 866–867.
28. Bechorner WE. Destruction of the intestinal mucosa after bone marrow transplantation and graft-versus-host disease. *Surv Synth Pathol Res* 1984; **3**: 264–274.
29. Epstein RJ, McDonald GB, Sale GE, Shulman HM and Thomas ED. The diagnostic accuracy of the rectal biopsy in acute graft-versus-host disease: a prospective study of thirteen patients. *Gastroenterology* 1980; **78**: 764–777.
30. Sloane JP and Norton J. The pathology of bone marrow transplantation. *Histopathology* 1993; **22**: 201–209.
31. Snover DC. Mucosal damage simulating acute graft-versus-host reaction in cytomegalovirus colitis. *Transplantation* 1985; **39**: 669–670.
32. McCarthy AL, Malik-Peiris JS, Taylor CE, Green MA, Sviland L, Pearson AD and Malcolm AJ. Increase in the severity of graft versus host disease by cytomegalovirus. *J Clin Pathol* 1992; **45**: 542–544.
33. Bombi JA, Nadal A, Carreras E, Ramirez J, Munoz J, Rozman C and Cardesa A. Assessment of the histopathologic changes in the colonic biopsy in acute graft-versus-host disease. *Am J Clin Pathol* 1995; **103**: 690–695.
34. Dilly SA and Sloane JP. Changes in rectal leucocytes after allogeneic bone marrow transplantation. *Clin Exp Immunol* 1987; **67**: 151–158.
35. Sviland L, Pearson ADJ, Eastham EJ, Green MA, Hamilton PJ, Proctor SJ and the Newcastle upon Tyne Bone Marrow Transplant Group. Class II antigen expression by keratinocytes and enterocytes – an early feature of graft-versus-host disease. *Transplantation* 1988; **46**: 402–406.
36. Nakhleh RE, Snover DC, Weisdorf S and Platt JL Immunopathology of graft-versus-host disease in the upper gastro-intestinal tract. *Transplantation* 1989; **48**: 61–65.
37. Sloane JP, Farthing MJG and Powles R. Histopathological changes in the liver after allogeneic bone marrow transplantation. *J Clin Pathol* 1980; **33**: 344–350.
38. Snover DC, Weisdorf SA, Ramsay NK, McGlave P and Kersey JH. Hepatic graft versus host disease: a study of the predictive value of liver biopsy in diagnosis. *Hepatology* 1984; **4**: 123–130.
39. Nonamura A, Mizukami Y, Matsubara F and Kobayashi K. Clinicopathological study of lymphocyte attachment to endothelial cells (endothelialitis) in various liver diseases. *Liver* 1991; **11**: 78–88.
40. Knapp AB, Crawford JM, Rappeport JM and Gollan JL. Cirrhosis as a consequence of graft-versus-host disease. *Gastroenterology* 1987; **92**: 513–519.
41. Holland NK, Wingard JR, Beschorner WE, Saral R and Santos GW. Bronchiolitis obliterans in bone marrow transplantation and its relationship to chronic graft-vs-host disease and low serum IgG. *Blood* 1988; **72**: 621–627.
42. Workman DL and Clancy J Jr. Interstitial pneumonitis and lymphocytic bronchiolitis/bronchitis as a direct result of acute lethal graft-versus-host disease duplicate the histopathology of lung allograft rejection. *Transplantation* 1994; **58**: 207–213.
43. Dilly SA and Sloane JP. Enlargement of the human spleen in graft-versus-host disease. *Transplantation* 1988; **45**: 741–743.
44. Tanaka J, Imamura M, Kasai M et al. Cytokine receptor gene expression in peripheral blood mononuclear cells during graft-versus-host disease after allogeneic bone marrow transplantation. *Leukaemia Lymphoma* 1995; **19**: 281–287.
45. van Dijken PJ, Wimperis J, Crawford JM and Ferrara JL. Effect of graft-versus-host disease on haematopoiesis after bone marrow transplantation in mice. *Blood* 1991; **78**: 2773–2779.
46. Muller-Hermelink HK and Sale GE. Pathological findings in human bone marrow transplantation. *Verh Dtsch Ges Pathol* 1983; **67**: 255–280.
47. Thomas JA, Sloane JP, Imrie SF, Ritter MA, Schuurman H-J and Huber J. Immunohistology of the thymus in bone marrow transplant recipients. *Am J Pathol* 1986; **122**: 531–540.
48. Sale GE, Schulman HM, Schubert MM et al. Oral and ophthalmic pathology of graft versus host disease in man: predictive value of the lip biopsy. *Hum Pathol* 1981; **12**: 1022–1030.
49. Foulis AK, Farquharson MA and Sale GE. The pancreas in acute graft versus host disease in man. *Histopathology* 1989; **14**: 121–128.

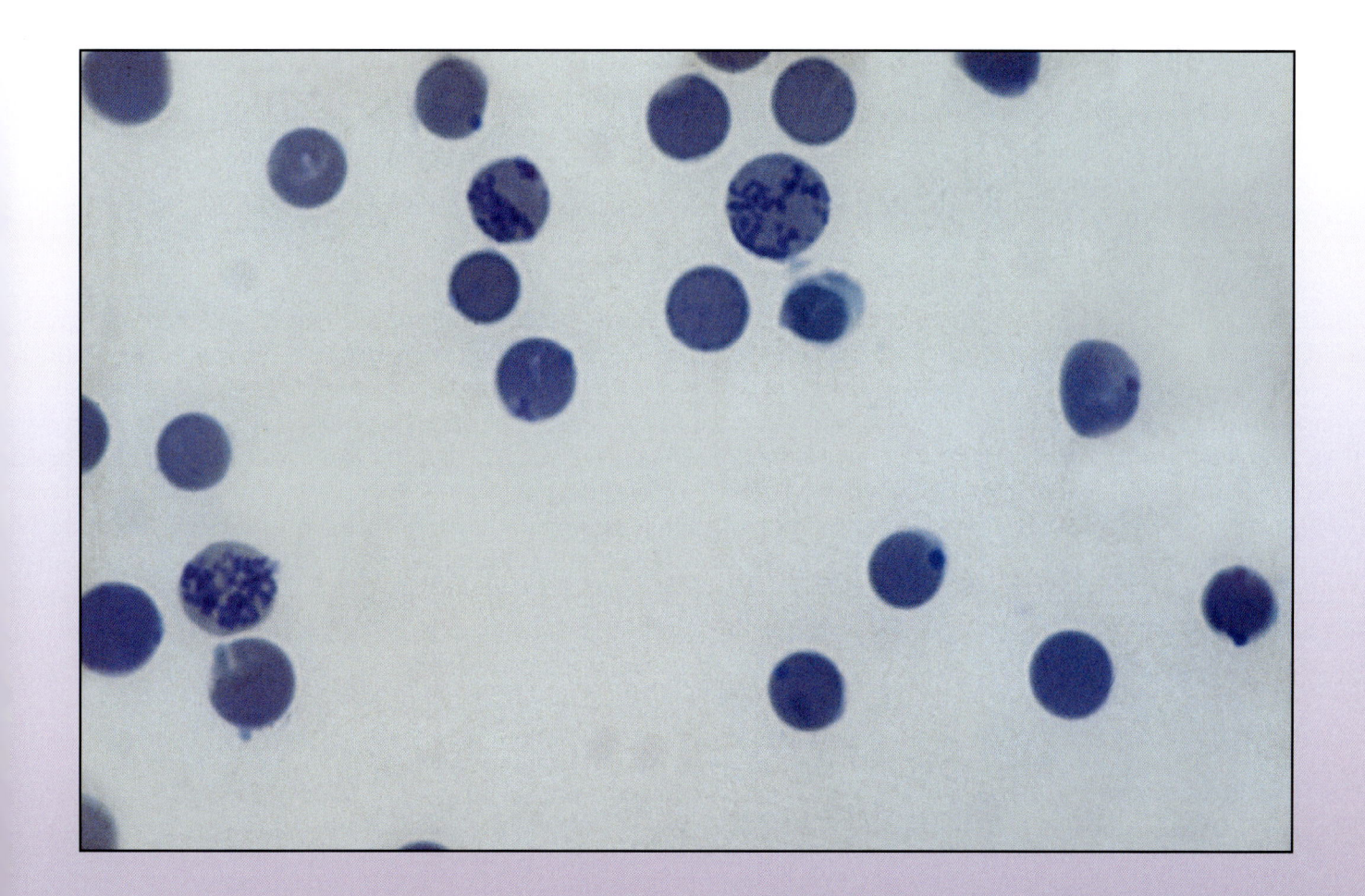

Chapter 40

Graft failure: diagnosis and management

Jayesh Mehta and Seema Singhal

Introduction

Pancytopenia as a result of myeloablative chemotherapy or chemoradiotherapy is universal after autologous or allogeneic blood or bone-marrow transplantation. However, the counts usually recover after a variable period of time depending upon a number of different disease-, patient-, donor-, graft- and treatment-related factors. Failure of sustained engraftment after transplantation is manifested by failure of peripheral blood counts to recover (primary failure of engraftment) or a fall in the counts after initial recovery (secondary or late failure of engraftment). Depending upon a combination of the above factors, the incidence of graft failure varies from <1% for non-T-cell-depleted HLA identical sibling allografts to almost 50% for T-cell-depleted HLA mismatched transplants [1–21]. Table 40.1 shows some of the causes of graft failure.

The term 'graft rejection' implies an active, immunologically-mediated process in the setting of allogeneic transplantation, where an otherwise adequate inoculum of cells from the donor is rejected by residual immune cells of host origin. The term 'graft failure', includes failure pf engraftment due to immune or non-immune causes, and includes graft rejection.

Definition

Failure to attain an absolute neutrophil count of 0.1, 0.2 or 0.5×10^9/litre by day 21–42 in association with a severely hypocellular marrow has been variously used to diagnose primary graft failure [1–12,16–18,20,23–27]. The clinical condition of transplanted patients who are persistently pancytopenic beyond three to four weeks often deteriorates sharply, due to serious opportunistic infections or haemorrhage. It is not known what proportion of these patients would ultimately recover haematopoiesis if they did not experience lethal complications (i.e. given an indefinite period of time to recover haematopoiesis). Therefore, graft failure has to

Table 40.1 Factors associated with predisposition to graft failure

Disease	Aplastic anaemia
	Marrow fibrosis
	Defective marrow microenvironment
Patient	Pretransplant sensitization
	Positive antidonor lymphocytotoxic cross-match
Donor	HLA-mismatch
	Unrelated
	Cord blood
Graft	T-cell depletion
	Low infused cell dose
	Pharmacological purging
	Damaged stem cells
Conditioning regimen	Inadequate immunosuppression
Post-transplant therapy	Inadequate immunosuppression
	Ganciclovir
	Histamine H_2-receptor blockers
	Other myelosuppressive drugs
Infections	Cytomegalovirus
	Other viral infections

be diagnosed in a somewhat arbitrary way on a set day after transplantation.

It may be advantageous to make the definition of primary graft failure flexible from the point of view of the management: in patients who are clinically unwell, graft failure may be diagnosed on day 21, whereas in patients who are clinically well and stable, one could delay the diagnosis until day 28. A low leukocyte count as early as two weeks post-transplant has been shown to be associated with an increased risk of subsequent graft failure and death due to complications of pancytopenia such as infections and haemorrhage [28]. Figures 40.1–40.3 show that a low leukocyte count on day 16 after allogeneic BMT, T-cell depleted grafts and transplants from unrelated or HLA-mismatched donors are associated with a significantly increased risk of subsequent graft failure or complications of pancytopenia [28]. Therefore, in patients at high risk of graft failure (Table 40.2), graft failure may be diagnosed in functional terms even earlier in order to institute management when the patient's clinical condition is good – and when intervention has a chance of succeeding.

Late graft failure has been defined as decline in the neutrophil count to less than 0.5×10^9/litre for three days in the absence of any obvious cause of myelosuppression or relapse after initially adequate recovery [8,23].

Bone-marrow findings

Severe pancytopenia is usual for the first week following BMT. The marrow during this period is usually extremely hypocellular or acellular. Discrete aggregates of haematopoietic cells are observed in the bone marrow at 14 days. In the third week, the cellularity is highly variable, and the localization of the various cell lineages and the ratios of myeloid cells to erythroid cells are abnormal [29]. Clustering of cells of the same lineage in the same stage of maturation is prominent. Absence of clustering of haematopoietic cells is often associated with either failure of engraftment or early leukaemic relapse. In addition to marked hypocellularity, the marrow may rarely show diffuse histiocytosis with foamy eosinophilic cytoplasm in delayed engraftment after autologous bone-marrow transplantation [30]. Lymphoid aggregates may be seen in immunologically-mediated graft rejection.

Immunologic graft rejection

In addition to infusion of an adequate number of haematopoietic progenitors, successful allo-

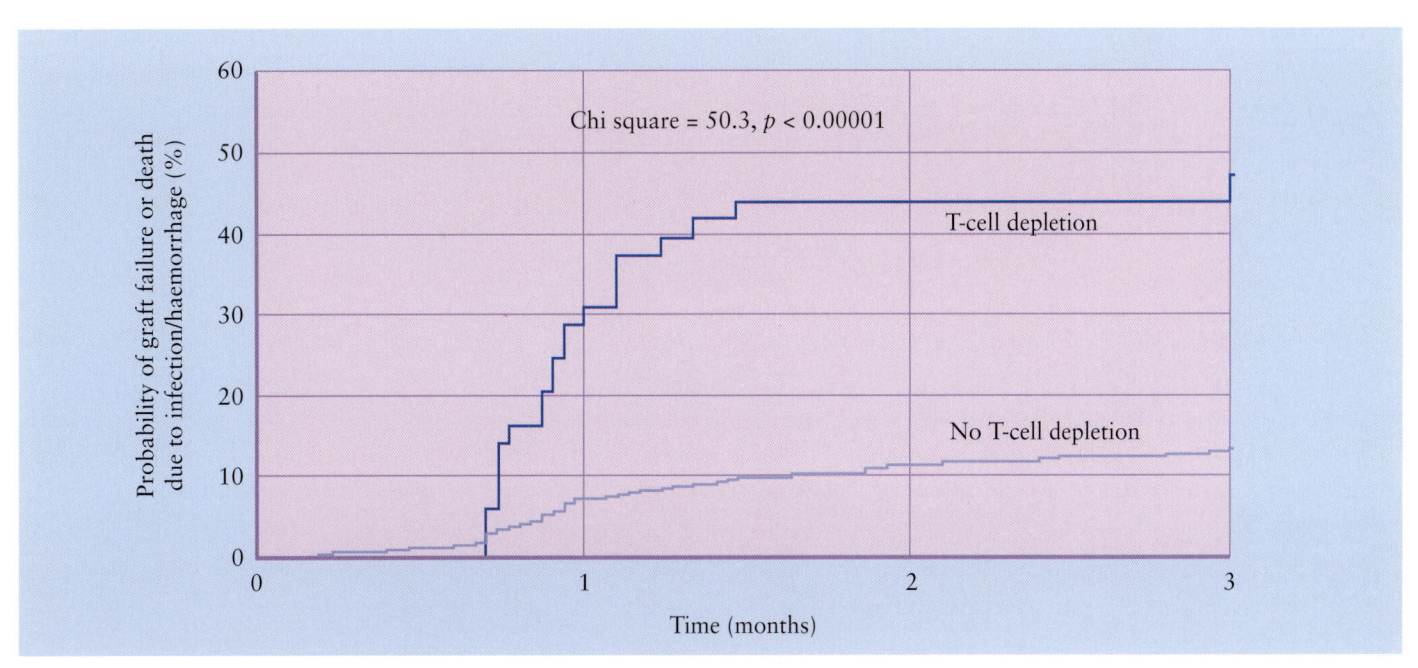

Figure 40.1 The effect of T-cell depletion on the probability of graft failure or death due to complications of pancytopenia amongst 712 allograft recipients with haematologic malignancies [28].

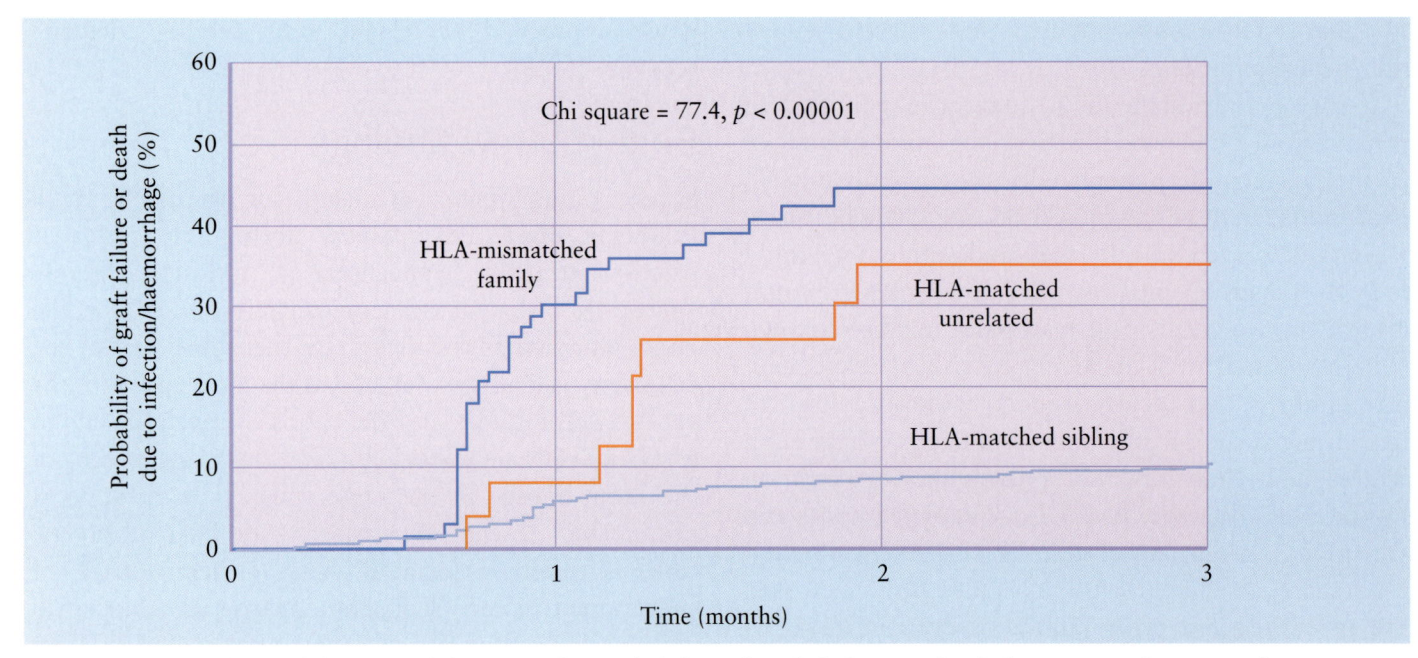

Figure 40.2 The effect of the type of donor on the probability of graft failure or death due to complications of pancytopenia amongst 712 allograft recipients with haematologic malignancies [28].

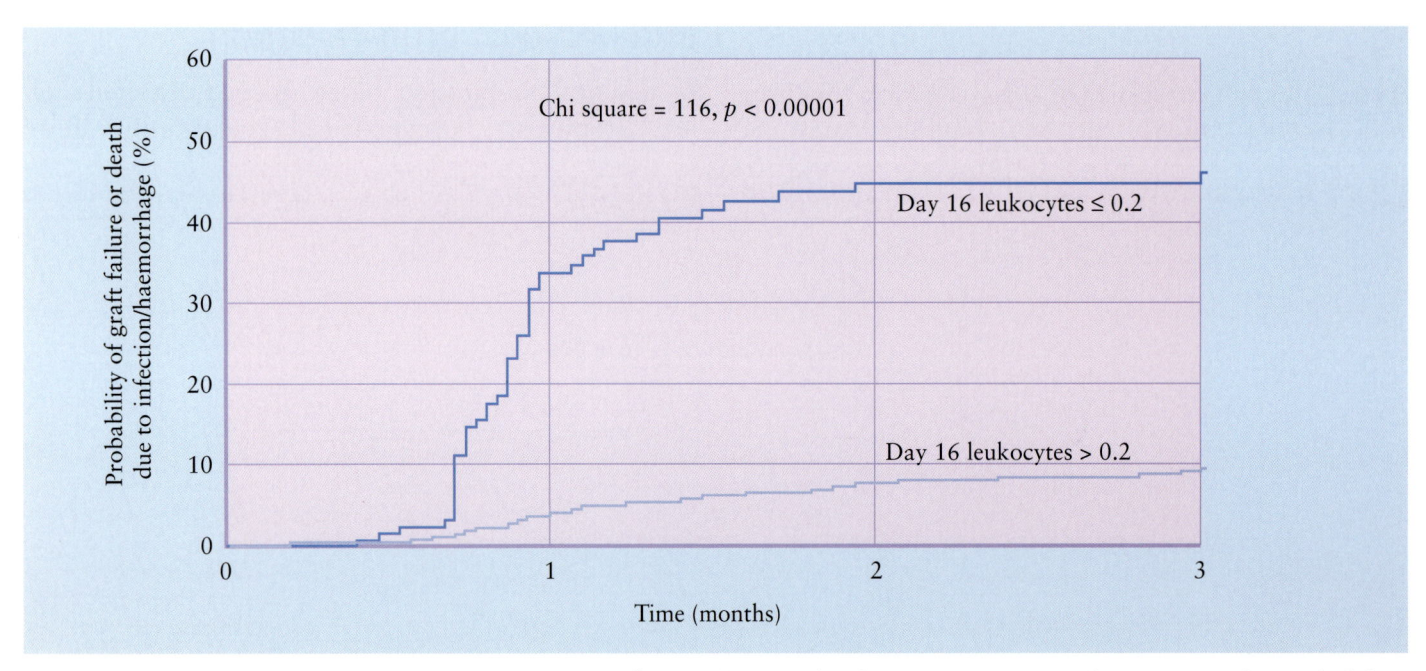

Figure 40.3 The effect of the total leukocyte count (10^9/L) on day 16 after bone-marrow transplantation on the probability of graft failure or death due to complications of pancytopenia among 712 allograft recipients with haematologic malignancies [28].

Table 40.2 *Prevention of graft rejection: approach to a high-risk allograft recipient*

Identification of patients at risk of rejection

- HLA-mismatched donor
- Positive antidonor lymphocytotoxic cross-match
- T-cell depletion
- Transfused aplastic anaemia
- Unrelated donor

Measures to minimize the possibility of rejection

- Ensure that the conditioning regimen is adequately immunosuppressive.
  Should contain at least one of the following major immunosuppressive agents: cyclophosphamide, melphalan, thiotepa or total body irradiation.

- Intensify pretransplant immunosuppression.
  Add at least one of the following supplementary agents, especially if only one of the major immunosuppressive agents is to be used: antilymphocyte globulin, campath-1G or other antilymphocyte monoclonal antibody, total lymphoid irradiation.

- Consider using G-CSF-mobilized peripheral blood stem cells an an alternative to or in addition to the marrow.

- Maximize the number of infused cells (the numbers represent the starting quantity prior to any *ex vivo* manipulation). At least 3×10^8 nucleated cells/kg for marrow, at least 5×10^8 mononuclear cells or 2×10^6 $CD34^+$ cells/kg for peripheral blood.

- Employ post-transplant immunosuppression (cyclosporin and/or methotrexate) even if T-cell depletion used for GvHD prophylaxis.

- Monitor methotrexate levels if there is renal dysfunction, and consider omitting the day 11 methotrexate in patients with significant renal dysfunction.

- Avoid all myelosuppressive drugs after transplantation.

Other measures

- Cryopreserve autologous marrow or blood stem cells pre-allograft if possible.
- Add G-CSF if the total leukocyte count is $\leq 0.1 \times 10^9$/litre on day 12 (if not on a growth factor already).
- Consider a second infusion of cells (allogeneic or autologous) if the total leukocyte count is $\leq 0.1 \times 10^9$/litre on day 14 and the bone marrow is severely hypocellular.
- Ensure that there is no folate or vitamin B_{12} deficiency.

engraftment requires a balance between immunocompetent host cells capable of rejecting the graft and immunocompetent donor cells facilitating engraftment. Conditioning regimens used prior to allogeneic transplantation should eliminate residual disease, ablate the host haematopoietic system to create 'space' for the donor marrow, and destroy the recipient's immune system to eliminate immunocompetent cells capable of causing rejection of the donor marrow. Adequate myeloablation and immunosuppression result in complete allo-engraftment, whereas inadequacy of both results in graft rejection with autologous reconstitution. Inadequate myeloablation results in mixed lymphohaematopoietic chimaerism, and inadequate immunosuppression results in mixed lymphoid chimaerism, both with an increased risk of relapse and late graft rejection. This may be an oversimplification of the actual process of allo-engraftment because recipient lymphohaematopoietic cells regularly survive myeloablative conditioning regimens including total body irradiation [31,32]. T-cells within the graft suppress rejection by causing an anti-host haematopoiesis effect which eliminates residual host cells [33]. This explains the increased risk of graft rejection with T-cell-depleted allografts. This risk can be decreased substantially by intensifying the conditioning regimen to eliminate host immunocompetent cells more effectively.

There are two different mechanisms underlying graft rejection: natural killer (NK) cell-mediated rejection [34] and T-cell-mediated rejection in the setting of minor or major histocompatibility antigen disparity or prior sensitization of the host to donor antigens [34–36]. The NK-mediated rejection is a form of allograft resistance seen amongst genotypically identical donor–recipient pairs, and has even been seen after syngeneic transplantation for aplastic anaemia [37]. The T-cells mediating rejection of genotypically non-identical marrow are cytotoxic cells of recipient origin expressing CD2, CD3, CD5, CD6, CD8 and Ia antigens [38]. There is evidence to suggest that graft failure observed in association with histocompatibility differences between donor and recipient may also be mediated by persistent host antibodies specific for donor antigens through antibody-dependent cell-mediated cytotoxicity or complement-mediated cytotoxicity [39]. Third-party-mediated graft rejection and GvHD due to transfused immunocompetent cells in inadequately irradiated blood products has also been described [40].

Graft rejection is usually characterized by transient occurrence of donor-derived haematopoiesis followed by a relative lymphocytosis of host origin, and then failure of all haematopoiesis or autologous recovery. Graft rejection is most commonly seen in previously transfused patients with aplastic anaemia who are conditioned with cyclophosphamide alone [3,9,17]. Graft rejection is also a major concern in HLA-mismatched transplants, especially if T-cell depletion is used to prevent graft-versus-host disease (GvHD).

The role of the bone-marrow microenvironment

There are anecdotal reports which suggest that recipient bone-marrow microenvironment damage contributes to graft failure. Marsh *et al.* described a 60-year-old woman with drug-induced aplastic anaemia who experienced graft failure four times after BMT from a healthy monozygotic twin despite increasingly intensive conditioning after each episode of graft failure [41]. *In vitro* studies showed no evidence of a recipient-derived cellular or humoral inhibitor of donor haematopoiesis, or of an intrinsic defect of donor stem-cell growth. Matthews *et al.* administered ^{131}I-labelled anti-CD45 monoclonal antibody to patients with acute leukaemia receiving a standard conditioning regimen to augment irradiation to haematopoietic tissues [42]. In this study, the patient receiving the highest total dose of irradiation (>3000 cGy) died of graft failure despite having been transplanted from an HLA-identical family member. It is possible that irradiation-induced damage to the stromal microenvironment could have contributed to graft failure.

The Seattle group initially reported that marrow fibrosis affected engraftment adversely [43], but subsequently found no significant effect of marrow fibrosis on engraftment [44]. Failed engraftment in patients with myelofibrosis has been in the setting of T-cell-depleted grafts, and it is likely that this was responsible for graft failure rather than marrow fibrosis [45]. Engraftment of autologous cells has been rapid in acute leukaemia with marrow fibrosis [46].

Drug-induced myelosuppression

Haematopoiesis in the regenerative post-transplant state may be more susceptible to the suppressive influence of various drugs, and potentially myelosuppressive drugs should be used very cautiously, if at all, to minimize the risk of drug-induced graft failure.

Ganciclovir is commonly used for the treatment of cytomegalovirus infections after bone-marrow transplantation and causes dose-dependent myelosuppression. Its use in patients prior to secure engraftment or its continued use in patients with ganciclovir-induced myelosuppression can result in graft failure [47]. If ganciclovir is used for prophylaxis of cytomegalovirus infections, it should not be commenced until the absolute neutrophil count is at least 0.5×10^9/litre on three consecutive days. Ganciclovir should be withheld if the absolute neutrophil count drops to less than 0.5×10^9/litre. In patients who have not engrafted or who have low counts, foscarnet is a useful substitute [47,48].

Although histamine H_2-receptor blocking agents are otherwise safe drugs, both cimetidine and ranitidine have been shown to cause myelosuppression after bone-marrow transplantation and should be avoided [49,50]. Adequate data are not available to establish whether other drugs of the same class such as famotidine and nizatidine are any safer. Omeprazole and sucralfate are probably safe alternatives. Chloramphenicol is associated with idiosyncratic or dose-dependent myelosuppression [51], and its use has been temporally associated with failure of allo-engraftment [52].

In patients with delayed engraftment with no obvious cause for low counts, it is prudent to review all drugs and discontinue all those which are not absolutely essential.

The patient with aplastic anaemia

Graft rejection is more common following BMT for severe aplastic anaemia compared with BMT for most other diseases, and its incidence is as high as 30% in previously transfused patients [3,9,17,53]. In a study of 233 patients allografted from HLA-identical siblings for severe aplastic anaemia after conditioning with 200 mg/kg cyclophosphamide as a single agent, 44 rejected their grafts [3]. Five risk factors were identified for graft rejection: earlier year of transplant, a large number of platelet transfusions prior to the transplant, a positive relative response in mixed leukocyte culture, a low marrow cell dose and omission of donor buffy coat cell infusion for transfused patients. The lower likelihood of graft rejection in patients transplanted more recently could have been related to improved transfusion practices. While a European Blood and Marrow Transplant group (EBMT) study confirmed this observation [17], an International Bone Marrow Transplant Registry (IBMTR) study [9] could find no effect of the year of transplant on rejection rates.

A more detailed examination of the effect of the marrow cell dose on engraftment [53] showed that in addition to lower rejection rates, higher marrow cell doses resulted in significantly faster granulocyte and platelet recovery and significantly improved survival due to the reduction in the incidence of graft rejection. Neither acute nor chronic GvHD were influenced by marrow cell dose. It is clearly very important to maximize the cell dose (minimum 3×10^8 nucleated marrow cells/kg recipient weight) in patients being allografted for severe aplastic anaemia.

In patients rejecting their first grafts, second grafts from the same or different donors are utilized with variable success after intensified conditioning, usually with cyclophosphamide and antilymphocyte globulin [9,17,54]. In patients who repeatedly reject their grafts, it may still be possible to attain sustained engraftment by maximizing immunosuppression [55]. It would clearly be best to identify patients at risk of graft rejection earlier on, and try to prevent rejection (Table 40.2).

The role of blood stem-cell allografts

Granulocyte colony-stimulating factor (G-CSF)-mobilized peripheral blood stem cells contain a large number of stem cells as well as T-cells, often as much as 1 log higher than in the marrow [56]. It is possible that G-CSF-mobilized blood stem cells may engraft when a marrow allograft from the same donor has failed [57,58]. Additionally, it has been shown that addition of G-CSF-mobilized T-cell-depleted peripheral blood stem cells to T-cell-depleted HLA-mismatched marrow results in much higher engraftment rates [59].

Conditioning regimens

Most commonly used conditioning regimens for allogeneic BMT contain total body irradiation, cyclophosphamide, or both, for their immunosuppressive properties [60–65]. Other agents used to enhance the immunosuppressive properties of conventional conditioning regimens or regimens thought to be inadequately immunosuppressive include total lymphoid irradiation, antilymphocyte globulin, monoclonal antibodies such as Campath and thiotepa [18,55,66–68]. Melphalan alone has been reported to result in allo-engraftment of marrow from HLA-identical sibling donors, but not from HLA-mismatched donors [52].

While 16 mg/kg of busulphan with 120 mg/kg of cyclophosphamide is sufficiently immunosuppressive to permit consistent engraftment of HLA-identical sibling marrow, it may not permit this with unrelated donor grafts [18]. It is possible that this lower cyclophosphamide dose [18] in combination with variable busulphan pharmacokinetics [69] may contribute to the increased incidence of graft failure. Amongst patients conditioned with busulphan and cyclophosphamide, Slattery et al. showed that the average steady-state busulphan concentration was the only significant determinant of graft rejection in multivariate analysis. An average concentration of at least 200 ng/ml was needed to avoid the rejection of HLA-identical sibling marrow, whereas 600 ng/ml was needed to avoid the rejection of HLA-mismatched related or HLA-matched unrelated marrow. Their data also showed variability in busulphan pharmacokinetics with age, suggesting that the use of a fixed dose for all ages and indications may not be appropriate [69].

Graft failure after autologous transplantation

Slow and incomplete engraftment is often a problem after autografting [22], especially with marrow as the source of stem cells [22], in patients with acute leukaemia [14,22], with extensive treatment prior to collection of cells [22], with antibody-mediated [70] or pharmacological [14] purging, and with low cell doses [22]. Graft failure has been noted to be a problem in chronic myeloid leukaemia patients who receive chemotherapy-mobilized Philadelphia chromosome-negative stem cells [21,71,72].

Infusion of a minimum of 2×10^8 nucleated cells/kg body weight has been associated with rapid neutrophil as well as platelet recovery in patients with acute leukaemia, and also with lower transplant-related mortality and better disease-free survival in acute myeloid leukaemia [73,74]. In order to prevent graft failure or incomplete/delayed engraftment, patients with lower cell yields should probably not be transplanted. The minimum number of peripheral blood stem cells that results in consistent (as opposed to rapid) engraftment is probably 1×10^6 CD34$^+$ cells/kg, below which engraftment may be incomplete or there may be failure of engraftment.

Prevention of graft failure

With established graft failure, immunologically mediated or otherwise, the mortality due to infections and haemorrhage is high. The best approach to successful management of graft failure is its prevention. Careful planning of all aspects of the transplant can minimize the risk of graft rejection or failure (Tables 40.2 and 40.3).

The role of growth factors

While the use of growth factors has been associated with more rapid neutrophil engraftment, there are no controlled data to support the use of growth factors in reducing the risk of graft failure [75]. However, starting growth factors in patients with delayed or failed engraftment is probably an appropriate step. The agents usually used have been granulocyte–macrophage colony-stimulating factor (GM-CSF) and G-CSF.

Nemunaitis et al. administered GM-CSF to 37 patients with graft failure after allogeneic (n = 15), autologous (n = 21) or syngeneic (n = 1) BMT at daily doses of 60–1000 µg/m^2 for 14 or 21 days [24]. Twenty-one patients reached an absolute neutrophil count of $\geq 0.5 \times 10^9$/litre within two weeks of starting therapy, while 16 did not. None of the 7 patients who received pharmacologically purged autografts responded. The survival of the GM-CSF-treated group was significantly better than that of a historical control group.

Weisdorf et al. compared GM-CSF administration for 14 days to sequential GM-CSF and G-CSF

Table 40.3 Prevention of graft failure: approach to a high-risk autograft recipient

Identification of patients at risk of graft failure

    Acute leukaemia (especially acute myeloid leukaemia)
    Advanced disease
    Chemotherapy-mobilized Philadelphia chromosome-negative blood stem cells
    Low cell dose
    Purged marrow

Measures to minimize the possiblity of rejection

- Consider using G-CSF-mobilized peripheral blood stem cells as an alternative to, or in addition to, the marrow if acceptable from the disease point of view.
- Maximize the number of infused cells (the numbers represent the starting quantity prior to any *ex vivo* manipulation). At least 2×10^8 nucleated cells/kg for marrow, or at least 5×10^8 mononuclear or 1×10^6 CD34$^+$ cells/kg for peripheral blood.
- Avoid all myelosuppressive drugs after transplantation.

Other measures

- Keep unmanipulated cells as back-up in case of purged or manipulated grafts.
- Cryopreserve additional autologous marrow or blood stem cells pretransplant if possible (especially patients in advanced remission in whom cells harvested in an earlier remission are being used, where recently-harvested cells may acceptable as back-up).
- Add G-CSF if the total leukocyte count is $\leq 0.1 \times 10^9$/litre on day 14 if not on a growth factor already.
- Consider infusing back-up cells if the total leukocyte count is $\leq 0.1 \times 10^9$/litre on day 21 and the bone marrow is severely hypocellular.
- Ensure that there is no folate or vitamin B_{12} deficiency.

administration for 7 days each in patients with primary or secondary graft failure after autologous or allogeneic BMT [26]. Patients receiving GM-CSF alone reached a neutrophil count of $\geq 0.5 \times 10^9$/litre at 2–61 days (median 8 days) after therapy, while those receiving sequential GM-CSF and G-CSF recovered at 1–36 days (median 6 days). Recovery times were comparable for autologous, related and unrelated grafts. Survival at 100 days after enrollment was superior after treatment with GM-CSF alone ($P = 0.026$); only 1 of 23 patients treated with GM-CSF died, versus 7 of 24 treated with sequential GM-CSF and G-CSF.

Second infusion of haematopoietic stem cells

In the absence of demonstrable immunological rejection, a second infusion of cells from the same donor can be used without further conditioning. If there is evidence of rejection, additional immunosuppression or use of a different donor may result in engraftment. G-CSF-mobilized peripheral blood stem cells have been successfully used to treat failure of marrow engraftment from the same donor [57,58]. Table 40.4 suggests guidelines for a second infusion of cells in case of delayed or failed engraftment. It is critical to consider second infusions early because of the logistic difficulties and delay involved in obtaining more cells, especially from unrelated donors.

The results of second allogeneic infusions are not very encouraging [23,25], but this does work in a selected group of patients. Mortality from infections and GvHD remains a problem. Bolger *et al.* [23] reinfused cells from the original donor without any further conditioning in 57 allografted patients who had persistently poor graft function in the absence of demonstrable rejection or persistent/recurrent disease. All 34 patients surviving more than one month after the second infusion achieved a neutrophil count of 0.5×10^9/litre, and 20 became independent of platelet transfusions. Acute GvHD occurred in 86% of patients, and chronic GvHD in all 20 patients surviving for at least five months; 10 patients became long-term survivors.

Davies *et al.* [25] infused marrow for a second time in 33 allografted patients who experienced primary ($n = 21$) or secondary ($n = 12$) graft failure. The second infusion resulted in engraftment in 57% of patients with primary and 33% of patients with secondary graft failure, with one-quarter of the patients in each group projected to be surviving at one year. Infection, predominantly fungal, was the most frequent cause of death, and GvHD developed in 52% of evaluable patients.

Infusion of cryopreserved autologous stem cells after failed allo-engraftment has been shown to result in consistent myeloid recovery and avoidance of the immediate infectious and haemorrhagic consequences of prolonged marrow aplasia [27]. Patients treated this way survive the transplant procedure and can at least be discharged from the hospital. Long-term outcome in such patients depends upon the underlying disease and the quality of autologous cells. Conversely, failure of autologous engraftment has been treated with an allograft [76].

Therapeutic graft rejection

Infusion of autologous cells in the relatively early stages after allogeneic transplantation is likely to result in rejection of allogeneic cells. This may be utilized as treatment of refractory, life-threatening GvHD. A

Table 40.4 Guidelines for a second infusion of cells in case of delayed or failed engraftment

Allografts

- Look for the origin of blood/marrow cells by DNA restriction fragment-length polymorphism (RFLP), variable number tandem repeats (VNTR), cytogenetic or HLA-typing studies: this is especially important in transplants where the risk of immunologically-mediated graft rejection is high.

- Increase immunosuppression with corticosteroids, antilymphocyte globulin, other antilymphocyte monoclonal antibodies, cyclophosphamide or total lymphoid irradiation (bearing in mind the risk of toxicity and infections) if there is evidence of host lymphocytosis with no persistent donor cells in the circulation.

- Infuse G-CSF-mobilized peripheral blood stem cells if the first graft was from bone marrow.

- Avoid T-cell depletion if the first graft was T-cell depleted.

- Consider using a different donor, especially if there is no evidence of persisting donor cells.

- Ensure adequate GvHD prophylaxis during and after the second infusion of allogeneic cells.

- Consider infusion of autologous cells if available.

Autografts

- Infuse unmanipulated cells if graft failure occurred after the infusion of purged or manipulated cells.

- Consider an infusion of allogeneic cells under appropriate circumstances.

syngeneic marrow infusion has been used to successfully treat refractory, progressive grade IV acute GvHD after allogeneic marrow transplantation [27]. The syngeneic marrow probably caused rejection of the allogeneic marrow, resulting in complete resolution of GvHD. Similarly, stored autologous marrow has been utilized for treatment of acute GvHD developing after liver transplantation, and infusion of allogeneic marrow from the liver donor for induction of specific transplantation tolerance [77].

Rejection and the basis of 'hit-and-run' immunotherapy

It is attractive to speculate that even the transient presence of immunocompetent allogeneic cells may result in a 'hit-and-run' graft-versus-tumour effect, whereby residual malignant cells escaping the effects of the conditioning regimen are eliminated by partially or fully HLA-matched allogeneic lymphocytes before the latter are rejected by the patient's immune system. This is being explored in two ways: allogeneic mini-transplants using moderately immunosuppressive but non-myeloablative regimens which permit complete allo-engraftment initially, but subsequent autologous recovery results in rejection of the allograft and elimination of the chimaerism. The second technique is to infuse a small number of haplo-identical or HLA-identical lymphocytes shortly after a conventional autograft [78]. These lymphocytes may remain in the circulation transiently and cause antitumour effects prior to being rejected. Occasional engraftment of allogeneic cells with severe GvHD is a problem. However, there are no data to support this approach at the moment [79].

References

1. Powles RL, Morgenstern GR, Kay HE et al. Mismatched family donors for bone-marrow transplantation as treatment for acute leukaemia. *Lancet* 1983; i: 612–615.
2. Bozdech MJ, Sondel PM, Trigg ME et al. Transplantation of HLA-haploidentical T-cell-depleted marrow for leukemia: addition of cytosine arabinoside to the pretransplant conditioning prevents rejection. *Exp Haematol* 1985; **13**: 1201–1210.
3. Deeg HJ, Self S, Storb R et al. Decreased incidence of marrow graft rejection in patients with severe aplastic anemia: changing impact of risk factors. *Blood* 1986; **68**: 1363–1368.
4. Patterson J, Prentice HG, Brenner MK et al. Graft rejection following HLA matched T-lymphocyte depleted bone marrow transplantation. *Br J Haematol* 1986; **63**: 221–230.
5. Martin PJ, Hansen JA, Torok-Storb B et al. Graft failure in patients receiving T-cell-depleted HLA-identical allogeneic marrow transplants. *Bone Marrow Transplant* 1988; **3**: 445–456.
6. Niederwieser D, Pepe M, Storb R, Loughran TP Jr and Longton G. Improvement in rejection, engraftment rate and survival without increase in graft-versus-host disease by high marrow cell dose in patients transplanted for aplastic anaemia. *Br J Haematol* 1988; **69**: 23–28.
7. Burnett AK, Hann IM, Robertson AG et al. Prevention of graft-versus-host disease by *ex vivo* T cell depletion: reduction in graft failure with augmented total body irradiation. *Leukaemia* 1988; **2**: 300–303.
8. Anasetti C, Amos D, Beatty PG et al. Effect of HLA compatibility on engraftment of bone marrow transplants in patients with leukemia or lymphoma. *New Engl J Med* 1989; **320**: 197–204.
9. Champlin RE, Horowitz MM, Van Bekkum DW et al. Graft failure following bone marrow transplantation for severe aplastic anemia: risk factors and treatment results. *Blood* 1989; **73**: 606–613.
10. Kernan NA, Bordignon C, Heller G et al. Graft failure after T-cell-depleted human leukocyte antigen identical marrow transplants for leukemia. I. Analysis of risk factors and results of secondary transplants. *Blood* 1989; **74**: 2227–2236.
11. Trigg ME, Gingrich R, Goeken N et al. Low rejection rate when using unrelated or haploidentical donors for children with leukemia undergoing marrow transplantation. *Bone Marrow Transplant* 1989; **4**: 431–437.
12. Ash RC, Casper JT, Chitambar CR et al. Successful allogeneic transplantation of T-cell-depleted bone marrow from closely HLA-matched unrelated donors. *New Engl J Med* 1990; **322**: 485–494.
13. Marmont AM, Horowitz MM, Gale RP et al. T-cell depletion of HLA-identical transplants in leukemia. *Blood* 1991; **78**: 2120–2130.
14. Rowley SD, Piantadosi S, Marcellus DC et al. Analysis of factors predicting speed of hematologic recovery after transplantation with 4-hydroperoxycyclophosphamide-purged autologous bone marrow grafts. *Bone Marrow Transplant* 1991; **7**: 183–191.
15. Kernan NA, Bartsch G, Ash RC et al. Analysis of 462 transplantations from unrelated donors facilitated by the National Marrow Donor Program. *New Engl J Med* 1993; **328**: 593–602.
16. Davies SM, Ramsay NKC, Haake RJ et al. Comparison of engraftment in recipients of matched sibling or unrelated donor marrow allografts. *Bone Marrow Transplant* 1994; **13**: 51–57.
17. McCann SR, Bacigalupo A, Gluckman E et al. Graft rejection and second bone marrow transplants for acquired aplastic anaemia: a report from the Aplastic Anaemia Working Party of the European Bone Marrow Transplant Group. *Bone Marrow Transplant* 1994; **13**: 233–237.
18. Mehta J, Powles RL, Mitchell P, Rege K, De Lord C and Treleaven J. Graft failure after bone marrow transplantation from unrelated donors using busulphan and cyclophosphamide for conditioning. *Bone Marrow Transplant* 1994; **13**: 583–587.

19. Hale G and Waldmann H. Control of graft-versus-host disease and graft rejection by T cell depletion of donor and recipient with Campath-1 antibodies. Results of matched sibling transplants for malignant diseases. *Bone Marrow Transplant* 1994; **13**: 597–611.
20. Schultz KR, Ratanatharathorn V, Abella E et al. Graft failure in children receiving HLA-mismatched marrow transplants with busulfan-containing regimens. *Bone Marrow Transplant* 1994; **13**: 817–822.
21. Mehta J, Mijovic A, Powles R et al. Myelosuppressive chemotherapy to mobilize normal stem cells in chronic myeloid leukemia. *Bone Marrow Transplant* 1996; **17**: 25–29.
22. Mehta J, Powles R, Horton C, Treleaven J and Singhal S. Factors affecting engraftment and hematopoietic recovery after unpurged autografting in acute leukemia. *Bone Marrow Transplant* 1996; **18**: 319–324.
23. Bolger GB, Sullivan KM, Storb R et al. Second marrow infusion for poor graft function after allogeneic marrow transplantation. *Bone Marrow Transplant* 1986; **1**: 21–30.
24. Nemunaitis J, Singer JW, Buckner CD et al. Use of recombinant human granulocyte–macrophage colony-stimulating factor in graft failure after bone marrow transplantation. *Blood* 1990; **76**: 245–253.
25. Davies SM, Weisdorf DJ, Haake RJ et al. Second infusion of bone marrow for treatment of graft failure after allogeneic bone marrow transplantation. *Bone Marrow Transplant* 1994; **14**: 73–77.
26. Weisdorf DJ, Verfaillie CM, Davies SM et al. Hematopoietic growth factors for graft failure after bone marrow transplantation: a randomized trial of granulocyte-macrophage colony-stimulating factor (GM-CSF) versus sequential GM-CSF plus granulocyte-CSF. *Blood* 1995; **85**: 3452–3456.
27. Mehta J, Powles R, Singhal S, Horton C and Treleaven J. Outcome of autologous rescue after failed engraftment of allogeneic marrow. *Bone Marrow Transplant* 1996; **17**: 213–217.
28. Mehta J, Powles R, Horton C et al. Early identification of patients at risk of death due to infections, hemorrhage, or graft failure after allogeneic bone marrow transplantation on the basis of the leukocyte counts. *Bone Marrow Transplant* 1997; **19**: 349–355.
29. Van den Berg H, Kluin PM and Vossen JM. Early reconstitution of haematopoiesis after allogeneic bone marrow transplantation: a prospective histopathological study of bone marrow biopsy specimens. *J Clin Pathol* 1990; **43**: 365–369.
30. Rosenthal NS and Farhi DC. Failure to engraft after bone marrow transplantation: bone marrow morphologic findings. *Am J Clin Pathol* 1994; **102**: 821–824.
31. Schwartz E, Lapidot T, Gozes D, Singer TS and Reisner Y. Abrogation of bone marrow allograft resistance in mice by increased total body irradiation correlates with eradication of host clonable T cells and alloreactive cytotoxic precursors. *J Immunol* 1987; **138**: 460–465.
32. Theobald M, Hoffmann T, Bunjes D and Heit W. Comparative analysis of *in vivo* T cell depletion with radiotherapy, combination chemotherapy, and the monoclonal antibody Campath-1G, using limiting dilution methodology. *Transplantation* 1990; **49**: 553–559.
33. Hakim FT and Shearer GM. Abrogation of hybrid resistance to bone marrow engraftment by graft-vs-host-induced immune deficiency. *J Immunol* 1986; **137**: 3109–3116.
34. Murphy WJ, Kumar V and Bennett M. Rejection of bone marrow allografts by mice with severe combined immune deficiency (SCID). Evidence that natural killer cells can mediate the specificity of marrow graft rejection. *J Exp Med* 1987; **165**: 1212–1217.
35. Bierer BE, Emerson SG, Antin J et al. Regulation of cytotoxic T lymphocyte-mediated graft rejection following bone marrow transplantation. *Transplantation* 1988; **46**: 835–839.
36. Voogt PJ, Fibbe WE, Marijt WA et al. Rejection of bone-marrow graft by recipient-derived cytotoxic T lymphocytes against minor histocompatibility antigens. *Lancet* 1990; **335**: 131–134.
37. Goss GD, Wittwer MA, Bezwoda WR et al. Effect of natural killer cells on syngeneic bone marrow: *in vitro* and *in vivo* studies demonstrating graft failure due to NK cells in an identical twin treated by bone marrow transplantation. *Blood* 1985; **66**: 1043–1046.
38. Bosserman LD, Murray C, Takvorian T et al. Mechanism of graft failure in HLA-matched and HLA-mismatched bone marrow transplant recipients. *Bone Marrow Transplant* 1989; **4**: 239–245.
39. Barge AJ, Johnson G, Witherspoon R and Torok-Storb B. Antibody-mediated marrow failure after allogeneic bone marrow transplantation. *Blood* 1989; **74**: 1477–1480.
40. Drobyski W, Thibodeau S, Truitt RL et al. Third-party-mediated graft rejection and graft-versus-host disease after T-cell-depleted bone marrow transplantation, as demonstrated by hypervariable DNA probes and HLA-DR polymorphism. *Blood* 1989; **74**: 2285–2294.
41. Marsh JCW, Harhalakis N, Dowding C, Laffan M, Gordon-Smith EC and Hows JM. Recurrent graft failure following syngeneic bone marrow transplantation for aplastic anaemia. *Bone Marrow Transplant* 1989; **4**: 581–585.
42. Matthews DC, Appelbaum FR, Eary JF et al. Development of a marrow transplant regimen for acute leukemia using targeted hematopoietic irradiation delivered by ^{131}I-labeled anti-CD45 antibody, combined with cyclophosphamide and total body irradiation. *Blood* 1995; **85**: 1122–1131.
43. Rajantie J, Sale GE, Deeg HJ et al. Adverse effect of severe marrow fibrosis on hematologic recovery after chemoradiotherapy and allogeneic bone marrow transplantation. *Blood* 1986; **67**: 1693–1697.
44. Soll E, Massumoto C, Clift RA et al. Relevance of marrow fibrosis in bone marrow transplantation – a retrospective analysis of engraftment. *Blood* 1995; **86**: 4667–4673.
45. Singhal S, Powles R, Treleaven J, Lumley H, Pollard C and Mehta J. Allogeneic bone marrow transplantation for primary myelofibrosis. *Bone Marrow Transplant* 1995; **16**: 743–746.
46. Mehta J, Powles RL, Shepherd V, Dainton M and Treleaven J. Transplantation of autologous peripheral blood stem cells mobilized using GM-CSF for acute leukemia with myelofibrosis. *Leukaemia Lymphoma* 1993; **11**: 157–158.
47. Singhal S, Mehta J, Powles R et al. Three weeks of ganciclovir for cytomegaloviraemia after allogeneic bone marrow transplantation. *Bone Marrow Transplant* 1995; **15**: 777–781.

48. Chang J, Powles R, Singhal S, Jameson B, Treleaven J and Mehta J. Foscarnet therapy for cytomegalovirus infection after allogeneic bone marrow transplantation. *Clin Infect Dis* 1996; **22**: 583–584.
49. Agura ED, Vila E, Petersen FB, Shields AF and Thomas ED. The use of ranitidine in bone marrow transplantation. A review of 223 cases. *Transplantation* 1988; **46**: 53–56.
50. Mehta J, Powles R, Treleaven J et al. Cimetidine-induced myelosuppression after bone marrow transplantation. *Leukaemia Lymphoma* 1994; **13**: 179–181.
51. Appelbaum FR and Fefer A. The pathogenesis of aplastic anemia. *Semin Hematol* 1981; **18**: 241–257.
52. Singhal S, Powles R, Treleaven J, Horton C and Mehta J. Melphalan alone prior to allogeneic bone marrow transplantation from HLA-identical sibling donors for hematologic malignancies: alloengraftment with potential preservation of fertility. *Bone Marrow Transplant* 1996; **18**(6): 1049–1057.
53. Niederwieser D, Pepe M, Storb R, Loughran TP Jr and Longton G. Improvement in rejection, engraftment rate and survival without increase in graft-versus-host disease by high marrow cell dose in patients transplanted for aplastic anaemia. *Br J Haematol* 1988; **69**: 23–28.
54. Storb R, Weiden PL, Sullivan KM et al. Second marrow transplants in patients with aplastic anemia rejecting the first graft: use of a conditioning regimen including cyclophosphamide and antithymocyte globulin. *Blood* 1987; **70**: 116–121.
55. Or R, Mehta J, Kapelushnik J et al. Total lymphoid irradiation, anti-lymphocyte globulin and Campath 1-G for immunosuppression prior to bone marrow transplantation for aplastic anemia after repeated graft rejection. *Bone Marrow Transplant* 1994; **13**: 97–99.
56. Singhal S, Powles R, Treleaven J, Long S, Rowland A and Mehta J. Comparison of cell yields in a double-blind randomized study of allogeneic marrow versus blood stem cell transplantation. *Br J Haematol* 1996; **93**(Suppl 1): 37.
57. Dreger P, Suttorp M, Haferlach T, Loffler H, Schmitz N and Schroyens W. Allogeneic granulocyte colony-stimulating factor-mobilized peripheral blood progenitor cells for treatment of engraftment failure after bone marrow transplantation. *Blood* 1993; **81**: 1404–1407.
58. Molina L, Chabannon C, Viret F et al. Granulocyte colony-stimulating factor-mobilized allogeneic peripheral blood stem cells for rescue graft failure after allogeneic bone marrow transplantation in two patients with acute myeloblastic leukemia in first complete remission. *Blood* 1995; **85**: 1678–1679.
59. Aversa F, Tabilio A, Terenzi A et al. Successful engraftment of T-cell-depleted haploidentical 'three-loci' incompatible transplants in leukemia patients by addition of recombinant human granulocyte colony-stimulating factor-mobilized peripheral blood progenitor cells to bone marrow inoculum. *Blood* 1994; **84**: 3948–3955.
60. Thomas ED, Storb R, Clift RA et al. Bone-marrow transplantation. *New Engl J Med* 1975; **292**: 832–843, 895–902.
61. Powles RL, Clink HM, Spence D et al. Cyclosporin A to prevent graft-versus-host disease in man after allogeneic bone-marrow transplantation. *Lancet* 1980; **i**: 327–329.
62. Santos GW, Tutschka PJ, Brookmeyer R et al. Marrow transplantation for acute nonlymphocytic leukemia after treatment with busulfan and cyclophosphamide. *New Engl J Med* 1983; **309**: 1347–1353.
63. Tutschka PJ, Copelan EA and Klein JP. Bone marrow transplantation for leukemia following a new busulfan and cyclophosphamide regimen. *Blood* 1987; **70**: 1382–1388.
64. Snyder DS, Chao NJ, Amylon MD et al. Fractionated total body irradiation and high-dose etoposide as a preparatory regimen for bone marrow transplantation for 99 patients with acute leukemia in first complete remission. *Blood* 1993; **82**: 2920–2928.
65. Spitzer TR, Peters C, Ortlieb M et al. Etoposide in combination with cyclophosphamide and total body irradiation or busulfan as conditioning for marrow transplantation in adults and children. *Int J Radiat Oncol Biol Phys* 1994; **29**: 39–44.
66. Slavin S, Naparstek E, Aker M et al. The use of total lymphoid irradiation (TLI) for prevention of rejection of T-lymphocyte depleted bone marrow allografts in non-malignant hematological disorders. *Transplant Proc* 1989; **21**: 3053–3054.
67. Przepiorka D, Dimopoulos M, Smith T et al. Thiotepa, busulfan, and cyclophosphamide as a preparative regimen for marrow transplantation: risk factors for early regimen-related toxicity. *Ann Haematol* 1994; **68**: 183–188.
68. Mehta J, Powles R, Singhal S et al. T-cell depleted allogeneic bone marrow transplantation from a partially HLA-mismatched unrelated donor for progressive chronic lymphocytic leukemia and fludarabine-induced bone marrow failure. *Bone Marrow Transplant* 1996; **17**: 881–883.
69. Slattery JT, Sanders JE, Buckner CD et al. Graft-rejection and toxicity following bone marrow transplantation in relation to busulfan pharmacokinetics. *Bone Marrow Transplant* 1995; **16**: 31–42.
70. Mehta J, Powles R, Singhal S et al. Autologous transplantation with CD52 monoclonal antibody-purged marrow for acute lymphoblastic leukemia: long-term follow-up. *Leukaemia Lymphoma* 1997; **25**: 479–486.
71. Carella AM, Pollicardo N, Pungolino E et al. Mobilization of cytogenetically 'normal' blood progenitors cells by intensive conventional chemotherapy for chronic myeloid and acute lymphoblastic leukemia. *Leukaemia Lymphoma* 1993; **9**: 477–483.
72. O'Brien SG, Rule S, Spencer A et al. Autografting in chronic phase CML using PBPCs mobilized by intermediate-dose chemotherapy. *Br J Haematol* 1995; **89**(Suppl 1): 39.
73. Mehta J, Powles R, Singhal S et al. Autologous bone marrow transplantation for acute myeloid leukemia in first remission: identification of modifiable prognostic factors. *Bone Marrow Transplant* 1995; **16**: 499–506.
74. Demirer T, Gooley T, Buckner CD et al. Influence of total nucleated cell dose from marrow harvests on outcome in patients with acute myelogenous leukemia undergoing autologous transplantation. *Bone Marrow Transplant* 1995; **15**: 907–913.
75. Anasetti C, Anderson G, Appelbaum FR et al. Phase III study of rhGM-CSF in allogeneic marrow transplantation from unrelated donors. *Blood* 1993; **82**(Suppl 1): 454a.

76. Finke J, Euchenhofer B, Zeller C et al. Successful allogenic transplantation after autologous graft failure. *Transplantation* 1994; **57**: 1265–1266.
77. Ricordi C, Tzakis AG, Zeevi A et al. Reversal of graft-versus-host disease with infusion of autologous bone marrow. *Cell Transplant* 1994; **3**: 187–192.
78. Nagler A, Ackerstein A, Or R et al. Adoptive immunotherapy with mismatched allogeneic peripheral blood lymphocytes (PBL) following autologous bone marrow transplantation (ABMT). *Exp Hematol* 1992; **20**: 705.
79. Singhal S, Mehta J, Hood S et al. Third transplants for myeloma relapsing after two prior autografts. *Blood* 1997; **90** (Suppl 1): In press.

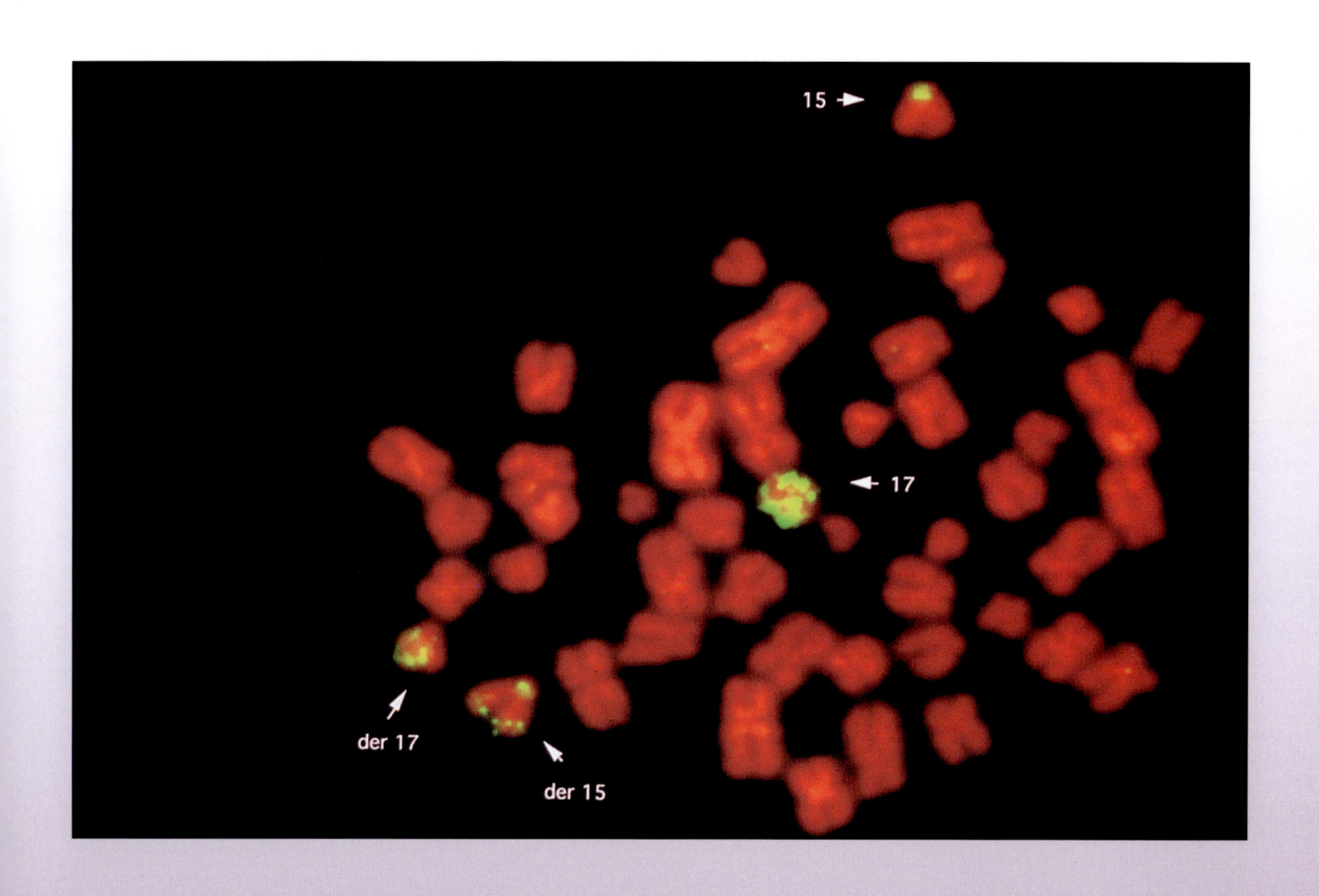

Chapter 41

Minimal residual disease in acute leukaemia

Jacques J.M. van Dongen, Tomasz Szczepañski
and Marja J. Pongers-Willemse

Introduction

The development of combination chemotherapy three decades ago with subsequent modifications, resulted in major progress in the treatment of acute leukaemias with induction of complete remission in most patients [1]. The burden of malignant cells at diagnosis is estimated at 1×10^{12}. Complete remission of disease is currently based on finding less than 5% of blasts in routine cytomorphologic preparation and thus theoretically occurs when tumour load has decreased to 1×10^{10}. Based on clinical experience, intensive and long-lasting chemotherapy is necessary to prolong complete remission into a five-year event-free survival. This may require bone-marrow transplantation in cases of high-risk acute lymphoblastic leukaemias and most acute myeloid leukaemias. Further intensification of treatment results in higher toxicity and increases the risk of developing secondary malignancies, usually with very poor prognosis [2]. Despite current aggressive therapy, many patients relapse, implying that the treatment does not kill all clonogenic leukaemic cells in every patient, and that surviving leukaemic cells remain undetectable by routine cytomorphology. Therefore, reliable and sensitive techniques are required to detect 'minimal residual disease' (MRD) to evaluate the effectiveness of the treatment in leukaemia patients, and to allow the prediction of impending relapse before its clinical manifestation.

During the last decade, several MRD detection methods have been evaluated. These include conventional cytogenetics, fluorescence *in situ* hybridization (FISH), cell-culture systems, immunophenotyping, Southern blotting and polymerase chain reaction (PCR) techniques. The detection limit of most of these methods is not lower than 1–5% malignant cells [3–6]. However, depending on the phenotype and genotype of the leukaemia, immunophenotyping techniques and PCR techniques are able to detect lower frequencies of leukaemic cells varying from 0.1 to 0.001% (Figure 41.1) [7–11].

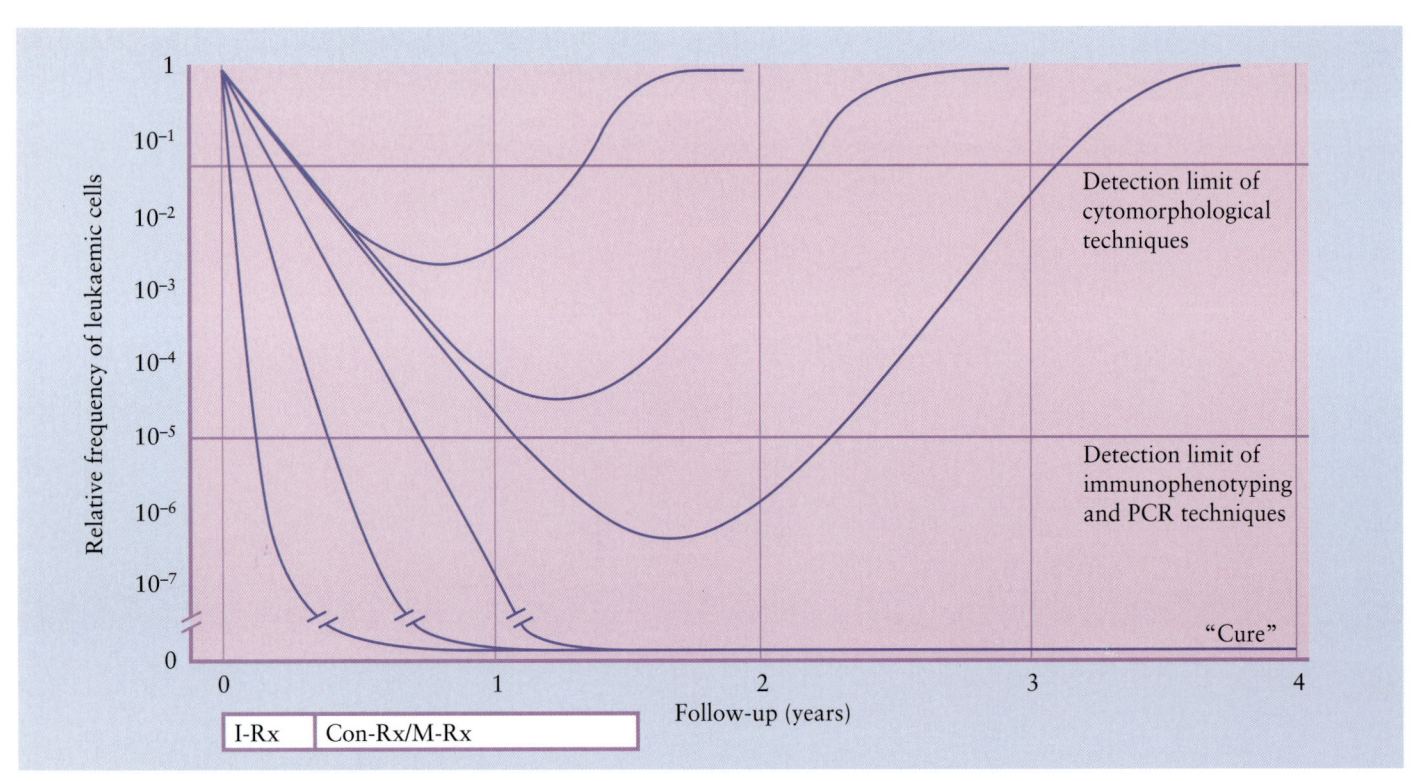

Figure 41.1 Hypothetical graph representing the putative relative frequencies of leukaemic cells in blood or bone marrow of acute leukaemia patients during and after chemotherapy and during development of relapse. The potential detection limit of cytomorphological techniques as well as that of immunophenotyping and PCR techniques are indicated. I-Rx = induction treatment, Con-Rx = consolidation treatment, M-Rx = maintenance treatment.

MRD detection by use of immunophenotyping

The immunological classification of acute leukaemias is based on the assumption that malignant cells are counterparts of normal immature haematopoietic cells. Most neoplastic lymphoblasts indeed have immunophenotypes comparable to normal immature lymphoid cells; the same applies to immunophenotypes of AML. Consequently, the background of normal haematopoietic cells limits the immunophenotypic detection of leukaemic cells [7–9,12–14]. However, leukaemias frequently display unusual or aberrant antigen expression, which allows MRD detection. These 'leukaemia-associated' immunophenotypes generally concern cross-lineage antigen expression, maturational asynchronic antigen expression, antigen overexpression and/or ectopic antigen expression (Figure 41.2) [9,13]. Ectopic antigen expression refers to detection of positive cells outside their normal breeding sites and homing areas, or the expression of antigens not found on normal haematopoietic cells. Although leukaemic phenotypes are detectable with microscopic double immunofluorescence stains, flow cytometry especially represents a powerful tool for detection of unusual and aberrant antigen expression. Current flow cytometers allow routine multiparameter analysis (two scatter parameters and three fluorochrome parameters) as well as simultaneous detection of surface membrane and intracellular antigens [15,16]. The ideal target for immunophenotypic MRD detection would be chimaeric proteins resulting from fusion genes of chromosomal translocations like BCR-ABL protein from t(9;22) and TEL-AML1 protein from t(12;21), since these are unique for the leukaemic cell population. Despite many efforts, monoclonal antibodies for reliable flow cytometric detection of these leukaemia-specific chimaeric proteins are not yet available.

Precursor B-cell acute lymphoblastic leukaemia

The background of normal terminal deoxynucleotidyl transferase-positive (TdT$^+$) and/or CD10$^+$ precursor B-cells in bone marrow (BM) (generally <10% of mononuclear cells) and peripheral blood (PB) (generally <0.4% of mononuclear cells) hampers the detection of MRD in precursor B-ALL patients by use of CD10/TdT double staining [8,17,18]. In bone marrow regenerating after chemotherapy or bone-marrow transplantation, the levels of normal TdT$^+$ precursor B-cells further increase and can even reach levels as high as 50% of mononuclear cells [8,19]. Nevertheless, a strong correlation was recently found between persisting increased percentages of CD10$^+$/CD19$^+$ and CD20$^-$/CD22$^+$ fractions of CD34$^+$

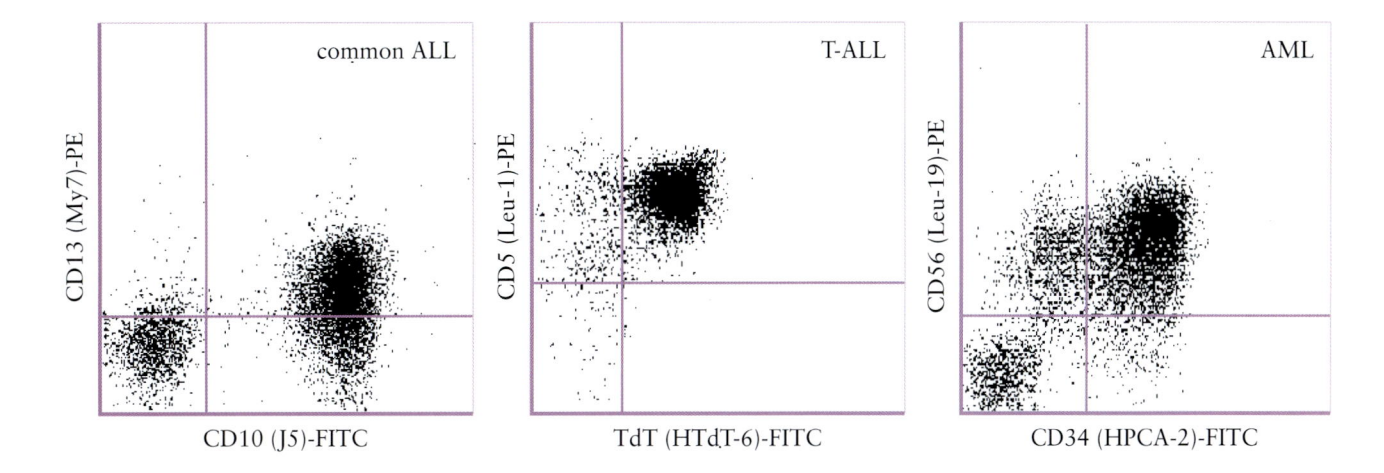

Figure 41.2 Examples of leukaemia-associated immunophenotypes in acute leukaemia. (Left) Weak cross-lineage CD13 expression in a patient with common-ALL. (Middle) Ectopic co-expression of the CD5 antigen and TdT, a typical characteristic of T-ALL, which is normally only found in the cortical thymus and not in extrathymic locations such as blood or bone marrow. (Right) Asynchronous expression of CD34 and CD56 in an AML patient.

cells in bone marrow and increased likelihood of relapse [20]. However, clinical importance of these findings and precise definition of clinically significant cut-off points for the subsets requires evaluation in future studies.

Several types of unusual or aberrant antigen expression are found in precursor B-ALL (Table 41.1). This mainly concerns cross-lineage expression of T-cell antigens (e.g. CD5 and CD7) or myeloid antigens (e.g. CD13, CD33 and CDw65), maturational asynchronic expression of antigens (e.g. expression of CD20 in CD45-negative blast cells, expression of CD21 in $CD10^+/TdT^+$ blasts) and antigen overexpression (especially the CD10 antigen) [21,22]. Such leukaemia-associated immunophenotypes are found in 70–80% of precursor B-ALL, but are generally restricted to a single unusual or aberrant antigen (Table 41.1). Recent studies indicate that ectopic surface membrane expression of chondroitin sulphate proteoglycan NG2 is found in precursor B-ALL with t(4;11) and t(11;19) [23]. This ectopic NG2 expression probably represents a true leukaemia characteristic, because it is not found in normal blood or bone-marrow cells [24]. Preliminary results of prospective clinical MRD studies using leukaemia-specific antigen combinations indicate that induction of morphological complete remission is frequently associated with persistence of immunologically detectable malignant blasts [11,25]. High precursor B-cell counts at disease presentation are particularly correlated with higher levels of MRD at the end of induction treatment. The presence of MRD during maintenance therapy or off treatment is uniformly associated with impending relapse. Some false-negative results have been observed due to immunophenotypic shifts at the time of relapse [11,25].

T-cell acute lymphoblastic leukaemia

Nearly all T-ALLs express TdT as well as the pan-T-cell antigens CD2, cytoplasmic CD3 (CyCD3), CD5 and CD7. Many of them express additional T-cell antigens such as CD1a, CD3, CD4 and/or CD8. In healthy individuals the T-cell antigen$^+$/TdT$^+$ immunophenotype is expressed by most cortical thymocytes, but in extrathymic locations such cells are absent or rare (<0.3% of mononuclear cells in BM and <0.02% in PB). If they occur, they generally only express the CD2 and/or CD7 antigens, but no other T-cell antigens such as CD1a, CD3, CD4 or CD8. Dilution experiments have demonstrated that the microscopic T-cell antigen/TdT double-labelling technique has a detection limit of 10^{-4} to 10^{-5} [8]. A prospective study on 35 T-ALL patients revealed that microscopic detection of 'ectopic' T-cell antigen$^+$/TdT$^+$ cells in BM and PB can indeed be used for evaluation of the effectiveness of the cytostatic treatment used [9]. Although T-ALL is frequently hyperleukocytic at presentation, there is probably no correlation between MRD levels at the end of induction treatment and initial white blood cell count (WBC). This observation is in agreement with the lack of prognostic value of the initial blast count in T-ALL patients [11,25].

In principle, the T-cell antigen/TdT double-labelling technique can also be performed by flow cytometry in

Table 41.1 Leukaemia-associated immunophenotypes in acute leukaemia.

Leukaemia-associated phenotype	Precursor B-ALL (%)	T-ALL (%)	AML (%)
Cross-lineage antigen expression	~50	~50	~70
Asynchronous antigen expression	~10	~25	~40
Overexpression or absence of antigen	~30	0	~15
Ectopic phenotype	~5*	~90	~10*
Total	70–80	90–100	70–80

*Based on ectopic NG2 expression in acute leukaemias with 11q23 translocations [23,24].

~90% of T-ALLs (Figure 41.2). Furthermore, cross-lineage antigen expression, asynchronous antigen expression and ectopic CD1 expression can be used for flow cytometric MRD detection in a proportion of T-ALL patients (Table 41.1).

Acute myeloid leukaemia

Cross-lineage antigen expression is found in approximately 70% of AMLs. This especially concerns TdT expression as well as expression of the T-cell antigens CD2 and CD7 and the B-cell antigen CD19. Also, maturational asynchronic antigen expression can be found in AML, for example, co-expression of CD15 and CD34, CD56 and CD34, and CD15 with CD117, combinations which are not seen in normal bone marrow [14,26–28]. Aberrant antigen overexpression can concern CD13, CD14 and CD34. Comparable to ALL with 11q23 translocations, in AML with 11q23 abnormalities, ectopic NG2 expression is also found, which probably represents an excellent leukaemia marker [24]. In the majority of AMLs, immunophenotypic subpopulations can be identified, in contrast to most ALLs. This also applies to the cross-lineage and asynchronic antigen expression.

Microscopic myeloid antigen/TdT double labelling was demonstrated to be useful for monitoring the effectiveness of treatment in TdT$^+$ AML patients, especially if TdT positivity at diagnosis encompassed more than 1% (preferably >10%) of the leukaemic cells; this is seen in around 60% of AML patients [29]. The preliminary results of MRD monitoring in AML patients after BMT demonstrated an unequivocal association between the detection of immunophenotypically abnormal cells and subsequent relapse. Furthermore, in AML patients subjected to autologous BMT, detection of leukaemia-specific phenotypes in harvested bone marrow was associated with treatment failure due to relapse [25].

Multiparameter flow cytometric detection of unusual or aberrant immunophenotypes can potentially be used for MRD detection in 70–80% of AML (Table 41.1). The detection limit of such multiparameter analyses is dependent upon the normal flow cytometric background and is estimated to be 10^{-3} to 10^{-4}, dependent on the type of triple labelling. In this context it should also be noted that immunophenotypic MRD studies in AML are hampered by the fact that generally only one subpopulation of the AML blast cells is monitored [29]. However, in most AMLs, multiple aberrant marker combinations can be used for MRD monitoring and no major changes of the aberrant immunophenotypes are found in AML at relapse [30].

Immunological MRD detection in cerebrospinal fluid

Despite the relatively low incidence of central nervous system (CNS) involvement as demonstrated by the presence of morphologically distinct blasts and/or increased cerebrospinal fluid (CSF) pleocytosis (>5 cells/ml), introduction of preventive therapy for CNS leukaemia was one of the most important improvements in treatment of leukaemia [31,32]. This indicates potential, subclinical, asymptomatic CNS involvement in the majority of leukaemia patients.

Normal CSF does not contain TdT$^+$ progenitor cells. They are apparently unable to migrate through the normal blood–brain barrier. The presence of TdT$^+$ cells in CSF (without PB contamination) at diagnosis is a high-risk factor for the development of CNS leukaemia [33].

MRD detection by use of PCR techniques

Amplification of a short DNA fragment or mRNA by use of PCR methodology allows the detection of low frequencies of malignant cells if the target DNA or mRNA sequences are tumour-specific. Two types of PCR targets have been widely used for MRD detection in leukaemia patients: junctional regions of rearranged immunoglobulin (Ig) and T-cell receptor (TCR) genes and breakpoint fusion regions of chromosome aberrations. Recently, increased levels of Wilms tumour (WT1) gene transcription were found to be another promising MRD target [34].

The theoretical detection limit of the PCR technique is approximately 10^{-6} if a DNA segment is used as a PCR target. This is based on the assumption that one cell contains around 10 pg DNA and that one PCR tube can maximally contain 10 μg DNA. Although this detection limit can indeed be reached, it generally varies between 10^{-3} and 10^{-6}, depending on the type of tumour-specific PCR target. Because of the extremely high sensitivity of PCR techniques, all possible precautions should be taken to prevent cross-contamination of PCR products between patient samples in PCR-mediated MRD studies.

Quantification of MRD by use of the PCR technique is difficult, because of the biphasic kinetics of amplification with an exponential phase followed by a plateau. Furthermore, minor variations in reverse transcription (RT) efficiency, annealing of primers, and primer extension processes can lead to major variations after 30–35 PCR cycles. These problems can be overcome when limiting dilution of the target DNA is performed. This is a very laborious procedure, but results in an accurate estimation of the tumour load [35]. Alternatively, the use of serial dilutions of DNA or RNA from the leukaemic cell sample at diagnosis in normal mononuclear cells DNA and the use of internal (co-amplified) controls generally allow a reasonable, at least semiquantitative, estimation of MRD levels. Nevertheless, it will be difficult to reach the accuracy of MRD detection obtained with immunophenotyping [36].

Junctional regions as PCR targets for MRD detection

Deletion and insertion of nucleotides during gene-rearrangement processes turn junctional regions of rearranged Ig and TCR genes into unique 'fingerprint-like' sequences, which are assumed to be different in each lymphocyte and thus also in each lymphoid leukaemia. Therefore, junctional regions can be used as leukaemia-patient-specific targets for MRD–PCR analysis, using primers at opposite sides. For this purpose the various Ig and/or TCR gene rearrangements should be identified in each leukaemia at initial diagnosis. One strategy, so-called 'gene fingerprinting' is based on analysis of the exact size of the monoclonal PCR product at presentation. Overrepresentation of PCR products of this size on the background of normal polyclonal PCR products during follow-up is consistent with persistence of MRD. This approach has a sensitivity between 10^{-3} and 10^{-4} [37,38]. Automated fluorescent, high-resolution PCR fragment analysis, so-called 'gene scanning', is an improved automated version of gene fingerprinting and is currently being evaluated for application in MRD monitoring [39,40].

The alternative, and certainly more sensitive approach, is to determine the precise nucleotide sequence of the junctional regions of the Ig and TCR gene rearrangements and to design junctional region-specific oligonucleotides, which can be used as patient-specific probes (or primers) for MRD detection during follow-up of the leukaemia patients.

In virtually all precursor B-ALL it is possible to find rearranged Ig heavy-chain (*IGH*) genes, and in most cases (80–90%) this concerns complete V$_H$–D$_H$–J$_H$ rearrangements on at least one allele. Ig kappa light chain (*IGK*) and Ig lambda light chain (*IGL*) gene rearrangements were found to occur in 60% and 20% of precursor B-ALL, respectively [41,42]. The vast majority (80%) of all *IGK* gene rearrangements in precursor B-ALL appear to represent so-called 'deletional rearrangements', i.e. deletions of the Cκ and/or Jκ-Cκ gene segments via rearrangement of the kappa-deleting element (Kde) [41]. Kde rearrangements occur in at least 50% of precursor B-ALL patients (Table 41.2).

TCR gene rearrangements occur at high frequencies in the total group of ALLs. Virtually all T-ALLs have rearranged TCR beta (*TCRB*), TCR gamma (*TCRG*), and/or TCR delta (*TCRD*) genes, while cross-lineage TCR gene rearrangements are found in most precursor B-ALLs (Table 41.2).

Junctional regions of *IGH*, *IGK* (especially Kde), *TCRG* and *TCRD* gene rearrangements are convenient MRD–PCR targets, because they require only a limited number of PCR primer sets. The vast majority (90%) of precursor B-ALL patients can be monitored by application of junctional regions of *IGH*, *IGK*, *TCRG* and/or *TCRD* gene rearrangements. In virtually all T-ALLs (95%) *TCRG* and/or *TCRD* junctional regions are good targets for MRD monitoring (Table 41.3).

Pitfalls of MRD detection by PCR analysis of junctional regions
Type of rearrangement and background of normal cells

The detection limit of the MRD–PCR technique is related to the size of the junctional region (i.e. the number of random deletions and insertions) and the background of normal cells with comparable Ig or TCR gene rearrangements. Junctional regions of complete V$_H$–D$_H$–J$_H$ and Vδ–Dδ–Jδ rearrangements or incomplete Dδ–Jδ rearrangements are extensive (mean of 20–30 nucleotides), whereas junctional regions of complete Vγ–Jγ and incomplete Vδ–Dδ and Dδ–Dδ

Table 41.2 Frequencies of Ig and TCR gene rearrangements and deletions in precursor-B-ALL and T-ALL*

	IGH (%)		IGK (%)**		IGL (%)	TCRB (%)	TCRG (%)	TCRD (%)	
	R	D	R	D	R	R	R	R	D
Precursor-B-ALL (n = 110)	96	3	30	30	20	36	57	50	40
T-ALL (n = 150)	20	0	0	0	0	90	93	70	25
Total ALL***	83	2	26	17	17	45	62	53	37

*Van Dongen et al., unpublished results. R = one or both alleles rearranged; D = both alleles deleted or one allele deleted with the other in germline configuration.
**Kde rearrangements are found in ~50% of precursor B-ALL [41].
***Calculated percentages, based on the fact that precursor B-ALL and T-ALL represent 80–85% and 15–20% of childhood ALL, respectively.

Table 41.3 Junctional regions of Ig or TCR genes as major PCR targets for MRD detection in acute leukaemias*

Gene	Rearrangement	Frequency of applicability (%)**	
		Precursor B-ALL	T-ALL
IGH	VH–DH–JH	80–90	NT***
IGK	Kde rearrangement	~50	0
TCRG	Vγ–Jγ	~55	~90
TCRD	Vδ2–Dδ3	~35	~5
	Dδ2–Dδ3	~5	~5
	Vδ1–Jδ1	0	~37
	Vδ2–Jδ1	0	~11
	Vδ3–Jδ1	0	~7
	Dδ2–Jδ1	0	~12
	All TCRD targets	~40	~52
At least one target		~95	>98
At least two targets		~90	~95
At least three targets		~65	~60

*The detection limit of PCR analysis of junctional regions of rearranged Ig and TCR genes varies from 10^{-3} to 10^{-6} and is dependent on normal background and the size of the junctional region.
**The indicated percentages represent frequencies within the different leukaemias.
***NT = not tested.

rearrangements are three to four times smaller (mean of 5–7 nucleotides) [9,43]. Incomplete *TCRD* gene rearrangements with short junctional regions are especially characteristic for precursor B-ALL, i.e. Vδ2–Dδ3 and Dδ2–Dδ3 (Table 41.3 and Figure 41.3). Normal cells can contain the same rearranged gene segments as the leukaemic cells. For instance Vδ1–Jδ1 rearrangements frequently occur in T-ALL, but also occur in a small fraction (0.1–3%) of normal blood T-cells. VγI–Jγ1.3 and VγI–Jγ2.3 rearrangements occur in both precursor B-ALL and T-ALL, but are also found in a large part of normal blood T-cells. Therefore, it is obvious that MRD–PCR analyses of long Vδ1–Jδ1 junctional regions in general will be more sensitive than MRD–PCR analyses of short Vγ–Jγ junctional regions [9] (Figure 41.4).

Subclone formation and clonal evolution

A prerequisite for the MRD–PCR technique is the stability of the PCR targets during the disease course in order to prevent false-negative MRD results. However, in 30–40% of precursor B-ALL, multiple *IGH* gene rearrangements are found at diagnosis [44]. They are caused by continuing rearrangements and secondary

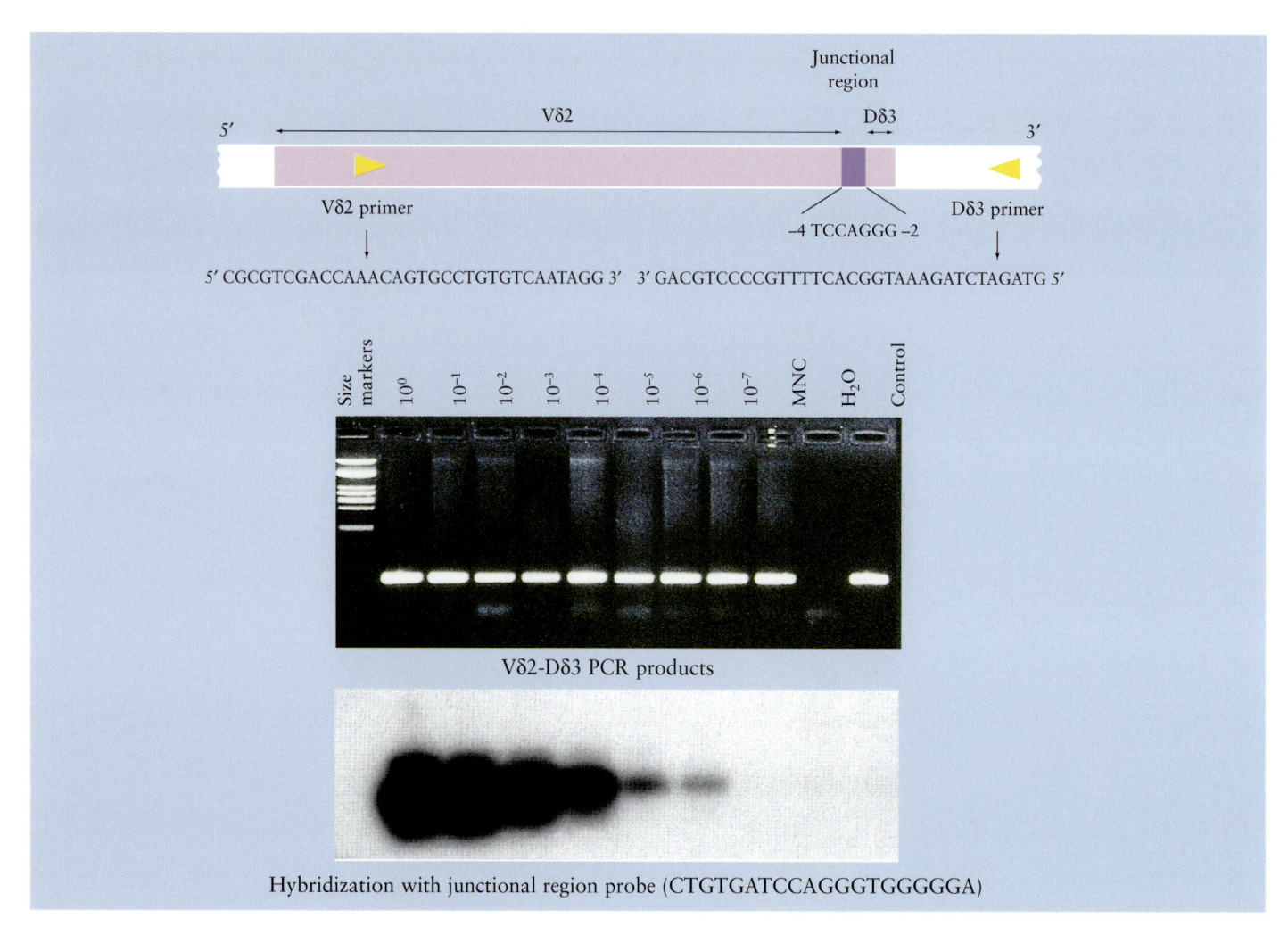

Figure 41.3 Precursor B-ALL patient with a Vδ2–Dδ3 rearrangement as PCR target for MRD detection. The specificity of the junctional region is based on the deletion of six nucleotides and the random insertion of seven nucleotides. This sequence information was used for the design of a patient-specific junctional region probe. DNA from the ALL cells was diluted into DNA from normal mononuclear blood cells (MNC) and subjected to PCR analysis with Vδ2 and Dδ3 primers, followed by size separation of the PCR products in an agarose gel, blotting onto a nylon membrane, and hybridization with the junctional region probe. In all dilution steps and in the MNC, Vδ2–Dδ3 PCR products were found, but only the first five dilution steps appeared to contain leukaemia-derived PCR products, i.e. a sensitivity of 10^{-5} was reached.

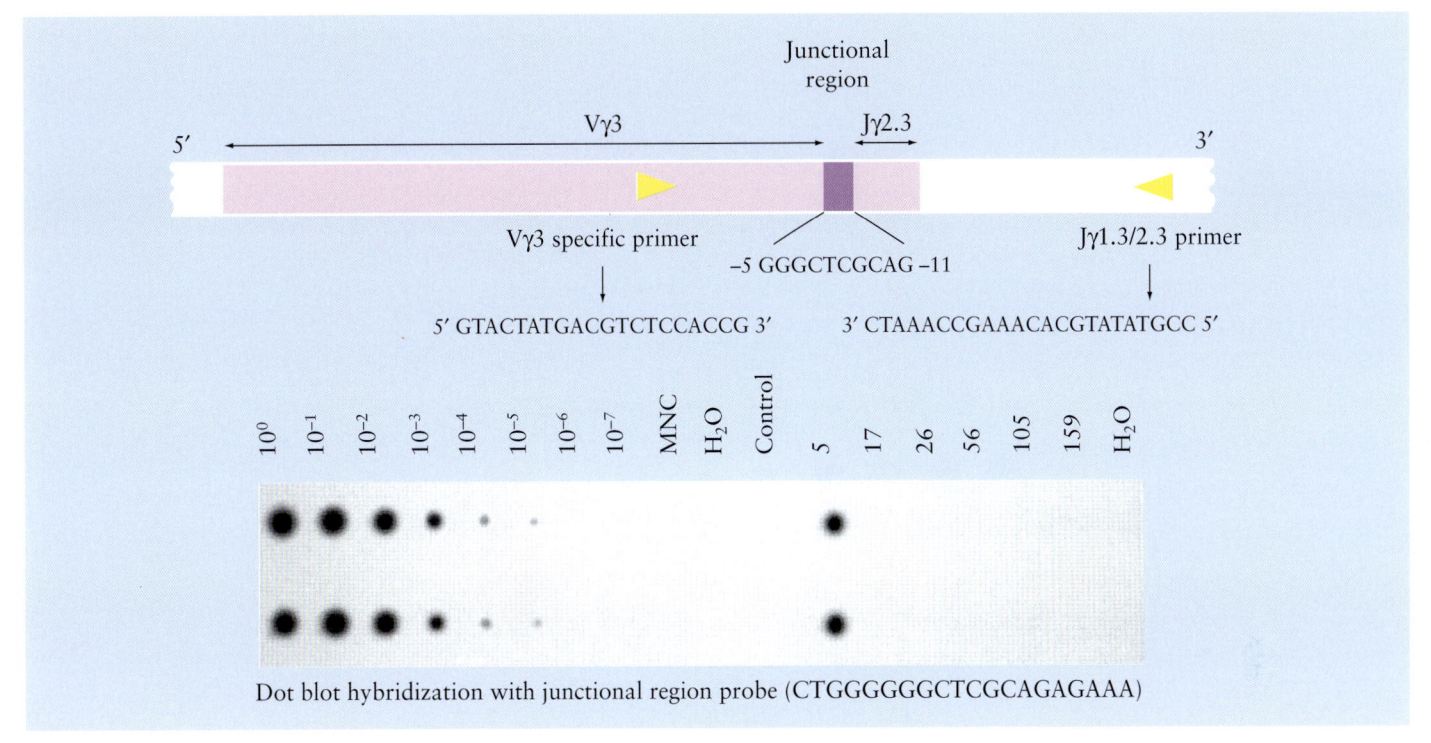

Figure 41.4 A Vγ3–Jγ2.3 rearrangement was used as MRD target to monitor a precursor B-ALL. The patient-specific probe was designed according to the junctional region sequence with a deletion of 16 nucleotides and insertion of 10 nucleotides. Tenfold dilutions were made of DNA from the leukaemic cells into DNA from MNC. PCR analysis with Vγ3 and Jγ1.3/2.3 primers was performed on the dilution samples and DNA samples from bone marrow during follow-up. The PCR products were blotted in duplicate on a nylon membrane and hybridized with the junctional region probe. The positive control for amplification of the Vγ3–Jγ2.3 rearrangement is not recognized by the patient-specific probe. The time points of the follow-up samples at the right side of the blot are given in weeks. The sensitivity of the MRD–PCR targets was 10^{-4}. The week 5 follow-up sample (end of induction therapy) was found positive and the tumour load was estimated to be 10^{-2}, based on comparison of the signal with that of the diluted DNA from diagnosis.

rearrangements which lead to subclone formation (bi-/oligoclonality). Such subclone formation at diagnosis is less frequent at the *TCRG* and *TCRD* gene level in T-ALL and Kde rearrangements in precursor B-ALL [45,46].

As a consequence of the subclone formation processes, changes in Ig and TCR gene-rearrangement patterns at relapse represent an important pitfall in MRD–PCR analysis of junctional regions. Changes in *IGH* gene-rearrangement patterns at relapse occur at high frequency in precursor B-ALL, especially when subclone formation is already present at diagnosis [45]. Most changes can be attributed to continuing rearrangements and secondary rearrangements, such as VH to D–JH rearrangements and VH replacements, respectively. One possibility for preventing false-negative results is to design D–N–J specific probes or primers, which remain unchanged during VH replacements and are independent of VH to D–J rearrangements [47–50].

Changes in *TCRG* and *TCRD* gene rearrangements at relapse are found in both precursor B-ALL and T-ALL, but generally concern only one allele [45]. In precursor B-ALL, changes in Vδ2–Dδ3 were found in at least 25% of cases, mostly because of continuing Vδ–Dδ to Jα rearrangements [50,51]. Preliminary results of MRD monitoring using Kde rearrangements describe rarely occurring clonal evolution; we found that in 16 out of 17 childhood ALL patients, the Kde rearrangments determined at diagnosis remained identical at relapse [52]. Nevertheless, it appears that the recombinase enzyme system remains continuously active in most ALLs. This is in line with the finding that the chance of changes in rearrangement patterns appears to increase with time (i.e. with remission duration) [45]. However, in patients with recurrence of disease, further clonal evolution is usually not observed from first relapse onwards [53]. Despite the high frequency of immunogenotypic changes in ALL at

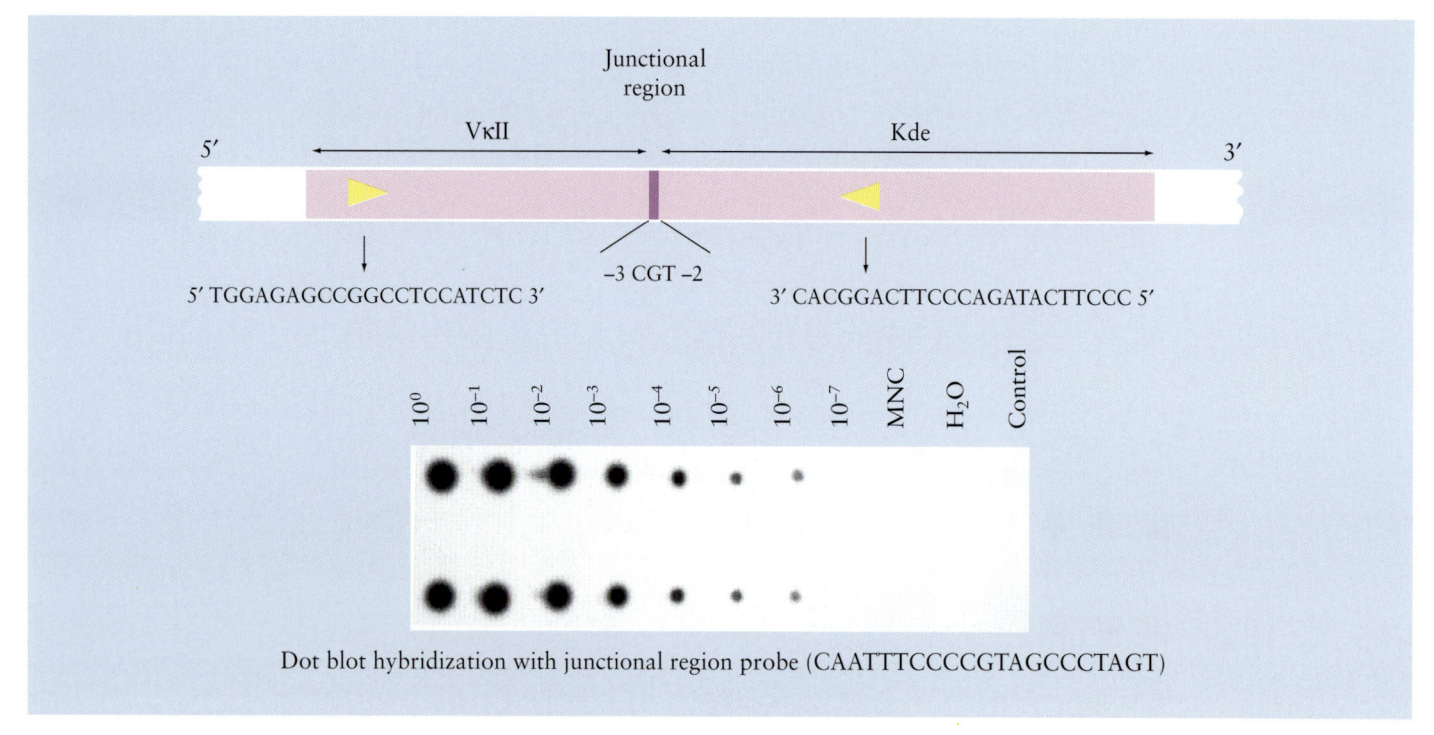

Figure 41.5 A sensitive IGK target for MRD monitoring is shown. DNA from a precursor B-ALL patient at diagnosis was diluted into MNC–DNA and PCR analysis performed with VκII and Kde primers. PCR products were dot blotted in duplicate and hybridized with the patient-specific probe. The VκII–Kde junctional region with only minor deletion and insertion reached a high sensitivity of 10^{-6}. Techniques and symbols are as described in Figure 41.4.

relapse, it was shown that at least one rearranged *IGH*, *TCRG* and/or *TCRD* allele remains stable in 90% of T-ALLs, in 90% of precursor B-ALL with monoclonal *IGH* genotype, and in 75% of precursor B-ALL with biclonal/oligoclonal *IGH* genotype at diagnosis [45]. These data indicate that MRD detection in ALL patients requires monitoring of two or more junctional regions of *IGH*, *TCRG* and/or *TCRD* genes in order to avoid false-negative results [45,46,48,50,53–55]. The application of Kde rearrangements may also be an important additional PCR target (Figure 41.5).

Preliminary results of clinical MRD studies in ALL using junctional regions as PCR targets

MRD studies using junctional regions as PCR targets mostly focused on childhood ALL patients. To date, several retrospective and some limited prospective studies in ALL patients have been published. Although the results of these clinical studies are not fully concordant, some preliminary conclusions can be drawn concerning the clinical value of MRD detection in ALL [35,53,56–70].

- Good clinical response to steroids with blast count in PB less than 1000 per μl after a week of single-agent steroid therapy, or absence of circulating blasts after 7 days of multi-agent induction chemotherapy were found to be important prognostic factors. As a logical continuation of clinical findings, low levels or absence of MRD after completion of induction therapy seems to predict good outcome. The level of PCR positivity after induction therapy seems to be an informative prognostic factor, independent of other clinically relevant risk factors.
- Steady decrease of MRD levels to negative PCR results during treatment is associated with favourable prognosis.
- Persistence of high MRD levels or steady increase of MRD levels generally leads to clinical relapse. In fact, PCR–MRD monitoring was shown to be effective for selecting the group of poor responders to chemotherapy with early relapse during maintenance treatment.
- Persisting MRD levels during treatment appear to be the best indicator of multidrug resistance.

- Low levels of MRD after therapy might be associated with development of late relapse.
- Absence of MRD at the end of treatment does not exclude recurrence of the disease.
- Sequential sampling generally shows positive MRD–PCR results prior to clinical relapse, unless false-negative results are obtained due to continuing or secondary rearrangements.
- 'Isolated' extramedullary relapse is usually associated with detectable MRD levels in bone marrow. This is in concordance with the clinical observation of the necessity for full systemic re-induction with chemotherapy in these patients to prevent impending haematological relapse. Nevertheless, some cases of isolated CNS relapse have been reported without detectable bone-marrow MRD.

These MRD–PCR results are in line with the immunophenotypic MRD results in T-ALL patients [9]. The emerging clinical application of autologous peripheral blood stem-cell transplantation following intensified chemotherapy requires careful control of the autologous graft for contamination with malignant cells. Detection of MRD in harvested graft material is associated with an increased risk of relapse following autologous transplantation [70].

Incomplete *TCRD* rearrangements have also been used in a pilot study as an MRD target for detection of CNS involvement in childhood precursor B-ALL. Identical rearrangements were found in BM and CSF in 43% of patients, which confirms the clinical assumption of much more frequent CNS involvement than diagnosed on the basis of morphological findings [71].

It can be expected that with the sensitive PCR assays presently available, residual leukaemic cells will be demonstrated in the majority of the patients at the end of induction therapy, but during further maintenance treatment PCR negativity will be reached in most patients. This stresses the importance of accurate quantitation of leukaemic cells during follow-up. By following the kinetics of the disappearance of leukaemic cells, especially during early phases of chemotherapy, it might be possible to recognize patients who do not optimally respond to therapy and therefore might have a higher chance of relapse.

In contrast to childhood ALL, adult ALL is characterized by a less favourable prognosis (cure rates of 20–35%) [72]. This is, on the one hand, explained by increased frequencies of high-risk features (age, high white blood cell count, high frequency of t(9;22) translocation, higher frequency of T-cell phenotype, etc.) and on the other hand by poorer treatment tolerance [73]. At present it is not known whether immunogenetics of adult ALL can explain the different immunobiology in comparison to childhood ALL. The preliminary results of MRD studies in adult ALL using junctional regions as MRD–PCR targets showed molecular response to chemotherapy to be similar to childhood ALL with higher frequencies of persistent MRD positivity in adults [74]. The levels of MRD in adult patients were, however, significantly higher than in comparably treated children. This points towards greater drug resistance in adult ALL, which has already been shown in studies on methotrexate metabolism [73,75].

Chromosome aberrations as PCR targets for MRD detection

In the first MRD–PCR studies, chromosome aberrations were used as PCR targets. For this purpose the oligonucleotide primers were designed at opposite sides of the breakpoint fusion region so that the PCR product contained the tumour-specific fusion sequences. In routinely performed MRD–PCR analysis, the PCR products should not exceed ~2 kb. Therefore, PCR-mediated amplification can only be used for chromosome aberrations in which the breakpoints of different malignancies cluster in a small area (total breakpoint area: preferably <2 kb), such as T-ALL-associated aberrations t(11;14)(p13;q11), t(1;14)(p34;q11), t(10;14)(q24;q11), where partner genes are juxtaposed to one of the segments of the *TCRA/D* locus, and the *TAL1* deletion. These translocations result from aberrant rearrangement processes and are comparable to the junctional regions of Ig and TCR genes in that the fusion regions of the breakpoints in these chromosome aberrations show deletion and random insertion of nucleotides. This implies that the fusion regions are different in each patient and therefore represent excellent patient-specific MRD–PCR targets [76–78].

In most translocations, the main consequence of fusion genes is subsequent synthesis of a chimaeric protein. The breakpoints are usually located in intronic DNA and spread over much larger areas than 2 kb.

Table 41.4 Chromosome aberrations as major PCR targets for MRD detection in acute leukaemias*

Aberration	Target (mRNA or DNA)	Frequency of applicability (%)**	
		Children	Adults
Precursor-B-ALL			
t(9;22)(q34;q11)	*BCR-ABL* (mRNA)	5–8	30–35
t(1;19)(q23;p13)	*E2A-PBX1* (mRNA)	5–8	<5
t(4;11)(q21;q23)	*MLL-AF4* (mRNA)	3c***	3–6
t(12;21)(p13;q22)	*TEL-AML1* (mRNA)	~30	1–3
T-ALL			
TAL1 deletion	*SIL-TAL1* (DNA)	10–25	
t(11;14)(p13;q11)	*RHOM2-TCRD* (DNA)	3–7	
t(1;14)(p34;q11)	*TAL1-TCRD* (DNA)	1–3	
t(10;14)(q24;q11)	*HOX11-TCRD* (DNA)	1–3	
AML			
t(8;21)(q22;q22)	*AML1-ETO* (mRNA)	5–8	
t(15;17)(q23;q21)	*PML-RARA* (mRNA)	5–10	
inv(16)(p13q22)	*CBFB-MYH11* (mRNA)	3–5	
11q23 aberrations	aberrant *MLL* (mRNA)	8–10	
t(9;22)(q34;q11)	*BCR-ABL* (mRNA)	1–3	

*The detection limit of PCR analysis of chromosome aberrations varies between 10^{-3} to 10^{-5}.
**The indicated percentages represent frequencies within the precursor B-ALL, T-ALL and AML groups.
***In infants the frequency of t(4;11) is ~60%.

This implies that the precise breakpoint recombination area has to be determined for each individual patient, which is laborious and time-consuming. However, a leukaemia-specific fusion mRNA, which is transcribed from a new leukaemia-specific fusion gene can be used as target for the MRD–PCR analysis after RT into cDNA. Examples are: *BCR-ABL* mRNA in cases with t(9;22), *E2A-PBX1* mRNA in most pre-B-ALL with t(1;19), *MLL/AF4* mRNA in null ALL with t(4;11), *TEL-AML1* mRNA in precursor B-ALL with t(12;21), *AML1-ETO* in AML with t(8;21) and *PML-RARA* in AML-M3 with t(15;17), *CBFB-MYH11* in AML-M4E0 with inv(16) [79–88] (Table 41.4).

An advantage of using specific chromosome translocations as tumour-specific markers is their stability during the disease course. However, only 20–40% of acute leukaemias have a specific, microscopically detectable chromosome aberration and in a proportion of these aberrations, the precise breakpoints are not yet known.

Pitfalls of MRD detection by RT-PCR of chromosome aberrations

In contrast to PCR products obtained from breakpoint fusion regions resulting from abnormal recombination processes (as in the *TAL1* deletion), RT-PCR products obtained from leukaemia-specific fusion mRNA are not patient-specific. Therefore, false-positive results due to cross-contamination of RT-PCR products between samples from different patients are difficult to recognize. Furthermore, very low levels of *BCR-ABL* mRNA have also been found in healthy individuals [89]. Finally, improper isolation of RNA may lead to false-negative results. All of these pitfalls should be considered before introducing the relatively easy RT-PCR technology into routine diagnostics.

Preliminary results of MRD studies in ALL using RT-PCR of chromosomal aberrations

The first studies on MRD detection in ALL based on RT-PCR concerned ALL with t(9;22). Long-term disease-free survival after intensive chemotherapy and/or bone-marrow transplantation was observed after eradication of clonogenic cells below the level of RT-PCR detectability [90–92]. However, due to the poor prognoses of ALL with t(9;22) and the very low frequency of complete cure, the above-mentioned results should be confirmed by large multicentre studies. The requirement of RT-PCR negativity as a *sine qua non* for cure was found in preliminary studies on MRD in ALL with t(4;11) and t(1;19) [93,94].

Recently, a new translocation has been described t(12;21) involving the *TEL* and *AML1* genes; this is the most frequently occurring recurrent abnormality in paediatric ALL [87]. The presence of this translocation is associated with a very good prognosis [86]. Preliminary results of MRD studies based on RT-PCR analysis of *TEL-AML1* transcripts suggest that the levels of MRD at the end of induction are below the threshold associated with a poor outcome [95,96].

MRD studies in AML using chromosomal translocations as RT-PCR targets

The best documented MRD studies in AML concern the monitoring of *PML-RARA* fusion mRNA in AML-M3 patients with t(15;17) and *AML1-ETO* fusion mRNA in AML-M2 patients with t(8;21).

The RT-PCR studies [82,97–107] in AML-M3 patients show that:

- PCR results are always positive at one month after diagnosis, probably due to remaining mature leukaemic cells; this finding did not correlate with outcome;
- treatment with all-*trans*-retinoic acid (ATRA) alone never eliminates all leukaemic cells;
- rapid loss of MRD–PCR positivity during the first three months of treatment correlates well with good outcome, whereas continuous positivity is associated with relapse;
- PCR negativity after completion of the treatment does not exclude relapse. Reappearance of detectable MRD usually precedes haematological relapse by two to three months. This is a much more sensitive predictive factor in comparison to the routinely used coagulation parameters;
- patients in long-term remission after chemotherapy or bone-marrow transplantation do not have detectable levels of MRD;
- patients with refractory AML-M3 are MRD positive even at the end of treatment intensification;
- peripheral blood stem-cell grafts with MRD positivity carry increased risk of subsequent relapse of disease.

The clinical value of the MRD–PCR studies in AML patients with t(8;21) is less certain. Several studies indicate that *AML1-ETO* fusion mRNA remains detectable in blood and bone marrow of patients in long-term remission after chemotherapy or allogeneic/autologous bone-marrow transplantation. It is not clear whether the detectability of *AML1-ETO* mRNA in these patients implies that the aberrant fusion protein is expressed and whether this is equivalent to the presence of clonogenic leukaemic cells [82,108–112]. However, a recent study reported disappearance of *AML1-ETO* mRNA in long-term survivors of leukaemia in complete remission over ten years [113].

Conclusion

Advanced diagnostic methods seem to have overcome the limitations of cytomorphology in follow-up of acute leukaemia patients. The use of double and triple immunolabelling techniques by flow cytometry permits the detection of uncommon or aberrant immunophenotypes at levels ranging from 10^{-3} to 10^{-5}. The PCR techniques allow detection of unique junctional regions of rearranged Ig and TCR genes (at the DNA level) and fusion regions of chromosome aberrations (at the DNA or mRNA/cDNA level) with detection limits from 10^{-3} to 10^{-6} [7,9,78].

In ALL and AML, immunophenotyping techniques as well as PCR analysis can be used for MRD detection (Table 41.5). Multiple MRD techniques can be used especially in the T-ALL group. Each MRD technique has its advantages and limitations, which have to be weighed carefully to make an appropriate choice [76].

Prospective multicentre studies on PCR-based MRD monitoring will hopefully answer several important questions:

1. Which techniques for MRD monitoring will be most suitable for each leukaemia subtype?
2. Is a sensitivity between 10^{-3} and 10^{-4} sufficient to obtain predictive information from MRD analysis?
3. Can MRD analysis be restricted to a single time point or a short time interval, or is prolonged sequential bone-marrow sampling required?

Table 41.5 Applicability of MRD techniques in acute leukaemias*

Types of acute leukaemia	Immunophenotyping Flow cytometry	PCR analysis Junctional regions of Ig/TCR genes	Chromosome aberrations
Precursor B-ALL	~80%	~90%	30–35% (childhood) 40–45% (adults)
T-ALL	>90%	~95%	10–25%
AML	~80%	~10%	25–40%

*The percentages indicate the applicability for MRD detection within each leukaemia group.

4. Will it be possible to restrict the MRD monitoring to blood samples or do we need to continue bone-marrow aspirations?

Despite the sensitivity of the MRD techniques, it should be realized that MRD negativity does not exclude the presence of leukaemic cells, because each MRD test only screens 10^5 to 10^6 cells, which represent a minor fraction of all BM and PB leukocytes in an individual. In addition, it might well be that the distribution of low numbers of leukaemic cells throughout the BM compartment is not homogeneous [114].

Finally, the clinical impact of MRD detection for the various subtypes of acute leukaemias is not fully established. The available data clearly indicate that the meaning of MRD positivity in ALL and AML-M3 is different from that in AML with t(8;21). However, the current prospective studies have to demonstrate the value of MRD detection for treatment of ALL and most AML patients, i.e. whether MRD information can be used for improved definition of remission and relapse criteria as well as for stratification of treatment protocols.

References

1. Rivera GK, Pinkel D, Simone JV, Hancock ML and Crist WM. Treatment of acute lymphoblastic leukemia. 30 years' experience at St Jude Children's Research Hospital. *New Engl J Med* 1993; **329**: 1289–1295.
2. Pui C-H, Relling MV, Rivera GK et al. Epipodophyllotoxin-related acute myeloid leukemia: a study of 35 cases. *Leukaemia* 1995; **9**: 1990–1996.
3. Van Dongen JJM and Wolvers-Tettero ILM. Analysis of immunoglobulin and T cell receptor genes. Part II. Possibilities and limitations in the diagnosis and management of lymphoproliferative diseases and related disorders. *Clin Chim Acta* 1991; **198**: 93–174.
4. Freireich EJ, Cork A, Stass SA et al. Cytogenetics for detection of minimal residual disease in acute myeloblastic leukemia. *Leukaemia* 1992; **6**: 500–506.
5. Heerema NA, Argyropoulos G, Weetman R, Tricot G and Secker-Walker LM. Interphase *in situ* hybridization reveals minimal residual disease in early remission and return of the diagnostic clone in karyotypically normal relapse of acute lymphoblastic leukemia. *Leukaemia* 1993; **7**: 537–543.
6. Nylund SJ, Ruutu T, Saarinen U, Larramendy ML and Knuutila S. Detection of minimal residual disease using fluorescence DNA *in situ* hybridization: a follow-up study in leukemia and lymphoma patients. *Leukaemia* 1994; **8**: 587–594.
7. Van Dongen JJM, Szczepanski T, de Bruijn MAC et al. Detection of minimal residual disease in acute leukemia patients. *Cytokines Molecular Therapy* 1996; **2**: 121–133.
8. Van Dongen JJM, Hooijkaas H, Adriaansen HJ, Hählen K and Van Zanen GE. Detection of minimal residual acute lymphoblastic leukemia by immunological marker analysis: Possibilities and limitations. In: *Minimal Residual Disease in Acute Leukemia*. A Hagenbeek and B Löwenberg (eds), 1986: 113–133 (Dordrecht: Nijhoff).
9. Van Dongen JJM, Breit TM, Adriaansen HJ, Beishuizen A and Hooijkaas H. Detection of minimal residual disease in acute leukemia by immunological marker analysis and polymerase chain reaction. *Leukaemia* 1992; **6S1**: 47–59.
10. Ito Y and Miyamura K. Clinical significance of minimal residual disease in leukemia detected by polymerase chain reaction. Is molecular remission a milestone for achieving a cure? *Leukemia Lymphoma* 1994; **16**: 57–64.
11. Campana D and Pui C-H. Detection of minimal residual disease in acute leukemia: methodologic advances and clinical significance. *Blood* 1995; **85**: 1416–1434.
12. Smith RG and Kitchens RL. Phenotypic heterogeneity of TDT+ cells in the blood and bone marrow: implications for surveillance of residual leukemia. *Blood* 1989; **74**: 312–319.
13. Campana D, Coustan-Smith E and Janossy G. The immunological detection of minimal residual disease in acute leukemia. *Blood* 1990; **76**: 163–171.

14. Macedo A, Orfao A, Ciudad J et al. Phenotypic analysis of CD34 subpopulations in normal human bone marrow and its application of the detection of minimal residual disease. *Leukaemia* 1995; **9**: 1896–1901.
15. Terstappen LWMM and Loken MR. Five-dimensional flow cytometry as a new approach for blood and bone marrow differentials. *Cytometry* 1988; **9**: 548–556.
16. Groeneveld K, Te Marvelde JG, Van den Beemd MWM, Hooijkaas H and Van Dongen JJM. Flow cytometric detection of intracellular antigens for immunophenotyping of normal and malignant leukocytes. *Leukaemia* 1996; **10**: 1383–1389.
17. Knulst AC, Adriaansen HJ, Hählen K et al. Early diagnosis of smoldering acute lymphoblastic leukemia using immunological marker analysis. *Leukaemia* 1993; **7**: 532–536.
18. Farahat H, Lens D, Zomas A, Morilla R, Matutes E and Catovsky D. Quantitative flow cytometry can distinguish between normal and leukaemic B-cell precursor. *Br J Haematol* 1995; **91**: 640–646.
19. Smedmyr B, Bengtsson M, Jakobsson A, Simonsson B, Öberg G and Tötterman TH. Regeneration of CALLA (CD10$^+$), TdT$^+$ and double-positive cells in the bone marrow and blood after autologous bone marrow transplantation. *Eur J Haematol* 1991; **46**: 146–151.
20. Vervoordeldonk SF, Merle PA, Behrendt H et al. Triple immunofluorescence staining for prediction of relapse in childhood B acute lymphoblastic leukaemia. *Br J Haematol* 1996; **92**: 922–928.
21. Drach J, Drach D, Glassl H, Gattringer C and Huber H. Flow cytometric determination of atypical antigen expression in acute leukemia for the study of minimal residual disease. *Cytometry* 1992; **13**: 893–901.
22. Hurwitz CA, Gore SD, Stone KD and Civin CI. Flow cytometric detection of rare normal human marrow cells with immunophenotypes characteristic of acute lymphoblastic leukemia cells. *Leukaemia* 1992; **6**: 233–239.
23. Behm FG, Smith FO, Raimondi SC, Pui C-H and Bernstein ID. Human homologue of the rat chondroitin sulfate proteoglycan, NG2, detected by monoclonal antibody 7.1, identifies childhood acute lymphoblastic leukemias with t(4;11)(q21;q23) or t(11;19)(q23;p13) and *MLL* gene rearrangements. *Blood* 1996; **87**: 1134–1139.
24. Smith FO, Rauch C, Williams DE et al. The human homologue of rat NG2, a chondroitin sulfate proteoglycan, is not expressed on the cell surface of normal hematopoietic cells but is expressed by acute myeloid leukemia blasts from poor-prognosis patients with abnormalities of chromosome band 11q23. *Blood* 1996; **87**: 1123–1133.
25. Campana D. Applications of cytometry to study acute leukemia: *in vitro* determination of drug sensitivity and detection of minimal residual disease. *Cytometry (Comm Clin Cytometry)* 1994; **18**: 68–74.
26. Reading CL, Estey EH, Huh YO et al. Expression of unusual immunophenotype combinations in acute myelogenous leukemia. *Blood* 1993; **81**: 3083–3090.
27. Macedo A, Orfao A, Gonzalez M et al. Expression of unusual immunophenotype combinations in acute myelogenous leukemia. *Blood* 1993; **81**: 3083–3090.
28. Macedo A, Orfao A, Martinez A, Vidriales MB, Valverde B, López-Berges MC and San Miguel JF. Immunophenotype of c-kit cells in normal human bone marrow: implications for the detection of minimal residual disease in AML. *Br J Haematol* 1996; **89**: 338–341.
29. Adriaansen HJ, Jacobs BC, Kappers-Klunne MC, Hählen K, Hooijkaas H and Van Dongen JJM. Detection of residual disease in AML patients by use of double immunological marker analysis for terminal deoxynucleotidyl transferase and myeloid markers. *Leukaemia* 1993; **7**: 472–481.
30. Macedo A, San Miguel JF, Vidriales MB et al. Phenotypic changes in acute myeloid leukaemia: implications in the detection of minimal residual disease. *J Clin Pathol* 1996; **49**: 15–18.
31. Mahmoud HH, Rivera GK, Hancock ML et al. Low leukocyte counts with blast cells in cerebrospinal fluid of children with newly diagnosed acute lymphoblastic leukemia. *New Engl J Med* 1993; **329**: 314–319.
32. Pinkel D and Woo S. Prevention and treatment of meningeal leukemia in children. *Blood* 1994; **84**: 355–366.
33. Hooijkaas H, Hählen K, Adriaansen HJ, Dekker I, Van Zanen GE and Van Dongen JJM. Terminal deoxynucleotidyl transferase (TdT)-positive cells in cerebrospinal fluid and development of overt CNS leukemia: a 5-year follow-up study in 113 children with a TdT-positive leukemia or non-Hodgkin's lymphoma. *Blood* 1989; **74**: 416–422.
34. Inoue K, Ogawa H, Yamagami T et al. Long-term follow-up of minimal residual disease in leukemia patients by monitoring *WT1* (Wilms tumor gene) expression levels. *Blood* 1996; **88**: 2267–2278.
35. Brisco MJ, Condon J, Hughes E et al. Outcome prediction in childhood acute lymphoblastic leukaemia by molecular quantification of residual disease at the end of induction. *Lancet* 1994; **343**: 196–200.
36. Cross NCP. Quantitative PCR techniques and applications. *Br J Haematol* 1995; **89**: 693–697.
37. Cole-Sinclair M, Foroni L and Hoffbrand AV. Genetic changes: relevance for diagnosis and detection of minimal residual disease in acute lymphoblastic leukaemia. *Baillière's Clin Haematol* 1994; **7**: 183–233.
38. Chim JCS, Coyle LA, Yaxley JC, Cole-Sinclair MF, Cannell PK, Hoffbrand AV and Foroni L. The use of IgH fingerprinting and ASO-dependent PCR for the investigation of residual disease (MRD) in ALL. *Br J Haematol* 1996; **92**: 104–115.
39. Kneba M, Bolz I, Linke B and Hiddemann W. Analysis of rearranged T-cell receptor b-chain genes by polymerase chain reaction (PCR) DNA sequencing and automated high resolution PCR fragment analysis. *Blood* 1995; **86**: 3930–3937.
40. Prevost-Blondel A, Ostankovitch M, Melle J, Pannetier C, Macintyre E, Dreyfus F and Guillet J-G. CDR3 size analysis of T-cell receptor V beta transcripts: follow-up study in a patient with T cell acute lymphoblastic leukemia. *Leukaemia* 1995; **9**: 1711–1717.
41. Beishuizen A, Verhoeven M-AJ, Mol EJ and Van Dongen JJM. Detection of immunoglobulin kappa light-chain gene rearrangement patterns by Southern blot analysis. *Leukaemia* 1994; **8**: 2228–2236.
42. Beishuizen A, Van Wering ER, Breit TM, Hählen K, Hooijkaas H and Van Dongen JJM. Molecular biology of acute lymphoblastic leukaemia: Implications for detection of minimal residual disease. In: *Acute Leukemias*. W Hiddeman, Th Büchner and B Wörmann (eds), 1996: 460–474 (Berlin: Springer-Verlag).

43. Breit TM and Van Dongen JJM. Unravelling human T-cell receptor junctional region sequences. *Thymus* 1994; **22**: 177–199.
44. Beishuizen A, Hählen K, Hagemeijer A *et al*. Multiple rearranged immunoglobulin genes in childhood acute lymphoblastic leukemia of precursor B-cell origin. *Leukaemia* 1991; **5**: 657–667.
45. Beishuizen A, Verhoeven M-AJ, Van Wering ER, Hählen K, Hooijkaas H and Van Dongen JJM. Analysis of immunoglobulin and T-cell receptor genes in 40 childhood acute lymphoblastic leukemias at diagnosis and subsequent relapse: implications for the detection of minimal residual disease by PCR analysis. *Blood* 1994; **83**; 2238–2247.
46. Ghali DW, Panzer S, Fischer S *et al*. Heterogeneity of the T-cell receptor δ gene indicating subclone formation in acute precursor B-cell leukemias. *Blood* 1995; **85**: 2795–2801.
47. Davi F, Gocke C, Smith S and Sklar J. Lymphocytic progenitor cell origin and clonal evolution of human B-lineage acute lymphoblastic leukemia. *Blood* 1996; **88**: 609–621.
48. Marshall GM, Kwan E, Habler M *et al*. Characterization of clonal immunoglobulin heavy chain and T cell receptor gene rearrangements during progression of childhood acute lymphoblastic leukemia. *Leukaemia* 1995; **9**: 1847–1850.
49. Steenbergen EJ, Verhagen OJ, Van Leeuwen EF, Von dem Borne AE and Van der Schoot CE. Distinct ongoing Ig heavy chain rearrangement processes in childhood B-precursor acute lymphoblastic leukemia. *Blood* 1993; **82**: 581–589.
50. Steward CG, Goulden NJ, Katz F *et al*. A polymerase chain reaction study of the stability of Ig heavy-chain and T-cell receptor δ gene rearrangements between presentation and relapse of childhood B-lineage acute lymphoblastic leukemia. *Blood* 1994; **83**: 1355–1362.
51. Steenbergen EJ, Verhagen OJ, Van Leeuwen EF, Van den Berg H, Von dem Borne AE and Van der Schoot CE. Frequent ongoing T-cell receptor rearrangements in childhood B-precursor acute lymphoblastic leukemia: implications for monitoring minimal residual disease. *Blood* 1995; **86**: 692–702.
52. De Bruijn MAC, Beishuizen A, Verhoeven M-AJ, de Bruin-Versteeg S, Van Wering ER and Van Dongen JJM. Stability of rearrangements of the immunoglobulin kappa deleting element in childhood precursor-B-acute lymphoblastic leukemia [Abstract 217]. *Br J Haematol* 1996; **93**(Suppl 2): 56.
53. Steenbergen EJ, Verhagen OJ, Van Leeuwen EF *et al*. Prolonged persistence of PCR-detectable minimal residual disease after diagnosis of first relapse predicts poor outcome in childhood B-precursor acute lymphoblastic leukemia. *Leukaemia* 1995; **9**: 1726–1734.
54. Taylor JJ, Rowe D, Kylefjord H, Chessells J, Katz F, Proctor SJ and Middleton PG. Characterisation of non-concordance in the T cell receptor γ-chain genes at presentation and clinical relapse in acute lymphoblastic leukemia. *Leukaemia* 1994; **8**: 60–66.
55. Baruchel A, Cayuela J-M, Macintyre E, Berger R and Sigaux F. Assessment of clonal evolution at Ig/TCR loci in acute lymphoblastic leukaemia by single-strand conformation polymorphism studies and highly resolutive PCR derived methods: implication for a general strategy of minimal residual disease detection. *Br J Haematol* 1995; **90**: 85–93.
56. Roberts WM, Estrov Z, Kitchingman GR and Zipf TF. The clinical significance of residual disease in childhood acute lymphoblastic leukemia as detected by polymerase chain reaction amplification of antigen–receptor gene sequences. *Leukaemia Lymphoma* 1996; **20**: 181–197.
57. Biondi A, Yokota S, Hansen-Hagge TE *et al*. Minimal residual disease in childhood acute lymphoblastic leukemia: analysis of patients in continuous complete remission or with consecutive relapse. *Leukaemia* 1992; **6**: 282–288.
58. Ito Y, Wasserman R, Galili N, Reichard BA, Shane S, Lange B and Rovera G. Molecular residual disease status at the end of chemotherapy fails to predict subsequent relapse in children with B-lineage acute lymphoblastic leukemia. *J Clin Oncol* 1993; **11**: 546–553.
59. Neale GAM, Menarguez J, Kitchingman GR, Fitzgerald TJ, Koehler M, Mirro J Jr and Goorha RM. Detection of minimal residual disease in T-cell acute lymphoblastic leukemia using polymerase chain reaction predicts impending relapse. *Blood* 1991; **78**: 739–747.
60. Nizet Y, Martiat P, Vaerman JL *et al*. Follow-up of residual disease (MRD) in B lineage acute leukemias using a simplified PCR strategy: evolution of MRD rather than its detection is correlated with clinical outcome. *Br J Haematol* 1991; **79**: 205–210.
61. Nizet Y, Van Daele S, Lewalle P *et al*. Long-term follow-up of residual disease in acute lymphoblastic leukemia patients in complete remission using clonogeneic IgH probes and the polymerase chain reaction. *Blood* 1993; **82**: 1618–1625.
62. Wasserman R, Galili N, Ito Y *et al*. Residual disease at the end of induction therapy as a predictor of relapse during therapy in childhood B-lineage acute lymphoblastic leukemia. *J Clin Oncol* 1992; **10**: 1879–1888.
63. Yamada M, Wasserman R, Lange B, Reichard BA, Womer RB and Rovera G. Minimal residual disease in childhood B-lineage lymphoblastic leukemia: persistence of leukemic cells during the first 18 months of treatment. *New Engl J Med* 1990; **323**: 448–455.
64. Yokota S, Hansen-Hagge TE, Ludwig W-D, Reiter A, Raghavachar A, Kleihauer E and Bartram CR. Use of polymerase chain reactions to monitor minimal residual disease in acute lymphoblastic leukemia patients. *Blood* 1991; **77**: 331–339.
65. Cavé H, Guidal C, Rohrlich *et al*. Prospective monitoring and quantitation of residual blasts in childhood acute lymphoblastic leukemia by polymerase chain reaction study of δ and γ T-cell receptor genes. *Blood* 1994; **83**: 1892–1902.
66. Goulden N, Langlands K, Steward C, Katz F, Potter M, Chessels J and Oakhill A. PCR assessment of bone marrow status in 'isolated' extramedullary relapse of childhood B-precursor acute lymphoblastic leukaemia. *Br J Haematol* 1994; **87**: 282–285.
67. Neale GAM, Pui C-H, Mahmoud HH, Mirro J Jr, Crist WM, Rivera GK and Goorha RM. Molecular evidence for minimal residual bone marrow disease in children with 'isolated' extra-medullary relapse of T-cell acute lymphoblastic leukaemia. *Leukaemia* 1994; **8**: 768–775.
68. O'Reilly J, Meyer B, Baker D, Herrmann R, Cannell P and Davies J. Correlation of bone marrow minimal residual disease and apparent isolated extramedullary relapse in childhood acute lymphoblastic leukaemia. *Leukaemia* 1995; **9**: 624–627.
69. Kitchingman GR. Residual disease detection in multiple follow-up samples in children with acute lymphoblastic leukemia. *Leukaemia* 1994; **8**: 395–401.

70. Seriu T, Yokota S, Nakao M et al. Prospective monitoring of minimal residual disease during the course of chemotherapy in patients with acute lymphoblastic leukemia, and detection of contaminating tumor cells in peripheral blood stem cells for autotransplantation. *Leukaemia* 1995; **9**: 615–623.
71. Januszkiewicz DA and Nowak JS. Molecular evidence for central nervous system involvement in children with newly diagnosed acute lymphoblastic leukemia. *Hematol Oncol* 1995; **13**: 201–206.
72. Cortes JE and Kantarjian HM. Acute lymphoblastic leukemia: a comprehensive review with emphasis on biology and therapy. *Cancer* 1995; **76**: 2393–2417.
73. Copelan EA and McGuire EA. The biology and treatment of acute lymphoblastic leukemia in adults. *Blood* 1995; **85**: 1151–1168.
74. Scholten C, Födinger M, Mitterbauer M et al. Kinetics of minimal residual disease during induction/consolidation therapy in standard-risk adult B-lineage acute lymphoblastic leukemia. *Ann Haematol* 1995; **71**: 155–160.
75. Brisco MJ, Hughes E, Neoh S-H et al. Relationship between minimal residual disease and outcome in adult acute lymphoblastic leukemia. *Blood* 1996; **87**: 5251–5256.
76. Van Dongen JJM and Adriaansen HJ. Immunobiology of leukemia. In: *Leukemia*, 6th edn. ES Henderson, TA Lister and MF Greaves (eds), 1996: 83–130 (Philadelphia: WB Saunders).
77. Breit TM, Mol EJ, Wolvers-Tettero ILM, Ludwig W-D, Van Wering ER and Van Dongen JJM. Site-specific deletions involving the *tal-1* and *sil* genes are restricted to cells of the T-cell receptor αβ lineage: T-cell receptor δ gene deletion mechanism affects multiple genes. *J Exp Med* 1993; **177**: 965–977.
78. Breit TM, Beishuizen A, Ludwig W-D et al. JJM. *tal-1* deletions in T-cell acute lymphoblastic leukemia as PCR target for detection of minimal residual disease. *Leukaemia* 1993; **7**: 2004–2011.
79. Rabbitts TH. Chromosomal translocations in human cancer. *Nature* 1994; **372**: 143–149.
80. Raimondi SC. Current status of cytogenetic research in childhood acute lymphoblastic leukemia. *Blood* 1993; **81**: 2237–2251.
81. The Groupe Français de Cytogénétique Hématologique. Cytogenetic abnormalities in adult acute lymphoblastic leukemia: correlations with hematologic findings and outcome. *Blood* 1996; **81**: 3135–3142.
82. Drexler HG, Borkhardt A and Janssen JWG. Detection of chromosomal translocations in leukemia–lymphoma cells by polymerase chain reaction. *Leukaemia Lymphoma* 1995; **19**: 359–380.
83. Hébert J, Cayuela J-M, Daniel M-T, Berger R and Sigaux F. Detection of minimal residual disease in acute myelomonocytic leukemia with abnormal marrow eosinophils by nested polymerase chain reaction with allele specific amplification. *Blood* 1994; **84**: 2291–2296.
84. Poirel H, Radford-Weiss I, Rack K et al. Detection of the chromosome 16 CBFb-MYH11 fusion transcript in myelomonocytic leukemias. *Blood* 1995; **85**: 1313–1322.
85. Privitera E, Rivolta A, Ronchetti D, Mosna G, Giudici G and Biondi A. Reverse transcriptase/polymerase chain reaction follow-up and minimal residual disease detection in t(1;19)-positive acute lymphoblastic leukaemia. *Br J Haematol* 1996; **92**: 653–658.
86. Shurtleff SA, Buijs A, Behm FG et al. TEL/AML1 fusion resulting from a cryptic t(12;21) is the most common genetic lesion in pediatric ALL and defines a subgroup of patients with an excellent prognosis. *Leukaemia* 1995; **9**: 1985–1989.
87. Romana SP, Poirel H, Leconiat M et al. High frequency of t(12;21) in childhood B-lineage acute lymphoblastic leukemia. *Blood* 1995; **86**: 4263–4269.
88. Raynaud S, Mauvieux L, Cayuela JM et al. TEL/AML1 fusion gene is a rare event in adult acute lymphoblastic leukemia. *Leukaemia* 1996; **10**: 1529–1530.
89. Biernaux C, Loos M, Sels A, Huez G and Stryckmans P. Detection of major bcr-abl gene expression at a very low level in blood cells of some healthy individuals. *Blood* 1995; **86**: 3118–3122.
90. Miyamura K, Tanimoto M, Morishima Y et al. Detection of Philadelphia chromosome-positive acute lymphoblastic leukemia by polymerase chain reaction: possible eradication of minimal residual disease by marrow transplantation. *Blood* 1992; **79**: 1366–1370.
91. Roberts WM, Rivera GK, Raimondi SC et al. Intensive chemotherapy for Philadelphia-chromosome-positive acute lymphoblastic leukaemia. *Lancet* 1994; **343**: 331–332.
92. Mitterbauer G, Födinger M, Scherrer R et al. PCR-monitoring of minimal residual leukaemia after conventional chemotherapy and bone marrow transplantation in BCR-ABL-positive acute lymphoblastic leukaemia. *Br J Haematol* 1995; **89**: 937–941.
93. Janssen JWG, Ludwig W-D, Borkhardt A et al. Pre-pre-B acute lymphoblastic leukemia: high frequency of alternatively spliced ALL1-AF4 transcripts and absence of minimal residual disease during complete remission. *Blood* 1994; **84**: 3835–3842.
94. Cimino G, Elia L, Rivolta A et al. Clinical relevance of residual disease monitoring by polymerase chain reaction in patients with ALL-1/AF-4 positive-acute lymphoblastic leukaemia. *Br J Haematol* 1996; **92**: 659–664.
95. Cayuela J-M, Baruchel A, Orange C et al. TEL/AML1 fusion RNA as a new target to detect minimal residual disease in pediatric B-cell precursor acute lymphoblastic leukemia. *Blood* 1996; **88**: 302–308.
96. Nakao M, Yokota S, Horiike S et al. Detection and quantification of TEL/AML1 fusion transcripts by polymerase chain reaction in childhood acute lymphoblastic leukemia. *Leukaemia* 1996; **10**: 1463–1470.
97. Diverio D, Pandolfi PP, Biondi A et al. Absence of reverse transcription-polymerase chain reaction detectable residual disease in patients with acute promyelocytic leukemia in long-term remission. *Blood* 1993; **82**: 3556–3559.
98. Huang W, Sun G-L, Li X-S et al. Acute promyelocytic leukemia: clinical relevance of two major PML-RARα isoforms and detection of minimal residual disease by retrotranscriptase/polymerase chain reaction to predict relapse. *Blood* 1993; **82**: 1264–1269.
99. Laczika K, Mitterbauer G, Korninger L et al. Rapid achievement of PML-RARα polymerase chain reaction (PCR)-negativity by combined treatment with all-*trans*-retinoic acid and chemotherapy in acute promyelocytic leukemia: a pilot study. *Leukaemia* 1994; **8**: 1–5.
100. Lo Coco F, Avvisati G, Diverio D et al. Molecular evaluation of response to all-*trans*-retinoic acid therapy in patients with acute promyelocytic leukemia. *Blood* 1991; **77**: 1657–1659.

101. Lo Coco F, Diverio D, Pandolfi PP et al. Molecular evaluation of residual disease as a predictor of relapse in acute promyelocytic leukaemia. Lancet 1992; 340: 1437–1438.
102. Miller Jr WH, Levine K, DeBlasio A et al. Detection of minimal residual disease in acute promyelocytic leukemia by a reverse transcription polymerase chain reaction assay for the PML/RAR-a fusion mRNA. Blood 1993; 82: 1689–1694.
103. Takatsuki H, Umemura T, Sadamura S et al. Detection of minimal residual disease by reverse transcriptase polymerase chain reaction for the PML/RAR-a fusion mRNA: a study in patients with acute promyelocytic leukaemia following peripheral stem cell transplantation. Leukemia 1995; 9: 889–892.
104. Martinelli G, Remiddi C, Visani G et al. Molecular analysis of PML-RARa fusion mRNA detected by reverse transcription-polymerase chain reaction assay in long-term disease-free acute promyelocytic leukaemia patients. Br J Haematol 1995; 90: 966–968.
105. Fukutani H, Naoe T, Ohno R et al. and the Leukemia Study Group of the Ministry of Health and Welfare (Kouseisho). Prognostic significance of the RT-PCR assay of PML-RARA transcripts in acute promyelocytic leukemia. Leukaemia 1995; 9: 588–593.
106. Korninger L, Knöbl P, Laczika K et al. PML-RARα PCR positivity in the bone marrow of patients with APL precedes haematological relapse by 2–3 months. Br J Haematol 1994; 88: 427–431.
107. Kane JR, Head DR, Balazs L et al. Molecular analysis of the PML-RARα chimeric gene in pediatric acute promyelocytic leukemia. Leukaemia 1996; 10: 1296–1302.
108. Nucifora G, Larson RA and Rowley JD. Persistence of the 8;21 translocation in patients with acute myeloid leukemia type M2 in long-term remission. Blood 1993; 82: 712–715.
109. Kusec R, Laczika K, Knöbl P et al. AML1/ETO fusion mRNA can be detected in remission blood samples of all patients with t(8;21) acute myeloid leukemia after chemotherapy or autologous bone marrow transplantation. Leukaemia 1994; 8: 735–739.
110. Nucifora G and Rowley JD. The AML1 and ETO genes in acute myeloid leukemia with a t(8;21). Leukaemia Lymphoma 1994; 14: 353–362.
111. Saunders MJ, Tobal K, Keeney S and Liu Jin JA. Expression of diverse AML1-MTG8 transcripts is a consistent feature in acute myeloid leukemia with t(8;21) irrespective of disease phase. Leukaemia 1996; 10: 1139–1142.
112. Jurlander J, Caligiuri MA, Ruutu T et al. Persistence of the AML1/ETO fusion transcript in patients treated with allogeneic bone marrow transplantation for t(8;21) leukemia. Blood 1996; 88: 2183–2191.
113. Satake N, Maseki N, Kozu T et al. Disappearance of AML1-MTG8(ETO) fusion transcript in acute myeloid leukaemia patients with t(8;21) in long-term remission. Br J Haematol 1995; 91: 892–898.
114. Martens AC, Schultz FW and Hagenbeek A. Nonhomogeneous distribution of leukemia in the bone marrow during minimal residual disease. Blood 1987; 70: 1073–1078.

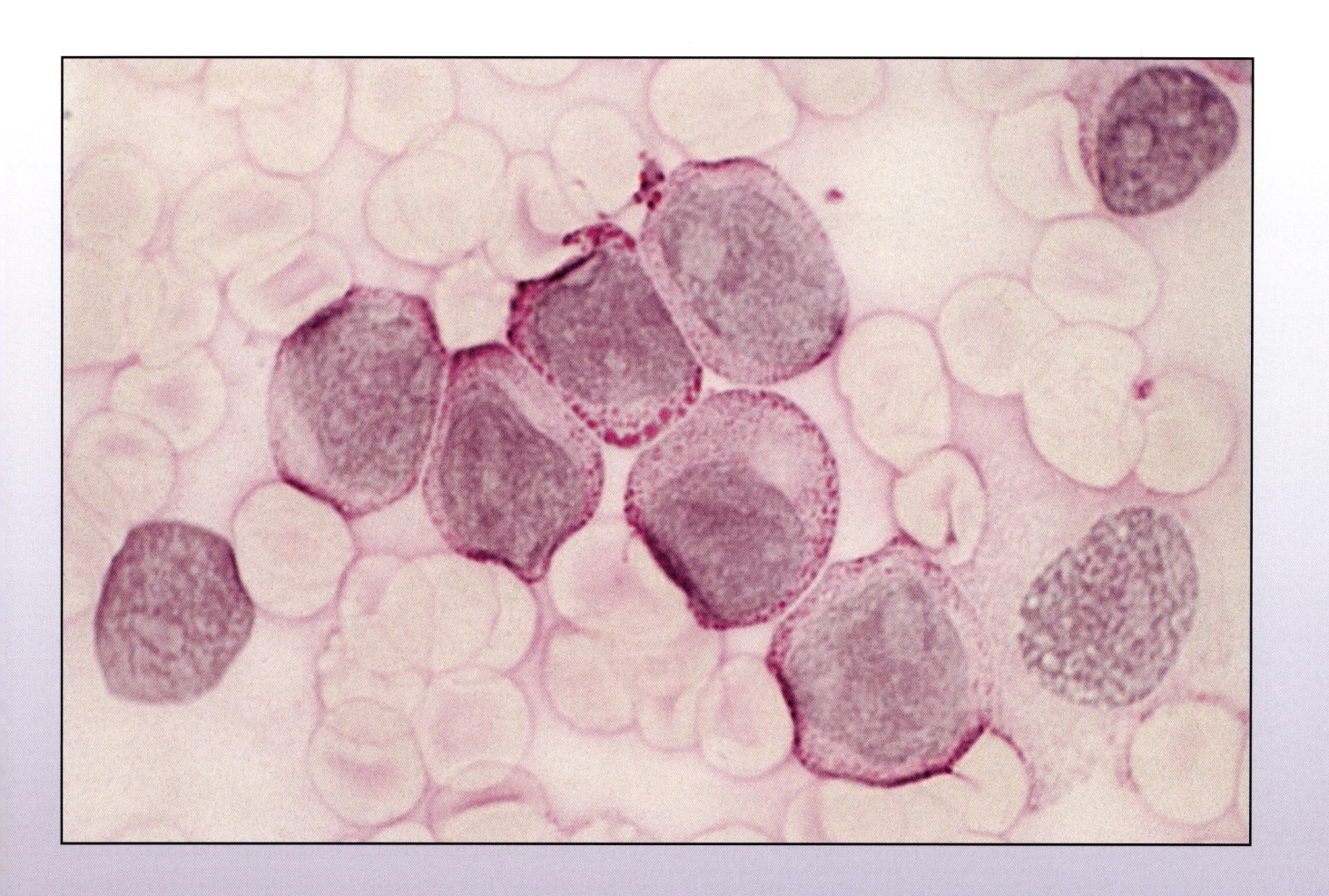

Chapter 42
Relapse and its management

Hans-Jochem Kolb and Johann Mittermüller

Introduction

Allogeneic bone-marrow transplantation has brought about remissions in haematopoietic malignancies which are otherwise refractory to treatment [1,2]. In a minority of these patients, remissions have persisted for more than a decade without further maintenance treatment, and some patients may be cured. However, relapse of the primary malignancy remains the most frequent cause of treatment failure for patients in both the early and more advanced stages of their disease. The three-year probability of relapse after allogeneic transplantation in early stages of leukaemia, i.e. first complete remission of acute leukaemia and chronic phase of chronic myelogenous leukaemia (CML) ranges from between 10 and 30% [3]. After transplantation in more advanced disease, the three-year probability of relapse is between 20 and 70% [4–7]. In patients surviving for more than three years after transplantation for acute leukaemia, the risk of relapse decreases, whereas for patients transplanted for CML in chronic phase, the relapse risk remains increased but may be lower in patients with human leukocyte antigen (HLA)-matched, unrelated donors. It is higher in patients with a syngeneic twin donor and after autografting. Relapse of leukaemia is the main cause of death after haematopoietic transplantation [5].

In general, risk factors predicting for a poor response to chemotherapy also apply to haematopoietic transplantation. The presence of cytogenetic abnormalities with a prognostic impact on remission rate and probability of relapse after chemotherapy are also associated with a higher probability of relapse after transplantation [3,5,8–11].

Nature of relapse and associated risk factors

Individual patients with evidence of recurrent leukaemia in donor cells have been reported [12–18], indicating the persistence of a leukaemogenic hazard. However, the great majority of leukaemic relapses occur in the recipient's cells. In these patients the leukaemic clone has not been eliminated by bone-marrow transplantation, and relapse results from the growth of the original clone.

Leukaemic relapse results from a minority of leukaemic cells endowed with extensive proliferative and self-renewal capacity which survive high-dose chemotherapy and radiotherapy [19]. Total body irradiation (TBI) and high doses of busulfan and melphalan are myeloablative and have their effect by eliminating haematopoietic stem cells. Their use in leukaemia therapy consequently requires infusion of haematopoietic stem cells. Several studies have compared the combination of cyclophosphamide and total body irradiation with that of busulfan and cyclophosphamide [20–22]. In CML, no differences were seen after TBI and busulfan [20]. The busulfan group fared less well in one study of patients with acute myeloid leukaemia (AML) [21] and in patients with advanced disease in the other study [22]. In a randomized European Bone Marrow Transplant (EBMT) study (unpublished), there were no differences in relapse rates and disease-free survival in either CML or AML. Higher radiation doses of 15.75 Gy were more effective in the eradication of AML and CML, but the overall survival was comparable to that of patients irradiated with 12 Gy only [23].

The use of etoposide in combination with TBI has been promising in patients with advanced disease [24]. However, most preparatory regimens failed to improve the disease-free survival of leukaemia patients after allogeneic transplantation. In a retrospective comparison of various radiation regimens, no difference was found in patients given unmanipulated bone marrow [25]. However, differences were observed in patients given T-cell-depleted marrow grafts. After T-cell depletion the relapse rate was higher in patients given lower doses of TBI or fractionated TBI. Therefore, the role of T-cells in the graft appears to be more important than variations in the conditioning regimen.

Allogeneic bone-marrow transplantation as a form of immunotherapy was first conceived by the Harwell group of scientists [26] and its potential for the treatment of leukaemia was investigated by Mathé and colleagues [27]. Only after the preconditions for successful marrow transplantation were known with regard to the selection of histocompatible donors, effective preparatory regimens and prophylaxis of acute graft-versus-host-disease (GvHD), could the effect of acute and chronic GvHD on leukaemia-free survival be evaluated [28]. In particular, chronic GvHD has a beneficial effect on relapse rate after transplantation. In patients with advanced disease, acute and chronic GvHD was beneficial for relapse-free survival [5]. Conversely, patients transplanted at an early stage of leukaemia had an increased risk of relapse if GvHD was absent [3]. Immunogenetically identical transplants from monozygotic twin donors are associated with an increased risk of relapse [29,30], and recipients of marrow from unrelated HLA-identical donors have a lower probability of relapse of leukaemia [31,32]. However, immunogenetic disparity may not by itself determine susceptibility to leukaemic relapse, but modification of the allogeneic immune reaction may influence the course of leukaemia [33–35]. Depletion of T-cells from the marrow graft for prevention of GvHD increases the probability of leukaemic relapse [3]. Obviously the graft-versus-leukaemia (GvL) effect is closely associated with the graft-versus-host reaction, but it may be separable in certain instances. One example is the probability of relapse in CML patients given T-cell-depleted marrow grafts: patients who develop GvHD despite T-cell depletion still have an increased risk of relapse [3]. T-cells may exert a graft-versus-leukaemia effect without inducing GvHD.

Forms of relapse

In leukaemia, relapse may be systemic, in many instances heralded by a drop in platelet count and sometimes improvement of GvHD. As a rule, progression is rapid, but the leukaemia may smoulder in some patients. Extramedullary relapses are fairly common after allogeneic marrow transplantation and about 13% of patients with AML and 24% of patients with acute lymphoid leukaemia (ALL) initially present with isolated extramedullary relapses [36,37]. Isolated extramedullary relapses tend to occur later than systemic relapses [36], many of these in testes and CNS. Most extramedullary relapses are followed by a systemic relapse.

In CML, cells carrying the Philadelphia chromosome may persist or recur after allogeneic marrow transplantation. Small amounts of Philadelphia-positive cells may disappear without therapeutic intervention in many patients [38,39]. Larger and increasing proportions of Philadelphia-positive cells may indicate persistence of the disease or cytogenetic relapse [40]. Cytogenetic relapses progress to haematological relapses unless they are treated.

A positive reverse transcriptase polymerase chain reaction (RT-PCR) for bcr/abl transcripts in CML patients after transplantation does not necessarily indicate recurrence of disease, since long-lived cells such as T-cells may persist without risk of relapse. An increasing signal in quantitative RT-PCR may predict relapse of CML [40].

Haematological relapse is characterized by recurrence of the clinical disease with reappearance of immature cells and basophils in the blood, leukocytosis and thrombocytosis unexplained by other causes such as infection or inflammatory response. Relapse of leukaemia with blasts and clinical signs of transformation is common after transplantation in accelerated and blastic phase of CML.

Treatment of relapse

There are several different ways to treat leukaemic relapses after haematopoietic transplantation and no single way is effective in all patients.

Withdrawal of immunosuppression

Successes have been reported for discontinuation of immunosuppressive therapy in single patients with CML, AML and ALL [33,35,41]. In particular, high doses of cyclosporin A have been associated with an increased incidence of relapse [42]. All patients who responded developed GvHD. If GvHD does not develop, the response may be only transient (personal observation). Abrupt discontinuation of cyclosporin A may be indicated as a first step in patients without severe GvHD.

Chemotherapy

Pace of the disease may dictate the treatment regimen used [12]. Most patients with acute leukaemia and transformed CML recurring after marrow transplantation need cytotoxic chemotherapy. In a retrospective analysis of 76 patients with ALL and 41 patients with AML, remissions were induced by conventional chemotherapy in about 40% of patients treated [43]. The median survival of responders was eight months in AML and 14 months in ALL, only 4 patients remaining in remission for more than two years. Patients with a longer duration of remission were more likely to respond to chemotherapy at relapse. The time interval from transplantation to relapse was important both in relation to leukaemia response and treatment-related toxicity [36]. Patients with leukaemia relapsing within 100 days of transplantation rarely achieved a remission, but suffered from severe toxicity. Remissions were more common in patients with a leukaemic relapse occurring more than a year after transplantation. Standard chemotherapy for re-induction and maintenance can improve survival and, in single patients, induce long-lasting remissions [44].

In patients with a slow disease pace and 'smouldering' forms of AML, low-dose cytosine arabinoside may be the treatment of choice [45,46]. Stabilization of the disease may be achieved for prolonged periods of time, and chemotherapy may be combined with adoptive immunotherapy. Rapidly progressive forms of relapse may not be controlled by treatment with low-dose cytosine arabinoside, and more intensive chemotherapy is required. Drug resistance should be considered in cases of early relapse [47].

Radiotherapy

Extramedullary relapses are common after allogeneic transplantation. They can involve any site of the body [48]. Isolated extramedullary relapses are rare, and in most cases multiple sites are infiltrated. Usually extramedullary relapses precede systemic recurrence. Combined treatment with radiation and chemotherapy may be indicated in symptomatic patients and in patients with large tumour masses. Leukaemic recurrences in the CNS and testes should be treated with radiation to the involved site together with systemic chemotherapy [49,50].

Little is known about radioresistance of leukaemia and its mechanisms. In T-lymphoblastic leukaemia, radioresistance appears to be associated with the CD3-positive immune phenotype [51].

Therapy with haematopoietic growth factors and cytokines

In recurrent AML, granulocytes of host type may be present [45] indicating differentiation of leukaemic blasts. Unfortunately, treatment with low-dose cytosine arabinoside has failed to support differentiation of blasts, haematopoietic recovery deriving exclusively from donor cells. Treatment with granulocyte colony-stimulating factor (G-CSF) has induced complete remissions for a prolonged period of time in 3 of 7 patients with leukaemic relapse [52]. Differentiation of the patient's blasts was not observed, but haematological recovery with donor cells occurred. Follow-up reports on this form of treatment have been less enthusiastic [53]. Granulocyte–monocyte colony-stimulating factor (GM-CSF) stimulates proliferation and differentiation of myelopoiesis [54], and more recently its immunomodulatory properties have aroused interest [55]. GM-CSF has not been studied systematically for the treatment of relapse. However, experience in single patients has not been promising (unpublished data).

Interferon-α has been used in the treatment of recurrent CML [56–58]. Its mechanism of action is a direct antiproliferative effect on the growth of CML cells, possibly by re-establishing a close contact with the supporting stroma [59], an immunomodulatory effect by upregulating the expression of cell-surface antigens such as HLA, and an activation of immune effector cells [60]. Various schedules for interferon-α therapy have been used, doses ranging from 1 to 5×10^6 U/m^2 daily, or 5×10^6 U/m^2 three times weekly. Haematological remissions were achieved in about 50% of patients and cytogenetic remissions in about 30% of patients with relapse in chronic phase of CML. In patients with cytogenetic relapse, complete cytogenetic remissions could be achieved in up to 30%. However, in a retrospective analysis involving multiple centres, interferon-α delayed progression of cytogenetic relapse to haematological relapse without improving cytogenetic response, as compared to untreated patients. Moreover, it improved survival of patients with advanced stage haematological relapse. In this multicentre study, the time of treatment with regard to the dynamics of the cytogenetic relapse could be taken into account.

Observations in single centres are consistent with long-lasting remissions in some patients with cytogenetic relapses treated with interferon-α. The role of interferon-α in the control of cytogenetic remission is only evaluable by a prospective randomized trial. However, this would expose the patient to the risk of progression to clinical disease.

The role of interferon-α in the treatment of AML and ALL is less well documented [61], but interferon-α may support immunotherapeutic approaches [62].

Interleukin-2 (IL-2) has been used more commonly in the treatment of acute leukaemia [63–67]. It enhances the antileukaemic activity of natural killer (NK) cells and cytotoxic T-cells [68] and has been used for prevention of leukaemic relapse in most studies [69,70]. Activity of IL-2 as a single agent has been reported in a few patients only [71,67,53], and its efficacy may be greater in conjunction with adoptive immunotherapy [65,72]. Larger studies on leukaemic relapses after allogeneic transplantation are required before its use can be recommended.

Second marrow transplants

Second bone-marrow transplants are the most intensive attempt to modify the disease course. Success depends very much on the time interval from the first transplant, the intensity of prior therapy, the disease stage and the performance status of the patient. Patients with advanced disease and early relapse have done poorly [12,73–88]. Second transplants undertaken less than one year after the first transplant in adults, and after less than six months in children are associated with a high transplant-related mortality [73,78,82,84,86]. The leukaemia-free survival more than three years after second transplantation is less than 20% in most larger series [78,84,86] and it is superior in patients with CML [82] and in those patients with a longer interval from the first transplant.

Most patients are chimaeric at the time of relapse. Immunosuppressive preparation is not required if the same allogeneic donor is used. In patients who were prepared with total body irradiation for the first transplant, busulfan alone [79], in combination with VP-16 [74], or in combination with cyclophosphamide [82,87], has been used for conditioning. Occasionally, patients with identical twin donors have been transplanted successfully the second time with marrow from an allogeneic HLA-identical sibling donor [78]. In several instances, allogeneic transplants have been performed after a first autologous transplant [87]. Transplantation from a matched unrelated donor after a first autologous transplant cannot be generally recommended.

The use of peripheral blood stem-cell transplants instead of marrow for second transplants has become more common [88]. It is not known whether the larger dose of lymphocytes administered with the blood stem-cell concentrate confers a greater antileukaemic effect.

Donor lymphocyte transfusions

The chimaeric state of patients with leukaemic relapses provides particular conditions for adoptive immunotherapy using lymphocytes and other immunocompetent cells from the marrow donor. Persistent chimaerism after discontinuation of immunosuppressive therapy indicates a state of tolerance which can not be abrogated by transfusion of lymphocytes from the donor [89]. Transplantation of T-cell-depleted bone marrow can induce mixed chimaerism in dog leukocyte antigen (DLA)-identical dogs. Transfusion of donor lymphocytes does not produce GvHD, if delayed for at least two months after transplantation. Nevertheless, chimaerism regresses to complete donor type [90]. In mice, the delayed transfusion can cure leukaemia without producing GvHD [91].

In accordance with the results of animal experiments, transfusion of donor lymphocytes has induced complete remissions in patients with recurrent CML [92]. A summary of the results obtained from EBMT centres demonstrates the response of more than 70% of patients with recurrent CML in haematological and cytogenetic relapse (Table 42.1) [62]. Responses were complete cytogenetic responses, and in most patients, molecular remissions with the absence of bcr/abl transcripts in a RT-PCR. Results are poor in patients with CML relapsing in the transformed phase.

Responses have been observed in a minority of patients with AML and myelodysplasia. They are rare in patients with ALL, multiple myeloma and lymphoma. However, single reports have described the response of multiple myeloma [93,94] to the transfusion of donor lymphocytes. Single patients with recurrent polycythaemia vera and refractory anaemia [95] have also responded to this form of adoptive immunotherapy.

In CML patients treated for cytogenetic or haematological relapse, the responses are quite durable (Figure 42.1). Second relapses have occurred, but remissions could be induced in many by repeated lymphocyte transfusions.

Responses have not been as durable in patients with recurrent acute leukaemia, but some patients with recurrent AML have survived for more than two years. In acute leukaemia, treatment has frequently included

Table 42.1 Graft-versus-leukaemia effect of donor lymphocyte transfusions – EBMT study follow-up (June 1996)

Diagnosis	Patients studied (n)	Patients evaluable (n)*	Complete remission (%)	
Chronic myelogenous leukaemia				
cytogenetic relapse	28	25	19	(76%)
haematological relapse	79	72	53	(74%)
transformed phase	20	14	1	(7%)
Polycythaemia vera	1	1	1	
Acute myeloid leukaemia	57	37	9	(24%)
Myelodysplastic syndrome	10	8	3	(38%)
Acute lymphoid leukaemia	40	20	2	(10%)
Non-Hodgkin's lymphoma	2	2	1	
Multiple myeloma (MMY)	8	7	1	(14%)

*Patients in remission after chemotherapy and patients surviving less than 30 days after donor lymphocyte transfusions were excluded from analysis.

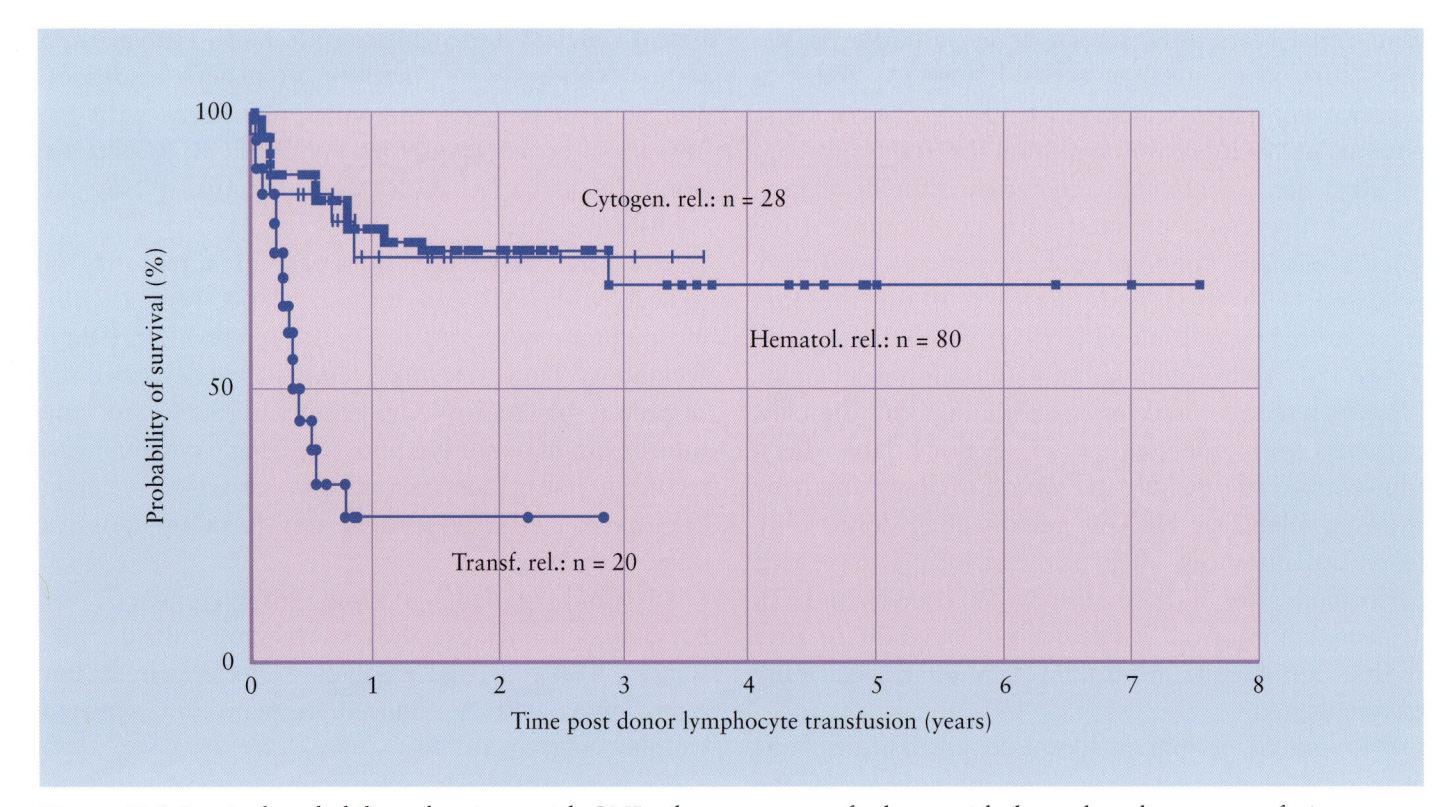

Figure 42.1 Survival probability of patients with CML after treatment of relapse with donor lymphocyte transfusion.

chemotherapy. Four groups of patients were definable: those treated with donor lymphocyte transfusions alone, patients treated with chemotherapy and donor lymphocyte transfusions together, patients treated with donor lymphocyte transfusions when they were in remission after chemotherapy, and patients treated with lymphocyte transfusions after chemotherapy had failed (Tables 42.2 and 42.3). Recurrent AML did respond to donor lymphocyte transfusions either without prior chemotherapy or after chemotherapy had failed (Table 42.2), and only two patients with relapsed ALL responded to lymphocyte transfusions without prior chemotherapy (Table 42.3).

The median number of mononuclear blood cells transfused was $3.5 \times 10^8/k$. An influence of the cell dose on response could not be evaluated, because several centres increased the dose of cells in a stepwise fashion. Two hundred and fifty-eight patients were reported, and of these, 118 died. In 9 patients the cause of death was not evaluated and 5 patients died early

Table 42.2 Graft-versus-leukaemia effect of donor lymphocyte transfusions – EBMT study follow-up (June 1996) Results in acute myeloid leukaemia

Treatment***	Studied	Patients evaluable* (n)	Complete remission (n) (%)	Remission duration (days)
DLT without chemotherapy	28	23	4 (17%)	301, 436, 969**, 1494**
DLT with chemotherapy	9	6	2 (33%)	237, 406**
DLT after CR with chemotherapy	10	8	8	59, 68, 159**, 201**, 312**, 324, 535**, 791**
DLT after failure to achieve CR with chemotherapy	9	7	3 (43%)	128**, 502**, 977

*Patients who survived at least 30 days after DLT.
**Indicates remission at the time reported.
***DLT = donor lymphocyte transfusions; CR = complete remission.

Table 42.3 Graft-versus-leukaemia effect of donor lymphocyte transfusions – EBMT study follow-up (June 1996) Results in acute lymphoid leukaemia

Treatment***	Studied	Patients evaluable* (n)	Complete remission (n) (%)	Remission duration (days)
DLT without chemotherapy	9	8	1 (12%)	460**
DLT with chemotherapy	11	8	1 (12%)	158**
DLT after CR with chemotherapy	14	14	13	21, 32, 47**, 71, 122**, 164, 185, 200, 255, 302**, 370**, 442**, 539
DLT after failure to achieve CR with chemotherapy	6	4	0	

*Patients who survived at least 30 days after DLT
**Indicates remission at the time reported.
***DLT = donor lymphocyte transfusions; CR = complete remission.

after treatment. Eighty-nine patients died of leukaemia and 15 patients died of causes other than leukaemia. Major complications of lymphocyte transfusion were GvHD and myelosuppression. GvHD of grade II and higher developed in about 60% of patients, and myelosuppression in 30–40%.

In most cases of myelosuppression, transfusion of stem cells from the donor, as either marrow or blood, led to the recovery of haematopoiesis. In some patients with severe chronic GvHD, haematopoiesis did not recover despite infusion of stem cells. The mechanism of myelosuppression is probably similar to that of transfusion-associated GvHD [96]. Transfused T-cells recognize haematopoietic cells of the recipient and eliminate them.

Prevention of myelosuppression secondary to donor lymphocyte transfusion has been attempted by transfusing peripheral blood stem cells with the lymphocytes [97]. However, myelosuppression was not preventable in all patients. Myelosuppression is less frequent in patients treated for cytogenetic relapse of CML than in those with haematological relapse. The best method of preventing myelosuppression may be an earlier transfusion of lymphocytes, before most of the haematopoiesis is produced by the CML.

Several approaches to preventing GvHD without losing the graft-versus-leukaemia effect have been explored. One approach is to transfuse small doses of cells, increasing the amount in a stepwise fashion until the disease responds or GvHD develops [98]. In some patients there is a therapeutic window, where a GvL reaction without GvHD occurs. Unfortunately, the GvL reaction may require several weeks or months to eliminate the leukaemic clone [99] and unless GvHD occurs it is difficult to assess the effects of increasing the cell dose early on.

Another approach is to deplete the CD8-positive T-cells from the inoculum [100] since CD4-positive T-cells may exert a GvL effect without producing GvHD [101]. In any case, patients treated with donor lymphocytes should be followed closely for evidence of GvHD and treated as clinically indicated.

The use of interferon-α in addition to lymphocyte transfusions was initiated in most patients as a primary method for treating CML relapse. In a retrospective analysis, interferon-α did not improve the response to donor lymphocyte transfusions. However, this situation cannot be assessed with a retrospective analysis, since many patients were only treated with donor lymphocytes after interferon-α had failed. In single patients, a response to donor lymphocytes has been observed after interferon-α alone was added. However, some patients only responded to the combination of donor lymphocytes with interferon-α and interleukin-2 [65,72].

The mechanism of the GvL reaction is unknown, but T-cells and NK cells may contribute to the effect [102]. Obviously, an alloimmune reaction is involved, because donor lymphocyte transfusions have failed to induce remissions in syngeneic twins [103], but the response was excellent in a few patients with matched unrelated donors. GvL effects have also been observed in patients with HLA-mismatched donors, but the numbers are too small to permit a meaningful evaluation. As in most cases the patient is HLA-identical with the donor, minor histocompatibility antigens may be involved in the reaction. However, the GvL reaction may be separable from a GvH reaction, because about 30% of patients without any signs of GvHD and 68% of patients with mild GvHD respond to the GvL reaction. A GvL reaction directed against potential leukaemia-specific antigens may exist. Cytotoxic T-cells have been produced against the bcr–abl fusion peptide [104,105], but their potential role in patient treatment has not been defined.

The spectrum of activity of transfusion-induced GvL reaction is consistent with a role for dendritic cells produced by the leukaemia. In CML and sometimes in AML, differentiation toward mature dendritic cells can occur. These cells are well able to stimulate and sustain a reaction against the leukaemia. It can be speculated that lymphoblastic leukaemias and lymphomas cannot generate dendritic cells as part of the leukaemic clone, which would account for the inferior results seen after relapse in these diseases when treated with donor lymphocyte infusions.

Outlook for graft-versus-leukaemia reactions

The possibility of treating leukaemia with lymphocytes from the marrow donor offers several new approaches in haematopoietic transplantation. Firstly, induction of tolerance by depletion of T-cells from the marrow graft may be associated with less acute GvHD and the incumbent complications. Secondly, donor lymphocytes could be transfused into high-risk patients earlier after transplantation, prior to leukaemia relapse. Thirdly, donor lymphocytes may be prepared by *ex vivo* co-cultivation with dendritic cells presenting the leukaemia specific antigen [104,105]. Another possibility concerns immunization against minor histocompatibility antigens as far as they are preferentially expressed on haematopoietic cells [106]. Finally, immunized T-cells can be transfected with a suicide gene which allows T-cells to be extinguished as soon as they attack the normal patient organs [107]. T-cells may also be used in this setting for the treatment of tumours as well as viral infections [108]. All of these new developments allow hope for patients with otherwise refractory disease.

References

1. Thomas ED, Storb R, Clift RA *et al.* Bone marrow transplantation. *New Engl J Med* 1975; **292**: 832–843.
2. Thomas ED, Buckner CD, Banaji M *et al.* One hundred patients with acute leukemia treated by chemotherapy, total body irradiation and allogeneic marrow transplantation. *Blood* 1977; **49**: 511–533.
3. Horowitz MM, Gale RP, Sondel PM *et al.* Graft-versus-leukemia reactions after bone marrow transplantation. *Blood* 1990; **75**: 555–562.
4. Horowitz MM. New IBMTR/ABMTR slides summarize current use and outcome of allogeneic and autologous transplants. *IBMTR Newsletter* 1995; **2**: 2–8 (Abstr).
5. Sullivan KM, Weiden PL, Storb R *et al.* Influence of acute and chronic graft-versus-host disease on relapse and survival after bone marrow transplantation from HLA-identical siblings as treatment of acute and chronic leukemia. *Blood* 1989; **73**: 1720–1728.
6. Barrett AJ, Horowitz MM, Gale RP, Biggs JC, Blume KG, Camitta BM *et al.* Bone marrow transplantation for acute lymphoblastic leukemia: factors influencing relapse and survival. *Blood* 1989; **74**: 862–871.
7. Gale RP, Butturini A and Horowitz MM. HLA-identical sibling bone marrow transplants for acute lymphoblastic leukemia. *Bone Marrow Transplant* 1995; **15**(Suppl 1): S199–S202.
8. Gale RP, Horowitz MM, Weiner RS *et al.* Impact of cytogenetic abnormalities on outcome of bone marrow transplantation in acute myelogenous leukemia in first remission. *Bone Marrow Transplant* 1995; **16**: 203–208.
9. Zander AR, Keating M, Dicke K *et al.* A comparison of marrow transplantation with chemotherapy for adults with acute leukemia of poor prognosis in first complete remission. *J Clin Oncol* 1988; **6**: 1548–1557.
10. Barrett AJ, Horowitz MM, Gale RP *et al.* Bone marrow transplantation for Philadelphia-chromosome positive acute lymphoblastic leukemia. *Blood* 1992; **79**: 3067–3070.
11. Goldman JM, Gale RP, Horowitz MM *et al.* Bone marrow transplantation for chronic myelogenous leukemia in chronic phase: increased risk of relapse associated with T-cell depletion. *Ann Intern Med* 1988; **108**: 806–814.
12. Barrett AJ, Joshi R and Tew C. How should acute lymphoblastic leukaemia relapsing after bone marrow transplantation be treated? *Lancet* 1985; **i**: 1188–1191.
13. Fialkow PJ, Thomas ED, Bryant JI and Neiman PE. Leukaemic transformation of engrafted human marrow cells *in vivo*. *Lancet* 1971; **1**: 251–255.
14. Thomas ED, Bryant JI, Buckner CD *et al.* Leukaemic transformation of engrafted human marrow cells *in vivo*. *Lancet* 1972; **1**: 1310–1313.
15. Goh K and Klemperer MR. *In vivo* leukemia transformation: cytogenetic evidence of *in vivo* leukemic transformation of engrafted marrow cells. *Am J Hematol* 1977; **2**: 283–290.
16. Elfenbein GJ, Brogaonkar DS, Bias WB *et al.* Cytogenetic evidence for recurrence of acute myelogenous leukemia after allogeneic bone marrow transplantation in donor hematopoietic cells. *Blood* 1978; **52**: 627–636.
17. Newburger PE, Latt SA, Pesando JM *et al.* Leukemia relapse in donor cells after allogeneic bone marrow transplantation. *New Engl J Med* 1981; **304**: 712–714.
18. Marmont AM, Frassoni F, Bacigalupo A *et al.* Recurrence of Philadelphia-positive leukemia in donor cells after marrow transplantation for chronic granulocytic leukemia. *New Engl J Med* 1984; **310**: 903–906.
19. Lapidot T, Sirard C, Vormoor J *et al.* A cell initiating human acute myeloid leukaemia after transplantation into SCID mice. *Nature* 1994; **367**: 645–648.
20. Buckner CD, Clift RA, Appelbaum F *et al.* A randomized study comparing two transplant regimens for CML in chronic phase. *Blood* 1992; **80**: 72 (Abstr).
21. Blaise D, Maraninchi D, Archimbaud E *et al.* Allogeneic bone marrow transplantation for acute myeloid leukemia in first remission. A randomized trial of busulfan–cytoxan versus cytoxan–total body irradiation as preparative regimen. A report of the Group d' Etudes de la Greffe de Moelle Osseuse. *Blood* 1992; **79**: 2578–2582.
22. Ringden O, Ruutu T, Nikoskelainen J *et al.* and the Nordic BMT Group. A randomized trial comparing busulfan with total body irradiation as conditioning in allogeneic bone marrow transplant recipients with leukemia. A report from the Nordic Bone Marrow Transplantation Group. *Blood* 1994; **83**: 2723–2730.
23. Clift RA, Buckner CD, Appelbaum F *et al.* Allogeneic marrow transplantation in patients with acute myeloid leukemia in first remission: a randomized trial of two radiation regimens. *Blood* 1990; **76**: 1867–1871.
24. Blume KG, Kopecky KJ, Henslee-Downey PJ. A prospective randomized comparison of total body irradiation-etoposide versus busulfan–cyclophosphamide as preparatory regimens for bone marrow transplantation in patients with leukemia who were not in first remission: a Southwest Oncology Group Study. *Blood* 1993; **81**: 2187–2193.
25. Marmont AM, Horowitz MM, Gale RP *et al.* T-cell depletion of HLA-identical transplants in leukemia. *Blood* 1991; **78**: 2120–2130.
26. Barnes DHW and Loutit JF. Treatment of murine leukaemia with X-rays and homologous bone marrow. *Br J Haematol* 1957; **3**: 241–252.
27. Mathé G, Amiel JL, Schwarzenberg L, Cattan A and Schneider M. Adoptive immunotherapy of acute leukemia:

Experimental and clinical results. *Cancer Res* 1965; **25**: 1525–1530.

28. Weiden PL, Sullivan KM, Flournoy N, Storb R, Thomas ED and The Seattle Marrow Transplant Team. Antileukemic effect of chronic graft-versus-host disease. Contribution to improved survival after allogeneic marrow transplantation. *New Engl J Med* 1981; **304**: 1529–1531.
29. Fefer A, Sullivan KM, Weiden PL, Buckner CD, Schoch G, Storb R and Thomas ED. Graft-versus-leukemia effect in man: the relapse rate of acute leukemia is lower after allogeneic than after syngeneic marrow transplantation. *Prog Clin Biol Res* 1987; **244**: 401–408.
30. Gale RP, Horowitz MM, Ash R *et al*. Identical twin bone marrow transplantation for leukemia. *Ann Intern Med* 1994; **120**: 646–652.
31. Kernan NA, Bartsch G, Ash RC *et al*. Analysis of 462 transplantations from unrelated donors facilitated by the National Marrow Donor Program. *New Engl J Med* 1993; **328**: 593–602.
32. McGlave P, Bartsch G, Anasetti C, Ash R, Beatty P, Gajewski J and Kernan NA. Unrelated donor marrow transplantation therapy for chronic myelogenous leukemia: initial experience of the National Marrow Donor Program. *Blood* 1993; **81**: 543–550.
33. Odom LF, August CS, Githens JH *et al*. Remission of relapsed leukemia during a graft-versus-host reaction. A graft-versus-leukemia reaction in man? *Lancet* 1978; **ii**: 537–540.
34. Collins RH, Rogers Z, Bennett M, Kumar V, Nikein A and Fay JW. Hematologic relapse of chronic myelogenous leukemia following allogeneic bone marrow transplantation: apparent graft-versus-leukemia effect following abrupt discontinuation of immunosuppression. *Bone Marrow Transplant* 1992; **10**: 391–395.
35. Higano CS, Brixey M, Bryant EM, Durnam DM, Doney K, Sullivan KM and Singer JW. Durable complete remission of acute nonlymphocytic leukemia associated with discontinuation of immunosuppression following relapse after allogeneic bone marrow transplantation. A case report of a probable graft-versus-leukemia effect. *Transplantation* 1990; **50**: 175–177.
36. Mortimer J, Blinder MA, Schulman S *et al*. Relapse of acute leukemia after marrow transplantation: natural history and results of subsequent therapy. *J Clin Oncol* 1989; **7**: 50–57.
37. Doney K, Fisher L, Appelbaum F *et al*. Treatment of adult acute lymphoblastic leukemia with allogeneic bone marrow transplantation. Multivariate analysis of factors affecting acute graft-versus-host disease, relapse and relapse-free survival. *Bone Marrow Transplant* 1991; **7**: 453–459.
38. Thomas ED, Clift RA, Fefer A *et al*. Marrow transplantation for the treatment of chronic myelogenous leukemia. *Ann Intern Med* 1986; **104**: 155–163.
39. Goldman JM, Apperley J, Jones L *et al*. Bone marrow transplantation for patients with chronic myeloid leukemia. *New Engl J Med* 1986; **314**: 202–207.
40. Lin F, van Rhee F, Goldman JM and Cross NCP. Kinetics of increasing BCR-ABL transcript numbers in chronic myeloid leukemia patients who relapse after bone marrow transplantation. *Blood* 1996; **87**: 4473–4478.
41. Collins RHJ, Rogers ZR, Bennett M, Kumar V, Nikein A and Fay JW. Hematologic relapse of chronic myelogenous leukemia following allogeneic bone marrow transplantation: apparent graft-versus-leukemia effect following abrupt discontinuation of immunosuppression. *Bone Marrow Transplant* 1992; **10**: 391–395.
42. Bacigalupo A, van Lint MT, Occhini D *et al*. Increased risk of leukemia relapse with high-dose cyclosporine A after allogeneic marrow transplantation for acute leukemia. *Blood* 1991; **77**: 1423–1428.
43. Frassoni F, Barrett AJ, Granena A *et al*. Relapse after allogeneic bone marrow transplantation for acute leukaemia: a survey by the EBMT of 117 cases. *Br J Haematol* 1988; **70**: 317–320.
44. Bostrom B, Woods WG, Nesbit ME *et al*. Successful reinduction of patients with acute lymphoblastic leukemia who relapse following bone marrow transplantation. *J Clin Oncol* 1987; **5**: 376–381.
45. Mittermüller J, Kolb HJ, Gerhartz HH and Wilmanns W. *In vivo* differentiation of leukemic blasts and effect of low dose ara-c in a marrow grafted patient with leukemic relapse. *Br J Haematol* 1986; **62**: 757–762.
46. Mittermüller J, Kolb HJ, Clemm C *et al*. Chimerism and treatment of recurrent leukemia after marrow transplantation. *J Cancer Res Clin Oncol* 1990; **116**: 577 (abstr).
47. Bertino JR and Goker E. Drug resistance in acute leukemia. *Leukaemia Lymphoma* 1993; **11**: 37–41.
48. Bekassy AN, Hermans J, Gorin NC and Gratwohl A. EBMT. Granulocytic sarcoma after allogeneic bone marrow transplantation: a retrospective European multicenter survey. *Bone Marrow Transplant* 1996; **17**: 801–808.
49. Chak LY, Sapozink MD and Cox R. Extramedullary lesions in non-lymphocytic leukemia: results of radiation therapy. *Int J Radiat Oncol Biol Phys* 1983; **9**: 1173–1176.
50. Bowman W, Aur R, Hustu H and Rivera G. Isolated testicular relapse relapse in acute lymphocytic leukemia of childhood: categories and influence on survival. *J Clin Oncol* 1984; **2**: 924–929.
51. Uckun F, Ramsay NKC, Waddick K *et al*. *In vitro* and *in vivo* radiation resistance associated with CD3 surface antigen expression in T-lineage acute lymphoblastic leukemia. *Blood* 1991; **78**: 2945–2955.
52. Giralt S, Escudier S, Kantarijan H *et al*. Preliminary results of treatment with filgastrim for relapse of leukemia and myelodysplasia after allogeneic bone marrow transplantation. *New Engl J Med* 1993; **329**: 757–761.
53. Giralt SA and Champlin RE. Leukemia relapse after allogeneic bone marrow transplantation: a review. *Blood* 1994; **84**: 3603–3612.
54. Metcalf D. Clonal analysis of the action of GM-CSF on the proliferation and differentiation of myelomonocytic leukemic cells. *Int J Cancer* 1979; **24**: 616–623.
55. Widmer-Pack MD, Olivier W, Valinski J, Schuler G and Steinman RM. Granulocyte–macrophage colony stimulating factor is essential for the viability and function of cultured murine epidermal Langerhans cells. *J Exp Med* 1987; **166**: 1494–1498.
56. Arcese W, Mauro FR, Alimena G *et al*. Interferon therapy for Ph1-positive CML patients relapsing after T-cell depleted allogeneic bone marrow transplantation. *Bone Marrow Transplant* 1990; **5**: 309–315.
57. Arcese W, Goldman JM, DArcangelo E *et al*. Outcome for patients who relapse after allogeneic bone marrow transplantation for chronic myeloid leukemia. *Blood* 1993; **82**: 3211–3219.

58. Higano CS, Raskind WH and Singer JW. Use of alpha interferon for the treatment of relapse of chronic myelogenous leukemia in chronic phase after allogeneic marrow transplantation. *Blood* 1992; **80**: 1437–1442.
59. Dowding C, Guo AP, Osterholz J, Siczkowski M, Goldman J and Gordon M. Interferon-alpha overrides the deficient adhesion of chronic myeloid leukemia primitive progenitor cells to bone marrow stromal cells. *Blood* 1991; **78**: 499–505.
60. Baron S, Tyring SK, Fleischmann WR et al. The interferons – mechanism of action and clinical applications. *J Am Med Ass* 1991; **266**: 1375–1383.
61. Palva IP, Almqvist A, Elonen E et al. Value of maintenance therapy with chemotherapy or interferon during remission of acute myeloid leukemia. *Eur J Haematol* 1991; **47**: 229–233.
62. Kolb HJ, Schattenberg A, Goldman JM et al. Graft-versus-leukemia effect of donor lymphocyte transfusions in marrow grafted patients. *Blood* 1995; **86**: 2041–2050.
63. Lotzova E, Savary CA and Herberman RB. Induction of NK cell activity against fresh human leukemia in culture with interleukin 2. *J Immunol* 1987; **138**: 2718–2727.
64. Charak BS, Brynes RK, Chogyoji M, Kortes V, Tefft M and Mazumder A. Graft versus leukemia effect after transplantation with interleukin-2-activated bone marrow. Correlation with eradication of residual disease. *Transplantation* 1993; **56**: 31–37.
65. Slavin S, Naparstek E, Nagler A et al. Allogeneic cell therapy with donor peripheral blood cells and recombinant human interleukin-2 to treat leukemia relapse after allogeneic bone marrow transplantation. *Blood* 1996; **87**: 2195–2204.
66. Soiffer R, Murray C, Cochran K et al. Clinical and immunological effects of prolonged infusions of low dose recombinant interleukin-2 after autologous and T-cell depleted allogeneic bone marrow transplantation. *Blood* 1992; **79**: 517–526.
67. Verdonck LF, van Heugten HG, Giltay J and Franks CR. Amplification of the graft-versus-leukemia effect in man by interleukin-2. *Transplantation* 1991; **51**: 1120–1124.
68. Charak BS, Choudary G, Tefft M and Mazumder A. Interleukin-2 in bone marrow transplantation: preclinical studies. *Bone Marrow Transplant* 1992; **10**: 103–111.
69. Fefer A, Benyunes MC, York A, Buckner CD and Thompson JA. Use of interleukin-2 after bone marrow transplantation. *Bone Marrow Transplant* 1995; **15**(Suppl 1): S162–S166.
70. Blaise D, Olive D, Stoppa A et al. Hematologic and immunologic effects of the systemic administration of recombinant interleukin-2 after autologous bone marrow transplantation for hematological malignancies. *Blood* 1990; **76**: 1092–1097.
71. Foa R, Meloni G, Tosti S, Novarino A, Fern S and Gavosta F. Treatment of acute myelogenous leukaemia patients with recombinant interleukin-2: a pilot study. *Br J Haematol* 1991; **77**: 491–496.
72. Lönnqvist B, Brune M and Ljungman P. Lymphoblastoid human interferon and low dose IL-2 combined with donor lymphocyte infusion as therapy of a third relapse of CML – a case report. *Bone Marrow Transplant* 1996; **18**: 241–242.
73. Wright SE, Thomas ED, Buckner CD, Clift RA and Fefer A. Experience with second marrow transplants. *Exp Haematol* 1976; **4**: 221–226.
74. Blume KG and Forman SJ. High dose busulfan/etoposide as a preparative regimen for second bone marrow transplants in hematologic malignancies. *Blut* 1987; **55**: 49–53.
75. Atkinson K, Biggs JC, Dodds A et al. Second marrow transplants for recurrence of haematological malignancy. *Bone Marrow Transplant* 1985; **1**: 159–166.
76. Champlin RE, Ho W, Lenarsky C, Mitsuyasu R, Feig S and Gale RP. Successful second bone marrow transplantation for AML or ALL. *Transplant Proc* 1985; **17**: 496–499.
77. Marmont AM, van Lint MT, Frassoni F and Bacigalupo A. Second bone marrow transplants for relapsed leukaemia after allogeneic bone marrow transplantation. *Bone Marrow Transplant* 1988; **3**(Suppl 1): 332–333.
78. Barrett AJ, Locatelli F, Treleaven JG, Gratwohl A, Szydlo R and Zwaan FE. Second transplants for leukaemic relapse after bone marrow transplantation: high early mortality but favorable effect of chronic GvHD on continued remission. *Br J Haematol* 1991; **79**: 567–574.
79. Cullis JO, Schwarer AP, Hughes TP et al. Second transplants for patients with chronic myeloid leukaemia in relapse after original transplant with T-depleted donor marrow: feasibility of using busulphan alone for re-conditioning. *Br J Haematol* 1992; **80**: 33–39.
80. Spinolo JA, Yau JC, Dicke KA et al. Second bone marrow transplants for relapsed leukemia. *Cancer* 1992; **69**: 405–409.
81. Hashimoto S, Nakaseko T, Asai T et al. Second bone marrow transplantation for hematological malignancies. *Exp Haematol* 1992; **20**: 715 (Abstr).
82. Wagner JE, Vogelsang GB, Zehnbauer BA et al. Relapse of leukemia after bone marrow transplantation: effect of second myeloablative therapy. *Bone Marrow Transplant* 1992; **9**: 205–209.
83. Shing MMK and Vowels MR. Role of second bone marrow transplants. *Bone Marrow Transplant* 1993; **12**: 21–25.
84. Radich JP, Sanders JE, Buckner CD et al. Second allogeneic marrow transplantation for patients with recurrent leukemia after initial transplant with total body irradiation-containing regimens. *J Clin Oncol* 1993; **11**: 304–313.
85. Lalit K. Leukemia: management of relapse after allogeneic bone marrow transplantation. *J Clin Oncol* 1994; **12**: 1710–1717.
86. Mrsic M, Horowitz MM, Atkinson K et al. Second HLA-identical sibling transplants for leukemia recurrence. *Bone Marrow Transplant* 1992; **9**: 269–275.
87. Chiang KY, Weisdorf D, Davies SM et al. Outcome of second bone marrow transplantation following a uniform conditioning regimen as therapy for malignant relapse. *Bone Marrow Transplant* 1996; **17**: 39–42.
88. Martinez JA, Picon I, Carral A, de la Rubia J, Sanz GF and Sanz MA. Allogeneic peripheral blood progenitor cells mobilized by G-CSF (filgastrim) for a second transplant in a patient with acute myeloid leukemia in relapse. *Bone Marrow Transplant* 1995; **15**: 149–151.
89. Weiden PL, Storb R, Tsoi M-S, Graham TC, Lerner KG and Thomas ED. Infusion of donor lymphocytes into stable canine radiation chimeras: implications for mechanism of transplantation tolerance. *J Immunol* 1976; **116**: 1212–1219.
90. Kolb HJ, Beisser K, Mittermueller J et al. Adoptive immunotherapy in human and canine chimeras. In: *Acute Leukemias – Pharmacokinetics*. W Hiddemann, T Büchner and W Plunkett et al. (eds), 1992: 595–600 (Berlin: Springer).

91. Johnson BD, Drobyski WR and Truitt RL. Delayed infusion of normal donor cells after MHC-matched bone marrow transplantation provides an antileukemia reaction without graft-versus-host disease. *Bone Marrow Transplant* 1993; **11**: 329–336.
92. Kolb HJ, Mittermueller J, Clemm C, Ledderose G, Brehm G, Heim M and Wilmanns W. Donor leukocyte transfusions for treatment of recurrent chronic myelogenous leukemia in marrow transplant patients. *Blood* 1990; **76**: 2462–2465.
93. Verdonck LF, Lokhorst HM, Dekker AW, Nieuwenhuis HK and Petersen EF. Graft-versus-myeloma effect in two cases. *Lancet* 1996; **347**: 800–801.
94. Tricot G, Vesole DH, Jagannath S, Hilton J, Munshi N and Barlogie B. Graft-versus-myeloma effect: Proof of principle. *Blood* 1996; **87**: 1196–1198.
95. Porter DL, Roth MS, Lee SJ, McGarigle C, Ferrara JLM and Antin JH. Adoptive immunotherapy with donor mononuclear cell infusions to treat relapse of acute leukemia or myelodysplasia after allogeneic bone marrow transplantation. *Bone Marrow Transplant* 1996; **18**: 975–980.
96. Anderson KC and Weinstein HJ. Transfusion-associated graft-versus-host disease. *New Engl J Med* 1990; **323**: 315–321.
97. Flowers M *et al*. Use of peripheral blood stem cells for immune therapy. *Blood* 1995 (Abstract).
98. Mackinnon S, Papadopoulos EB, Carabasi MH *et al*. Adoptive immunotherapy evaluating escalating doses of donor leukocytes for relapse of chronic myeloid leukemia after bone marrow transplantation: separation of graft-versus-leukemia responses from graft-versus-host disease. *Blood* 1995; **86**: 1261–1268.
99. van Rhee F and Goldman JM. Donor lymphocyte therapy in bone marrow transplantation. In: *Cell Therapy – Stem Cell Transplantation, Gene Therapy, and Cellular Immunotherapy*. G Morstyn and W Sheridan (eds), 1996: 550–567 (Cambridge: Cambridge University Press).
100. Giralt S, Hester J, Huh Y *et al*. CD8-depleted donor lymphocyte infusion as treatment for relapsed chronic myelogenous leukemia after allogeneic bone marrow transplantation. *Blood* 1995; **86**: 4337–4343.
101. Alyea EP, Canning C, Collins H *et al*. Efficacy and toxicity of CD4 positive donor T-lymphocyte transfusion for treatment of relapsed chronic myelogenous leukemia (CML) after allogeneic BMT. *Blood* 1996; **88**(Suppl 1): 682 (Abstr).
102. Jiang YZ, Cullis JO, Kanfer EJ, Goldman JM and Barrett AJ. T-cell and NK cell mediated graft-versus-leukaemia reactivity following donor buffy coat transfusion to treat relapse after marrow transplantation for chronic myeloid leukaemia. *Bone Marrow Transplant* 1993; **11**: 133–138.
103. Bunjes D, Hertenstein B, Wiesneth M, Novotny J, Frickhofen N, Arnold R and Heimpel H. Donor lymphocyte transfusions and low-dose interleukin-2 in 2 patients with relapsed CML after syngeneic BMT. *Bone Marrow Transplant* 1996; **17**(Suppl 1): S9 (Abstr).
104. Bocchia M, Korontsvit T, Xu Q, Mackinnon S, Yang SY, Sette A and Scheinberg DA. Specific human cellular immunity to *bcr–abl* oncogene-derived peptides. *Blood* 1996; **87**: 3587–3592.
105. Mannering SI, McKenzie JL and Hart DN. Generation of T-lymphocyte clones specific for the BCR–ABL fusion peptide presented by dendritic cells and other antigen presenting cells. *Bone Marrow Transplant* 1996; **17**(Suppl 1): S59 (Abstr).
106. Voogt PJ, Goulmy E, Veenhof WFJ, Hamilton M, Fibbe WE, Van Rood JJ and Falkenburg JHF. Cellularly defined minor histocompatibility antigens are differentially expressed on human hematopoietic progenitor cells. *J Exp Med* 1988; **168**: 2337–2347.
107. Bonini C, Ferrari G, Verzelletti S *et al*. HSV-TK Gene transfer into donor lymphocytes for control of allogenic graft-versus-leukaemia. *Science* 1997; **276**: 1719–1724.
108. Rooney CM, Smith CA, Ng CYC, Loftin SK, Li CL, Krance RA, Brenner MK and Heslop HE. Use of gene-modified virus-specific T lymphocytes to control Epstein–Barr-virus-related lymphoproliferation. *Lancet* 1995; **345**: 9–13.

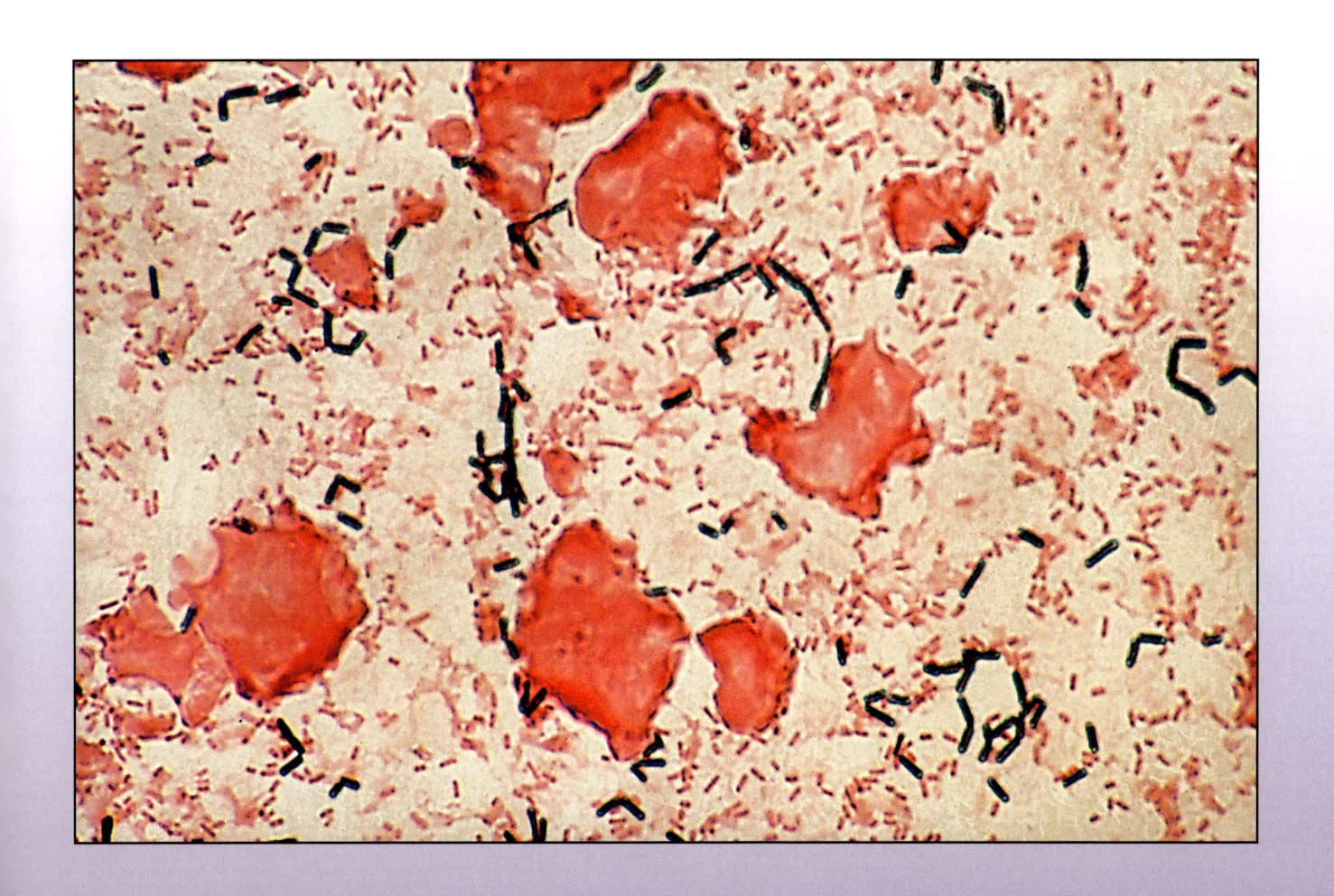

Chapter 43
Bacterial infections

Unell Riley

Introduction

Infection is one of the most significant complications of bone-marrow transplantation. The bone-marrow transplant recipient is immunocompromised for a number of reasons (Table 43.1), the most important in the early phase of transplantation being neutropenia and anatomic-barrier disruption of mucosal surfaces and the integument.

Table 43.1 Factors involved in immunosuppression in bone-marrow transplantation

- Disruption of the anatomic barrier
- Neutropenia
- Dysfunction of cellular immunity
- Dysfunction of humoral immunity
- Hyposplenism

Anatomic-barrier disruption

The intact skin and mucosa are vital for the protection of the individual from bacterial infection and this barrier can be disrupted in a number of ways (Table 43.2). Cytotoxic agents and irradiation can lead to mucositis and also ciliary dysfunction which predisposes to pneumonia [1–3]. Iatrogenic causes of skin disruption are becoming more common with the universal use of long-term tunnelled venous catheters in the management of these patients. These devices have distinct advantages for patients and medical and nursing staff, but there are many complications, the most important of which is infection. Portals of entry

Table 43.2 Causes of skin and mucosa disruption

- Damage to skin by venepuncture or bone-marrow aspiration
- Indwelling intravenous catheters
- Mucosal damage by bronchoscopy/endoscopy
- Mucosal damage by cytotoxic agents or irradiation

Table 43.3 Possible sites for entry of infection with central venous catheters

- Catheter exit sites
- Catheter/giving set junction
- During change of intravenous fluid container
- Contamination of Y-junction, heparinized flush solution, etc.
- Contaminated fluid container

for infection are listed in Table 43.3, but the most important is the catheter insertion site. These infections manifest themselves in three ways:
- exit site infection.
- tunnel infection.
- catheter-associated bacteraemia or septicaemia.

Neutropenia

It has been known for some time that neutropenia is associated with an increased risk of bacterial infection [4]; this is particularly true after the total neutrophil count has fallen below 0.5×10^9/litre. The risk is greater still if neutropenia is prolonged (more than seven days), profound ($<0.1 \times 10^9$/litre) and if the fall in the neutrophil count is rapid, all of which occur in bone-marrow transplantation [5].

The combination of neutropenia and anatomic-barrier disruption allow bacteria to cross damaged mucosa and skin and cause localized or disseminated infection. The most common sites for entrance and localized infection are the skin, peri-anal area, distal oesophagus, colon, periodontium, oropharynx and lung (Table 43.4).

The organisms

The usual source of infecting organisms is from established colonization, often from the patient's endogenous flora, or from bacteria acquired in the hospital environment [6,7]; 50% of infections are due to hospital-acquired organisms. This is especially true if the patient has already received broad-spectrum antibiotics. There is some evidence that previous antibiotics can reduce the protective function of

Table 43.4 Common sites for entrance of infection and localized infection

- Skin
- Peri-anal area
- Distal oesophagus
- Colon
- Periodontium
- Oropharynx
- Lung

anaerobes in the gut lumen and allow more antimicrobial-resistant, nosocomial bacteria to colonize and translocate across the gut wall in the presence of an intact mucosa [8,9].

The majority of infections in neutropenic, mucosa-damaged patients are caused by *Pseudomonas aeruginosa*, *Escherichia coli*, *Klebsiella* spp., coagulase-negative staphylococci, *Staphylococcus aureus* and *Streptococcus* spp.

Sepsis caused by aerobic gram-negative bacilli such as the Enterobacteriaceae and *Pseudomonas aeruginosa* have traditionally been the most feared type of infection with their propensity to cause overwhelming sepsis, leading to toxaemia, in a neutropenic patient. However, since the 1980s there has been a shift in the spectrum of bacterial infections such that infections due to Gram-positive bacteria have become more common than those due to Gram-negative bacilli [10]. This is probably due to a number of factors including the widespread use of central venous catheters, possibly the greater use of cytotoxic agents causing more mucositis, and increased use of fluoroquinolones as prophylaxis. Some centres have also reported a reduced incidence of infection due to *Pseudomonas aeruginosa*.

Gram-negative infection usually manifests itself as a septicaemia-like illness. However, Enterobacteriaceae, in particular, can cause localized infection in the peri-anal area and repeated localized sepsis should prompt a search for peri-anal lesions such as peri-anal fissures or haemorrhoids. The most serious localized infection in bone-marrow transplantation is that due to *Pseudomonas aeruginosa*. This can take a number of forms, the most common being ecthyma gangrenosum lesions which are vasculitic skin lesions with a necrotic centre, caused by subcutaneous invasion by the organism [11]. They can occur as a metastatic manifestation of *Pseudomonas aeruginosa* septicaemia, or as a primary skin lesion. Similar lesions have been produced by *Aspergillus* spp. [12,13], mucormycosis [14] and *Candida* spp. [15] *Pseudomonas aeroginosa* has also been associated with buccal and orbital cellulitis.

Gram-positive bacterial isolates are now the most common during the neutropenia following bone-marrow transplantation. Most commonly they are due to *Staphylococcus epidermidis*, and this is thought to be due to wide use of long-term central venous catheters. *Staphylococcus epidermidis* can readily colonize these devices producing a very thick glycocalyx [16] which is protective and makes eradication of the bacteria from the line by antibiotics very difficult. Although usually considered of low virulence, in this setting they can produce repeated bacteraemias, tunnel catheter infections and even progress to large-vein thrombophlebitis with occlusion, and bacterial endocarditis.

Other causes of line-associated infection are *Staphylococcus aureus*, *Corynebacterium jeikeium* and *Bacillus* spp. which can also cause serious sepsis in neutropenic patients. *Staphylococcus aureus* is an important cause of sepsis, as it can gain access through broken skin and mucosa, and can cause septicaemia as well as localized lesions in the line, skin or in the lungs. It is important to note that although most infections caused by *Staphylococcus aureus* are acquired by patients endogenously, they can also acquire *Staphylococcus aureus* readily from exogenous sources in the form of a hospital-acquired infection. These organisms are commonly more resistant, such as methicillin-resistant *Staphylococcus aureus* (MRSA).

Line infection with *Corynebacterium jeikeium* can lead to metastatic abscesses in the subcutaneous soft tissue and muscle [17–20], which can be difficult to treat since these bacteria are intrinsically highly resistant. The environmental pseudomonads can also cause line infections. These organisms are often multiply resistant to antibiotics. For example, *Stenotrophomonas maltophilia* [21] is intrinsically resistant to carbapenems.

Alpha-haemolytic streptococci are now being increasingly recognized as a significant cause of sepsis in the neutropenic patient [22-25]. *Streptococcus mitis* has been associated with adult respiratory distress syndrome (ARDS) and a septic shock syndrome [2,26,27]. *Streptococcus sanguis* has been associated with severe oral mucositis. There is particular concern that these types of infections are often seen in patients receiving prophylaxis with ciprofloxacin [28,29].

Diagnosis of infection

Diagnosis is particularly difficult in bone-marrow transplant patients due to the lack of clinical signs and symptoms [30]. In severe neutropenia, there may be no abscess formation, pus or inflammation where there is a localized infection. In the management of infection in the bone-marrow transplant patient, the results of clinical examination and history-taking, in addition to microbiological findings, are important. Fever still remains the main indicator for initiation of antibiotic therapy. The degree of fever which should trigger antibiotic treatment is ill-defined but in general, a single axillary temperature of 38.5°C, or two consecutive temperatures of >37.5°C when blood products have not been given should lead to initiation of therapy. Clinical evidence of an infection site should also be sought, particularly in known risk areas such as the peri-anal area, lungs, skin, central venous catheter exit site and the oropharynx. Tachycardia, breathlessness and inadequate organ function can also be indicators of infection. Adult respiratory distress syndrome can be a manifestation of sepsis. A chest X-ray taken at the onset of fever may not always show lung infiltrates and should therefore be repeated in cases of persistent fever [31]. C-reactive protein may help in the differentiation of fever due to bacterial and fungal infection rather than other causes [32,33]. C-reactive protein is usually specific for bacterial and fungal infections, and thus a fall in C-reactive protein may indicate a response to treatment, and a rise, a persistent secondary infection or non-response to empirical therapy.

Microbiological investigation should include taking blood cultures. Ideally at least 20 ml of blood should be taken to detect low levels of bacteraemia. The specificity of the blood culture may be reduced if taken through a catheter which may be colonized by coagulase-negative staphylococci. Sets of blood cultures should be taken, peripherally and from each lumen of the central venous catheter, before commencement of empirical therapy.

Quantitative blood culture methods may be useful for differentiating bacteraemia due to the central venous catheter or from a tissue source; however, this requires labour-intensive methods and is expensive [34]. Microbiological samples should also be taken from suspected sites of infection and may include exit site swabs, urine samples and sputum samples.

The role of surveillance cultures

Surveillance cultures have sometimes been used to monitor infection problems in bone-marrow transplant patients. Since there is evidence that colonization precedes infection [35], it is to be expected that surveillance cultures are able to predict causative organisms, influence empirical regimens which are used for treatment of febrile neutropenia, detect the presence of multiple resistant organisms (including MRSA and vancomycin-resistant enterococci) and to monitor the efficacy of gut decontamination. However, information gained from surveillance has proved disappointing in that the causative agent of infection is rarely predicted [36]. Routine surveillance cultures are also time-consuming and expensive if performed properly and can escalate to a large number of samples being sent weekly from the same patient.

The isolation of *Pseudomonas aeruginosa*, *Aspergillus* and non-albicans *Candida* spp. [37,38], however, may be helpful in the management of the neutropenic patient. Therefore, surveillance cultures should probably be limited to weekly samples from the nose to detect colonization due to *Staphylococcus aureus* and *Aspergillus* spp., catheter exit site swabs to detect heavy growth of staphylococci or environmental pseudomonads, and throat and stool samples to detect colonization with *Candida* spp., to check the efficacy of gut decontamination and to monitor the resistance patterns of any isolated aerobic Gram-negative bacilli.

Empirical antimicrobial chemotherapy

Since the 1960s, it has been realized that there can be significant mortality due to Gram-negative sepsis in the neutropenic patient if antibiotic therapy is delayed.

With the introduction of effective empirical therapy promptly at the onset of fever, a marked reduction in mortality rates has occurred [39,40]. The antibiotic regimen chosen should be bactericidal and also broad spectrum to provide cover for the aerobic Gram-negative bacilli such as *Pseudomonas aeruginosa*, *Klebsiella pneumoniae* and *Escherichia coli*, which are the most feared and can cause mortality in this situation.

A number of empirical regimens have been evaluated in clinical trials. The earliest used, and probably still the most popular, is a beta-lactam with anti-pseudomonal activity, in combination with an aminoglycoside [39–42]. The first beta-lactams used consisted of ureidopenicillins, such as piperacillin, but now also include highly active beta-lactams which are also more stable against beta-lactamases. These include third-generation cephalosporins such as ceftazidime, and the carbapenems such as imipenem and meropenem.

This combination has the advantage that it may provide a bactericidal synergy and also reduce the emergence of resistance. However, disadvantages include the nephrotoxicity and toxicity associated aminoglycosides, and the cost and inconvenience of monitoring levels. However, most toxicity has occurred with the traditional method of multidose administration of aminoglycosides, and there is recent evidence showing that once-daily aminoglycoside dosing is as effective as multiple dosing, while producing less nephrotoxicity [43]. Although there is little documented evidence of any efficacy in bone-marrow transplant recipients, this mode of administration may represent an advance [44].

Double beta-lactam combinations have also been used [45]. Here, the main concerns revolve around development of resistance, since the site of action within the antibiotics is the same, and certain beta-lactam combinations can actually be antagonistic for particular Enterobacteriaceae [46,47]. This may potentially be overcome by the combination of a beta-lactam with a quinolone such as ciprofloxacin [48].

There has been increasing interest in the use of monotherapy for the treatment of febrile neutropenia. A number of studies, with the help of meta-analysis, have shown that ceftazidime has an equivalent efficacy in treatment as compared with combination therapy [49]. This has also been shown in other trials for imipenem [45], meropenem [50] and ceftazidime [51]. However, most of these studies have not been conducted on bone-marrow transplant recipients where the degree of neutropenia is more severe, and length of neutropenia is much longer. Thus, the efficacy of monotherapy in bone-marrow transplant patients is still questioned.

There are conflicting ideas concerning the use of intravenous ciprofloxacin empirically, although a randomized study showed reasonable efficacy of monotherapy [52]. However, the European Organisation for Research and Treatment of Cancer had to discontinue a study due to an unacceptably high mortality rate and most failings were due to Gram-positive infections [53]. These problems may be overcome by combining ciprofloxacin with either a glycopeptide or a ureidopenicillin [48] The use of ciprofloxacin for empirical therapy will always be constrained by its use as a prophylactic agent.

With the increasing incidence of Gram-positive infections in the febrile neutropenic patient, glycopeptide treatment has been advocated as having a role to play in initial empirical therapy. A number of randomized clinical trials have shown that there is no survival advantage with the addition of a glycopeptide, such as vancomycin, to the initial therapy in febrile neutropenia [54–56].

A further consideration is the increase in vancomycin-resistant enterococci in oncology and bone-marrow transplant units [57]. These organisms are generally multiresistant and there are very few antibiotic treatment options if they cause clinical infection. There appears to be an association between heavy vancomycin usage and an increased incidence of vancomycin-resistant enterococci [57,58]. It is felt that use of these antibiotics in empirical therapy can still be reserved for suspected line and skin sepsis or where a particular institution has a high incidence of MRSA or *Streptococcus mitis* infection [59].

Ultimately, the choice of an empirical regimen depends upon the presentation of infections and the resistance patterns of the organisms commonly seen in a particular institution. Modifications to the empirical therapy regimen may be needed depending upon the nature of the infection and fever presentation. For example, in severe gingivitis or peridontal infection, addition of an anti-anaerobic agent may be appropriate, whereas a glycopeptide may be indicated for a catheter-associated infection. However, use as empirical therapy of a beta-lactam agent such as imipenem which possesses anaerobic activity in addition to anti-staphylococcal activity, may make this unnecessary.

After empirical therapy has been started, it should only be modified when there is a clearly defined reason for so doing, such as no improvement in fever despite proper antibiotic dosing, persistent clinical signs or symptoms, clinical deterioration or the isolation of pathogens which are either resistant to empirical therapy or persist despite empirical therapy. The decision for change should also be made on the basis of daily evaluation of the patient. When there is microbiological evidence for the cause of infection, treatment should be tailored to treat this specifically when sensitivities are available. Again, modification in treatment depends upon the isolate and the suspected site of infection. For instance, in *Staphylococcus aureus* septicaemia, treatment should include a specific anti-staphylococcal agent for 14 days [60,61]. If there is no microbiological isolate, a decision should be made concerning the changing or modification of empirical therapy. Although it may take four days for a sensitive infection to respond to treatment during neutropenia, 72 hours is a reasonable time to try an empiric regimen and to await positive microbiology results. A change to a different broad spectrum antibacterial agent may be considered, but this should be dependent upon organisms and resistance patterns in individual institutions.

Since non-bacterial causes of infection, particularly fungal, are also common in immunosuppressed patients, the addition of a non-bacterial agent should be considered. It should also be remembered in bone-marrow transplantation, where prolonged neutropenia is the norm, that patients often have more than one febrile episode, commonly originating from a different site or being caused by more resistant organisms than those which led to the initial febrile episode. Strategies for empirical antibiotic therapy must take all these factors into account.

Duration of treatment in patients with fever of unknown origin who have shown a good response to antimicrobials is also a contentious issue. Some would suggest continuing antibiotic therapy for 14 days or until the patient's neutrophil count rises above 0.5×10^9/litre. This, however, leaves the patient at risk of toxicity secondary to the antibiotic therapy and many would advocate a minimum of seven days treatment with four consecutive afebrile days and with no residual evidence of localized infection.

References

1. Dyhedal I and Lamvik J. Respiratory insufficiency in acute leukaemia following treatment with cytosine arabinoside and septicaemia with *Streptococcus viridans*. *Eur J Haematol* 1989; **42**: 405–406.
2. Arning M, Gehrt A, Aul C et al. Septicaemia due to *Streptococcus mitis* in neutropenic patients in acute leukaemia. *Blut* 1990; **61**: 364–368.
3. Kern W, Jurrie E and Schmeiser T. Streptococcal bacteraemia in adult patients with leukaemia undergoing aggressive chemotherapy: a review of 55 cases. *Infection* 1990; **18**: 138–145.
4. Bodey GP, Buckley M, Sathe YS et al. Qualitative relationship between circulating leucocytes and infections in patients with acute leukaemia. *Ann Intern Med* 1966; **64**: 328–340.
5. Schimpff SC. Therapy of infection in patients with granulocytopenia. *Med Clin North Am* 1978; **61**: 1101–1118.
6. Pizzo PA Robichaud KJ, Wesley R et al. Fever in the paediatric and young adult patient with cancer: a prospective study of 1001 episodes. *Medicine* 1982; **61**: 153.
7. Schimpff SC, Young VM, Greene WH et al. Origin of infection in acute non-lymphocytic leukaemia: significance of hospital acquisition of potential pathogens. *Ann Intern Med* 1972; **77**: 707–714.
8. Van der Waagi DD, Berghuis J and Lekkerkerk JEC. Colonization resistance of the digestive tract of mice during systemic antibiotic therapy: *J Hyg (Camb)* 1972; **70**: 605–610.
9. Deitch EA, Winterton J and Berg R. Effect of starvation, malnutrition and trauma on the gastrointestinal tract flora and bacterial translocation. *Arch Surg* 1987; **122**: 1019–1024.
10. Pizzo PA, Ladisch S, Simon R et al. Increasing incidence of Gram-positive sepsis in cancer patients. *Med Paed Oncol* 1978; **5**: 241–244.
11. Bodey GP, Jadeja L and Elting L. *Pseudomonas* bacteraemia: a retrospective analysis of 410 episodes. *Ann Intern Med* 1985; **145**: 1621–1629.
12. Walmsley S, Devi S, King S et al. Invasive *Aspergillus* infections in a paediatric hospital: a ten year review. *Pediatr Infect Dis* 1993; **12**: 673–682.
13. Allo MA, Miller J, Townsend T et al. Primary cutaneous aspergillosis associated with Hickman intravenous catheters. *New Engl J Med* 1987; **317**: 1105–1108.
14. Anaissie E. Opportunistic mycoses in the immunocompromised host: experience at a cancer centre and review. *Clin Infect Dis* 1992; **14**(Suppl 1): S43–S53.
15. Fine JD, Miller JA, Harrist TJ et al. Cutaneous lesions in disseminated candidiasis mimicking ecthyma gangrenosum *Am J Med* 1981; **70**: 1133–1135.
16. Tenney JH, Moody MR, Newman KA et al. Adherent micro-organisms on luminal surfaces of long-term intravenous catheters: importance of *Staphylococcus epidermidis* in patients with cancer. *Ann Intern Med* 1986; **146**: 1949–1954.

17. Pearson TA, Braine HG and Rathbarn HK. *Corynebacterium* species in oncology patients. *J Am Med Ass* 1997; **238**: 1737–1740.
18. Gill VJ, Manning C, Lumsom M *et al.* Antibiotic-resistant group JK bacteria in hospitals. *J Clin Microbiol* 1981; **13**: 472–477.
19. Stamm WE, Tompkins LS, Wagner KF *et al.* Infection due to *Corynebacterium* species in marrow transplant patients. *Ann Intern Med* 1979; **91**: 167–173.
20. Dan M, Somer I, Knobel B *et al.* Cutaneous manifestations of infection with *Corynebacterium* JK. *Rev Infect Dis* 1988; **10**: 1204–1207.
21. Khadori N, Elting L, Wong E, Schable B and Bodey GP. Nosocomial infection due to *Xanthomonas maltophila* (*Pseudomonas maltophila*) in patients with cancer. *Rev Infect Dis* 1990; **12**: 997–1003.
22. Awada A, van der Auwera P, Meunier F *et al.* Streptococcal and enterococcal bacteraemia in patients with cancer. *Clin Infect Dis* 1992; **15**: 33–48.
23. Richard V, Meurnier F, van der Auwera P *et al.* Pneumococcal bacteraemia in cancer patients. *Eur J Epidemiol* 1988; **4**: 242–245.
24. Valteau D, Hartmann O, Brugieres L, Vassal G *et al.* Streptococcal septicaemia following autologous bone marrow transplantation in children treated with high-dose chemotherapy. *Bone Marrow Transplant* 1991; **7**: 415–419.
25. Villablenca JG, Steiner M, Kersey J *et al.* The clinical spectrum of infection with viridans streptococci in bone marrow transplant patients. *Bone Marrow Transplant* 1990; **6**: 387–393.
26. Elting LS, Bodey GP and Keefe BH. Septicaemia and shock syndrome due to viridans streptococci: a case control study of predisposing factors. *Clin Infect Dis* 1992; **14**: 1201–1207.
27. McWhinney DHM, Gillespie SH, Kibbler CC, Hoffbrand AV and Prentice HG. Streptococcus mitis and ARDS in neutropenic patients: *Lancet* 1991; **337**: 429 (Letter).
28. Karp JE, Merz WG, Hendicksen C *et al.* Oral norfloxacin for prevention of Gram-negative bacterial infection in patients with acute leukaemia and granulocytopenia. *Ann Intern Med* 1987; **106**: 1–7.
29. Dekker AW, Rozenberg Arsaka M and Verhoef J. Infection prophylaxis in acute leukaemia: a comparison of ciprofloxacin with trimethoprim-sulphamethoxazole and colistin. *Ann Intern Med* 1987; **106**: 7–12.
30. Sickles EA, Green WH and Wiemak PT. Clinical presentation of infection in granulocytopenic patients. *Arch Intern Med* 1975; **135**: 715–719.
31. Dorowitz GR, Harman C, Pope T and Stewart M. The role of the roentengram in the febrile neutropenic patients. *Arch Intern Med* 1991; **151**: 701–704.
32. Lightenborg PC, Hoepelman IM, Oude Sogtoen GAC, Dekker AW, van der Tweel I, Rozenberg-Arsaka M and Verhoef J. C-reactive protein in the diagnosis and management of infections in granulocytopenic and non-granulocytopenic patients. *Eur J Clin Microbiol Infect Dis* 1991; **10**: 25–31.
33. De Bel C, Gerritson E, de Maaker G, Moolenaar A and Vossen J. C-reactive protein in the management of children with fever after allogenic bone marrow transplantation. *Infection* 1991; **19**: 92–96.
34. Kiehn TE and Armstrong D. Changes in the spectrum of organisms causing bacteraemia and fungaemia in immunocompromised patients due to venous access devices. *Eur J Clin Microbiol Infect Dis* 1990; **9**: 869–872.
35. Schimpff SC. Surveillance cultures. *J Infect Dis* 1981; **144**: 81–84.
36. Kramer BS, Pizzo PA, Robichaud KJ *et al.* Role of serial microbiological surveillance and clinical evaluation in the management of cancer patients with fever and granulocytopenia. *Am J Med* 1982; **72**: 561–568.
37. Aisner J, Murillo J, Schimpff SC *et al.* Invasive aspergillosis in acute leukaemia: correlation with more cultures and antibiotics use. *Ann Intern Med* 1979; **90**: 4–9.
38. Wells CL, Ferrieri P, Weisdorf DJ *et al.* The importance of surveillance stool cultures during periods of severe neutropenia. *Infect Control* 1987; **8**: 317–319.
39. Schimpff, SC, Saterlee W, Young VM *et al.* Empirical therapy with carbenicillin and gentamicin for febrile patients with cancer and granulocytopenia. *New Engl J Med* 1971; **284**: 1061–1065.
40. Love LJ Schimpff SC, Schiffer CA *et al.* Improved prognosis of granulocytopenic patients with Gram-negative bacteraemia. *Am J Med* 1980; **68**: 643–648.
41. The EORTC International Antimicrobial Therapy Co-operative Group. Ceftazidime combined with short and long course amikacin for empirical therapy of Gram-negative bacteraemia in cancer patients with granulocytopenia. *New Engl J Med* 1987; **317**: 1692–1698.
42. Working Committee, Infectious Disease Society of America. Hughes WT, Armstrong D, Bodey GP *et al.* Guidelines for the use of antimicrobial agents in neutropenic patients with unexplained fever. *J Infect Dis* 1990; **161**: 381–396.
43. Barza M, Ioannidis JPA, Cappelleri JC and Lau J. Single or multiple daily doses of aminoglycosides: a meta-analysis. *Br Med J* 1996; **312**: 338–344.
44. EORTC International Antimicrobial Therapy Co-operative Group. Single daily dosing of amikacin and ceftriaxone is an efficacious and no more toxic than multiple daily dosing of amikacin and ceftazidime. *Ann Intern Med* 1993; **115**: 584–593.
45. Winston DJ, Ho WG, Bruckner DA *et al.* Beta-lactam antibiotic therapy in febrile granulocytopenic patients: a randomized trial comparing cefoperazone plus piperacillin, ceftazidime plus piperacillin, and imipenem alone. *Ann Intern Med* 1991; **115**: 849–859.
46. Bodey GP. Evolution of antibiotic therapy for infection in neutropenic patients: studies at MD Anderson Hospital. *Rev Infect Dis* 1989; **1**(Suppl 7): S1582–S1590.
47. Bodey GP, Fainstein V, Elting LS *et al.* Beta-lactam regimens for the febrile neutropenic patient. *Cancer* 1990; **65**: 9–16.
48. Philpott-Howard JN, Barker KF, Wade JJ, Kaczmarski RS, Smelley JC and Mufti GJ. Randomised multi-centre study of ciprofloxacin plus azlocillin versus gentamicin and azlocillin in the treatment of febrile neutropenia patients. *J Antimicrob Chemother* 1990; **26**: 549–559.
49. Sanders JW, Pave NR and Moore RD. Ceftazidime monotherapy for empiric treatment of febrile neutropenic patients – a meta-analysis. *J Infect Dis* 1991; **164**: 907–916.
50. Canetta A, Calandra T, Gaya H, Zinner SH *et al.* Monotherapy with meropenem versus combination therapy with ceftazidime plus amikacin in empirical therapy for fever in granulocytopenic patients with cancer. *Antimicrob Agents Chemother* 1996; **40**: 1108–1115.

51. Novokova IRO, Donnelly JP and DePauw BE. Ceftazidime as monotherapy or combined with teicoplanin for initial empiric treatment of presumed bacteraemia in febrile granulocytopenic patients. *Antimicrob Agents Chemother* 1991; **35**: 672–678.
52. Johnson PRE, Liu Yin JA and Tooth JA. High-dose intravenous ciprofloxacin in febrile neutropenic patients. *J Antimicrob Chemother* 1990; **26**: 101–107.
53. Meunier F, Zinner SH, Gaya H, Calandra T, Viscoli C, Klastersky J and Glauser M. Prospective randomised evaluation of ciprofloxacin versus piperacillin plus amikacin for empiric antibiotic therapy for febrile granulocytopenic cancer patients with lymphoma and solid tumours. *Antimicrob Agents Chemother* 1991; **35**: 872–878.
54. Attal M, Schalaifer D, Richie H et al. Prevention of Gram-positive infection after bone marrow transplantation by systemic vancomycin: a prospective, randomised trial. *J Clin Oncol* 1991; **9**: 865–870.
55. Shenep JL, Hughes WT, Robertson PK et al. Vancomycin, ticarcillin and amikacin compared with ticarcillin–clavulanate and amikacin in the empirical treatment of febrile, neutropenia children with cancer. *New Engl J Med* 1988; **319**: 1053–1058.
56. Rubin M, Hathorn JW, Marshall D et al. Gram-positive infections and the use of vancomycin in 550 episodes of fever and neutropenia. *Ann Intern Med* 1988; **108**: 30–35.
57. Montecalvo MA, Horowitz H, Gedris C et al. Outbreak of vancomycin-, ampicillin-, and aminoglycoside-resistant *Enterococcus faecium* bacteraemia in an adult oncology unit. *Antimicrob Agents Chemother* 1994; **38**: 1363–1367.
58. Hospital Infection Control Practices Advisory Committee. Recommendations for the prevention of spread of vancomycin resistance. *Infect Control Hosp Epidemiol* 1995; **16**: 1105–1113.
59. The EORTC International Antimicrobial Therapy Cooperative Group and the National Cancer Institute of Canada-Clinical Trials Group. Vancomycin added to empirical antibiotic therapy for fever in granulocytopenic cancer patients. *J Infect Dis* 1991; **161**: 951–958 (Erratum: *J Infect Dis* 1991; **164**: 832).
60. Nolan CM and Beaty HN. *Staphylococcus aureus* bacteraemia: current clinical problems. *Am J Med* 1976; **60**: 495.
61. Iannini PB and Grossley K. Therapy of *Staphylococcus aureus* bacteraemia associated with a removal focus of infection. *Ann Intern Med* 1976; **84**: 558–560.

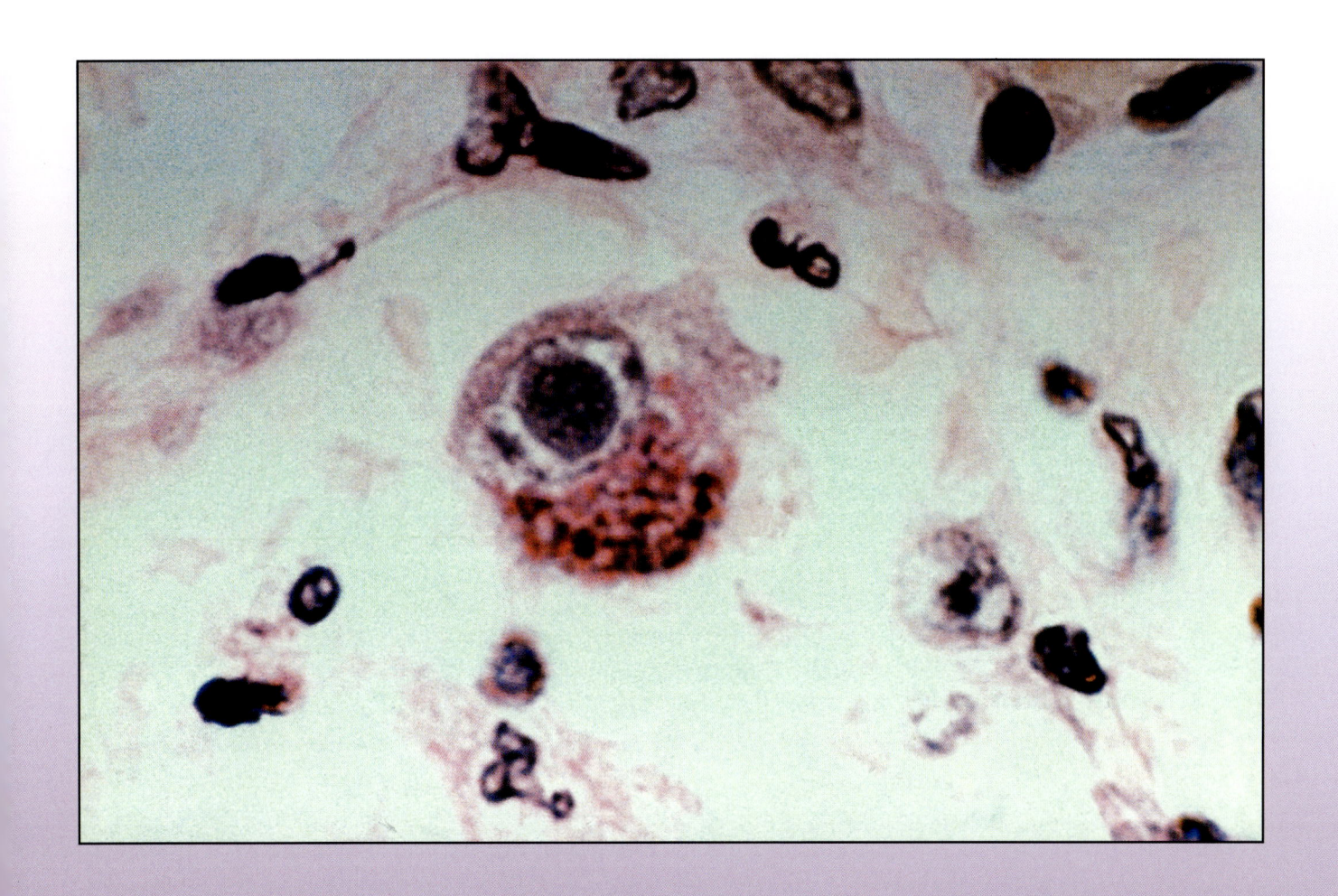

Chapter 44

Cytomegalovirus

Grant Prentice, Jane E. Grundy and Pearl Kho

Introduction

Cytomegalovirus (CMV), a member of the herpes virus family, causes an increasingly well characterized spectrum of disease. Although CMV can co-exist in remarkable symbiosis in those with a normal immune system, CMV disease is well established as causing life-threatening pathology in those who are immunocompromised, none more so than the recipient of an allogeneic stem-cell transplant, either bone-marrow transplant (BMT) or peripheral blood stem-cell (PBSC) transplant.

Although the rate of CMV reactivation (infection) is almost as high in recipients of autologous stem cells, the rate of disease is very low. The clinical features of CMV disease of lung, gastrointestinal tract, liver, retina and CMV syndrome are well known to transplant physicians and are not covered in this chapter. Here we deal with diagnosis, prevention and treatment, all rapidly evolving topics.

Definitions

Considerable confusion surrounds the terminology related to CMV and the following guide is designed to clarify this.

Latency: The presence of non-replicating CMV DNA in tissue or cells.

Infection: The presence of replicating virus; found in monocytes, this is not synonymous with disease.

Disease: Tissue damage is present and can reasonably be attributed to the virus shown to be present at that site. The diagnosis of CMV must be based on the isolation of virus from that site and not from a peripheral site of shedding, for example, on liver biopsy for CMV hepatitis [1].

Types of CMV infection

- *Primary infection* occurs when a seronegative individual becomes infected with CMV for the first time. Most primary infection, documented by the demonstration of antibody, occurs in childhood but continues to be acquired throughout life in the non-immune individual. In seronegative bone-marrow transplant recipients, the source of virus is usually from administered blood products, although marrow has also been shown to transmit CMV infection.
- *secondary infection* is a term used to denote infection of a previously seropositive individual, and can be of two different types: reinfection and reactivation.
- *reinfection* can occur when a seropositive individual is infected with a new exogenous strain of CMV introduced from another source, such as blood products or donor marrow.
- *reactivation* in a previously seropositive individual is due to secondary infection with the host's latent endogenous strain of CMV.

The virus is not usually eliminated from the body following primary infection, but persists throughout life, either in a latent state or at low levels of virus replication. Thus, latent or persistent infection can be reactivated, particularly following immunosuppressive therapy. In cases where a seropositive individual receives blood products or transplanted cells/tissues from seropositive donors, it is not usually possible to determine whether subsequent CMV infection is due to reactivation of latent endogenous recipient virus, or to reinfection with a new strain of CMV, and in such cases the term 'secondary infection' should be used.

Diagnosis of CMV

Diagnosis of CMV infection

CMV infection is best diagnosed by isolation of the virus or by detection of viral nucleic acid or proteins, rather than on serological criteria, especially in immunocompromised hosts. Although seroconversion can be used to detect primary CMV infection, this can be delayed in the immunocompromised, particularly in bone-marrow transplant recipients [2]. In addition, there can be problems because of the detection of passive antibody from administered blood products. IgM as well as IgG responses may be delayed during primary infection in the immunocompromised [2]. Similarly, the detection of a rise in antibody level in a seropositive patient may be delayed in the immunocompromised state. Thus, in immunocompromised hosts the detection of virus, rather than antibody, is the method of choice.

Serology does, however, have a place in the management of immunocompromised patients, since an accurate determination of the serological status of the patient and, in the case of a transplant recipient, the donor, is necessary in order to distinguish between the different types of CMV infection. Thus, seronegative recipients can be given screened blood products from seronegative donors in order to prevent primary CMV infection in the recipient. In addition, CMV seropositive recipients, who are at high risk of reactivating their latent virus, can be identified and possibly enrolled into prophylactic programmes or monitored closely for evidence of reactivation, and entered into pre-emptive therapy programmes.

Diagnosis of CMV disease

The diagnosis of CMV disease at a particular site must be based on the detection or isolation of the virus at that site. It is not possible to diagnose CMV pneumonitis, hepatitis or gastrointestinal disease based on the detection of peripheral virus shedding; demonstration of CMV infection at the appropriate site is an absolute requirement [1].

Laboratory diagnosis

Viraemia

In the blood, CMV is predominantly associated with leukocytes. In acute infection, both neutrophils and monocytes contain viral DNA [3] although more infectious virus is associated with the neutrophils than the monocytes. Until recently, the problems of detecting CMV in the blood of patients with low leukocyte counts was largely ignored, and there is a clear need to relate any diagnostic test on blood samples to the number of leukocytes present [4]. The conventional method for detection of CMV in blood has been the isolation of the virus in susceptible cells *in vitro*, usually human fibroblasts. The presence of the virus is then usually demonstrated by the appearance of a typical cytopathic effect. However, the isolate should be confirmed as being CMV by immununostaining with CMV-specific monoclonal antibodies. Because of the slow growth of clinical isolates of CMV in culture, a more rapid diagnosis can be made by staining the cells approximately 24 hours after inoculation with monoclonal antibodies to CMV immediate, early, or early proteins (the basis of the so-called Shell Vial or detection of early antigen fluorescent foci (DEAFF) assays) [5,6] Many centres, however, incubate the inoculated cells for up to three or even five days before staining to increase sensitivity,

since the amount of CMV in the blood is very low compared to the amount found in other types of clinical samples.

There is considerable variation in the way all of these culture-based assays are performed in different laboratories. No standard agreed amount of sample is added to a particular number of cells, and some centres inoculate the cells with whole blood, while others use buffy coat. In addition, different cell lines have different sensitivities for CMV replication. Furthermore, attention has not been paid to the leukocyte count and therefore to the number of leukocytes inoculated. Thus, while virus isolation has often been considered to be the 'gold standard', in practice this method has never been used in a standard manner at all.

The low sensitivity of a culture-based method for detecting CMV in the blood has led to the development of more sensitive assays such as the antigenaemia test or polymerase chain reaction (PCR)-based methods. The antigenaemia test relies upon the detection of the CMV tegument phosphoprotein pp65 (or more recently the phosphoprotein pp150) in peripheral blood neutrophils [7]. The neutrophils are harvested on dextran or metrizoate gradients, and a set number of cells are cytocentrifuged onto microscope slides, before fixing and staining by immunofluorescence- or immunoperoxidase-based methods. The number of positive cells per a set number of cells examined, for example 200 000 cells, is determined. This method thus has the advantage that it controls for any difference in leukocyte count and it is also semiquantitative. The sensitivity of the antigenaemia test has been shown to be affected by the length of time taken to process the sample, the type of fixative and the antibodies used [8]. It has been generally agreed that paraformaldehyde, and not acetone, is the fixative of choice [9]. Variation occurs in the way different laboratories report results, because some use the number of cells added to the cytocentrifuge per slide, while others actually count the number of cells on the slide, which is much fewer cells than are lost during the cytocentrifugation procedure. Thus, it is recommended that results are reported as the number of positive cells per defined number of cells actually on the slide.

The most commonly used PCR-based method for the detection of CMV in blood is the detection of viral DNA in the leukocyte fraction [4,10,11]. The detection of viral DNA in plasma [12,13] and viral mRNA in leukocytes has also been used, but the clinical significance of these tests awaits evaluation. Some protocols used for the detection of CMV DNA in leukocytes would also detect CMV DNA in plasma, since the leukocytes are not separated from the plasma before DNA extraction. Due to the previous lack of commercially available kits for CMV DNA detection by PCR, laboratories developed widely varying protocols for 'in-house' assays which can have very different sensitivities. As with the other methods for detecting CMV in blood, it is particularly important to control for the number of leukocytes analyzed. The Infectious Disease Working Party of the European Group for Blood and Marrow Transplantation (EBMT) recently recommended the following guidelines for the detection of CMV DNA in leukocytes by PCR [4]:

1. Blood should be collected into EDTA (heparin inhibits the PCR reaction, especially in stored samples) [4].
2. A standard number of leukocytes (probably 200,000) should be processed.
3. DNA from a standard number of leukocyte equivalents should be added per PCR reaction.
4. Primers in a region of the CMV genome shown to be conserved among clinical CMV isolates should be employed (a single base change can alter amplification of PCR products by 2–3 logs) [14].
5. A control cellular gene should be included to verify that the sample has amplifiable DNA.
6. A specificity step should be included to verify that the amplified product is CMV DNA, usually a second hybridization step or the use of a nested PCR. If a standard number of leukocytes is used for the DNA extraction, it is then recommended that a standard amount of DNA is added per PCR reaction, in order to control for differences in the extraction process.

Bronchoalveolar lavage fluid

CMV has been reported to be present in both the fluid and cellular fractions of bronchoalveolar lavage [15]. The virus is usually detected by either virus isolation or by the appearance of immediate early antigen in inoculated cell cultures (Shell Vial or DEAFF assays) as discussed for blood above. The usual practice is to inoculate both the fluid and cellular fractions. The use of PCR for the detection of CMV in bronchoalveolar lavage is still under investigation and should not be accepted as a diagnostic criterion at present. A standard amount of fluid should be instilled into the lungs.

Saliva or urine

CMV is usually detected in saliva/throat washings or urine using the same methods as those described above for bronchoalveolar lavage, as well as by the detection of viral DNA by PCR. The latter should follow points 3–6 in the recommendations described above for the detection of CMV by PCR in blood and, in addition, a standard method for collection of the sample, and a standard volume of sample should be processed and added per PCR reaction. It should also be noted that the detection of CMV in urine samples by certain methods may be affected by the pH of urine, which can vary considerably. This should therefore be taken into account when designing protocols.

Biopsy/autopsy specimens

The methods available include the detection of viral antigens by immunostaining [16] or the detection of viral nucleic acid by *in situ* hybridization [17,18] on fixed sections from biopsy or autopsy tissue. The detection of cells bearing characteristic intranuclear inclusions by conventional histology is also often taken as being diagnostic for CMV, but if possible, a more specific method should be used. In addition to the above methods, biopsy or autopsy tissue can be homogenized, and the virus detected by inoculation into susceptible cells or the viral DNA or mRNA detected in the homogenate by PCR. Methods are currently being developed for *in situ* PCR. It is important to realize that these various methods are not measuring the same parameters. In addition, the use of antibodies against different viral proteins for immunostaining tissue sections is a further source of variation, since those against immediate early proteins will pick up abortive as well as productive infection, while those against early or late proteins will detect only productive infection. *In situ* hybridization for viral DNA will detect predominantly replicating virus, although non-replicating virus present inside phagocytic cells could possibly also be detected, whilst hybridization for mRNA could pick up both abortive and/or productive replication depending upon the choice of immediate early or early/late probes, respectively. The choice of PCR primers will determine which type of infection can be detected in homogenized tissue or by *in situ* PCR. There is clearly a need for standardization of methodology between centres, particularly for clinical trials.

The need for standardization of diagnostic methods

Variations in the methods used to detect CMV, and in their sensitivities in difference centres, make it difficult to compare the results obtained in different centres, and to apply the findings obtained in one centre to those found in another. As much of the antiviral therapy used in marrow and stem-cell transplant recipients currently relies upon the detection of CMV, usually in the blood, it follows that, even when using the same treatment protocol, patients will be treated differently in different centres. Furthermore, the techniques used to diagnose CMV disease, for example detection of CMV in bronchoalveolar lavage or in tissue sections, are also widely different in different centres, so that the outcome of treatment protocols will be perceived to be different in different centres. Future studies, especially multicentre clinical trials, should standardize the methods used. Only one method should be used to detect CMV in a particular type of specimen, for example blood. If two methods are used, then the data from such trials must be analyzed separately. Trial protocols should standardize the protocols and reagents used, and verify that the sensitivity of the assay chosen is equivalent in different centres.

Prevention and treatment of CMV

Potential diagnostic problems associated with the use of antiviral agents

An important consideration is that attention must be paid to the possible effects of any antiviral agent given to the patient on the ability to diagnose CMV infection/disease. Attention should thus be paid to the mechanism of action of the agent given and the appropriateness of the detection method used. Firstly, the possible effects of the presence of an antiviral agent in the clinical sample on the ability to detect the virus in that sample must be considered. For example, it may not be possible to detect the CMV present in a clinical sample by methods which rely upon the ability of the virus to infect susceptible cells in culture, if the sample also contains sufficient levels of an antiviral agent to prevent CMV infection *in vitro*. Thus, the method of detection of CMV must be shown not to be affected by the presence of the antiviral agent itself in a clinical sample, or false-negative results could occur.

It should be considered that antiviral treatment might affect different methods of CMV detection differently. For example, if an antiviral agent blocks viral DNA synthesis, and hence late protein synthesis too, detection methods based on late proteins or their mRNA would be expected to show a decrease in CMV detection following effective antiviral therapy, while those based on immediate early or early antigen/gene detection might show less or no effect of the treatment. Thus, if the diagnostic results are being used to monitor therapy and to make further decisions on treatment regimens, care should be taken in the choice of the diagnostic test employed.

The possible effect of antiviral agents on the cell types carrying virus must also be considered. As mentioned above, in clinical specimens such as blood, CMV is predominantly associated with leukocytes. Account must therefore be taken of the possible effects of antiviral agents on leukocytes. For example, the anti-CMV drug, ganciclovir, is often associated with neutropenia, and therefore when using diagnostic tests to detect the presence of CMV in the blood of patients receiving ganciclovir, methods must be adjusted for neutrophil count. If not, false-negative results for CMV detection will occur because there were not enough neutrophils present in the sample.

Strategies for prevention of CMV disease in the BMT recipient

Four clinical strategies are currently used in the management of CMV disease: prophylaxis, suppression, pre-emptive therapy and treatment [19]. The degree of risk of developing CMV disease and the safety profile of the presently available drugs are employed in determining which is most appropriate. Symptomatic CMV infection (CMV disease), particularly CMV pneumonia in these patients, is often fatal. The mortality rate of patients with untreated CMV pneumonia is approximately 85% [20].

The use of CMV seronegative (or leukocyte-depleted) blood products for CMV seronegative BMT patients receiving marrow from CMV-seronegative donors prevents CMV disease [21]. However, this is relevant to only a minority of BMT recipients. Immunoglobulin prophylaxis, either hyperimmune to CMV or standard, has proven generally disappointing. Antiviral agents have been employed in an attempt to prevent the development of CMV infection and disease where either donor or recipient are seropositive.

Prophylaxis
Antiviral agents are administered to all BMT recipients at risk of developing CMV disease. Therapy is started prior to any detection of CMV.

Suppression
Antiviral agents are administered to BMT recipients when CMV is detected in peripheral sites such as the urine or throat washings, but prior to the development of any clinical symptoms of CMV disease.

Pre-emptive therapy
Antiviral agents are given to BMT patients when CMV is detected systemically such as in the blood or bronchoalveolar lavage, but prior to the development of symptoms of CMV disease.

Treatment
Antiviral agents are given when clinical symptoms and signs are evident. Established CMV disease includes: interstitial pneumonia, oesophagitis, gastritis, hepatitis, encephalitis, vasculitis and CMV-associated syndrome (fever and cytopenia with CMV viraemia).

Regimens used to manage CMV
Some of the larger prophylactic studies and outcomes are illustrated in Table 44.1.

Prophylaxis
Meyers et al. [22] gave intravenous aciclovir, 500 mg/m^2 three × daily to BMT recipients who were herpes simplex virus and CMV seropositive from five days prior to 30 days after transplant or until hospital discharge. Herpes simplex virus seronegative patients were followed as untreated controls. In a study by Prentice et al. [23], patients were randomized to receive one of three prophylactic regimens: i.v. aciclovir 500 mg/m^2 three × daily from five days before transplant to 30 days after transplant, followed by oral aciclovir 800 mg q.d.s. for a further six months; i.v. aciclovir at the same dose from day −5 to day +30 followed by placebo for a further six months; or oral aciclovir 200 (children) to 400 mg (adults) four × daily from day −5 to day +30, followed by placebo until seven months post-transplant (control group). Patients developing CMV viraemia were treated (pre-emptive) with ganciclovir, with or without immunoglobulin, at the discretion of the physician.

Table 44.1 A summary of results of prophylactic studies at 100 days post-transplant*†

Parameter	Meyers et al. [22]		Prentice et al. [23]			Goodrich et al. [24]		Winston et al. [25]	
	Aciclovir (i.v.)	None	Aciclovir (i.v.), aciclovir (p.o.)	Aciclovir (i.v.), PCB	Aciclovir (p.o.), PCB	Aciclovir (i.v.), GCV	Aciclovir (i.v.), PCB	GCV	PCB
Patients (n)	86	65	105	103	102	33	31	40	45
CMV infection (%)	59	75	40	40	55	3	45	20	43
CDM disease (%)	22	38	7	15	11	0	29	10	24
CMV death (%)	16	28	0	6	6	3	6	8	9
Survival (%)	71	46	88	74	72	88	81	70	64

*For a more detailed analysis of these studies see HG Prentice and P Kho [19].
†PCB = placebo; GCV = ganciclovir.

Goodrich et al. [24] gave i.v. aciclovir 500 mg/m² three × daily from the start of the pretransplant conditioning regimen until myeloid engraftment to all patients. At engraftment, patients were randomized to have either i.v. ganciclovir 5 mg/kg or placebo twice daily for five days, and then the same dose once a day until 100 days post-BMT. All patients who excreted CMV were removed from the study and treated with ganciclovir.

Winston et al. [25] randomized patients seven days prior to bone-marrow transplant to receive either i.v. ganciclovir 2.5 mg/kg three × daily or placebo. Ganciclovir prophylaxis was stopped on the day before transplantation and restarted at engraftment at a dose of 6 mg/kg once a day for five days per week until day +120. Patients who became neutropenic temporarily discontinued the drug until neutrophil recovery was $>1.0 \times 10^9$/litre, when ganciclovir was restarted at a dose of 6 mg/kg once a day on every other day. Patients who developed CMV disease were treated with ganciclovir at the discretion of the physician.

Atkinson et al. [26] gave ganciclovir to CMV-seropositive recipients at a dose of 5 mg/kg twice daily from day −8 to day +1 for all patients. Aciclovir 200 mg three × daily was given orally from day 0 until day +20. Ganciclovir prophylaxis was restarted on day +21 and continued until day +84, at 5 mg/kg three times per week. The results were compared with historical controls not receiving prophylactic ganciclovir.

Von Bueltzingsloewen et al., in an historical-controlled study, gave CMV-seropositive patients ganciclovir pretransplant at a daily dose of 6 mg/kg from day −10 to day −4. All patients were then given intravenous aciclovir at a daily dose of 1.5 g/m² in four divided doses, from three days pretransplant to 29 days post-transplant. From day +30 to day +90, i.v. ganciclovir was given at a daily dose of 6 mg/kg/day for five days each week in the absence of neutropenia, on three consecutive days. The historical control group received intravenous aciclovir prophylactically [27].

Suppression/pre-emptive therapy

Provided they had marrow engraftment, Goodrich et al. randomized patients in whom CMV was detected in the blood, urine, throat washings or bronchoalveolar lavage fluid, despite i.v. aciclovir prophylaxis at a dose of 500 mg/m² three × daily, to receive either placebo or i.v. ganciclovir 5 mg/kg twice daily for seven days and then the same dose once a day until 100 days post-BMT or until they were discharged from the hospital [28].

Schmidt et al. [29] randomized patients who were seropositive for CMV or who were receiving a graft from a CMV-positive donor and had CMV isolated from bronchoalveolar lavage on days 35 and 49 to receive ganciclovir or to be monitored without specific treatment. The dosage of i.v. ganciclovir given was 5 mg/kg twice daily for two weeks, followed by 5 mg/kg once a day for five days each week until 120 days after transplant. Patients who developed CMV pneumonia were treated with aciclovir and i.v. immune globulin. Although no controlled trials or pre-emptive treatment for CMV viraemia using ganciclovir are reported, a survey from the EBMT showed that 49 of the 70 participating centres used ganciclovir, either alone or combined with immunoglobulin, for pre-emptive treatment [12].

Treatment of established disease

A number of small, open studies have shown ganciclovir [30] alone to be suboptimal in treating established CMV pneumonia, with the mortality rate in patients treated with 2.5 mg/kg ganciclovir ranging from 50 to 90% [31–33]. Increasing the dose from 2.5 mg/kg three times to 5 mg/kg twice daily did not improve patient survival [34]. However, in an open study, Emmanuel et al. [35] reported a mortality rate of 30% at 10 months in patients treated with 2.5 mg/kg ganciclovir three times a day combined with intravenous immune globulin. Reed and colleagues [36] used CMV immune globulin and showed a mortality rate of 48%. In Europe, most BMT centres use ganciclovir together with intravenous immune globulin, with no apparent benefit attributable to the choice of CMV immune or conventional globulin seen, nor indeed to the dose of ganciclovir [34]. There is, as yet, no clear consensus on the role of immune globulin in the treatment or established disease, but it seems reasonable, on balance, to add this to the antiviral drugs. [37].

A non-randomized study suggested that the benefit of foscarnet is similar to that of ganciclovir [38]. A large randomized European multicentre study comparing the efficacy and safety of ganciclovir with foscarnet for the treatment of CMV disease is under way.

Analysis of the outcome of prophylactic strategies on infection, disease and survival
CMV infection

In most studies, CMV infection is usually defined as the isolation of CMV from an appropriate site, but in some reports an antibody response [25] or the presence of typical CMV inclusion bodies in a tissue specimen is the definition of CMV infection.

Results of the various prophylaxis studies are summarized in Table 44.1. The most effective drug for reducing the risk of CMV infection is ganciclovir although it has not increased survival. Ganciclovir given during conditioning and restarted at the time of engraftment reduced the incidence of CMV infection from 43% in the placebo group to 20% in the ganciclovir group [25]. By the use of i.v. aciclovir prophylaxis followed by ganciclovir from engraftment until 100 days post-BMT, Goodrich et al. [24] reduced the incidence from 45% in the aciclovir alone control group to 3% with aciclovir followed by ganciclovir. A further study of prophylactic aciclovir followed by ganciclovir again showed a substantial reduction in the incidence of CMV infection from a historical rate of 72% to 7.5% [27].

High-dose i.v. aciclovir given from the time of conditioning for approximately one month reduced the CMV infection rate by approximately 15% from that seen with either placebo or oral aciclovir [22,23].

Prevention of CMV disease by different prophylactic strategies

Meyers et al. [22] showed first that aciclovir alone given from conditioning until 30 days post-BMT could reduce the incidence of CMV disease. This effect could not be confirmed in a large randomized multicentre European study [23], perhaps because of the use of pre-emptive treatment, mainly ganciclovir, for CMV viraemia in approximately 20% of patients. High-dose i.v. aciclovir for 35 days followed by oral aciclovir 800 mg four times a day for a further six months also failed to significantly reduce the risk of CMV disease although only 1 of 7 patients who developed CMV pneumonia died (14%) employing this strategy. In contrast, 8 of the 11 patients in the i.v. aciclovir alone group and 6 of 6 in the control (p.o. aciclovir) group died. Goodrich et al. [24] showed that high-dose i.v. aciclovir given prior to BMT and continued until engraftment, followed by i.v. ganciclovir until 100 days post-BMT, completely prevented disease. This study allowed patients who excreted CMV while on aciclovir to be treated pre-emptively with ganciclovir. This impressive observation has been confirmed by Atkinson et al. [26] and Von Bueltzingsloewen et al. [27]. Winston et al. [25] showed that ganciclovir given prior to BMT and again at engraftment, resulted in a significant reduction in the incidence of CMV disease.

Pre-emptive treatment

In one study, patients who had CMV detected in bronchoalveolar lavage were treated with ganciclovir reducing the probability of CMV pneumonia from 70% in the control group to 10% [29]. Goodrich et al. [28] demonstrated that when ganciclovir was administered to patients who had had virus detected in blood, urine, throat washings or bronchoalveolar lavage fluid, treatment with ganciclovir reduced the incidence of CMV disease from 43% to 3%. However, negative surveillance failed to predict disease in 12%.

Foscarnet, given at a dose of 100 mg/kg/day, cleared viraemia in 7 of 10 patients, with 5 remaining disease-free at a median of seven months [39]. In a randomized study, 25 patients received either ganciclovir or foscarnet as pre-emptive treatment for CMV antigenaemia. No difference was found in the clearance of CMV antigenaemia, incidence of disease or survival [40].

Survival

The effects of prophylaxis on survival are summarized in Table 44.1. Meyers et al. [22] demonstrated a significant reduction in 100-day mortality using a short course of high-dose aciclovir, and although not confirmed by Prentice et al. [23], the latter study showed a reduction in mortality at 210 days, subsequently confirmed to be sustained at one year [41] in recipients of high-dose i.v. aciclovir followed by oral aciclovir for seven months. In this study, 100-day mortality was reduced from 28% in the control group to 12% in the recipients of i.v. plus oral aciclovir. The one-year survival rate was increased from 49% in recipients of low-dose aciclovir to 68% [41]. This benefit was not seen in the Goodrich et al. [24] study despite the clear anti-CMV effect of the ganciclovir (180-day mortality 26% in aciclovir recipients versus 30% in recipients of aciclovir and ganciclovir).

Winston et al. [25] studied the effect of administering i.v. ganciclovir or placebo prior to transplant and again at engraftment, but failed to show a reduction in mortality with ganciclovir (30% versus 36%).

Goodrich et al. [28] showed a significant reduction in 100-day mortality (17% versus placebo 3%) when CMV excretion was treated with ganciclovir. There were no deaths due to CMV in the ganciclovir group, compared to six CMV-associated deaths in the placebo group. Why survival benefit is seen with aciclovir and ganciclovir is not clear, but the myelosuppressive effects of ganciclovir may play a role.

Eleven of 37 patients (30%) who were receiving pre-emptive therapy with ganciclovir developed neutropenia requiring cessation of the drug [28] (3%, $P = 0.003$). Prophylactic i.v. aciclovir followed by ganciclovir is also associated with a higher incidence of neutropenia (30% versus 0%, $P = 0.0001$) compared to i.v. aciclovir alone [24], thus increasing the risk of bacterial infection. Although Winston et al. [25] administered ganciclovir only prior to BMT and then at engraftment, 58% of the ganciclovir and 28% of placebo recipients developed neutropenia requiring discontinuation of the study drug ($P = 0.005$).

Detection of CMV in the blood and bronchoalveolar lavage has been reported as a good predictor of CMV disease, and particularly for CMV pneumonia [42]. In such circumstances, the most effective anti-CMV therapy should be given, and at present this is either ganciclovir or foscarnet, despite their known toxicities.

The sensitivity of detecting CMV may be improved by using the CMV antigenaemia assay or by testing for the presence of CMV DNA using the polymerase chain reaction (PCR). However, the methods require standardization, given the current large variability. In addition, clinical correlates of the test results require validation before treatment regimens can be compared using these assays. It seems probable that a quantitative PCR method will prove the best method for achieving a high positive predictive value [43,44].

Prophylaxis potentially confers protection to all patients. It does, of course, involve drug administration to all patients, including those who might never suffer CMV disease. As such, a drug with little or no toxicity is preferable. Since survival benefit has been shown with aciclovir, it is the drug of choice despite having modest anti-CMV activity until an agent with greater activity and equivalent low toxicity becomes available.

Mortality without prophylaxis was 53%. This was reduced by half when aciclovir was given prior to transplant and continued until 30 days post-BMT. The largest reduction in mortality was reported in recipients of i.v. aciclovir followed by either ganciclovir [24] or oral aciclovir [23]. Ganciclovir, by contrast, administered pretransplant and again from engraftment, did not reduce this (mortality 54%). What is not yet clear is whether substitution of prophylaxis by close monitoring and pre-emptive therapy will achieve the same result. This is presently the standard practice in several centres, particularly in the USA.

Cellular therapy as prophylaxis and recent developments in drugs used for treatment

The cause of CMV reactivation and disease after BMT is the relative or absolute deficiency of anti-CMV cellular effectors. It is logical that the administration of cytotoxic T-cells, and ideally also memory T-cells, might prevent reactivation. Indeed, our group has previously demonstrated the protective role of a seropositive donor, where the recipient is also seropositive [45]. Proof of principle has been established in an elegant series of studies by Riddell and colleagues in Seattle [46]. In the absence of an effective and non-toxic conveniently administered drug, this approach will become favoured.

Several new, promising and potentially less toxic drugs are in an advanced stage of development or in early clinical trials. These include lobucavir [47] 1263W94 [48] and antisense oligonucleotides [49].

Conclusion

Since even the presently available best treatment for established disease has had limited success, a strategy of prophylaxis, linked to accurate detection, with frequent sampling for infection followed by pre-emptive therapy is preferred. This might include the use of some of the newer agents detailed above. We believe that the best strategy will involve techniques currently under development to avoid post-transplant antiviral immunosuppression and to leave the donor anti-CMV cellular repertoire intact by intelligent graft engineering [50,51]. Where the donor is not immune and vaccination is impractical, then *ex vivo* induction and expansion of anti-CMV effectors or an effective and non-toxic drug will be indicated.

References

1. Lungman P and Plotkin SA. Workshop of CMV Disease: Definitions, clinical severity scores and new syndromes. *Scand J Infect Dis* 1995; Suppl 99: 87–89.
2. Panjwani DD, Ball MG, Berry NJ et al. Virological and serological diagnosis of cytomegalovirus infection in bone marrow allograft recipients. *J Med Virol* 1985; **16**: 357–365.
3. Turtlinen LW, Salzman R, Jordan MC and Haase AT. Interactions of human cytomegalovirus with leucocytes *in vivo*: analysis by *in situ* hybridisation. *Microb Pathogen* 1987; **3**: 287–297.
4. Grundy JE, Ehrnst A, Einsele H, Emery VC, Hebart H, Prentice HG and Ljungman P. A three centre European external quality control study of PCR for the detection of cytomegalovirus DNA in blood. *J Clin Microbiol* 1996; **34**: 1166–1170.
5. Gleaves CA, Smith TF, Shuster EA and Pearson GR. Comparison of standard tube and Shell Vial cell culture techniques for the detection of cytomegalovirus in clinical specimens. *J Clin Microbiol* 1985; **21**: 217–221.
6. Griffiths PD, Panjwani DD, Stirk PR et al. Rapid diagnosis of cytomegalovirus infection in immunocompromised patients by detection of early antigen fluorescent foci. *Lancet* 1984; **ii**: 1242–1245.
7. van der Bij, van-Son WJ, van-der Berg AP, Tegzess AM, Torensma R and The TH. Cytomegalovirus (CMV) antigenemia: rapid diagnosis and relationship with CMV-associated clinical syndromes in renal allograft recipients. *Transplant Proc* 1989; **21**: 2061–2064.
8. Gema G, Revelio MG, Percivalle E and Morini F. Comparison of different immunostaining techniques and monoclonal antibodies to the lower matrix phosphoprotein (pp65) for optimal quantitation of human cytomegalovirus antigenemia. *J Clin Microbiol* 1992; **30**: 1232–1237.
9. The TH, van den Berg AP, Harmsen MC, van der Bij W and van Son WJ. The cytomegalovirus antigenemia assay: a plea for standarization. [Review.] *Scand J Infect Dis* 1995; 99(Suppl): 25–29.
10. Einsele H, Steidle M, Vallbracht A, Saal JG, Ehninger G and Muller CA. Early occurrence of human cytomegalovirus infection after bone marrow transplantation as demonstrated by the polymerase chain reaction technique. *Blood* 1991; **77**: 1104–1110.
11. Hebart H, Muller C, Loffler Jahn G and Einsele H. Monitoring of CMV infection: a comparison of PCR from whole blood, plasma PCR, pp65 antigenemia and virus culture in patients after bone marrow transplantation. *Bone Marrow Transplant* 1996; **17**: 861–868.
12. Ljungman P, de Bock R, Cordonnier C et al. Practices for cytomegalovirus diagnosis, prophylaxis and treatment in allogeneic bone marrow transplant recipients: a report from the Working Party for Infectious Diseases of the EBMT. *Bone Marrow Transplant* 1993; **12**: 39–403.
13. Link H, Battmer K, Stumme C et al. Cytomegalovirus infection in leucocytes after bone marrow transplantation demonstrated by mRNA *in situ* hybridisation. *Br J Haematol* 1993; **85**: 573–677.
14. Chou S. Effect of interstrain variation on diagnostic DNA amplification of the cytomegalovirus major immediate–early gene region. *J Clin Microbiol* 1992; **30**: 2307–2310.
15. Storch GA, Ettinger NA, Ockner D et al. Quantitative cultures of the cell fraction and supernatant of bronchoalveolar lavage fluid for the diagnosis of cytomegalovirus pneumonitis in lung transplant recipients. *J Infect Dis* 1993; **168**: 1502–1506.
16. Theise ND, Haber MM and Grimes MM. Detection of cytomegalovirus in lung allografts. Comparison of histologic and immunohistochemical findings. *Am J Clin Pathol* 1991; **96**: 762–766.
17. Genta RM, Bleyzer I, Cate TR, Tandon AK and Yoffe B. In situ hybridization and immunohistochemical analysis of cytomegalovirus-associated ileal perforation. *Gastroenterology* 1993; **104**: 1822–1827.
18. Rimsza LM, Vela EE, Frutiger YM et al. Rapid automated combined *in situ* hybrization and immunohistochemistry for sensitive detection of cytomegalovirus in paraffin embedded tissue biopsies. *Am J Clin Pathol* 1996; **106**: 544–548.
19. Prentice HG and Kho P. Clinical strategies for the management of cytomegalovirus infection and disease in allogeneic bone marrow transplant. *Bone Marrow Transplant* 1997; **19**: 135–142.
20. Meyers JD, Flournoy N and Thomas ED. Risk factor for cytomegalovirus infection after human marrow transplantation. *J Infect Dis* 1986; **153**: 478–488.
21. Bowden RA, Sayers M, Flournoy N et al. Cytomegalovirus immune globulin and seronegative blood. *New Engl J Med* 1986; **314**: 1006–1010.
22. Meyers J, Reed EC, Shepp DH et al. Acyclovir for prevention of cytomegalovirus infection and disease after allogeneic marrow transplantation. *New Engl J Med* 1988; **318**: 70–75.
23. Prentice HG, Gluckman E, Powles RL et al. The impact of long term acyclovir on cytomegalovirus infection and survival in allogeneic bone marrow transplantation. *Lancet* 1994; **343**: 749–753.
24. Goodrich JM, Bowden RA, Fisher L et al. Ganciclovir prophylaxis to prevent cytomegalovirus disease after allogeneic marrow transplant. *Ann Intern Med* 1993; **118**: 173–178.
25. Winston DJ, Ho WG, Bartoni RN et al. Ganciclovir prophylaxis of cytomegalovirus infection and disease in allogeneic bone marrow transplant recipients. *Ann Intern Med* 1993; **118**: 179–184.
26. Atkinson K, Downs K, Golena M et al. Prophylactic use of ganciclovir in allogeneic bone marrow transplantation: absence of clinical cytomegalovirus infection. *Br J Haematol* 1991; **79**: 57–62.
27. Von Bueltzingsloewen A, Bordigoni P, Witz F et al. Prophylactic use of ganciclovir for allogeneic bone marrow transplant recipients. *Bone Marrow Transplant* 1993; **12**: 197–202.
28. Goodrich JM, Mori M, Gleaves CA et al. Early treatment with ganciclovir to prevent cytomegalovirus disease after allogeneic bone marrow transplantation. *New Engl J Med* 1991; **325**: 1601–1607.
29. Schmidt GM, Horak DA, Niland JC, Duncan SR, Forman SJ and Zaia JA. A randomised, controlled trial of prophylactic ganciclovir for cytomegalovirus pulmonary infection in recipients of allogeneic bone marrow transplant. *New Engl J Med* 1991; **324**: 1005–1011.

30. Shepp DH, Dandliker PS, de Miranda P *et al.* Activity of 9-(2-hydroxy-1 (hydroxymethyl)ethoxymethyl)guanine in the treatment of cytomegalovirus pneumonia. *Ann Intern Med* 1985; **103**: 368–373.
31. Ettinger NA, Selby P, Powles R *et al.* Cytomegalovirus pneumonia: the use of ganciclovir in marrow transplant recipients. *J Antimicrob Chemother* 1989; **24**: 53–62.
32. Selby P, Powles RL, Jameson B *et al.* Treatment of cytomegalovirus pneumonia after bone marrow transplantation with 9-(2-hydroxy-1-(hydroxymethyl)-ethoxymethyl)guanine. *Lancet* 1986; **i**: 1377–1378.
33. Crumpacker C, Marlowe S, Zhang JL *et al.* Treatment of cytomegalovirus pneumonia. *Rev Infect Dis* 1988; **10**(Suppl 3): 538–546.
34. Ljungman P, Engelhard D, Link H *et al.* Treatment of interstitial pneumonitis due to cytomegalovirus with ganciclovir and intravenous immune globulin: Experience of European Bone Marrow Transplant Group. *Clin Infect Dis* 1992; **14**: 831–835.
35. Emmanuel D, Cunningham I, Jules-Elysee K *et al.* Cytomegalovirus pneumonia after bone marrow transplantation successfully treated with the combination of ganciclovir and high-dose intravenous immune globulin. *Ann Intern Med* 1988; **109**: 777–782.
36. Reed EC, Bowden RA, Dandliker PS *et al.* Treatment of cytomegalovirus pneumonia with ganciclovir and intravenous cytomegalovirus immunoglobulin in patients with bone marrow transplant. *Ann Intern Med* 1988; **109**: 783–788.
37. Crumpacker CS. Ganciclovir. *New Engl J Med* 1996; **335**: 721–729.
38. Aschan J, Ringden O, Ljungman P *et al.* Foscarnet for treatment of cytomegalovirus infection in bone marrow transplant recipients. *Scand J Infect Dis* 1992; **24**: 143–150.
39. Chang J, Powles R and Mehta J. Foscarnet treatment for CMV viremia in allo-BMT recipients. *Br J Cancer* 1995; **71**: 69.
40. Bacigalupo A, Tedone E, Van Lint MT *et al.* CMV prophylaxis with foscarnet in allogeneic bone marrow transplant recipients at high risk of developing CMV infections. *Bone Marrow Transplant* 1994; **13**: 783–788.
41. Prentice HG, Gluckman E, Powles RL *et al.* Long term survival in allogeneic bone marrow transplant recipients following acyclovir prophylaxis for CMV infection. *Bone Marrow Transplant* 1997; **19**: 129–133.
42. Meyers. JD, Ljungman P and Fisher LD. Cytomegalovirus excretion as a predictor of cytomegalovirus disease after marrow transplantation: the importance of cytomegalovirus viraemia. *J Infect Dis* 1990; **162**: 373–380.
43. Fox JC, Griffiths PD and Emery VC. Quantification of human cytomegalovirus DNA using the polymerase chain reaction. *J Gen Virol* 1992; **73**: 2405–2408.
44. Fox JC, Kidd M, Grifflths PD, Sweny P and Emery VC. Longitudinal analysis of cytomegalovirus in renal transplant recipients using a quantitative polymerase chain reaction: correlation with disease. *J Gen Virol* 1995; **76**: 309–319.
45. Grob JP, Grundy JE, Prentice HG *et al.* Immune donors can protect marrow transplant recipients from severe cytomegalovirus infections. *Lancet* 1987; **i**: 774–776.
46. Riddell SF; Watanbe KS, Goodrich JM et aI. Restoration of viral immunity in immunodeficient humans by the adoptive transfer of T-cell clones. *Science* 1992; **257**: 238–241.
47. Drew WL. Lalezari J Jourdan C *et al. In vivo* anti-cytomegalovirus activity and safety of oral lobucavir in HIV patients. In: *Proceedings of the Tenth International Conference on Antiviral Research*, 1987 (Abstr 14).
48. Wang LH, Peck R, Chan PQ *et al.* A phase I tolerability and pharmacokinetic (PK) trial of 1263W4 a novel anti-HCMV agent, in HIV infected volunteers. In: *Proceedings of the 6th International Cytomegalovirus Workshop*, 1997.
49. Pari GS, Field AK and Smith JE. Potent antiviral activity of an antisense oligonucleotide complementary to the intron–exon boundary of human cytomegalovirus genes *UL36* and *UIL37*. *Antimicrob Agents Chemother* 1995; 1157–1161.
50. Mavroudis DA, Jiang YZ, Hensel N *et al.* Specific depletion of alloreactivity against haplotype mismatched related individuals by a recombinant immunotoxin: a new approach to graft-versus-host disease prophylaxis in haplo-identical bone marrow transplantation. *Bone Marrow Transplant* 1996; **17**: 793–799.
51. Lowdell M, Koh M and Prentioe HG. Selective removal of alloreactive Iymphocytes from peripheral blood mononuclear cell preparations. *Br J Haematol* 1997; **97**(Suppl 1): 147.

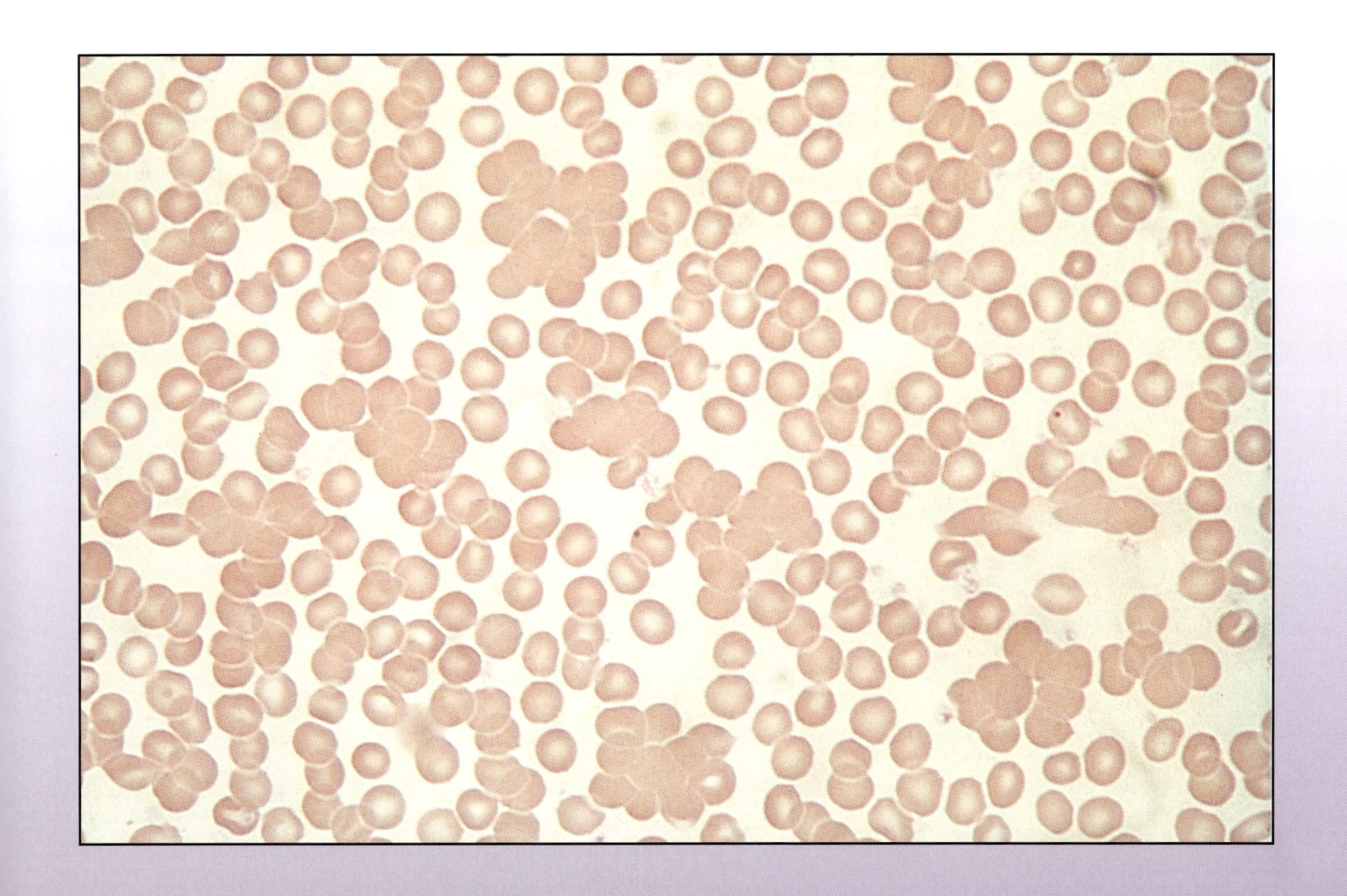

Chapter 45

Other viral infections

Diana Westmoreland

Introduction

Recovery from viral disease depends crucially upon the immunocompetence of the infected individual. Although the number of antiviral drugs available for use has increased during the last decade, few compare with good antibiotics either in efficacy or lack of toxicity, and for healthy individuals, recovery from virus disease is accomplished without the aid of specific treatment. Because there is rarely place for antiviral therapy in otherwise healthy people, specific diagnosis of virus infections has historically been of much less concern than of bacterial infections. Diagnostic techniques traditionally employed methods which were slow or depended upon the detection of antibody to the relevant virus pathogen.

It is important to recognize also that recovery from acute virus disease in healthy individuals is not always accompanied by elimination of the causative virus. Many viruses, particularly those of the herpes group, establish long-term (life-long in many cases) latent infections after recovery from initial disease. Such latent infections are kept under immune control with occasional (often symptomatic) periods of virus reactivation and shedding.

The immunocompromised patient, particularly those with the degree of immunosuppression needed post stem-cell transplant, is therefore particularly vulnerable to virus disease – so much so that treatments of limited effectiveness and significant toxicity are used in order to control infection.

The need for specific therapies has driven not only greater efforts by industry to produce more and better antiviral drugs but has also required rapid and reliable tests of specific virus infection from the diagnostic laboratory, which do not depend upon the individual's ability to mount a detectable immune response.

This chapter describes some of the diseases caused by viruses which are particularly troublesome in stem-cell transplant patients, their diagnosis and management.

Source of infection

Environmental

Stem-cell transplant patients are, like all of us, susceptible to virus acquisition from the community in which they live. Respiratory tract pathogens, diarrhoeal diseases and primary infections with childhood diseases can all cause severe illness in the immunocompromised host. Not only is the patient at risk in the community at large, but while in hospital he is at risk of nosocomial acquisition of pathogens in season when infected non-immunocompromised patients have required hospital admission, for example, respiratory syncytial virus (RSV) on paediatric units.

For each of these situations, prevention is better than cure, and cross-infection prevention and control are of paramount importance both in hospital and after the patient has been discharged. Avoidance of all infection is, however, probably an unrealistic goal, and for contact with some infections, prophylaxis using specific immunoglobulin is advised (e.g. chickenpox, measles).

The important infections in this category are summarised in Table 45.1.

Transfusion/blood product/donor tissue-associated infections

Stem-cell transplant recipients are potentially vulnerable to any blood-borne virus infection. The important infections are summarized in Table 45.2. Because of the recipient's immunocompromise and the potentially large infecting dose of virus, the consequence of such infections can be severe. Effort has been directed towards prevention of infection by screening donors of tissues, organs and blood for evidence of infection with blood-borne viruses. In some cases it is possible to treat blood products with chemicals or heat which inactivate infectious viruses without compromising biological activity. However, such screening can only be a partial solution. For some infections such as parvovirus B19, screening methods are not yet available; for others such as hepatitis G virus (HGV), reliable diagnostic methods have yet to be developed. There also remains a risk, albeit low, from as yet undiscovered viruses and from any disease which has an asymptomatic viraemic phase unless subsequent blood product processing has a viricidal phase.

Endogenous viral reactivation

Because of immunocompromise, stem-cell transplant recipients fail adequately to control their latent virus 'commensals'. The important infections are summarized in Table 45.3.

Table 45.1 Environmentally acquired virus infections after stem-cell transplant

Virus	Clinical presentation*	Treatment	Prognosis	Specific prophylaxis
Measles	Atypical rash, giant-cell pneumonia	None	Fatal	Immunization**
Primary varicella (chickenpox)	Severe chickenpox, necrotic lesions Pneumonitis	Acyclovir i.v. 10 mg/kg/t.d.s.	Good with prompt treatment	Zoster immune globulin (ZIG) immunization Acyclovir
Adenoviruses	URTI, LRTI, pneumonia	None	Variable	None
Respiratory syncytial virus	LRTI, pneumonia	Ribavirin (i.v. immunoglobulin)	Poor if pneumonia develops	None
Influenza	LRTI, pneumonia	Amantadine for influenza A	Poor if pneumonia develops	Amantadine for influenza immunization

*URTI = upper respiratory track infection; LRTI = lower respiratory tract infection.
**Immunization of household contacts as well as index patient before immunosuppression.

Table 45.2 Transfusion/donor-related infections

Virus	Clinical presentation*	Treatment	Prognosis	Specific prophylaxis
Hepatitis B	Non-icteric, icteric hepatic failure	Interferon	Poor	Donor screen (antigen test)**
Hepatitis C	Chronic liver disease. Veno-occlusive disease	Interferon	Poor	Donor screen (antibody test)**
HIV	AIDS	Azathioprine, didanosine	Poor	Donor screen (antibody test)**
Cytomegalovirus	Colitis, hepatitis, etc. Pneumonitis	Ganciclovir, foscarnet, ganciclovir, CMV hyperimmune globulin	Poor if pneumonia	Donor screen (antibody test)**, acyclovir, ganciclovir
Parvovirus B19	Aplastic anaemia, bone-marrow failure	i.v. immunoglobulin	Variable	None
HGV and other new hepatitis viruses	?	?	?	None
HTLV-1 and -2	Adult T-cell lymphoma Tropical spastic paraparesis Donor screen	–	–	Donor screen (antibody test)*,**
Other viraemia	–	–	–	None

*Only for hepatitis B does the screening test measure virus directly; all other viruses, screening tests are for antibody. Thus, a 'window period' may occur.
**Not routinely performed.

Table 45.3 Endogenous virus reactivations

Virus	Latency site	Clinical presentation	Treatment	Prognosis	Specific prophylaxis
Herpes simplex virus	CNS	Mucosal lesions/oral/genital, mucositis without demarked lesions, hepatitis, pneumonia	i.v. acyclovir, at least 5–10 mg/kg t.d.s.	Good for superficial lesions. Poor for hepatitis and pneumonia	Oral acyclovir
Varicella-zoster virus	CNS	Typical or atypical (disseminated) zoster	i.v. acyclovir, at least 10 mg/kg t.d.s.	Good	Long-term acyclovir
Cytomegalovirus (CMV)		See Table 45.2, and Chapter 44			
Epstein–Barr virus (EBV)	Peripheral blood lymphocytes	Polyclonal lymphoma (rare)	Chemotherapy donor lymphocyte infusion (DLI)	Poor but may respond to DLI	None
Human herpes, type 6	Peripheral blood lymphocytes	Possible copathogen in pneumonia	?Acyclovir ?Foscarnet		None
Human papilloma virus	Skin	Multiple warts, potential for malignant change	Topical therapy	Good	None
BK virus	Bladder	Haemorrhagic cystitis	None	Good	None
JC Virus	CNS	Progressive multifocal leukoencephalopathy	None	Fatal	None
Hepatitis B	Liver	Hepatitis, liver failure	Interferon, HBIG	Poor	HBIG, immunization
Hepatitis C	Liver	Chronic liver disease, veno-occlusive disease	Interferon, ribavirin	Poor	None

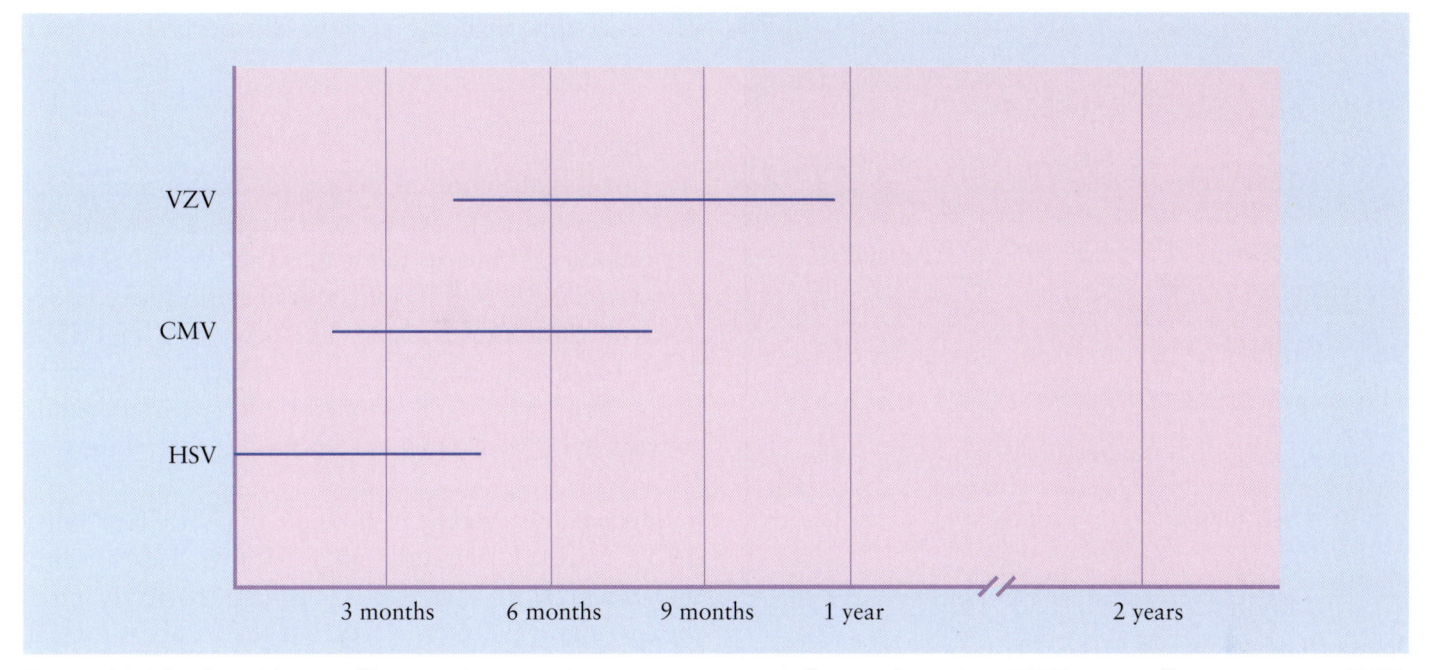

Figure 45.1 Peak incidence of herpes virus reactivations post stem-cell transplantation. VZV = varicella-zoster virus; CMV = cytomegalovirus; HSV = herpes simplex virus.

Many of the viruses are latent in the majority of the population and reactivation is an expected part of the post-transplant course. Although reactivations can occur at any time, perhaps surprisingly, many follow a predictable time course with a peak period post transplant where a particular reactivation is most common. This is illustrated in Figure 45.1. Several important endogenous infections are caused by herpes viruses, and for some, both effective treatment and prophylaxis are available. Other endogenous infections may be ubiquitous (BK virus, Epstein–Barr virus) but rarely cause disease even in transplant patients. If disease develops, however, there is no effective therapy and the patient may succumb.

Specific infections

Herpes simplex virus (HSV)
Clinical aspects

Reactivation lesions in immunocompromised patients may be more severe and protracted than in normal individuals. Chronic large ulcerated lesions persisting for weeks to years have been described [1,2]. Visceral dissemination may occur and mortality varies from 10 to 50% [3]. Skin lesions may appear atypical and be present at unusual sites. Involvement of the tracheobronchial tree may occur as part of local or disseminated disease. Pneumonia can result from contiguous spread of virus or can be secondary to local trauma caused by endotracheal incubation [2]. Oesophagitis is also common, and *Candida* oesophagitis frequently co-exists. Local trauma induced by nasogastric tubing is thought to be contributory. Widespread visceral involvement of liver, lungs, adrenals, gastrointestinal tract, the CNS and skin can occur, and under these circumstances the prognosis is poor. [4–7]. For diagnosis, see Table 45.4.

The prevalence of latent HSV infection varies in different communities; in the UK, about half the population is infected. A proportion of these latently infected individuals have a history of herpetic lesions (usually orofacial or genital) and all have detectable IgG antibody to the virus. (Note: A more sensitive method than complement fixation testing is needed to detect antibody reliably; commercially available IgG enzyme-linked immunosorbent assays (ELISA) are currently most widely used.) Demonstration of IgG antibody, indicating latent infection, can be used to identify those patients at risk of developing HSV mucositis post-transplant, enabling clinicians to cover the most vulnerable period for severe disease (0–2 months post-transplant) with prophylactic acyclovir [8].

Table 45.4 Diagnosis of herpes simplex virus infection post stem-cell transplant

Test	Speed	Sensitivity/specificity
Direct antigen detection	< 30 min	High/high
Electron microscopy	< 30 min	High/low
Histology/cytology	Several hours	Low/low
Virus isolation	24–48 hours	High/high
Serology for IgM/IgG Antibody rise		Of no value

After transplantation, serology has no role to play in the diagnosis of HSV disease. The virus can be easily isolated from lesions or swabs of the oral or genital area. Isolation can take several days and a rapid and reliable alternative is to examine clinical material from suspect lesions by direct immunofluorescence using commercially prepared directly labelled monoclonal antibodies to either HSV-1 or HSV-2 (Figure 45.2) (electron microscopy, whilst providing a same-day diagnosis of 'herpes virus', cannot distinguish between HSV and varicella-zoster virus and is thus less valuable). Direct immunofluorescence provides the clinician with a diagnosis within 30 minutes of receipt of the sample, enabling prompt appropriate acyclovir therapy.

Management

Acyclovir is the drug of choice for both prophylaxis and therapy of HSV infections in high-risk immunocompromised patients. The value of both intravenous and oral prophylaxis in seropositive bone-marrow transplant patients has been well described [8,9], but it may be that not all such patients require prophylaxis, and that a more cost-effective approach is to treat only those patients with proven reactivation of HSV.

Intravenous therapy is the route of choice (see Table 45.5) as oral bioavailability is low (20%) and unpredictable in stem-cell transplant patients. Oral therapy has a place, however, but the value of topical therapy is much more doubtful. The new product, valaciclovir will probably replace oral acyclovir because of its much greater bioavailability [10], and famciclovir (the oral preparation of penciclovir) has also been licensed for use in the treatment of herpes simplex reactivations.

Varicella-zoster virus (VZV)
Clinical aspects
Primary varicella (chickenpox)
This is a potentially lethal disease in stem-cell transplant recipients. All patients (especially children) who are to receive stem-cell transplants should have their immunity to VZV assessed. Seronegative patients

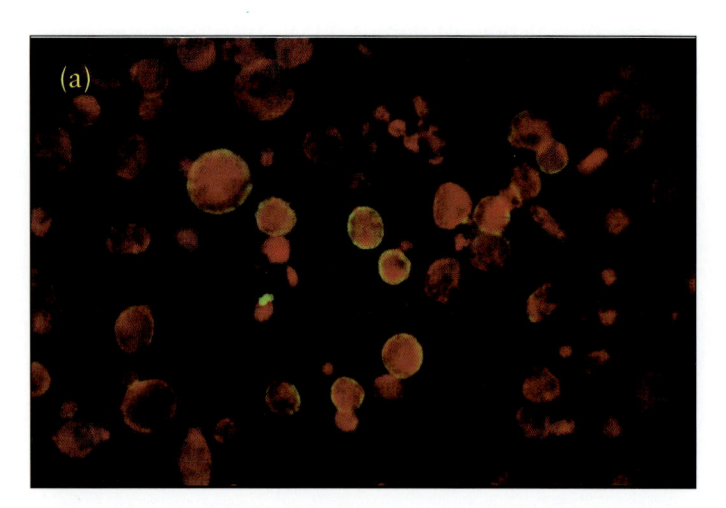

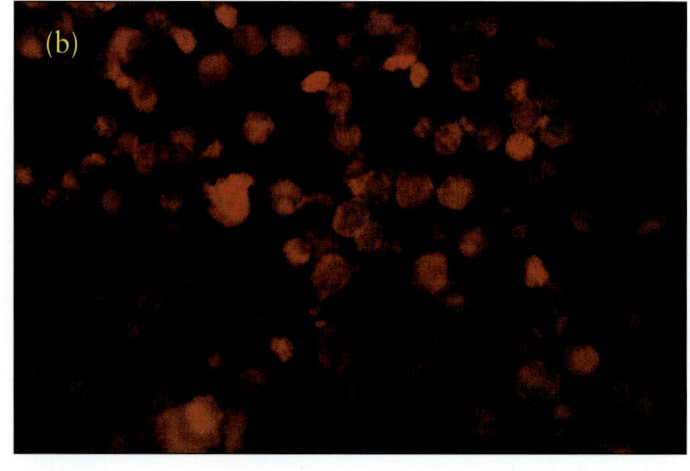

Figure 45.2 (a) Herpes simplex virus antigens in infected cells detected using direct fluorescein-labelled monoclonal antibody to HSV-1 proteins. (b) Uninfected cells showing no HSV-specific innumofluorescence.

Table 45.5 Management of herpes simplex and varicella-zoster post stem-cell transplant

Clinical presentation	Treatment
None – well patient previously HSV-antibody positive	Consider oral acyclovir prophylaxis four times daily for 1–3 months
Recurrent HSV mucosal lesions	Intravenous acyclovir 5 mg/kg t.d.s. for at least 48 hours (oral drug 400 mg five times daily may be preferred if patient out of hospital and systemically well)
Chickenpox (primary varicella-zoster virus)	Intravenous acyclovir, at least 10 mg/kg t.d.s. for 10–14 days
Zoster (shingles) (reactivation varicella-zoster virus)	Oral acyclovir (valaciclovir or Famvir) if patient out of hospital and systemically well. If patient unwell or lesions extensive, intravenous acyclovir at least 10 mg/kg t.d.s. for 10–14 days

are at risk of severe chickenpox as long as they remain on immunosuppressive therapy. If such patients are in contact with chickenpox, it is recommended that they receive passive antibody prophylaxis, intramuscular zoster immune globulin (ZIG) [11]. There is an accumulating body of evidence [12,13] that effective prophylaxis against disease is possible using acyclovir. If, as seems likely, it is possible to use this drug to decrease or abolish symptoms without preventing the development of natural immunity, this would be of great benefit.

Treatment of severe chickenpox in the immunocompromised patient requires acyclovir at high doses (see Table 45.5).

Reactivation zoster (shingles)

Following recovery from chickenpox at any time of life, varicella zoster virus remains latent in the dorsal root ganglia of the spinal cord. Shingles (herpes zoster) is due to reactivation of virus in the nerves supplying a particular dermatome or small group of adjacent dermatomes. Lesions erupt on the skin in a pattern dictated by its innervation. In otherwise healthy people there is little spread of virus but in stem-cell transplant patients local lesion extension, satellite lesions and visceral dissemination can all occur.

Zoster recurrences are most frequent several months after stem-cell transplantation, usually within the first year and repeated attacks can occur. For diagnosis see Table 45.6.

As for herpes simplex, direct antigen detection in clinical samples (lesion fluid, skin impression smears or BAL as appropriate) is the best method of diagnosis. Virus growth in culture is too slow to be of clinical value and serology has no place at all.

Table 45.6 Diagnosis of varicella-zoster-virus infection post stem-cell transplant

Test	Speed	Sensitivity/specificity
Direct antigen detection	< 30 mins	High/high
Electron microscopy	< 30 mins	High/low
Histology/cytology	Hours – days	Low/low
Virus isolation	2 – 3 weeks	High/high
Serology for IgM/IgG antibody rise		Of no value

Management

Varicella-zoster is sensitive to acyclovir and to the related drug penciclovir (the latter given orally as the pro-drug famciclovir). Higher doses of acyclovir are required than for HSV treatment (see Table 45.5). Therapy normally involves an initial period of intravenous followed by oral administration.

Of particular concern are heavily immuno-compromised patients immediately post stem-cell replacement. They have effectively no immunological resistance to VZV, and if in contact with chickenpox require prophylaxis with acyclovir (and ZIG) whatever their pretransplant immune status to VZV.

The new Herpes viruses (HHV6, HHV8)

The role of these viruses as causes of disease in stem-cell transplant recipients has yet to be established although there have been case reports of HHV6 reactivation associated with encephalitis, pneumonitis and graft suppression [14,15].

Diagnostic strategies are not well worked out. HHV6 is ubiquitous and its demonstration in diseased tissue by isolation, antigen detection or molecular methods such as the polymerase chain reaction (PCR) fail unequivocally to prove that the virus has a pathogenic role. Assessment of actively replicating virus, e.g. by Nucleic acid sequence based analysis (NASBA) technology, may be useful in the future.

HHV8 has been associated with body-cavity lymphomas in patients immunocompromised due to human immunodeficiency virus (HIV) infection. Whether there is a parallel disease in stem-cell recipients is, as yet, unclear.

Treatment of infections whose contribution to disease is unclear may be inappropriate. Appleton and coworkers suggest [16] that HHV6 reactivation may exacerbate graft-versus-host disease (GvHD) resulting in GvHD which is refractory to conventional management.

Epstein–Barr virus (EBV)

Clinical aspects

Primary EBV infection in transplant recipients has been described presenting typically as heterophile-positive mononucleosis or, atypically, even causing pneumonia resembling that caused by CMV [17]. Reactivation of EBV occurs commonly in transplant patients [18,19] usually without any associated symptoms. Very rarely in immuno-compromised patients, EBV may induce B-cell lymphoproliferative disease. These lymphomas are polyclonal or oligoclonal B-cell tumours which may evolve to monoclonal origin. In bone-marrow transplant recipients, such disease is generally confined the group who receive T-cell-depleted allografts.

Diagnosis

Because EBV is rarely a clinical problem in stem-cell transplant patients, development of diagnostic methods is not as advanced as for the other herpes viruses. Antibody responses are non-contributory in most cases. Direct antigen-detection methods are not available and would be difficult to interpret in view of the ubiquitous distribution of this infection. Virus isolation is very slow and currently not performed by most diagnostic virus laboratories.

Management

In most cases, treatment is unnecessary. Interferon and acyclovir have both been claimed to have a beneficial effect, but the evidence for this is very limited [20]. Management of EBV-related lymphoproliferative disease is unsatisfactory. Chemotherapy and radiotherapy are ineffective [20] and the most promising approach seems to be the infusion of donor EBV-specific cytotoxic T-cells [21].

Adenoviruses

Members of this virus group are common causes of respiratory and gastrointestinal illness in children, and of acute febrile illness in young adults. Severe morbidity and mortality can occur in transplant recipients. Pneumonia is probably the most frequently recognized problem [22–24], and may have an undulant or rapidly fatal course. Generalized infection is almost always associated with hepatitis and often diarrhoea, and the problems are much more frequent in the paediatric patient population. Haemorrhagic cystitis and renal damage have been described [25,26], particularly in association with adenovirus type 11.

Diagnosis is made by direct antigen detection from appropriate specimens (e.g. BAL), virus isolation (which takes several days) or molecular methods [24]. There is no specific therapy available, although ribavirin and intravenous immunoglobulin have been suggested [20,25,27], as has donor leukocyte infusion [25].

Papovaviruses (JC/BK/HPV)

There is a well established association between BK virus reactivation and chronic haemorrhagic cystitis post stem-cell transplant; however, only 25% of BK reactivations lead to haemorrhagic symptoms and busulphan and/or cyclophosphamide chemotherapy are probable cofactors [28,29]. The virus persists as a latent infection of the kidney and reactivates following immunosuppression. Diagnosis depends largely on molecular technology – PCR on urine being the method most often used to detect virus DNA. Virus isolation in culture is slow and not of great value diagnostically. Treatment is not well established but there are reports of success using vidarabine [28,30] and topical prostaglandin E_2 (PGE_2).

The closely related JC virus is rarely found in urine post bone-marrow transplant. JC reactivation in the CNS is associated with progressive multifocal leukoencephalopathy (PML) a fortunately rare, invariably fatal, progressive neurological degeneration for which there is no specific therapy.

Human papilloma viruses cause warts which are usually trivial in the immunocompetent. Stem-cell recipients may suffer from aggressive and florid wart proliferation which is both unsightly and presents a risk of malignant change in the skin. Wherever possible, such lesions should be ablated by local therapy.

Measles

In the past, measles was a much feared infection which had a high mortality in immunocompromised patients (particularly children being treated for leukaemia). Excess mortality was due mainly to giant-cell pneumonitis, but fatal encephalitis was also common. Specific therapy was not available, nor is it today. Measles has become a very rare infection in the UK as a result of widespread immunization. Pre-existing immunity in donors and recipients of stem-cell transplants is almost universal, and the virus is no longer circulating within the community.

Diagnosis of giant-cell pneumonitis was by direct detection of measles antigen using immunofluorescence antibody or by histological demonstration of typical syncytia which are the 'giant cells'.

Respiratory tract infections (RSV, influenza A and B, parainfluenza 1–3)

Pneumonia due to each of these viral pathogens has been described post stem-cell transplant. Virus circulation in the community is seasonal, and infections in transplant patients occur during periods of high incidence in the community. RSV is a particular problem, affecting 1–3% of patients after transplantation [31,32] and it is not confined to the extremes of life as in immunocompetent individuals.

Rapid diagnosis of each of these infections is possible using direct antigen detection by monoclonal fluorescein-labelled antibody. Suitable specimens include nasopharyngeal aspirates (from babies) or broncheoalveolar lavage material from patients with lower respiratory tract infection or pneumonia.

Clinical trials have shown ribavirin to be of benefit in treating immunocompetent infants infected with RSV, but post transplant, results have been disappointing, with a reported mortality of 50% despite aerosolized ribavirin for 10 days [31]. Ribavirin has also been used in stem-cell transplant patients with parainfluenza pneumonia (Figure 45.3) but its efficacy is doubtful [31,32].

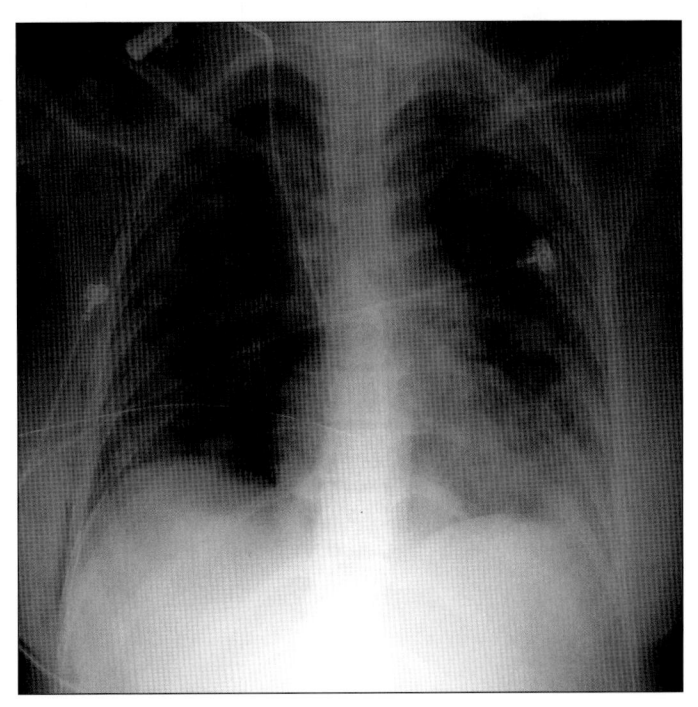

Figure 45.3 Chest radiograph of a young woman post stem-cell transplant with parainfluenza virus type 3 pneumonia.

Influenza A and B can cause mild or severe disease. In some studies clinical benefit has been claimed for the use of amantadine to treat influenza A pneumonia [31].

Enteroviruses

This group of viruses includes polio viruses, the coxsackievirus and echovirus groups, as well as many others. There has been a small number of outbreaks of enterovirus infections in stem-cell transplant units with a high patient morbidity and mortality. Such problems are, however, very rare. Oral polio vaccine should be avoided by immunocompromised patients, as this has been associated with a substantial risk of paralytic poliomyelitis. Family contacts of post stem-cell transplant patients should be immunized with live attenuated polio virus only if strict measures can be taken to prevent spread of the virus within the family.

Diagnosis of enterovirus infection still depends predominantly on virus isolation in cell culture, although immunofluorescence reagents are available. Specific management of such infections is limited. Intravenous immunoglobulin has been shown to be of benefit in hypogammaglobulaemic patients.

Gastroenteritis viruses

There is a variety of viruses (rotavirus, enteric adenoviruses, Norwalk-like agents, etc.) which cause gastroenteritis in both immunocompetent and immunocompromised individuals. Infection in the latter can be prolonged and associated with severe symptoms. Diagnosis is based on antigen detection or electron microscopy of stool; there is no specific treatment. The best option for post stem-cell transplant patients is prevention by meticulous cross-infection control measures and avoidance of 'high-risk' foods (e.g. shellfish).

Hepatitis B (HBV)

Screening of blood and organ donors and the exclusion of hepatitis B surface antigen-positive products has virtually abolished the problem of transfusion-related HBV infection post stem-cell transplant in the UK.

Patients with a history of hepatitis B infection, either resolved, or persisting in the 'carrier' state are at risk of reactivation of hepatitis B during post stem-cell transplant immune suppression. Reactivation may be subclinical, accompanied by mild hepatitis, or may lead to fulminant hepatic failure [33].

Diagnosis depends upon the detection of hepatitis B surface antigen, 'e' antigen and possibly HBV DNA in serum. Treatment with interferon may be of some benefit. Such a patient's family contacts should be immunized against hepatitis B.

Hepatitis C (HCV)

As for hepatitis B, the risk in the UK from transfusion-related hepatitis C should now be small because of donor screening. Patients who have acquired HCV infection prior to stem-cell transplant have a high incidence of post-transplant complications, not only chronic hepatitis and cirrhosis but also veno-occlusive disease. The risk of veno-occlusive disease in HCV antibody positive individuals is 82% compared with 32% in patients without HCV infection [34,35].

Diagnosis requires detection of HCV RNA rather than antibody in these immunocompromised patients. Reverse transcriptase PCR not only gives a direct assessment of whether the patient is viraemic but also, if quantitative, can indicate the viral load.

Specific treatment for HCV infection post-transplant is not established. Some encouraging results have been obtained using interferon post liver transplantation and ribavirin may be used on a compassionate use basis.

Finally, acute liver failure related to exacerbation of pre-existing HCV infection has been described in association with the withdrawal of immunosuppressive therapy post bone-marrow transplant [36]. The management of HCV-infected stem-cell transplant patients remains a challenge.

Parvovirus B19

This virus causes 'slapped cheek' or 'fifth' disease in immunocompetent children. It infects erythroid stem cells, and in immunocompromised individuals causes chronic anaemia due to the failure of immune elimination of the virus. Diagnosis is by means of DNA detection (PCR or dot blot), and therapy depends upon infusion of immunoglobulin containing anti-B19 antibodies. The infection may be prolonged, requiring repeated immunoglobulin infusions.

Figures 45.4–45.8 summarize the viruses which may affect a particular body site after transplantation, and which should therefore be screened for if there are clinical grounds to suspect that they are present.

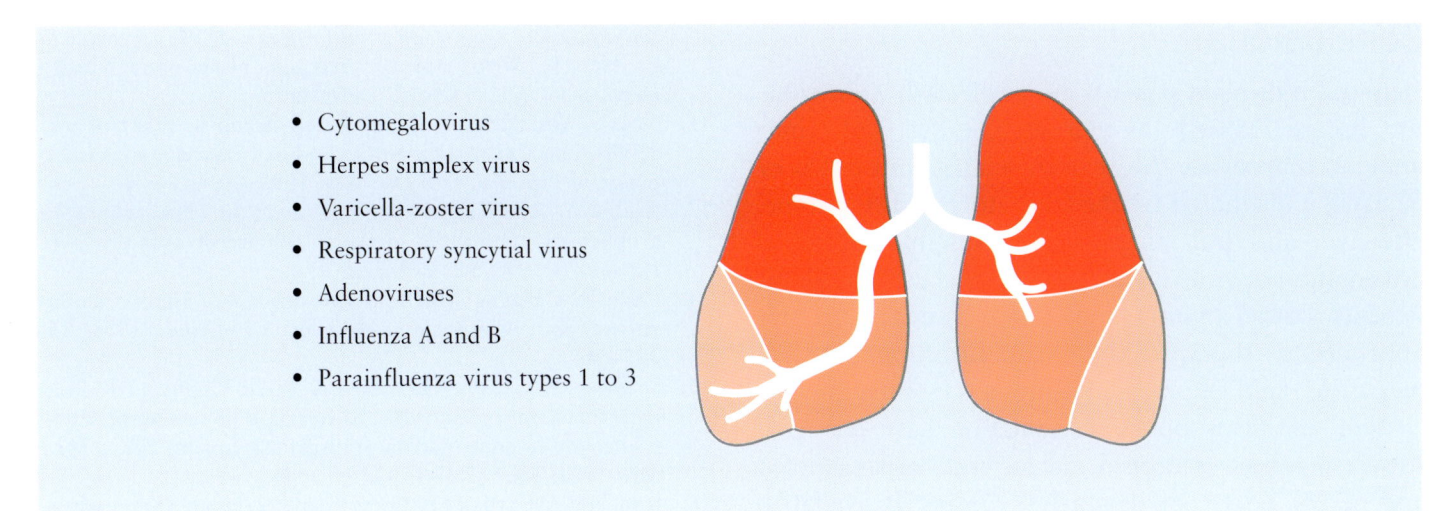

- Cytomegalovirus
- Herpes simplex virus
- Varicella-zoster virus
- Respiratory syncytial virus
- Adenoviruses
- Influenza A and B
- Parainfluenza virus types 1 to 3

Figure 45.4 Virus infections of the chest post stem-cell transplant

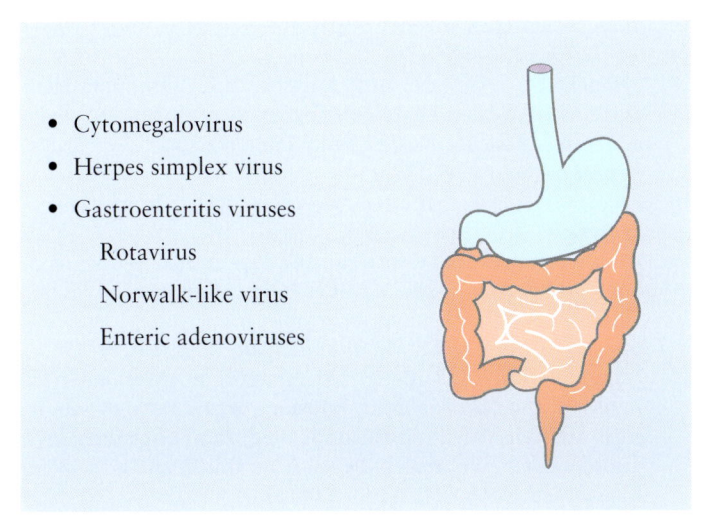

- Cytomegalovirus
- Herpes simplex virus
- Gastroenteritis viruses
  Rotavirus
  Norwalk-like virus
  Enteric adenoviruses

Figure 45.5 Virus infections of the gastrointestinal tract post stem-cell transplant

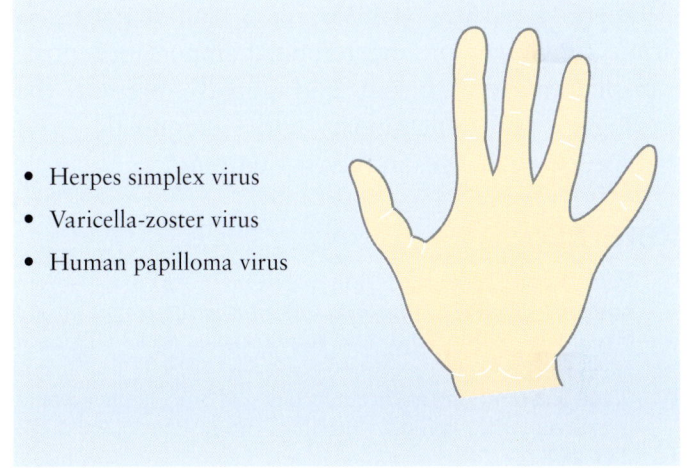

- Herpes simplex virus
- Varicella-zoster virus
- Human papilloma virus

Figure 45.7 Virus infections of the skin post stem-cell transplant

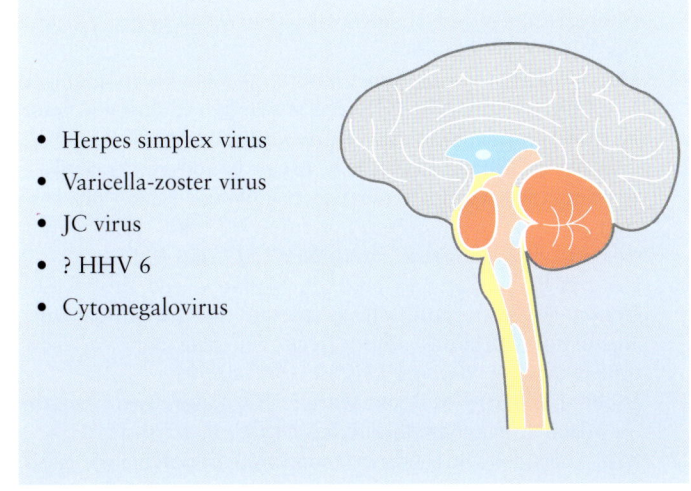

- Herpes simplex virus
- Varicella-zoster virus
- JC virus
- ? HHV 6
- Cytomegalovirus

Figure 45.6 Virus infections of the brain post stem-cell transplant

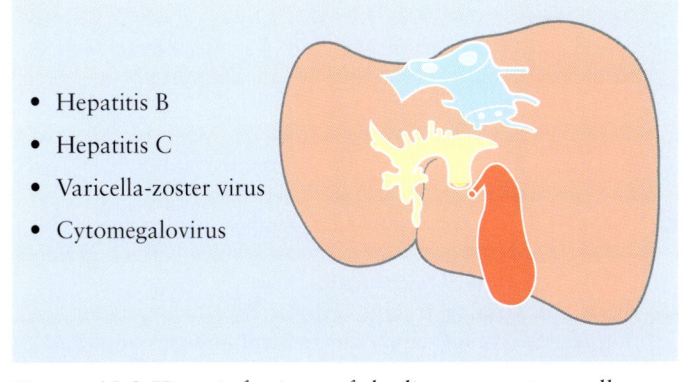

- Hepatitis B
- Hepatitis C
- Varicella-zoster virus
- Cytomegalovirus

Figure 45.8 Virus infections of the liver post stem-cell transplant

Conclusions

Stem-cell transplant patients are particularly vulnerable to disease caused by viruses because of their immunocompromise. Most of these infections can now be rapidly diagnosed by the laboratory and, for some, effective antiviral therapy is available. Clinical presentation of virus disease in post stem-cell transplant patients is often atypical, and in order to ensure prompt appropriate therapy and cross-infection control measures, rapid laboratory diagnosis is essential.

Viral problems post-transplantation have changed. Measles has been controlled, and for both herpes simplex and herpes zoster, good antiviral therapy is available. Newer problems such as hepatitis C should diminish in importance as less of the transplant population has received unscreened blood product support.

Emerging viruses (HHV6, 7, 8 and hepatitis G virus) are as yet of undetermined importance post-transplantation and will undoubtedly present the virologist and oncologist with diagnostic and therapeutic challenges in the coming years.

References

1. Hirsch M. Herpes group virus infections in the compromised host. In: *Clinical approach to infection in the compromised host.* RH Rubin and LS Young (eds), 1988 (Plenum Medical).
2. Nash G. Necrotising tracheobronchitis and bronchopneumonia consistent with herpetic infection. *Hum Pathol* 1972; 3: 283–291.
3. Wong K and Hirsh M. Herpes virus infections in patients with neoplastic disease: diagnosis and therapy. *Am J Med* 1984; 76: 464–478.
4. Elliot WC, Houghton DC, Bryant RE et al. Herpes simplex type 1 hepatitis in renal transplantation. *Arch Intern Med* 1980; 140: 1656–1660.
5. Douglas RG, Anderson MC and Weg JG. Herpes simplex virus pneumonia, occurrence in an allotransplanted lung. *J Am Med Ass* 1969; 210: 902–904.
6. Linneman CC, First MR and Alvira MM. Herpes virus hominis type 2 meningoencephalitis following renal transplantation. *Am J Med* 1976; 61: 703–708.
7. Naik HR and Chandrasekar PH. Herpes simplex virus (HSV) colitis in a bone marrow transplant recipient. *Bone Marrow Transplant* 1996; 17: 285–286.
8. Berry NJ, Grundy JE and Griffiths PD. Radioimmunoassay for detection of IgG antibodies to herpes simplex virus and its use as a prognostic indicator of HSV excretion in transplant patient. *J Med Virology* 1987; 21: 147–154.
9. McNeeley DF. Prophylaxis in patients with cancer. *Infect Med* 1995; 12: 203–210.
10. Crooks RJ and Murray A. Valaciclovir – a review of a promising new antiherpes agent. *Antiviral Chem Chemother* 1994; 5(Suppl 1): 31–37.
11. *Immunisation against Infectious Disease 1992.* Department of Health, Welsh Office, Scottish Home and Health Department, DHSS (Northern Ireland).
12. Suga S, Yoshikawa T, Ozaki T and Asano Y. Effect of oral acyclovir against primary and secondary viraemia in incubation period of varicella. *Arch Dis Child* 1993; 69: 639–643.
13. Asano Y, Yoshikawa T, Suga S et al. Post exposure prophylaxis of varicella in family contact by oral acyclovir. *Paediatrics* 1993; 92: 219–222.
14. Cone RN, Haung MW and Hackman RC. Human herpes virus 6 and pneumonia. *Leukaemia Lymphoma* 1994; 15: 235–241.
15. Drobyski WR, Knox KK, Majewski D and Carrigan DR. Brief report: fatal encephalitis due to variant B human herpesvirus-6 infection in bone marrow transplant recipient. *New Engl J Med* 1994; 330: 1357–1360.
16. Appleton AL, Sviland L, Peiris JSM et al. Human herpesvirus-6 infection in marrow graft-versus-host disease. *Bone Marrow Transplant* 1995; 16: 777–782.
17. Grose C, Henle W and Horwitz MS. Primary Epstein–Barr virus infection in a renal transplant recipient. *South Med J* 1977; 70: 1276–1278.
18. Strauch B, Seigel N and Andrews LL. Oropharyngeal excretion of Epstein–Barr virus by renal transplant recipients and other patients treated with immunosuppressive drugs. *Lancet* 1974; i: 234–237.
19. Chang RS, Lewis JP and Reynolds RD. Oropharyngeal excretion of Epstein–Barr virus by patients with lymphoproliferative disorders and by recipients of renal homografts. *Ann Intern Med* 1978; 88: 34–40.
20. Ward KN. Viral complications after bone marrow transplantation. *PHLS Microbiol Digest* 1996; 13: 16–19.
21. Papadopoulos EB, Ladanyi M, Emanuel D, Mackinnon S, Boulad F and Carabasi MH. Infusions of donor leukocytes to treat Epstein–Barr virus associated lymphoproliferative disorder after allogenic bone marrow transplantation. *New Engl J Med* 1994; 330: 1185–1191.
22. Shields AF, Hackman RC, Fife KH, Corey L and Myers J. Adenovirus infections in patients undergoing bone marrow transplantation. *New Engl J Med* 1985; 21: 529–533.
23. Neiman PE, Reeves W, Ray G. et al. A prospective analysis of intestitial viral pneumonia and opportunistic viral infections among recipients of allogeneic bone marrow grafts. *J Infect Dis* 1977; 136: 754–767.
24. Matsuse T, Matsui H, Shu CY et al. Adenovirus pulmonary infections identified by PCR and *in situ* hybridisation in bone marrow transplant patients. *J Clin Pathol* 1994; 47: 973–977.
25. Liles WC, Cushing H, Holt S. Bryan C and Hackman RC. Severe adenoviral nephritis following bone marrow transplantation. Successful treatment with intravenous ribavirin. *Bone Marrow Transplant* 1993; 12: 409.
26. Hromas R, Cornetta K, Stout E, Blauke C and Brown ER. Donor leukocyte infusion as therapy of life threatening adenoviral infections after T-cell depleted bone marrow transplantation. *Blood* 1994; 84: 1689–1690.
27. Buchold RM, Taylor P and Warmer JO. Neutralised ribavirin for adenovirus pneumonia. *Lancet* 1985; ii: 1070–1071.
28. Azzi A, Fanci R, Bosi A et al. Monitoring of polyomavirus BK viraemia in bone marrow transplantation patients by DNA hybridization assay and by polymerase chain reaction: an approach to assess the relationship between BK viraemia and

haemorrhagic cystitis. *Bone Marrow Transplant* 1994; **14**: 235–240.
29. Schneider EM and Dorries K. High frequency of polyomavirus infection in lymphoid cell preparations after allogenic bone marrow transplantation. *Transplant Proc* 1993; **25**: 1271–1273.
30. Chapman C, Flower AJE and Durrant STS. The use of vidarabine in the treatment of human polymavirus associated acute haemorrhagic cystitis. *Bone Marrow Transplant* 1991; **7**: 481–483.
31. Sable CA and Hayden FG. Orthomyxoviral and paramyxoviral infections in transplant patients. *Infect Dis Clin North Am* 1995; **9**: 987–1003.
32. Wendt CM and Hertz MI. Respiratory syncytial virus and parainfluenza virus infections in the immunocompromised host. *Semin Resp Infect* 1995; **10**: 224–231.
33. Martin BA, Lowe JM, Konicles PA and DiPersio JF. Hepatitis B reactivation following allogeneic bone marrow transplantation: case report and review of the literature. *Bone Marrow Transplant* 1995; **15**: 145–148.
34. Terrault NA, Wright TL and Pereira BJ. Hepatitis C infection in the transplant patient. *Infect Dis Clin North Am* 1995; **9**: 943–963.
35. Shuhart MC, Myerson D, Childs BH *et al*. Marrow transplant from hepatitis C seropositive donors: transmission rate and clinical course. *Blood* 1994; **84**: 3229–3235.
36. Kanamoni H, Kukawa H, Maruta A *et al*. Fulminant hepatitis C viral infection after allogenic bone marrow transplantation. *Am J Med Sci* **303**: 109–111.

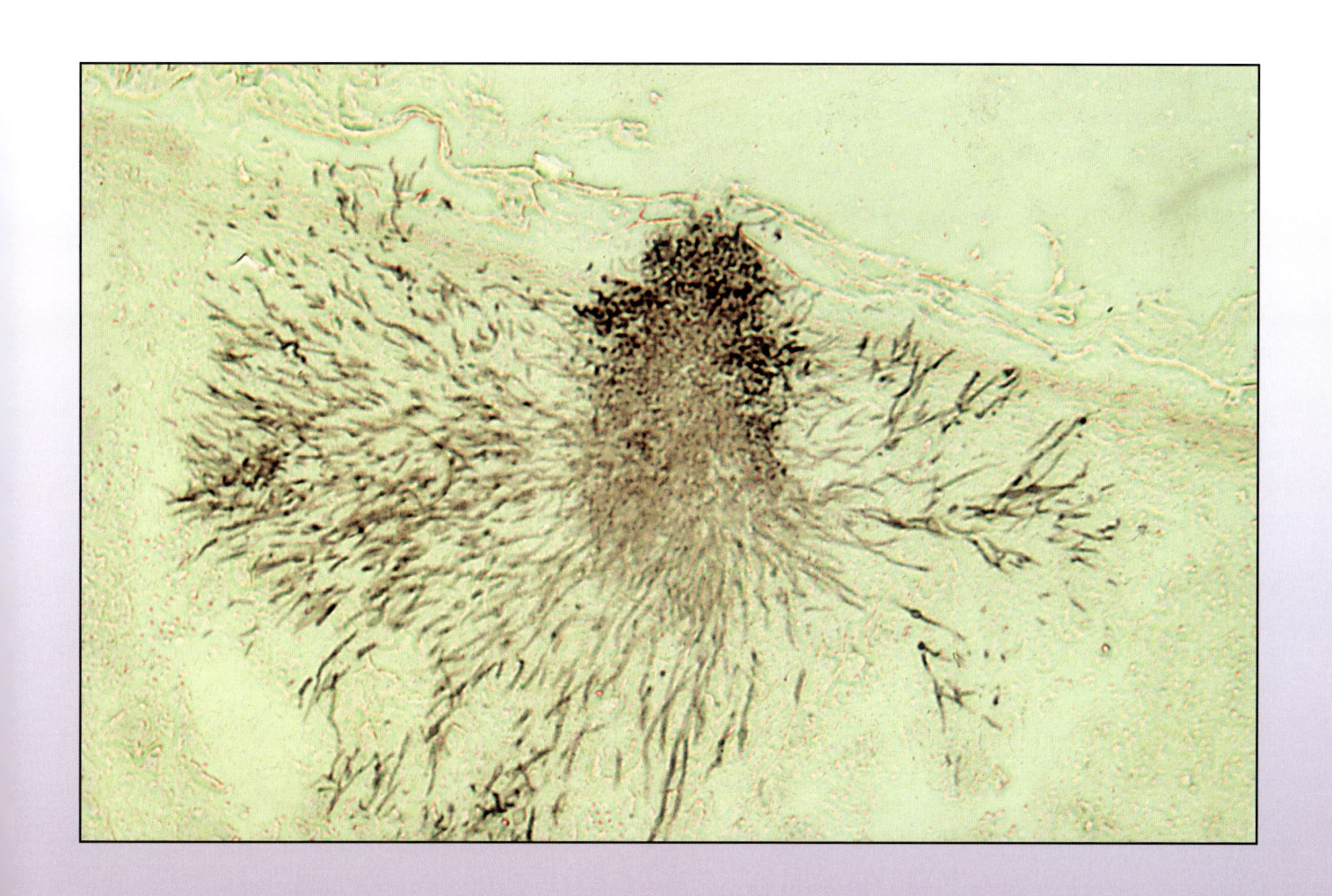

Chapter 46

Fungal infections

Rosemary A. Barnes

Introduction

Of all infectious complications, fungal infections remain the most problematic and are associated with serious morbidity in the bone-marrow transplant (BMT)/peripheral blood stem-cell (PBSC) transplant patient population. Fungal infection has been found in up to 25% of autopsies from patients with acute leukaemia [1] and higher rates have been reported from smaller studies on BMT patients [2]. Also, the risk of mortality in this patient group is higher than for other immunocompromised patients [3]. Even within the transplant population, a changing pattern of systemic mycoses is emerging with shifts in the population of potential hosts and emergence of resistance.

Candida and *Aspergillus* infections are the most common, but the list of emerging fungal pathogens is increasing rapidly [4] (Table 46.1). More significant is the 'pathogen shift' reported in systemic *Candida* infections. One study reported a decrease in the proportion of *C. albicans* infections from 87 to 31% of all yeast blood culture isolates over a five-year period [5] and similar trends with the emergence of non-*albicans* species such as *C. tropicalis*, *C. parapsilosis*, *C. glabrata* and *C. krusei* have been reported elsewhere. The widespread use of azoles has been implicated [6,7] in this trend but does not fully explain the shift and other factors such as the increased use of intravenous long-lines, total parenteral nutrition and severe mucositis which are probably involved [8].

Recent taxonomic changes based on ribosomsal RNA sequencing have led to the reclassification of some organisms, most notably *Pneumocystis carinii*, as fungi [9]. While some scepticism exists, regarding inclusion of this organism into the realms of mycology based on its apparent lack of a free-living form and ergosterol-free cell membranes, molecular and ultrastructural evidence compels its inclusion here [10].

The range of clinical presentation of fungal infections in PBSC transplants patients is shown in Table 46.2.

Table 46.1 Fungal pathogens in BMT patients

Classical fungal opportunists	Emerging fungal pathogens
Candida albicans	Candida spp.
Aspergillus fumigatus	Candida tropicalis
Aspergillus flavus	Candida parapsilosis
	Candida krusei
	Candida glabrata (Torulopsis)
	Candida lusitaniae
Mucorales (zygomycetes)	Other yeasts and yeast-like fungi
Absidia spp.	Rhodotorula spp.
Rhizopus spp.	Trichosporon beigelii
Rhizomucor spp.	Malassezia furfur
Mucor spp.	Saccharomyces cerevisciae
	Hansenula anomala
Cryptococcus neoformans	Filamentous fungi
	Fusarium spp.
Pneumocystis carinii	Acremonium spp.
	Paecilomyces spp.
	Scedosprorium spp.
	Penicillium spp.

Table 46.2 Spectrum of fungal infections

Disease	Common manifestations	Rare manifestations

Candidosis	Superficial mucositis
	Oesophagitis
	Fungaemia:
	  Catheter-related
	  + skin and muscle involvement
	Renal
	Acute disseminated candidosis
	Chronic disseminated candidosis
		Gastritis
		
		Ophthalmitis

Aspergillosis	Invasive pulmonary aspergillosis (IPA) with or without dissemination	Rhinocerebral disease Obstructive tracheobronchitis
Cryptococcosis	Meningitis	Primary cutaneous Pneumonia Skin lesions
Zygomycosis	Rhinocerebral disease	Pneumonia
Pneumocystosis	PCP pneumonia	
Fusariosis	Fungaemia Nodular skin lesions	Sinusitis
Trichosporosis	Fungaemia	Pneumonia Gastric lesions

Risk factors for fungal infection

Neutropenia is the major risk factor for all invasive fungal infections, with the degree of risk being determined by the duration and extent of neutropenia. Reduction in the period of neutropenia associated with the increased use of PBSC transplant and also haemopoietic growth factors might be expected to decrease the incidence of invasive fungal infections in these patients. Although there is some preliminary evidence to support a reduction in episodes of interstitial pneumonitis and fungal infection in PBSC transplant patients compared to an autologous BMT [11], this has not been widely substantiated, probably because of increases in other risk factors.

Broad-spectrum antibiotics predispose to yeast infections, with both the duration of usage and the number of agents determining the risk. Suppression of gastrointestinal flora combined with mucosal damage significantly enhances the risk of invasive *C. tropicalis* infections arising from the gut [12]. Central venous catheters and total parenteral nutrition are risk factors for non-*albicans* yeast infections with *C. parapsilosis* frequently implicated [13].

Following transplantation, impaired cell-mediated immunity and reduced immunoglobulin levels/subclass disturbances may result in cryptococcal infections and *Pneumocystis carinii* pneumonia. After allogeneic transplantation, graft rejection and graft-versus-host disease (GvHD) may pose a significant risk factor for aspergillosis and other filamentous fungi that may extend well into the post-transplant period [14]. Steroid use, whether as part of the conditioning regimen or as treatment of GvHD, affects cell-mediated immunity and may lead to cytokine imbalances that predispose to deep-seated fungal infection.

Exogenous factors may also contribute to the risk of nosocomial infection. Building and renovation work and contaminated ventilation systems have been implicated in outbreaks of aspergillosis [15]. There is some evidence for cross-infection with *Candida* spp. via the hands of healthcare workers and other exogenous sources such as contaminated infusates and prosthetic devices [16].

Diagnosis

Signs and symptoms of fungal infection are often absent or non-specific. Refractory fever unresponsive to broad-spectrum antibiotics may be the only manifestation. Isolation of fungus from blood cultures and other clinical specimens is rarely successful and 'response' to empirical amphotericin treatment is used as an inadequate marker of fungal infection. Detection of antibodies is unreliable in this patient population and seroconversion, if detected, occurs late in the course of disease and is of prognostic significance with a limited role in diagnosis [17]. Detection of fungal components or metabolites in body fluids has been a major area of interest. Antigen detection is well established in the diagnosis of cryptococcosis but has been less successful in other fungal infections. A wide variety of antigens is known to circulate in systemic candidosis and *Aspergillus* infections. Most attention has focused on the detection of circulating mannan or galactomannan in these respective conditions. The immunodominant epitopes have been characterized and the development of monoclonal antibodies has enabled their incorporation into commercially available latex agglutination kits. Although early studies were promising, further evaluations in neutropenic patients have been disappointing; the positive predictive value of the *Aspergillus* antigen test is 53% when serial samples are analyzed but falls to less than 12% if only single serum samples are available [18]. In another study, the mean number of serial samples required to obtain at least one positive test in proven aspergillosis was 13.7 [19]. This apparent lack of sensitivity has been attributed to the fluctuating levels of the low-molecular-weight antigens and the rapid clearance of mannan and galactomannan from the circulation, with the net result that frequent testing of patients (two to three times a week) is necessary if the test is to have a useful clinical application. This is a costly undertaking in a large group of patients. Attempts to improve sensitivity of fungal antigens continue [20] and the development of a commercial enzyme-linked immunosorbent assay (ELISA) to replace the latex agglutination test will assist in this goal, as will the characterization of other antigens as potential targets for detection [21,22].

Other fungal metabolites, such as mannitol and arabinitol, can be detected in fungal infection, and elevated serum D-arabinotol; creatinine ratios have been reported in the patients with deep-seated candidosis [23] but the routine use of these diagnostic tests is not widespread. Recently, it was reported that $(1\rightarrow 3)$-β-D-glucan, a characteristic fungal cell wall constituent, could be rapidly detected in invasive fungal infection using a modification of the chromogenic *Limulus* lysate test [24].

Molecular techniques have opened the way for rapid and sensitive diagnosis of a variety of opportunist pathogens but progress with the detection of fungal DNA by the polymerase chain reaction (PCR) has been hampered by problems with extracting fungal DNA from human samples. With the exception of *Pneumocystis carinii* infection, where DNA-amplification techniques have led to the development of highly sensitive PCR assays [25,26], the molecular diagnoses of fungal infections have been disappointing to date. A variety of *Candida* genes have been identified as targets for amplification including heat-shock protein (HSP)-90 [27], actin [28] and cytochrome P-450 lanosterol-α-demethylase genes [29] but few if any have succeeded in detecting less than 10 CFU/ml particularly in biological specimens. *Aspergillus* gene targets have included the 26S intergenic spacer gene of the rDNA complex [30], and the alkaline protease gene [31]. Most exciting is the possibility of screening specimens using a 'universal' fungal primer to amplify ribosomal DNA followed by differentiating by hybridization using species-specific probes. Early studies using this technique reported it to be highly sensitive (1 CFU/ml blood) and with high specificity for a wide range of fungal pathogens including *P. carinii* [32]. Larger studies to confirm the usefulness of this approach in the rapid diagnosis of infection are awaited.

Candidosis

Candidosis is the most common fungal infection seen following transplantation. Infections may be superficial, mucocutaneous or deep-seated. There is a wide variety of clinical presentations of deep fungal infection (Table 46.2), ranging from fungaemia, which is often catheter-related and may be complicated by haematogenous spread with skin and muscle involvement, to deep organ infection. Organ involvement may be single (e.g. renal candidosis) or multiple in the case of disseminated disease. *Candida* pneumonia is extremely rare unless part of the manifestation of disseminated disease, despite the relatively frequent isolation of yeasts from respiratory specimens. A characteristic syndrome of chronic mucocutaneous candidosis has been recognized with increasing frequency. This manifestation, previously known as 'hepatosplenic candidosis' presents during the period of neutrophil regeneration.

Mucosal candidosis occurs early following transplantation. Oral manifestations are commoner than oesophageal candidosis although both may precede invasive infection. Chronic intestinal candidosis can occur in patients with chronic GvHD. Regular surveillance cultures from skin and mucosal sites may be useful in transplant patients [33]. Although unable to differentiate between colonization and infection, the positive predictive value of the isolation of certain species such as *C. tropicalis* [34] is high and may be the trigger for pre-emptive therapy.

Infection associated with intravascular devices should be considered an absolute indication for line removal in addition to systemic antifungal treatment [35]. Lower-dose amphotericin B (0.7 mg/kg/day) is as effective as high dose in the treatment of candidaemia, and fluconazole is a therapeutic option [36] although few comparative trials in transplant patients have been performed and it should not be recommended for infections caused by *C. krusei* or *C. glabrata*. Acute disseminated candidosis is a life-threatening condition. Involvement of the skin is common with widespread tender macular erythematous lesions, and microabscesses may develop in the kidney and other organs. Ocular candidosis and ophthalmitis is surprisingly rare in this patient group even in the presence of disseminated disease.

Chronic disseminated candidosis is an extremely interesting condition that affects individuals following marrow recovery. A characteristic syndrome develops (Table 46.3) with non-specific early symptoms of refractory fever with sterile blood cultures, normal or mildly abnormal liver function tests and an elevated C-reactive protein. There are few localizing features at this stage and abdominal ultrasound and computed tomography (CT) scans performed in the first few weeks are usually grossly normal [37]. As the disease progresses into chronicity, liver tenderness and splenomegaly increase with marked nausea, anorexia and weight loss. The alkaline phosphatase elevation is disproportionate to that of the other liver enzymes. Computed tomography and magnetic resonance imaging (MRI) scans become markedly abnormal with multiple microabscesses scattered throughout the liver and spleen [38] (Figure 46.1). Other organs such as the

Table 46.3 Features of chronic disseminated candidosis	
Early	Late
Fever unresponsive to antibiotics	Abdominal tenderness and hepatosplenomegaly
Negative blood cultures	Anorexia, nausea and weight loss
Few localizing signs	Persistent fever up to 40°C
Normal or mildly abnormal liver enzymes	Alkaline phosphatase raised disproportionately to other enzymes
Normal ultrasound scan	Characteristic CT/MRI changes
C-reactive protein grossly elevated	Liver biopsy occasionally positive Response to antifungals poor Seroconversion unreliable

lungs and peritoneum may also be affected (Figure 46.2) demonstrating the true dissemination of the condition. Needle biopsy of the lesions may be positive histologically but microbiological documentation is rare. Laparoscopic biopsy of the lesions may be a more reliable diagnostic procedure. Response to antifungal agents is poor. The underlying pathogenesis is unclear but there is some evidence from animal models of immune disregulation, with cytokine-induced disturbance of T helper-1 (Th-1) and T helper-2 (Th-2) lymphocytes determining a non-healing pattern of disease [39] with impaired macrophage-dependent candicidal mechanisms. It is possible that the mannoprotein constituents of the *Candida* cell wall can control this downregulation of the immune response [40] which may be reversible with stimulatory (Th-1) cytokines such as interleukins IL-2 and IL-12, and interferon-γ [41].

Aspergillosis

Aspergillus spp. are ubiquitous saprophytic fungi which cause invasive disease predominantly during the neutropenic period. Corticosteroid usage and GvHD prolong the risk [14]. Invasive disease is acquired via the respiratory route, with the lungs representing the primary site of infection, although the upper airways and paranasal sinuses may be involved in rhinocerebral disease. Recently, a condition of *Aspergillus* tracheobronchitis or obstructive bronchial aspergillosis has been described in haematological malignancies [42] and transplantation patients [43]. First described in acquired immune deficiency syndrome (AIDS) patients, this condition manifests as respiratory obstruction with localized pseudomembranous destructive ulceration of the bronchial mucosa; pulmonary infiltrates are usually absent.

Cutaneous lesions are commonly a manifestation of disseminated disease, but occasional cases of primary infections associated with intravenous catheter sites have been reported [44].

Most commonly, *Aspergillus* infection presents as invasive pulmonary aspergillosis (IPA) with thrombotic and haemorrhagic lung infection. Pleuritic chest pain and cough are ominous features but chest radiographic findings are non-specific and variable and may be normal even in the terminal stages of the disease [45]. Pneumonia-like opacities or nodular opacities may be visible on chest X-ray, but cavitation requires the presence of neutrophils and this is a very late radiographic feature often heralding onset of resolution [46] (Figure 46.3).

Dissemination to any organ can occur, but the brain, liver and skin are common sites. In the brain, disseminated lesions may present as areas of infarction. Embolic cerebrovascular accidents are rare in thrombocytopenic patients following transplantation, and CNS infarction, particularly multiple lesions, should alert the clinician to the possibility of invasive fungal disease. Skin lesions often appear as ecthyma gangrenosum-like lesions.

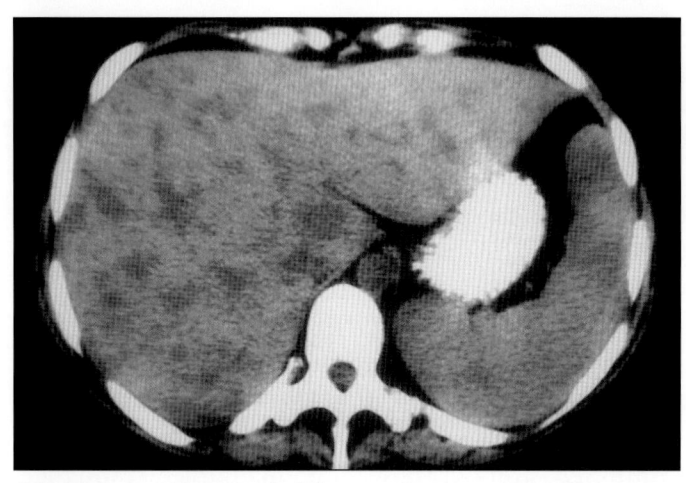

Figure 46.1 CT scan of abdomen showing multiple microabscesses throughout the liver and spleen in chronic disseminated candidosis.

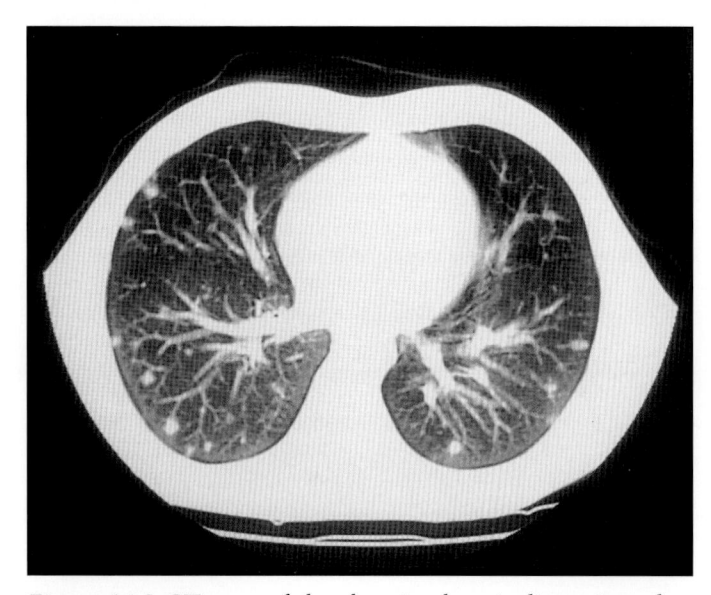

Figure 46.2 CT scan of the chest in chronic disseminated candidosis showing micronodular miliary distribution of lesions.

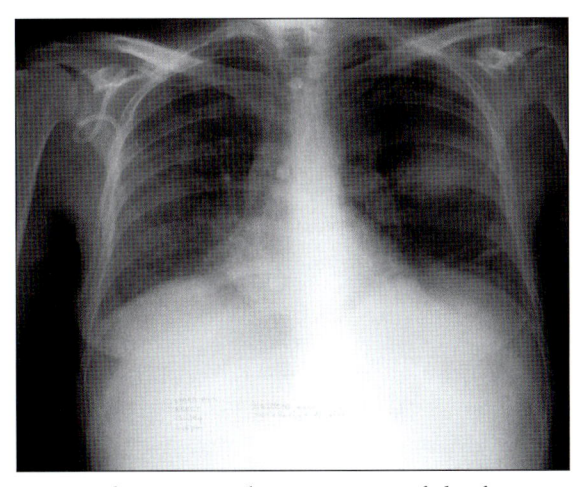

Figure 46.3 Chest X-ray showing some of the features of pulmonary aspergillosis.

Blood cultures are negative, except occasionally in cases of *Aspergillus* endocarditis. Invasive procedures to establish a definitive histological diagnosis carry a high risk of complications and are rarely performed. Mortality remains very high in transplant patients although there is some evidence that early initiation of high-dose amphotericin (before the appearance of pulmonary infiltrates), improves outcome [47]. Isolation from respiratory specimens including bronchoalveolar lavage (BAL) is specific but relatively insensitive [48]. Recently, it has been shown that isolation of *Aspergillus* spp. from specimens including sputa, BAL and endotracheal aspirates has a positive predictive value of 82% in BMT patients [49].

High-resolution CT scans of the chest are now considered the investigation of choice in the diagnosis of IPA. The presence of single or multiple enhancing nodules with cavitation, air crescent formation or the early CT-halo sign are strongly suggestive of filamentous fungal infection of which IPA remains by far the most common [46,50]. The proximity of lesions to major structures such as the pulmonary artery, risk of haemorrhage and the feasibility of surgery can also be assessed. Since other opportunist infections (notably fusariosis, pseudallescheriosis, nocardiosis) may occasionally give rise to similar CT appearances, diagnostic bronchoalveolar lavage remains a useful tool for attempted isolation of the organism, but cultures may be negative especially in focal disease [14]. If lesions or infiltrates are peripherally situated, a lung biopsy may be considered. Transthoracic fine-needle biopsies have been performed, but open-lung biopsy is probably safer and yields a better specimen. The investigations are complementary but it is sometimes prudent to perform the CT scan first, as significant desaturation following the BAL procedure, or pneumothoraces following biopsy, may cause a deterioration of the patient's condition such that a CT scan can no longer be adequately performed.

Computed tomography of the head and neck is also useful in the diagnosis of fungal sinusitis and rhinocerebral disease. Frequently, the diagnosis of aspergillosis is only established at autopsy. Even then, histology alone cannot reliably distinguish the branching septate hyphae of *Aspergillus* spp. from the morphologically similar fungal elements of other members of the hyalohyphomycosis family unless specialized immunohistological stains are used.

Other fungal infections
Cryptococcosis

In the UK, this is a rare condition following transplantation but may be commoner in developing countries [51]. Meningitis is the commonest manifestation but since the primary route of infection is via the lung, pulmonary infection may been seen in approximately 25% of cases. Occasionally, cutaneous infections are described. These present as multiple waxy, nodular lesions with necrotic ulcerating centres. Budding yeast forms with thick capsules are visible on skin biopsy (Figure 46.4). Cerebrospinal fluid (CSF) examination including India ink staining and antigen detection on CSF and serum are reliable diagnostic techniques [51].

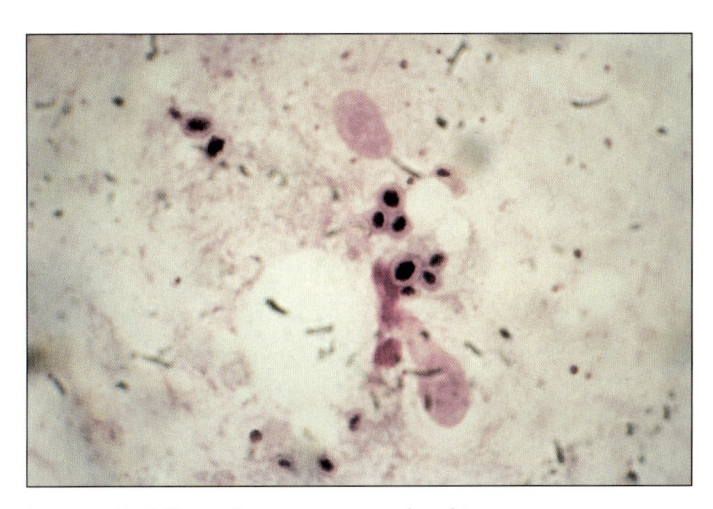

Figure 46.4 Capsular yeasts in a skin biopsy in cutaneous cryptococcosis.

Zygomycosis

Zygomycosis, often referred to as mucormycosis, is caused by the mucorales, which include *Absidia*, *Rhizopus*, *Rhizomucor* and other species [52]. Rhinocerebral disease is the most recognized manifestation in leukaemic and diabetic patients but is rarely reported after transplantation [53]. In this group of patients, sinonasal disease with pain, epistaxis and congestion is the usual presentation, but pulmonary disease and disseminated disease resembling aspergillosis may occur. Desferrioxamine therapy is a specific risk factor for these infections. Definitive diagnosis depends on biopsy-proven tissue invasion. The presence of broad, irregular hyphae with non-dichotomous branching (Figure 46.5) provides evidence of disease. High-dose amphotericin B is the treatment of choice, but response to antifungals is very poor, and extensive surgical debridement may be required but is frequently inappropriate for these particular patients.

Trichosporinosis

This yeast-like infection, predominantly caused by *T. begelii*, presents as disseminated infection similar to acute candidosis. The organism is widely distributed in the environment and may be part of the normal flora of the skin or mucous membranes. Maculopapular skin lesions are common, and blood cultures are frequently positive [54]. Funguria, pulmonary infiltrates and renal involvement can occur. Susceptibility to amphotericin B is variable and response to antifungal treatment is poor. The organism shares polysaccharide antigen determinants with the capsular antigen of *Cryptococcus neoformans*, and antigen testing using the cryptococcal latex agglutination kit may be positive in disseminated trichosporinosis. It is likely that this same antigen also functions as a major virulence determinant by interfering with neutrophil-mediated killing [55].

Fusariosis

This filamentous fungus often presents as pyrexia of unknown origin (PUO), although blood cultures may be positive and skin lesions are a common feature [56]. Skin lesions usually take the form of multiple firm erythematous nodules, but ecthyma gangrenosum-like lesions have also been reported [57]. Histologically, the fungus resembles *Aspergillus* spp. and culture is necessary for accurate diagnosis. Prognosis is poor in disseminated diseases as most isolates are resistant to conventional dosages of amphotericin B. Some isolated reports of clinical response to fluconazole have been published, but *in vitro* susceptibility testing is very variable.

Numerous other fungal infections including those caused by *Alternaria*, *Penicillium*, *Paecilomyces*, *Scopulariopsis*, *Malassezia* and other species can occur and appear regularly in the literature as isolated case reports. Unexplained skin lesions and rashes should always be biopsied and cultured, even though the diagnostic use of this remains disappointingly low [58]. In addition, histoplasmosis and coccidioidosis should be considered in the differential diagnosis in transplant patients from endemic areas.

Treatment

For many years, amphotericin B was the only parenteral antifungal agent suitable for the treatment of systemic fungal infections. Severe toxicities, primarily nephrotoxicity, are often dose-limiting and restrict the clinical usefulness of this broad-spectrum antifungal agent. However, the last decade has seen the introduction of newer antifungal agents such as the triazoles including fluconazole and itraconazole, and more recently voriconazole, in addition to a number of lipid-associated preparations of amphotericin B.

Azoles and triazoles

Ketoconazole and miconazole are unsuitable for use in neutropenic transplant patients because of toxicities

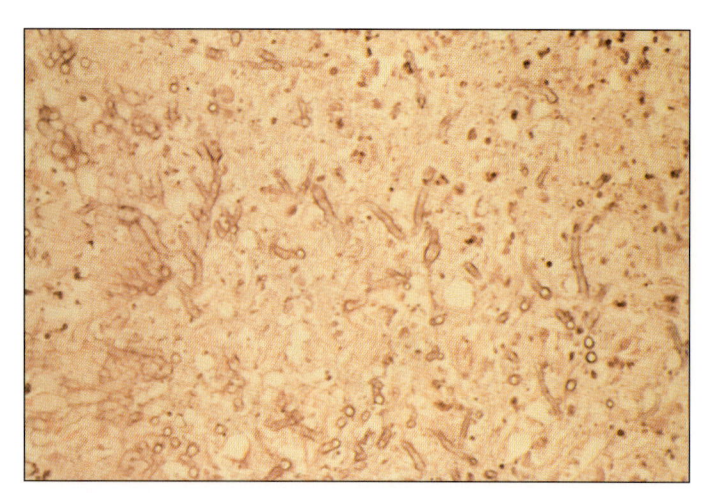

Figure 46.5 Broad irregular hyphae with wide angle branching in brain tissue in mucormycosis. (Haematoxylin & Eosin stain.)

and interactions with cyclosporin A. Fluconazole has been widely used in the treatment of *Candida* infections but relatively few randomized prospective trials of fluconazole versus amphotericin B as empirical therapy have been performed in neutropenic patients [59]. Studies in non-neutropenic patients [36] suggest it may be suitable in the treatment of known candidosis. However, the spectrum of activity is limited and fluconazole has no activity against most filamentous fungi and some non-*albicans* species (*C. krusei*) are intrinsically resistant and some, for example *C. glabrata*, may rapidly acquire resistance. Other species such as *C. tropicalis* show variable susceptibility patterns. For this reason, despite its excellent safety and tolerability profile, fluconazole cannot be recommended as a first-line agent in empirical treatment or in the treatment of documented yeast infections until speciation and susceptibility testing have been performed. Most *C. albicans* strains remain susceptible to fluconazole and it has been used successfully in these infections, as well as in chronic disseminated candidiasis [60,61], although often at dosages exceeding those recommended on the data sheet (≥ 800 mg/day).

Itraconazole is the other triazole agent currently available. In terms of spectrum of activity, itraconazole is superior to fluconazole and is active against *Candida* and *Aspergillus* spp. and other filamentous and dimorphic fungi. It has been used successfully in the treatment of invasive aspergillosis, although BMT patients responded less well than solid-organ transplant patients [62]. Drawbacks to itraconazole treatment have included the lack of an intravenous preparation and variable absorption of the oral capsular form, particularly in BMT patients. The forthcoming availability of an intravenous preparation and the development of an oral solution which has been shown to give reliable serum concentrations [63] have gone a long way in overcoming these problems. However, it is still necessary to 'load' patients for several days before steady-state concentrations are achieved, and it is advisable to monitor serum itraconazole to ensure that therapeutic levels are achieved.

New triazoles are under development. Voriconazole is currently under evaluation in phase III trials. Results from phase II studies are encouraging, and the agent has a broad spectrum of activity including fungicidal activity *in vitro* against *Aspergillus* spp.

Amphotericin B

Amphotericin B remains the drug of choice for empirical treatment, non-*albicans* yeast infections, aspergillosis, cryptococcosis and most other fungal infections due to its broad spectrum of activity. Dosages of 1 mg/kg/day are generally used for empirical treatment, 0.7 mg/kg/day is usually adequate for most yeast infections, although *C. lusitaniae* may rapidly acquire resistance, whereas dosages ≥ 1.5 mg/kg are required to treat many filamentous fungal infections such as zygomycoses and many cases of aspergillosis (Table 46.4). These higher levels are not readily achievable using conventional amphotericin deoxycholate.

The drug is given in 5% dextrose by slow intravenous infusion. Anaphylaxis can occur, and a test dose of 1 mg in 50 ml of dextrose over 2 hours is advisable. This is unnecessary in patients who have received amphotericin previously, but careful monitoring during the early stages of the infusion is required. Slow escalation of the dose over several days is not recommended in neutropenic patients with suspected fungal infection who should receive full dosage wuthin the first 24 hours. The drug is stable on exposure to light and infusion bags do not need covering. Early reactions such as chills and fevers ('shakes and bakes') are common and mediated by

Table 46.4 Fungal minimum inhibitory concentrations and minimum fungicidal concentrations

Fungus	Concentration (mg/litre)
Candida albicans	0.25–1
Candida spp.	0.25–2
Aspergillus spp.	0.05–2.5*
Trichosporon begelii	0.25–10
Rhizopus spp.	0.10–>100*
Pseudallescheria boydii	2.0–>100*
Fusarium spp.	0.6–10*

*Fungicidal concentrations may not be achievable using conventional amphotericin B.

cytokine and prostaglandin release. Such reactions may be self-limiting and disappear if treatment is continued. They may be ameliorated with pethidine or antihistamines, but corticosteroids, which are frequently recommended for these side-effects are best avoided in an immunocompromised patient with infection. Other acute reactions such as severe hypotension, cyanosis or bradycardia can occur and are indications for switching to a lipid preparation.

Renal toxicity is the major side-effect of conventional amphotericin treatment. Virtually all patients experience a decrease in glomerular filtration and a tubular defect resulting in severe electrolyte loss and a rising creatinine. Although usually reversible provided total cumulative doses do not exceed 4 g, it may take many months for renal function to return to normal, and concomitant therapies such as aminoglycosides or cyclosporin may exacerbate the toxicity. Intravenous supplements of potassium and magnesium are frequently required, and amiloride may be used to block the tubular loss of these electrolytes but is seldom completely effective.

A switch to a lipid preparation is necessary when the serum creatinine exceeds threefold its pretreatment baseline or 250 µmol/litre in an adult. The threshold in children is considerably lower than this, and the creatinine should not be allowed to rise above 150 µmol/litre.

Lipid preparations of amphotericin B

A variety of liposomes and lipid complexes have been developed to carry the insoluble amphotericin B within a biodegradable vesicle or lipid bilayer. Three commercial preparations are available: AmBisome, the only true liposomal preparation, amphotericin B colloidal dispersion (ABCD, Amphocil) and amphotericin B lipid complex (ABLC, Abelcet) [64]. These presentations are expensive, and consequently suspensions of amphotericin B in 20% Intralipid have been used. This is outside the product licence of either product, and results do not support this practice [65]. The pharmacokinetics of the different licensed preparations depend on the size, charge, stability and clearance of the lipid complex/liposome (Table 46.5). The increased selectivity of the lipid preparations for fungal ergosterol is thought to account for the decreased toxicity associated with these products (Figure 46.6), but efficacy is not necessarily increased. The improved therapeutic index that has been reported comes from the feasibility of administering much higher dosages of the drug, and possibly from selective targeting of the liposome through uptake by

Table 46.5 Lipid-containing preparations*

Parameter	Fungizone	AmBisome	Amphocil	ABLC	AmBisome–Intralipid emulsion
Shape	Micelles	SUV	discs	sheets	Micelles
Diameter (µm)	<0.4	0.08	0.12	1.6–11	Variable
AmBisome (%)	34	10	50	35	Variable
Toxicity					
renal	=	↓↓↓	↓↓	↓	=
immediate	=	↓↓	=	↑	=
C_{max}	=	↑	↓	↓	Variable
Area under the curve (related to Fungizone)	=	↑	=	↓	Variable

*SUV = small unilamellar liposomes; = = equivalent to fungizone; ↓ = decreased compared to fungizone; ↑ = increased compared to fungizone.

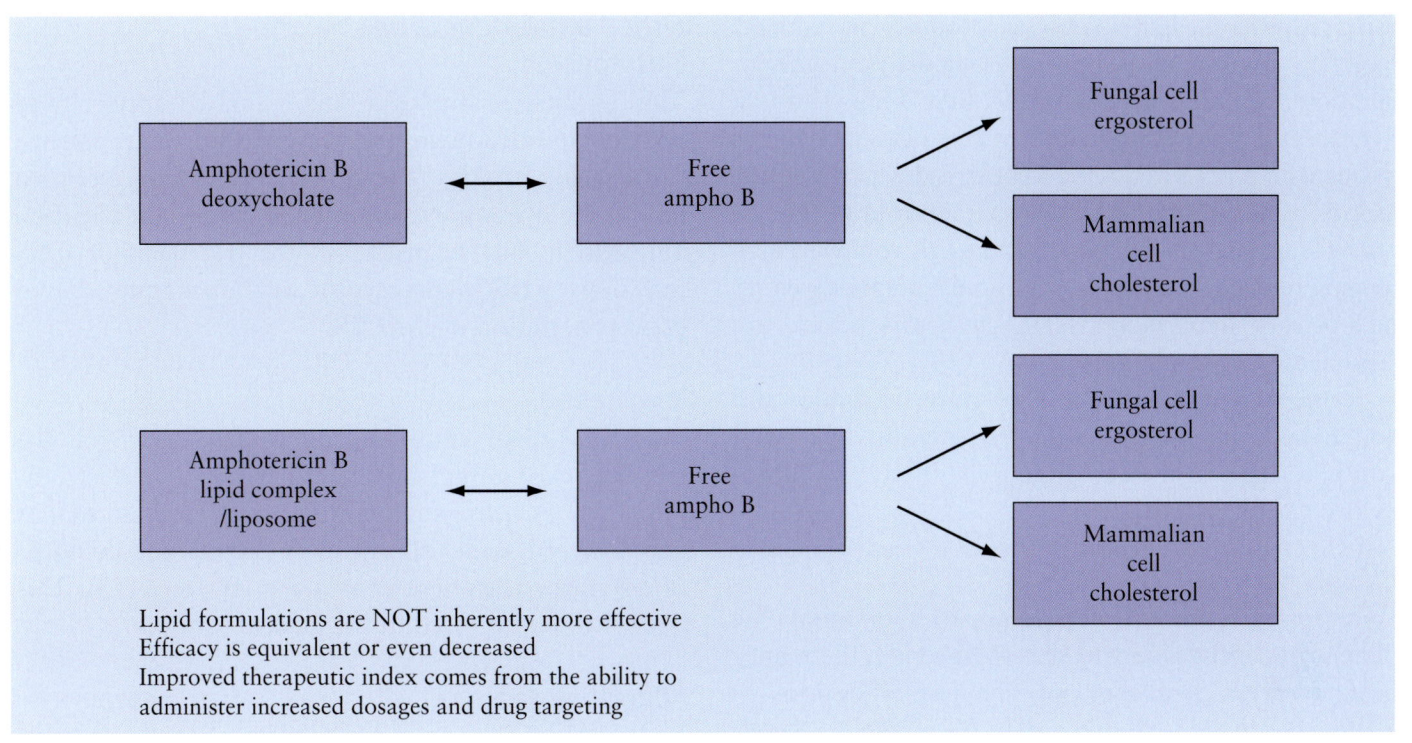

Figure 46.6 Improved selective toxicity of lipid preparations of amphotericin B.

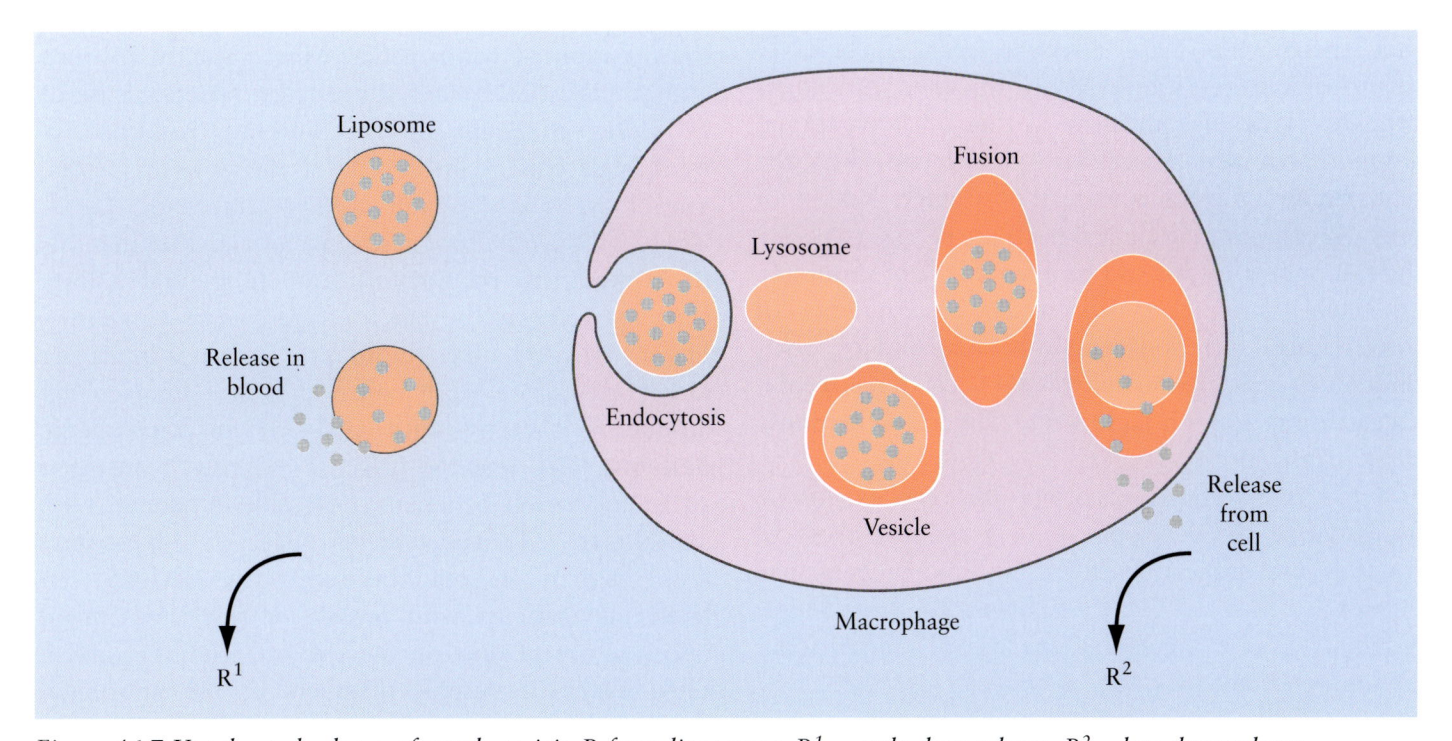

Figure 46.7 Uptake and release of amphotericin B from liposomes. R^1 = early drug release; R^2 = late drug release.

macrophages. The drug is then concentrated in the reticulo-endothelial system (Figure 46.7) and borne to sites of infection, or in the case of AmBisome, to the fungal cell wall [66].

All the commercially prepared lipid-associated preparations induce markedly less renal toxicity, and doses of 3–5 mg/kg/day can be given in the face of deteriorating renal function. However, the rationale for using expensive lipid-associated products in patients receiving total renal support (haemodialysis, haemofiltration) is dubious, especially since little is known about clearance of lipid preparations in these situations. The mechanism for reduced renal toxicity is due partly to the lack of concentration of lipid preparations in phagocyte poor tissues such as the kidney, and partly to preferential binding of negatively charged liposomal amphotericin to high-density lipoprotein (HDL) receptors which are lacking in renal tissue [67].

Immediate side-effects are more variable and anaphylaxis has been reported. Generally, liposomal amphotericin is better tolerated than the lipid-associated forms.

Efficacy data

Since lipid preparations depend in part upon uptake by phagocytes and delivery to sites of infection, there have been concerns that they may be less efficacious in leukopenic patients. Limited data from animal models seem to support this theory [68,69]. However, clinical experience [70–72] and anecdotal case reports suggest that these agents are effective even in severely neutropenic patients and are well tolerated. Efficacy is probably roughly equivalent to that of conventional amphotericin on a weight-for-weight basis. Thus, the higher dose regimens confer an advantage. Results of ongoing comparative clinical trials are necessary before the full impact of this can be assessed. Care should be taken when interpreting these studies, since numbers of proven fungal infections tend to be small and it is often difficult to separate the individual effects of neutrophil regeneration, growth factors and surgery on response rates.

Lipid preparations of drugs are very expensive, necessitating the development of a rational protocol for their use. Indications for using lipid preparations include:
- renal toxicity precluding the use of conventional amphotericin;
- severe immediate toxicity to amphotericin;
- infections where the fungicidal minimum inhibitory concentration is not readily achievable using conventional amphotericin;
- infections involving the reticulo endothelial system (liver and spleen particularly).

Increasingly, patient preference is a factor determining the use of lipid preparations.

Other antifungal drugs

Flucytosine

This pyrimidine analogue has a limited spectrum of activity confined mainly to yeast species and resistance can develop rapidly. The drug is myelosuppressive so its routine use is not advocated in transplant patients, although it may be useful in the treatment of CNS infections, particularly cryptococcal meningitis, due to good penetration of the CSF.

Terbinafine

This allylamine compound is widely used for the treatment of superficial dermatophyte infections. However, *in vitro* susceptibility data suggest that it may have a broader spectrum of activity and could be of use in the treatment of systemic mycoses [73]. This has yet to be explored in the clinical setting.

Adjunctive therapy

Biological response modifiers such as cytokines and growth factors have been used prophylactically in PBSC transplant for some time in attempts to shorten the duration of neutropenia. More recently, *in vitro* and animal studies have suggested a beneficial use of cytokines to augment the immune response in established fungal infection. Of the growth factors, granulocyte–macrophage colony-stimulating factor (GM-CSF) has the broadest range of activities in terms of stimulating phagocytes and fungicidal killing capacity, followed by macrophage colony-stimulating factor (M-CSF) and granulocyte colony-stimulating factor (G-CSF) [74]. Clinical data are limited, but adjunctive therapy with GM-CSF in neutropenic patients [75] and M-CSF in marrow transplant patients [76] was beneficial, especially in patients with candidosis. Prospective trials of liposomal amphotericin in combination with GM-CSF in leukaemic patients with proven or suspected fungal infection are planned in the UK and should establish these agents as useful members of the antifungal armamentarium. In addition, they will explore the possibility that growth factors and antifungal agents, particularly lipid preparations, could act synergically.

Other cytokines such as interleukins and interferons are also potential adjunctive therapies [41]. Gamma-interferon is established as a useful agent in the prevention of fungal and other infections in patients with chronic granulomatous disease [77] and is effective in a mouse model of disseminated candidosis [78]. It is likely to be of benefit in patients with chronic infections such as CDC [79], and in patients with impaired T-cell-mediated immunity where other agents such as IL-12, anti-IL-4 and anti-IL-10 alone or in combination, may also have a role.

Other factors

Attempts to reduce corticosteroid and other immunosuppressive therapies to a minimum are an essential part of the treatment of fungal infection in transplant patients. Removal of intravenous catheters in patients with candidaemia and other blood-borne fungal infection is mandatory. Surgery should also be considered in zygomycotic infections and in some patients with nodular aspergillosis. Finally, granulocyte transfusions may be useful in fungal infections in patients with prolonged neutropenia, especially if donors are used who have been primed with colony-stimulating factors [80].

Prevention and prophylaxis

Prevention of acquisition is of major importance in transplant patients. Potted plants, flowers and some foodstuffs such as pepper, may be the source of fungal spores and should be avoided during the neutropenic period. Laminar airflow (LAF) rooms with high-efficiency particulate air (HEPA) filters are effective in preventing the nosocomial acquisition of aspergillosis. It must be remembered that protection cannot be guaranteed for the small numbers of patients who are already colonized prior to admission or who leave the protected environment for radiological or other diagnostic procedures. These rooms are expensive to maintain and are often reserved for high-risk allogeneic transplant patients and for those undergoing matched unrelated donor transplantation. The majority of *Candida* infections are endogenous, with colonization preceding infection. Exogenous acquisition can be minimized by strict aseptic technique and maintenance of mucosal and skin barriers.

Chemoprophylaxis has long been used in neutropenia [81], but experts are divided in their opinion between the use of topical non-absorbable preparations and systemic azoles. The ideal antifungal for prophylaxis should be broad spectrum, fungicidal, well tolerated and cheap with good bioavailability and a low association with development of resistance. Unfortunately, few if any of the currently available preparations fulfil these criteria. Randomized studies have suggested that azoles are superior to topical agents in the prevention of superficial and systemic infections and fluconazole is most frequently used in this situation. Doses used vary widely. The British Society for Antimicrobial Chemotherapy Antifungal Working Party recommended 50 mg/day [82] whereas Goodman and colleagues demonstrated a beneficial effect of 400 mg/day in a randomized placebo-controlled trial [83]. Another study has shown that fluconazole is as effective but better tolerated than amphotericin B treatment at 0.5 mg/kg three times a week [84]. Concerns about the limited spectrum of fluconazole and the risk of resistant strains emerging have restricted its prophylactic use in some centres. More recently, fluconazole has been compared with itraconazole oral solution as prophylaxis in neutropenia, and the latter seems to be of additional benefit in preventing *Aspergillus* infections [85]. To date, fluconazole is the only agent that has been proven to be cost-effective as prophylaxis in BMT patients, as defined by avoidance of infection or colonization and the ability to continue prophylaxis [86]. Against this is the study by Schaffner and Schaffner which suggested that fluconazole prophylaxis increased the duration of neutropenia and infection-related health care costs [87].

Amphotericin B has been used in a variety of prophylactic schedules ranging from 0.1 mg/kg/day to 1 mg/kg weekly [84,88], but a definite benefit has not been established and the deoxycholate preparations are poorly tolerated.

Liposomal amphotericin has been used in some small studies [89] but it is difficult to justify this expense without more conclusive data on efficacy. Nasal administration and aerosol delivery of amphotericin [90,91] have been attempted with conflicting results. Given the size of particles in the colloidal suspension of amphotericin B deoxycholate, it is unlikely that inhaled drug reaches the terminal airways in humans, although there may be some benefit in reducing sino-nasal disease.

Caution must be used when interpreting the results of these trials, as many of the endpoints (reduction in colonization, reduction of superficial infection, reduction of systemic infection, improved survival) are flawed by our inability to diagnose infection or distinguish colonization from infection. Consequently, the numbers of proven systemic infections in these studies tend to be small and some of the diagnostic criteria used are suspect. Few studies have employed a reduction of empirical amphotericin B usage as an endpoint, although trials looking at this are now underway.

Prophylaxis should be commenced before the onset of neutropenia and should be continued until marrow recovery. In patients with GvHD, the risk period is prolonged and prophylaxis should be extended.

Secondary prophylaxis is essential in patients with a previous history of fungal infection because of the risk of reactivation during transplantation. Patients with a previous history of aspergillosis should be considered for surgical resection of any remaining mycotic lung sequestrum. Thereafter, full-dose amphotericin B treatment is recommended on alternate days throughout the period of immune suppression.

Pneumocystis carinii

Despite its reclassification as a fungus, *Pneumocystis carinii* does not sit completely at ease in this group and many aspects of its lifestyle, diagnosis and treatment fit in more closely with protozoan infection. Infections usually occur after engraftment as a result of the post-transplant T-cell defect, but certain underlying diseases (acute lymphoblastic leukaemia, lymphoma), conditioning regimens (cytosine arabinoside) and corticosteroids are additional specific risk factors. The presentation of illness is more acute in this group of patients than in HIV-infected individuals, but recurrences are less frequent [92].

Infection usually presents as an interstitial pneumonitis, but features can vary considerably. Progressive dyspnoea and a dry cough are the commonest presenting symptoms but *Pneumocystis carinii* pneumonia (PCP) can also present as a fulminant infection mimicking bacterial sepsis. Fever is usually, but not invariably present. Chest radiographs show interstitial or acinar infiltrates but may be normal in the early stages [93]. Hypoxia is a feature in more than 90% of patients at presentation, and may worsen rapidly on exercise and as the patient progresses to respiratory failure. Extrapulmonary pneumocystosis has been reported occasionally.

It is unclear whether PCP is a primary infection arising *de novo*, or reactivation of previous asymptomatic infection. Seroprevalence studies tend to support the reactivation theory [94] but post-mortem studies using sensitive PCR techniques have failed to find evidence of *P. carinii* in the lungs of asymptomatic individuals [95]. Clusters of cases of PCP representing apparent point-source outbreaks have also been reported and support the argument for *de novo* infection [94]. Until it is possible to cultivate the organism reliably and identify environmental reservoirs, it is unlikely that these controversies will be resolved. Meanwhile, it may be advisable to isolate patients with PCP to prevent patient-to-patient transmission via the respiratory route.

Diagnosis

Pneumocystis carinii pneumonia must be distinguished from other causes of respiratory infection. Induced sputum examination has proved useful in the human immunodeficiency virus (HIV)-positive setting, but the differential diagnosis tends to be wider in transplant patients and the cyst/trophozoite load is less, such that BAL is the preferred diagnostic procedure in this group. Diagnosis depends on demonstration of the organism in the BAL fluid using a variety of staining techniques: Giemsa and Gomori's methenamine silver staining are simple to perform but relatively insensitive. Immunofluorescence methods using direct or indirect staining with monoclonal antibodies improve sensitivity (Figure 46.8) but require extensive washing stages to avoid non-specific fluorescence. Molecular diagnosis by PCR is highly sensitive and specific, but the test is not rapidly available at every centre and so has a limited role in clinical management of the patient.

Treatment and prevention

Trimethoprim-sulphamethoxazole (TMP-SMZ, 20 mg/kg trimethoprim) remains the treatment of choice for PCP and it may take several days for a response to become apparent. Patients can be switched to oral therapy after 7–10 days if they are responding. Pentamidine, clindamycin–primaquine and atovaquone are all suitable agents for patients unable to tolerate TMP-SMZ. The addition of corticosteroids is beneficial in the treatment of severe PCP in AIDS but efficacy has not been proven outside of this patient group. Although the use of steroids in PCP in transplant

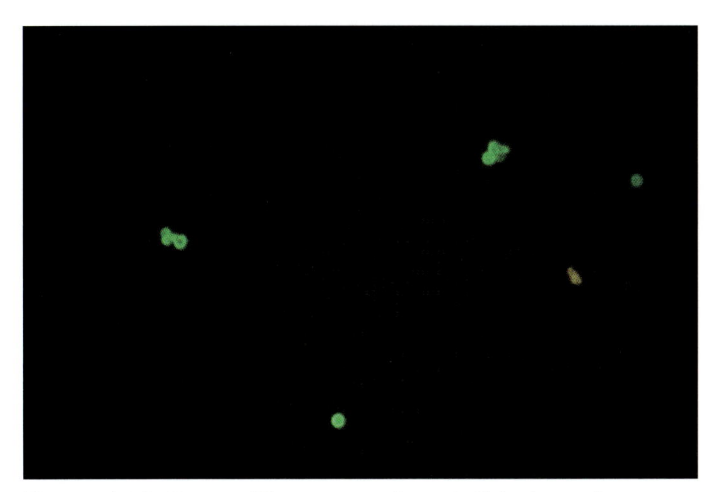

Figure 46.8 Cysts of Pneumocystis carinii *in bronchoalveolar lavage fluid stained by immunofluorescence.*

recipients may be rational, care must be taken before extrapolating from results from HIV-positive patients.

Low-dose TMP-SMZ (twice daily, three times a week) provides excellent prophylaxis and should be continued for 200 days after transplantation. Monthly aerosolized pentamidine may also be used for prevention, and is of use while patients have a suboptimal peripheral blood count after transplantation because it does not cause the marrow suppression associated with TMP-SMZ.

References

1. Bodey G, Bueltmann NB, Duguid W et al. Fungal infections in cancer patients: an international autopsy survey. *Eur J Clin Microbiol* 1992; **11**: 99–109.
2. Chandrasekar PH, Weinmann A, Shearer C and the Bone Marrow Transplant Team. Autopsy-identified infections among bone marrow transplant recipients: a clinicopathological study of 56 patients. *Bone Marrow Transplant* 1995; **16**: 675–681.
3. De Bock R. Epidemiology of invasive fungal infection in bone marrow transplantation. *Bone Marrow Transplant* 1994; **14**(Suppl 5): S1–S2.
4. Anaissie EJ, Bodey GP and Rinaldi MG. Emerging fungal pathogens. *Eur J Clin Microbiol Infect Dis* 1989; **8**: 323–330.
5. Price MF, LaRocca MT and Gentry LO. Fluconazole susceptibilities of *Candida* species and distribution of species recovered from blood cultures over a 5-year period. *Antimicrob Agents Chemother* 1994; **38**: 1422–1424.
6. Wingard JR, Merz WG, Rinaldi MG, Johnson TR, Karp JE and Saral R. Increase in *Candida krusei* infection among patients with bone marrow transplantation and neutropenia treated prophylactically with fluconazole. *New Engl J Med* 1991; **325**: 1274–1277.
7. Wingard JR, Merz WG, Rinaldi MG, Miller CB, Karp JE and Saral R. Association of *Torulopsis glabrata* infections with fluconazole prophylaxis in neutropenic bone marrow transplant patients. *Antimicrob Agents Chemother* 1993; **37**: 1847–1849.
8. Iwen PC, Kelly DM, Reed EC and Hinrichs SH. Invasive infection due to *Candida krusei* in immunocompromised patients not treated with fluconazole. *Clin Infect Dis* 1995; **20**: 342–347.
9. Edman JC, Kovacs JA, Masur H, Santi DV, Elwood HJ and Sogin ML. Ribosomal RNA sequence shows *Pneumocystis carinii* to be a member of the fungi. *Nature* 1988; **334**: 519–522.
10. Kwon-Chung KJ. Phylogenetic spectrum of fungi that are pathogenic to man. *Clin Infect Dis* 1996; **19**(Suppl 1): S1–S7.
11. Liberti G, Pearce R, Taghipour G, Majolino I and Goldstone AH. Comparison of peripheral blood stem-cell and autologous transplantation for lymphoma patients. *Ann Oncol* 1994; **5**(Suppl 2): 151–153.
12. Walsh TJ and Merz WG. Pathologic features in the human alimentary tract associated with invasiveness of *Candida tropicalis*. *Am J Clin Pathol* 1986; **85**: 498–502.
13. Martino P, Girmenia C, Micozzi A, Raccah R, Gentile G, Venditti M and Mandelli F. Fungaemia in patients with leukemia. *Am J Med Sci* 1993; **306**: 225–232.
14. McWhinney PHM, Kibbler CC, Hamon MD et al. Progress in the diagnosis and management of aspergillosis in bone marrow transplantation: 13 years experience. *Clin Infect Dis* 1993; **17**: 397–404.
15. Rhame FS. Prevention of nosocomial aspergillosis. *J Hosp Infect* 1991; **18**(Suppl A): 466–472.
16. Pfaller MA. Epidemiology of candidiasis. *J Hosp Infect* 1995; **30**(Suppl): 329–338.
17. Burnie JP. Early diagnosis of fungal infection. *Curr Opin Infect Dis* 1995; **8**: 258–260.
18. Ansorg R, Von Heinegg EH and Rath PM. *Aspergillus* antigenuria compared to antigenaemia in bone marrow transplant patients. *Eur J Clin Microbiol Infect Dis* 1994; **13**: 582–589.
19. Haynes KA and Rogers TR. Retrospective evaluation of a latex agglutination test for diagnosis of invasive aspergillosis in immunocompromised patients. *Eur J Clin Microbiol Infect Dis* 1994; **13**: 670–674.
20. Grundy MA, Coakley WT and Barnes RA. Highly sensitive detection of fungal antigens by ultrasound-enhanced latex agglutination. *J Med Vet Mycol* 1995; **33**: 201–203.
21. Walsh TJ, Heythorne JW and Seville JD. Detection of circulating *Candida* enolase by immunoassay in patients with cancer and invasive candidiasis. *New Engl J Med* 1991; **324**: 1026–1031.
22. Barnes RA. *Aspergillus* infection: does serodiagnosis work? *Serodiagn Immunother Infect Dis* 1993; **5**: 135–138.
23. Reiss E and Morrison CJ. Nonculture methods for diagnosis of disseminated candidiasis. *Clin Microbiol Rev* 1993; **6**: 311–323.
24. Obayashi T, Yoshida M, Mori T et al. Plasma (1-3)-beta-D-glucan measurement in diagnosis of invasive deep mycosis and fungal febrile episodes. *Lancet* 1995; **345**: 17–20.
25. Wakefield AE, Pixley FJ, Banerji S, Sinclair K, Miller RF and Moxon ER. Detection of *Pneumocystis carinii* with DNA amplification. *Lancet* 1990; **336**: 451–453.
26. Peters SE, Wakefield AE, Banerji S and Hopkin JM. Quantification of the detection of *Pneumocystis carinii* by DNA amplification. *Mol Cell Probes* 1992; **6**: 115–117.

27. Crampin AC and Matthews RC. Application of the polymerase chain reaction to the diagnosis of candidosis by amplification of a *HSP90* gene fragment. *J Med Microbiol* 1993; **39**: 233–238.
28. Kan VL. Polymerase chain reaction for the diagnosis of candidemia. *J Infect Dis* 1993; **168**: 779–783.
29. Burgener-Kairuz P, Zuber J-P, Jaunin P, Buchman TG, Bille J and Rossier M. Rapid detection and identification of *Candida albicans* and *Torulopsis (Candida) glabrata* in clinical specimens by species-specific nested PCR-amplification of a cytochrome P-450 lanosterol-alpha-demethylase (L1A1) gene fragment. *J Clin Microbiol* 1994; **32**: 1902–1907.
30. Spreadbury C, Holden D, Aufaure-Brown A, Bainbridge B and Cohen J. Detection of *Aspergillus fumigatus* by polymerase chain reaction. *J Clin Microbiol* 1993; **31**: 615–621.
31. Tang CM, Holden DW, Aufauvre-Brown and Cohen J. Detection of *Aspergillus* spp. by the polymerase chain reaction and its evaluation in bronchoalveolar fluid. *Am Rev Resp Dis* 1993; **148**: 1313–1317.
32. Einsele H, Hebart H, Roller G et al. Detection and identification of fungal pathogens in blood using molecular probes. *J Clin Microbiol* 1997; **35**: 1353–1360.
33. Riley DK, Pavia AT, Beatty PG, Denton D and Carroll KC. Surveillance cultures in bone marrow transplant recipients: worthwhile or wasteful? *Bone Marrow Transplant* 1995; **15**: 469–473.
34. Pfaller M, Cabezudo I, Koontz F, Bale M and Gingrich R. Predictive value of surveillance cultures for systemic infection due to *Candida* species. *Eur J Clin Microbiol* 1987; **6**: 628–633.
35. Nguyen MH, Peacock JE, Tanner DC et al. Therapeutic approaches to patients with candidaemia. *Arch Intern Med* 1995; **155**: 2429–2435.
36. Rex JH, Bennett JE, Sugar AM et al. A randomized trial comparing fluconazole with amphotericin B for the treatment of candidemia in patients without neutropenia. *New Engl J Med* 1994; **331**: 1325–1330.
37. Anttila VJ, Ruutu P, Bondestam S et al. Hepatosplenic yeast infection in patients with acute leukemia: a diagnostic problem. *Clin Infect Dis* 1994; **18**: 979–981.
38. Gorg C, Weide R, Schwerk WB, Koppler H and Havemann K. Ultrasound evaluation of hepatic and splenic microabscesses in the immunocompromised patient: sonographic patterns, differential diagnosis, and follow-up. *J Clin Ultrasound* 1994; **22**: 525–529.
39. Romani L, Mencacci A, Tonnetti L et al. IL-12 is required and prognostic *in vivo* for T helper type 1 differentiation in murine candidiasis. *J Immunol* 1994; **153**: 5167–5175.
40. Mencacci A, Torosantucci A, Spaccapelo R, Romani L, Bistoni F and Cassone A. A mannoprotein constituent of *Candida albicans* that elicits different levels of delayed-type hypersensitivity, cytokine production and anticandicidal protection in mice. *Infect Immun* 1994; **62**: 5353–5360.
41. Kullberg BJ and van't Wout JW. Cytokines in the treatment of fungal disease. *Biotherapy* 1994; **7**: 195–210.
42. Tait RC, O'Driscoll BR and Denning DW. Unilateral wheeze caused by pseudomembranous *Aspergillus* tracheobronchitis in the immunocompromised patients. *Thorax* 1993; **48**: 1285–1287.
43. Hummel M, Schuler S, Hempel S, Rees W and Hetzer R. Obstructive bronchial aspergillosis after heart transplantation. *Mycoses* 1993; **36**: 425–428.
44. Romero LS and Hunt SJ. Hickman catheter-associated primary cutaneous aspergillosis in a patient with acquired immunodeficiency syndrome. *Int J Dermatol* 1995; **34**: 551–553.
45. Young RC, Bennett JE, Vogel CL, Carbone PP and de Vita VT. Aspergillosis: the spectrum of disease in 98 patients. *Medicine (Baltimore)* 1970; **49**: 147–173.
46. Winer-Muram HT, Gurney JW, Bozeman PM and Krance RA. Pulmonary complications after bone marrow transplantation. *Radiol Clin N Am* 1996; **34**: 97–118.
47. Shpilberg O, Douer D, Goldschmied-Reouven A, Block C, Ben-Bassat I and Ramot B. Invasive aspergillosis in patients with acute leukemia. *Leukaemia Lymphoma* 1991; **4**: 257–262.
48. Von Eiff M, Roos N, Fegeler W, Von Eiff C, Zuhlsdorf M, Glaser J and Van der Loo J. Pulmonary fungal infections in immunocompromised patients: incidence and risk factors. *Mycoses* 1994; **37**: 329–335.
49. Horvath JA and Dummer S. The use of respiratory-tract cultures in the diagnosis of invasive pulmonary aspergillosis. *Am J Med* 1996; **100**: 171–178.
50. Barloon TJ, Galvin RG, Mori M, Stanford W and Gingrich RD. High-resolution ultrafast chest CT in the clinical management of febrile bone marrow transplant patients with normal or non-specific chest roentgenograms. *Chest* 1991; **99**: 928–933.
51. Khanna N, Chandramuki A, Deasai A and Ravi V. Cryptococcal infections of the central nervous system: an analysis of predisposing factors, laboratory findings and outcome in patients from South India with special reference to HIV infection. *J Med Microbiol* 1996; **45**: 376–379.
52. Sugar AM. Mucormycosis. *Clin Infect Dis* 1992; **14**(Suppl 1): S126–129.
53. Morrison VA and McGlave PB. Mucormycosis in the BMT population. *Bone Marrow Transplant* 1993; **11**: 383–388.
54. Anaissie E and Bodey GP. Disseminated trichosporinosis: meeting the challenge. *Eur J Clin Microbiol Infect Dis* 1991; **10**: 711–713.
55. Lyman CA, Walsh TJ, Pizzo PA, Devil SJN, Nathanson J and Frasch CE. Detection and quantitation of the glucuronoxylomannan-like polysaccharide antigen from clinical and non-clinical isolates of *Trichosporon begelii* and implications for pathogenicity. *J Clin Microbiol* 1995; **33**: 126–130.
56. Rabodonirina M, Piens MA, Monier MF, Gueho E, Fiere D and Mojon M. *Fusarium* infections in immunocompromised patients: case reports and literature review. *Eur J Clin Microbiol Infect Dis* 1994; **13**: 152–161.
57. Prins C, Chavaz P. Tamm K and Hauser C. Ecthyma gangrenosum-like lesions: a sign of disseminated *Fusarium* infection in the neutropenic patient. *Clin Exp Dermatol* 1995; **20**: 428–430.
58. Chren M-M, Lazarus HM, Salata RA and Landefeld S. Cultures from skin biopsy tissue from immunocompromised patients with cancer and rashes. *Arch Dermatol* 1995; **131**: 552–555.
59. Anaisse EJ, Darouiche RO, Abi-Said D et al. Management of invasive candidal infections: results of a prosepctive randomised multicenter study of fluconazole versus amphotencin B and review of the literature. *Clin Infect Dis* 1996; **23**: 964–997.

60. Kauffman CA, Bradley SF, Ross SE and Weber DR. Hepatosplenic candidosis: successful treatment with fluconazole. *Am J Med* 1991; **92**(2): 137–141.
61. Anaissie E, Bodey GP, Kantarjian H *et al*. Fluconazole therapy for chronic disseminated candidiasis in patients with leukaemia and prior amphotericin B treatment. *Am J Med* 1991; **91**: 1452.
62. Denning DW, Lee JY, Hostetler JS *et al*. NIAID Mycoses Study Group Multicenter trial of oral itraconazole therapy for invasive aspergillosis. *Am J Med* 1994; **97**: 135–144.
63. Prentice AG, Warnock DW, Johnson SAN, Phillips MJ and Olliver DA. Multiple dose pharmacokinetics of oral solution of itraconazole in autologous bone marrow transplant patients. *J Antimicrob Chemother* 1994; **34**: 247–252.
64. van Burik JH and Bowden RA. Standard antifungal treatment, including role of alternative modalities to administer amphotericin B. *Baillière's Clin Infect Dis* 1995; **2**: 89–109.
65. Moreau P, Milpied N, Fayette N, Ramee J-F and Harousseau J-L. Reduced renal toxicity and improved clinical tolerance of amphotericin B in neutropenic patients. *J Antimicrob Chemother* 1992; **30**: 535–541.
66. Adler-Moore JP and Proffitt RT. Development, characterization, efficacy and mode of action of AmBisome, a unilamellar liposomal formulation of amphotericin B. *J Liposome Res* 1993; **3**: 429–450.
67. Wasan KM, Motron RE, Rosenblum MG and Lopez-Berestein G. Decreased toxicity of liposomal amphotericin B due to association of amphotericin B with high-density lipoproteins: role of lipid transfer protein. *J Pharmaceut Sci* 1994; **83**: 1006–1010.
68. Moonis M, Ahmad I and Bachhawat BK. Effect of elimination of phagocytic cells by liposomal dichloromethylene diphosphonate on *Aspergillosis* virulence and toxicity of liposomal amphotericin B in mice. *J Antimicrob Chemother* 1994; **33**: 571–583.
69. Van Etten EWM, van den Heuvelde-de Groot C and Bakker-Woudenberg IAJM. Efficacies of amphotericin B deoxycholate (Fungizone), liposomal amphotericin B (AmBisome) and fluconazole in the treatment of systemic candidosis in immunocompetent and leucopenic mice. *J Antimicrob Chemother* 1993; **32**: 723–739.
70. Mills W, Chopra R, Linch DC and Goldstone AH. Liposomal amphotericin B in the treatment of fungal infections in neutropenic patients: a single centre experience of 133 episodes in 116 patients. *Br J Haematol* 1994; **86**: 754–760.
71. Oppenheim BA, Herbrecht R and Kusne S. The safety and efficacy of amphotericin B colloidal dispersion in the treatment of invasive mycoses. *Clin Infect Dis* 1995; **21**: 1145–1153.
72. Oravcova E, Mistrik M, Sakalova A *et al*. Amphotericin B lipid complex to treat invasive fungal infections in cancer patients: report of efficacy and safety in 20 patients. *Chemotherapy* 1995; **41**: 473–476.
73. Balfour JA and Faulds D. Terbinafine: a review of its pharmacodynamic and pharmacokinetic properties and therapeutic potential in superficial mycoses. *Drugs* 1992; **43**: 259–284.
74. Roilides E, Walsh TJ and Pizzo PA. Clinical use of cytokines during fungal infection. In: *Hemopoietic Growth Factors and Mononuclear Phagocytes*. R Van Furth (ed.), 1993: 90–97 (Basel: Karger).
75. Bodey GP, Anaissie E, Gutterman J and Vadhan-Raj S. Role of granulocyte–macrophage colony-stimulating factor as adjuvant therapy for fungal infection in patients with cancer. *Clin Infect Dis* 1993; **17**: 705–707.
76. Nemunaitis J, Shannon-Dorcy K and Appelbaum FR. Long-term follow-up of patients with invasive fungal disease who received adjunctive therapy with recombinant human macrophage colony-stimulating factor. *Blood* 1993; **82**: 1422–1427.
77. Gallin JI, Malech HL, Weening RS, Curnutte JT, Quie PG, Jaffe HS and Ezekowitz RAB. The International Chronic Granulomatous Disease Cooperative Study Group. A controlled trial of interferon gamma to prevent infection in chronic granulomatous disease. *New Engl J Med* 1991; **324**: 509–516.
78. Kullberg BJ, van't Wout JW and Hoogstraten C. Recombinant interferon gamma enhances resistance to acute disseminated *Candida albicans* infection in mice. *J Infect Dis* 1993; **168**: 436–443.
79. Poynton CH, Barnes RA and Rees J. Interferon gamma in the treatment of deep seated fungal infection in acute leukaemia. *Clin Infect Dis* 1998 (in press Jan edition).
80. Clarke K, Szer J, Shelton M, Coghlan D and Grigg A. Multiple granulocyte transfusions facilitating successful unrelated bone marrow transplantation in a patient with very severe aplastic anemia complicated by suspected fungal infection. *Bone Marrow Transplant* 1995; **16**: 723–726.
81. Uzun O and Anaissie EJ. Antifungal prophylaxis in patients with haematological malignancies: a reappraisal. *Blood* 1995; **86**: 2063–2072.
82. Working Party for the British Society of Antimicrobial Chemotherapy. Chemoprophylaxis for candidosis and aspergillosis in neutropenia and transplantation: a review and recommendations. *J Antimicrob Chemother* 1993; **32**: 5–21.
83. Goodman JL, Winston DJ, Greenfield RA *et al*. A controlled trial of fluconazole to prevent fungal infections in patients undergoing bone marrow transplantation. *New Engl J Med* 1992; **326**: 845–851.
84. Bodey GP, Anaissie EJ, Etling LS, Estey E, O'Broen S and Kantarjian H. Antifungal prophylaxis during remission-induction chemotherapy for acute leukemia: fluconazole versus amphotericin B. *Cancer* 1994; **73**: 2099–2106.
85. Morgenstern GR, Prentice AG, Prentice HG, Popuer JE, Schey SA and Warnock DW. Itraconazole oral solution vs fluconazole suspension for antifungal prophylaxis in neutropenic patients. 36th Interscience Conference of Antimicrobiol Agents and Chemotherapy, New Orleans 1996 Abstr LM 34, 286.
86. Stewart A, Powles R, Hewetson M, Antrum J, Richardson C and Mehta J. Costs of antifungal prophylaxis after bone marrow transplantation: a model comparing oral fluconazole, liposomal amphotericin and oral polyenes as prophylaxis against oropharyngeal infections. *PharmacoEconomics* 1995; **8**: 350–361.
87. Schaffner A and Schaffner M. Effect of prophylactic fluconazole on the frequency of fungal infections, amphotericin B use and health care costs in patients undergoing intensive chemotherapy for hematologic neoplasias. *J Infect Dis* 1995; **172**: 1035–1041.
88. Riley DK, Pavia AT, Beatty PG, Petersen FB, Spruance JL, Stokes R and Evans TG. The prophylactic use of low-dose

amphotericin B in bone marrow transplant patients. *Am J Med* 1994; **97**: 509–514.

89. Tollemar J, Ringden O, Andersson S, Sundberg, Ljungman P, Sparrelid E and Tyden G. Prophylactic use of liposomal amphotericin (AmBisome) against fungal infections: a randomised trial in bone marrow transplant recipients. *Transplant Proc* 1993; **25**: 1495–1497.

90. Beyer J, Schwartz S, Heinemann V and Siegent W. Strategies in prevention of invasive pulmonary aspergillosis in immunocompromised or neutropenic patients. *Antimicrob Agents Chemother* 1994; **38**: 911–917.

91. Conneally E, Cafferkey MT, Daly PA, Keane CT and McCann SR. Nebulized amphotericin B as prophylaxis against aspergillosis in granulocytopenic patients. *Bone Marrow Transplant* 1990; **5**: 403–406.

92. Sepkowitz KA. *Pneumocystis carinii* pneumonia in patients without AIDS. *Clin Infect Dis* 1993; **17**(Suppl 2): S416–422.

93. Opravil M, Marincek B, Fuchs WA *et al*. Shortcomings of chest radiography in detecting *Pneumocystis carinii* pneumonia. *J Acquired Immune Deficiency Syndromes* 1994; **7**: 39–45.

94. Peglow SL, Smulian AG, Linke MJ *et al*. Serologic response to *Pneumocystis carinii* antigens in health and disease. *J Infect Dis* 1990; **161**: 296–306.

95. Peters SE, Wakefield AE, Sinclair K, Millard PR and Hopkin JM. A search for *Pneumocystis carinii* in post-mortem lungs by DNA amplification. *J Pathol* 1992; **166**: 195–198.

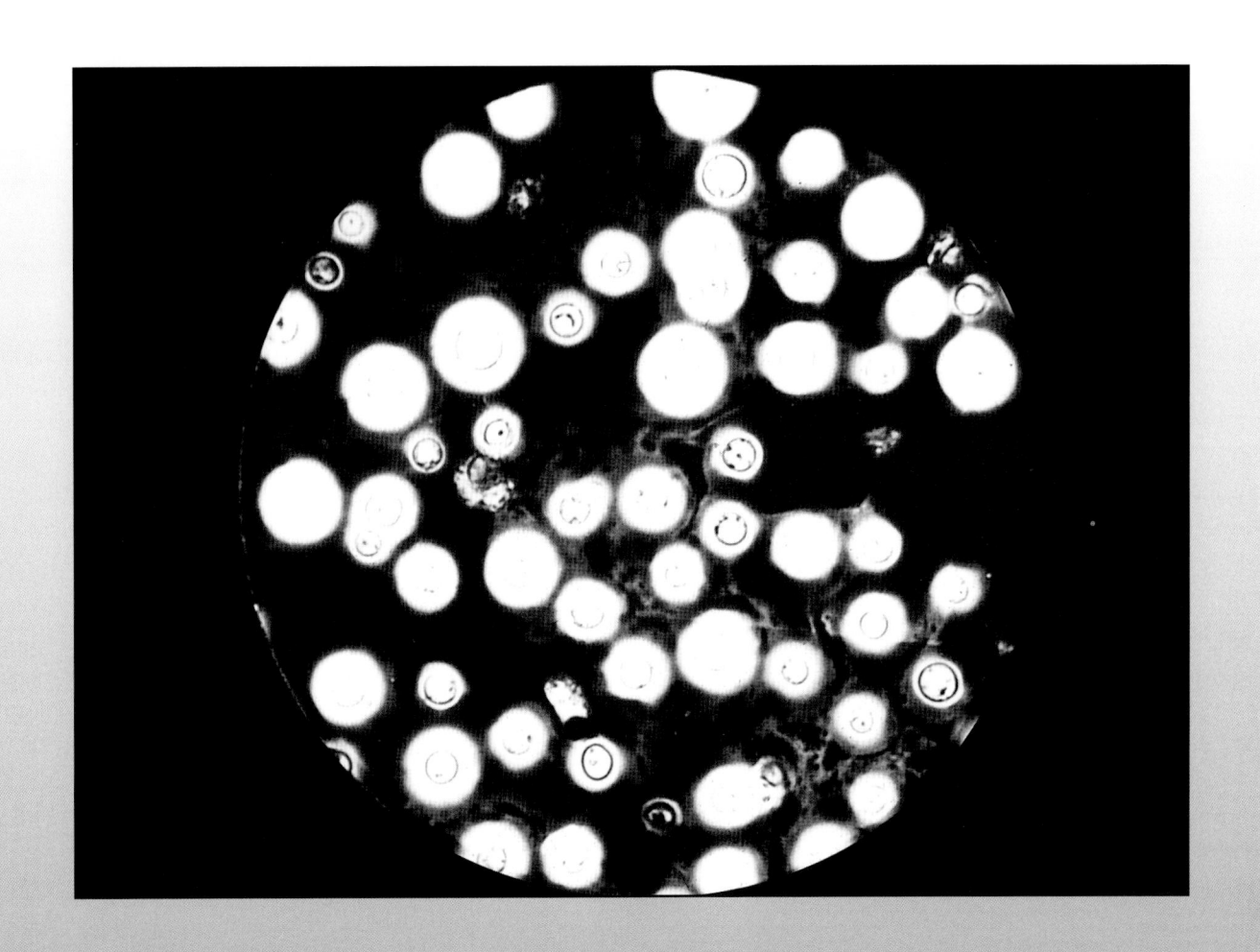

Chapter 47
Other infections

Rosemary A. Barnes

Introduction

Other infections occur sporadically following transplantation and the number of case reports describing rare and emerging pathogens is growing exponentially. Protozoan infections are relatively infrequent. *Toxoplasma gondii* is the major pathogen in this group but meningoencephalitis caused by *Acanthamoeba* [1] and *Naegleria* spp. [2] have been reported occasionally following exposure to contaminated water. Protozoan infections such as malaria and babesiosis may be more severe in immunocompromised patients especially if functional hyposplenism is a feature [3]. In endemic areas such as South America and Africa, typanosomal infection can occur and acute, transfusion-associated Chagas' disease has been reported after bone-marrow transplantation (BMT) [4].

Cryptosporidiosis (Figure 47.1) may cause severe diarrhoea complicated by villous atrophy and lactose intolerance. Most infections are self-limiting but symptoms may be intractable in immunosuppressed patients. There is no effective antimicrobial treatment but a lactose-free diet and bile acid-binding agents such as cholestyramine bring some symptomatic improvement in prolonged infections.

Nematodes are not normally associated with opportunist infections with the exception of *Strongyloides stercolis* infection which can occur in patients from endemic areas. Massive hyperinfection of the lungs and gastrointestinal system with dissemination to other organs can follow immunosuppression [5]. *Nocardia* [6] and *Actinomycetes* spp. infections [7], although rare, are a recognized problem and frequently occur in mixed infections with other recognized pathogens such as *Aspergillus* spp. and cytomegalovirus (CMV).

Toxoplasma gondii

Human infection with the intracellular parasite *T. gondii* occurs worldwide. Infection in immuno-competent individuals is usually asymptomatic or associated with mild fever and lymphadenopathy. By contrast, immunocompromised individuals such as transplant and human immunodeficiency virus (HIV)-infected patients, can present with fulminant disseminated infection. Infection is thought to result from reactivation of latent cysts and most cases have been reported following allogeneic transplantation in seropositive recipients although infection following autologous transplant can occur [8]. Parenteral transmission via blood transfusion has also been reported [9]. The incidence following peripheral blood stem cell (PBSC) transplant is unknown. The risk of infection is related to seroprevalence. In the UK and North America, incidence is low but rises in countries with endemicity such as France, and may be as high as 5% [10].

Most cases occur within six months of transplantation with the critical period being between 30 and 90 days. Reactivation of ocular toxoplasmosis (retinochoroiditis) may present earlier [11] and late infections more than one year post-BMT can occur [12]. Manifestations include fever, lymphadenopathy and hepatosplenomegaly. Cerebral localization with space-occupying lesions in the basal ganglia results in focal neurological signs but interstitial pneumonitis or pronounced dissemination to muscle including cardiac involvement are other manifestations. Mortality in BMT recipients with disseminated disease is very high and exceeds 70%. Diagnosis may be made by demonstration of the trophozoites (Figure 47.2) or tachyzoites within blood, bone marrow or bronchoalveolar lavage fluid or demonstration of cysts in tissue biopsies. Serological demonstration of specific IgG antibodies by dye test, latex agglutination or enzyme-linked immunosorbent assay (ELISA) may be used but these tests lack sensitivity for the detection of acute disease in immunocompromised patients and are more useful for identifying patients at risk of

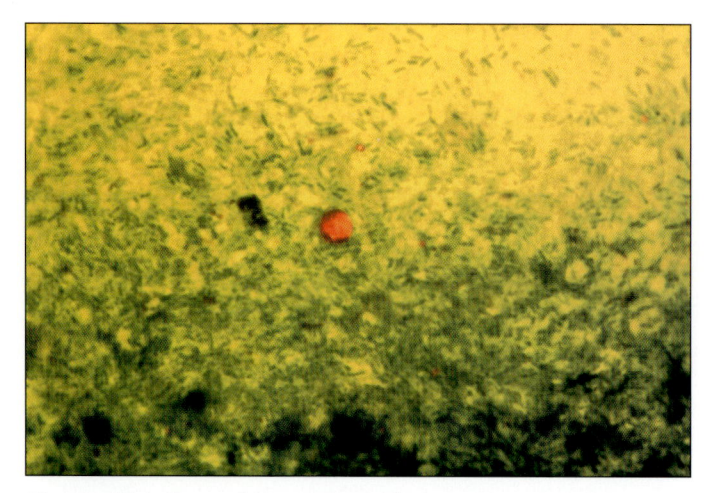

Figure 47.1 Cyst of Cryptosporidium parvum on faeces (modified Ziehl–Neelsen stain).

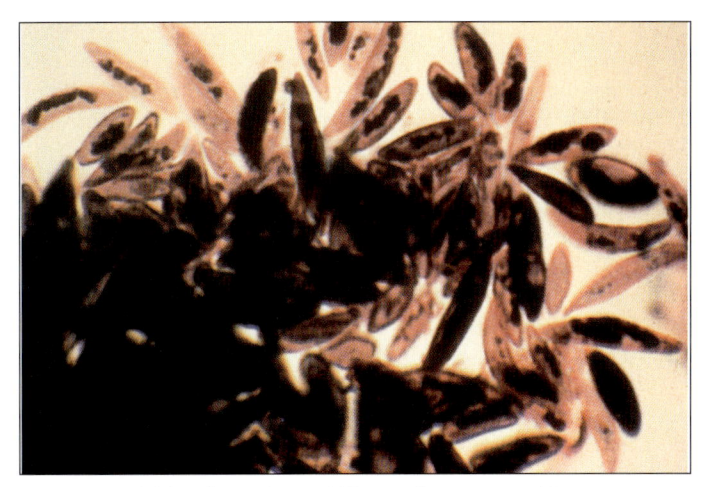

Figure 47.2 Trophozoites of *Toxoplasma gondii*.

reactivation. An immunosorbent agglutination assay (ISAGA) can detect IgM antibodies in acute disease but may be negative during reactivation. More recently, detection of specific DNA by the polymerase chain reaction (PCR) has been used successfully to diagnose human toxoplasmosis [10,13]. No antimicrobial agent has activity against the tissue cyst form but pyrimethamine and sulphonamides are active against trophozoites. These agents act synergistically and are used in combination (e.g. Fansidar) for periods of at least one month. Much longer courses of maintenance treatment may be required for patients with continued immunosuppression. Other antimicrobials such as clindamycin and spiramycin also have activity and may be used, often in combination with pyrimethamine, in patients allergic to sulphonamides. In countries with high endemic levels of toxoplasmosis, pretransplant screening of patients and prophylactic treatment of seropositive individuals may be cost-effective [10,11].

Nocardia infections

Nocardia species are saprophytic aerobic branching bacteria related to mycobacteria and the actinomycetes. They are ubiquitous in the environment and may cause sporadic infection in individuals with outdoor exposure to dust and soil but outbreaks of disease in solid organ transplant patients have been associated with building construction and renovation. Occasionally infection results from direct cutaneous implantation [14] but most often the agent is inhaled and causes pulmonary disease with dissemination to the central nervous system, skin and other organs. Infection usually occurs in the post-engraftment period often associated with acute or chronic graft-versus-host disease and corticosteroid usage. Fever, cough and pleuritic chest pain are the commonest presenting features and chest radiographs may show pulmonary infiltrates, consolidation, cavitating nodules and pleural effusions [6]. Enhancing lesions on computed tomography of the head may be found in patients with CNS disease. Symptoms are similar to invasive aspergillosis and indeed, 40% of reported cases had concomitant invasive fungal infection [6] indicating the degree of immunosuppression and exposure to similar point-sources of infection. Diagnosis is made by isolation of the organism from BAL fluid, sputum, tissue biopsies and occasionally blood cultures. Treatment is with trimethoprim-sulphamethoxazole (TMP-SMX) although low-dose intermittent prophylaxis for *Pneumocystis carinii* pneumonia prevention is ineffective in preventing *Nocardia* infection [15]. Some resistance to TMP-SMX has been reported and other agents such as minocycline, amikacin and imipenem are alternatives. Despite this, mortality remains high in this patient population.

Finally, as bone marrow and peripheral blood stem-cell transplantation become more widely available throughout the world, and as international travel continues to increase, the range of infectious complications will rise in parallel. Unusual infections will arise outside endemic areas in transplant recipients returning from abroad. All patients who wish to travel abroad particularly to the tropics and developing countries require individual advice on risks and available prophylactic measures [16].

References

1. Anderlini P, Przepiorka D, Luna M. Langford L, Andreeff M, Claxton D and Diesseroth AB. Acanthamoeba meningoencephalitis after bone marrow transplantation. *Bone Marrow Transplant* 1994; **14**: 459–461.
2. Ma P, Visvesvara GS, Martinez AJ, Theodore FH, Dagget P-M and Sawyer TK. Naegleria and acanthamoeba infections: review. *Rev Infect Dis* 1990; **12**: 490–513.
3. Baddely PG, Barnes RA, Finn AHR *et al*. Working Party of the British Committee for Standards in Haematology. Guidelines for the Prevention of Infection in the Patient with an Absent or Dysfunctional Spleen. *Br Med J* 1996; **321**: 430–434.
4. Altclas J, Jaimovich G, Milovic V, Klein F and Feldman L. Chagas' disease after bone marrow transplantation. *Bone Marrow Transplant* 1996; **18**: 447–448.

5. Bannon JP, Fater M and Solit R. Intestinal ileus secondary to Strongyloides stercolis infection: case report and review of the literature. *Am Surg* 1995; **61**: 377–380.
6. Choucino C, Goodman SA, Greer JP, Stein RS, Wolff SN and Dummer JS. Nocardia infections in bone marrow transplant recipients. *Clin Infect Dis* 1996; **23**: 1012–1029.
7. Hovi L, Saarinen UM, Donner U and Lindqvist C. Opportunistic osteomyelitis in the jaws of children on immunosuppressive chemotherapy. *J Pediatr Hematol Oncol* 1996; **18**: 90–94.
8. Geissmann F, Derouin F, Marolleau JP, Gisselbrecht C and Brice P. Disseminated toxoplasmosis following autologous bone marrow transplantation. *Clin Infect Dis* 1994; **19**: 800–801.
9. Saad R, Vincent JF, Cimon B, de Gentile L, Francois S, Bouachour G and Ifrah N. Pulmonary toxoplasmosis after allogeneic bone marrow transplantation: case report and review. *Bone Marrow Transplant* 1996; **18**: 211–212.
10. Foot ABM, Garin YJF, Ribaud P, Devergie A, Derouin F and Gluckman E. Prophylaxis of toxoplasmosis infection with pyrimethamine/sulfadoxine (fansidar) in bone marrow transplant recipients. *Bone Marrow Transplant* 1994; **14**: 241–245.
11. Peacock JE, Greven CM, Cruz JM and Hurd DD. Reactivation toxoplasmic retinochoroiditis in patients undergoing bone marrow transplantation: is there a role for chemoprophylaxis? *Bone Marrow Transplant* 1995; **15**: 983–987.
12. Bretagne S, Costa JM, Kuentz M, Simon D, Fortel I, Vernant JP and Cordonnier C. Late toxoplasmosis evidenced by PCR in a marrow transplant recipient. *Bone Marrow Transplant* 1995; **15**: 809–811.
13. Johnson JD, Butcher PD, Savva D and Holliman RE. Application of the polymerase chain reaction to the diagnosis of human toxoplasmosis. *J Infect* 1993; **26**: 147–158.
14. Freites V, Sumoza A, Bisotti R *et al.* Subcutaneous Nocardia asteroides abscess in a bone marrow transplant recipient. *Bone Marrow Transplant* 1995; **15**: 135–136.
15. Shearer C, Chandrasekar PH and the Bone Marrow Transplant Team. Pulmonary nocardiosis in a patient with a bone marrow transplant. *Bone Marrow Transplant* 1995; **15**: 479–481.
16. Conlon CP. The immunocompromised traveller. *Br Med Bull* 1993; **49**: 412–422.

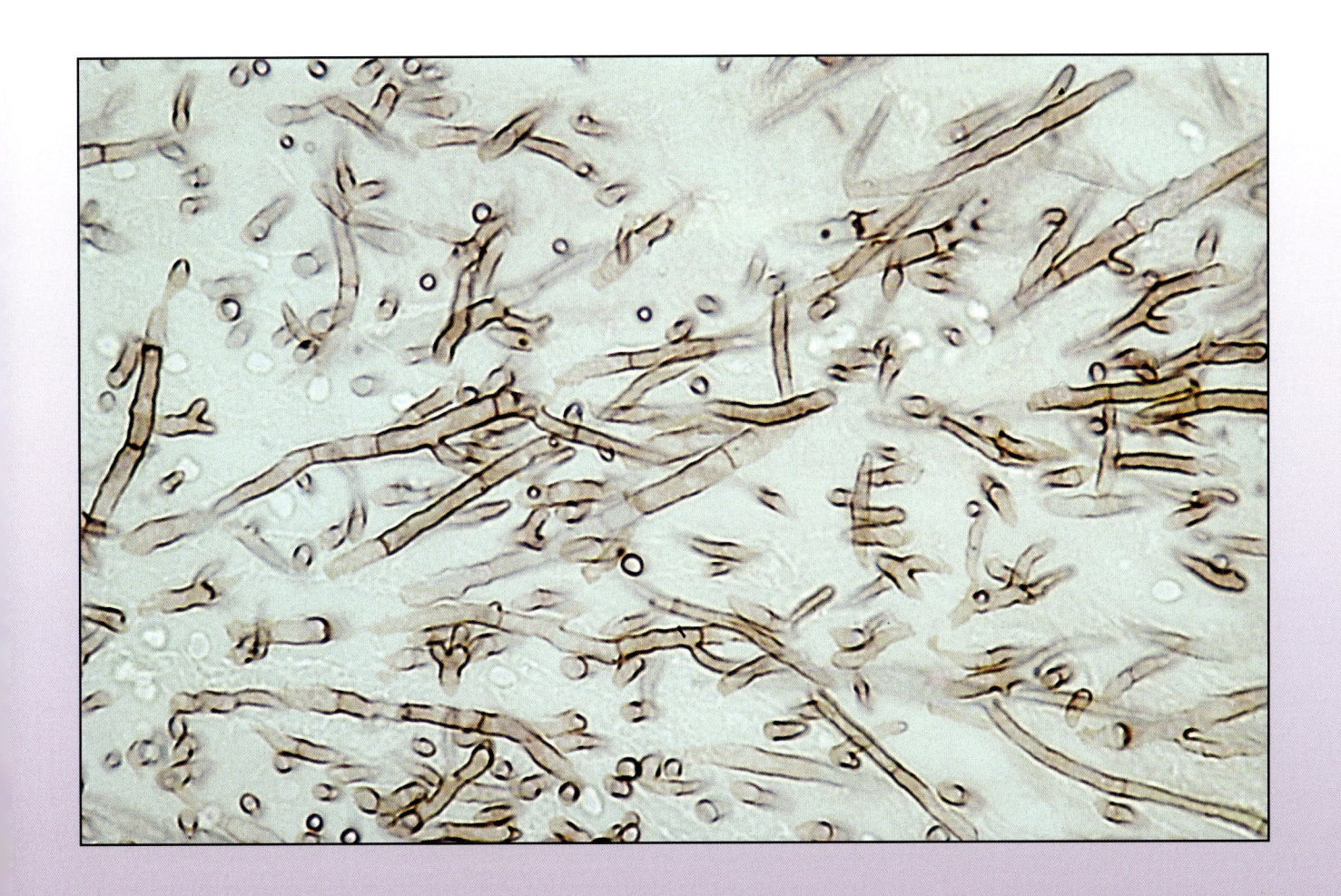

Chapter 48
Reimmunization after transplantation

Seema Singhal and Jayesh Mehta

Introduction

Immunization represents one of the most cost-effective means of preventing serious infectious diseases. The antigens available for routine or widespread use in children include diphtheria–pertussis–tetanus (DPT), trivalent polio, measles–mumps–rubella (MMR), *Haemophilus influenzae* type b (Hib), hepatitis B and tuberculosis (bacille Calmette–Guérin, BCG). Adult vaccines include diphtheria–tetanus (DT), hepatitis B, influenza virus and *Pneumococcus*. A number of other vaccines are available for special circumstances [1]. While the terms 'vaccination' and 'immunization' are often used interchangeably, 'immunization' refers to the provision of immunity by any means, active or passive. 'Passive immunization' refers to administration of antibody-containing immunoglobulin preparations to provide temporary protection. 'Active immunization' refers to the administration of a vaccine or a toxoid and is analogous to vaccination [1].

With time, most allograft and a large proportion of autograft recipients lose their immunity to poliovirus, tetanus, diphtheria and measles [2–8]. Additionally, transplant recipients are at increased risk of developing infections with organisms such as *H. influenzae* and *S. pneumoniae* for which vaccines are available [9–11]. For these reasons, it is essential to reimmunize blood- or bone-marrow transplant (BMT) recipients at appropriate times following the transplant [12,13].

Systematic reimmunization after BMT is a relatively neglected area. A survey of reimmunization practices in Europe found wide variations [12]. Tetanus toxoid vaccination was the most common practice, with 65% of the surveyed centres adminstering this to allograft recipients and 37% to autograft recipients. On the other hand, pertussis vaccination was the least common practice, with only one centre practising this [12].

Principles of vaccinating blood or marrow transplant recipients

Immune reconstitution after marrow transplantation follows a general pattern developing from immature to mature immune functions [14–20]. Immune reactivity during the first month post-graft is extremely low. Cytotoxic and phagocytic functions recover by day 100, but the more specialized functions of T- and B-lymphocytes may remain impaired for a year or even longer. After a period of time, the various components of the immune systems of most healthy marrow recipients begin to work synchronously, whereas the immune systems of patients with chronic graft-versus-host disease (GvHD) remain suppressed.

There are preliminary data showing faster immune reconstitution after autologous [21] as well as allogeneic [22] peripheral blood stem-cell transplantation compared with marrow. Because of this and the significantly larger inoculum of cells infused during blood stem-cell transplantation [23], it is possible that blood stem-cell graft recipients may have an earlier and better response to vaccines. However, all the data available so far on post-transplant immunization have been gathered on recipients of marrow grafts, and it is probably reasonable to treat blood stem-cell transplant recipients in the same way as marrow transplant recipients for the purposes of post-transplant reimmunization.

The most important factor which needs to be taken into account while considering vaccination after BMT is the immune status of the individual. Inactive, subunit or recombinant vaccines may be, at the worst, ineffective in BMT recipients, whereas live vaccines may be dangerous in immunocompromised patients (Table 48.1).

The amount of information available on reimmunization after BMT is still limited, and there are limited data on the effect of donor age, recipient age, disease and conditioning regimen on the need for immunization and its outcome. The general principles underlying vaccination of BMT recipients are shown in Table 48.2.

Live vaccines that are contraindicated in immunocompromised patients are:
- Adenovirus
- BCG
- Oral polio
- Measles–mumps–rubella
- Typhoid (Ty21a)
- Yellow fever

Table 48.1 Patients who should not be considered eligible for live vaccination after blood or marrow transplantation

All autograft recipients for two years*
All allograft recipients for two years*,**
Patients on immunosuppressive therapy for any reason
Patients suffering from chronic graft-versus-host disease, whether requiring therapy or not
Patients suffering from recurrent malignancy after transplantation

*These recommendations are based upon patients transplanted using marrow. Preliminary data suggest that immune reconstitution is faster in patients transplanted using blood stem cells. However, until more data and longer follow-up are available on immune function in patients transplanted using blood stem cells, the same guidelines should be followed for these patients.

**It is possible that immune recovery may take longer in recipients of T-cell depleted, human leukocyte antigen (HLA)-mismatched, or unrelated donor transplants. If there is any question about immune competence, serum immunoglobulin levels and the number of $CD4^+$ and $CD8^+$ cells should be determined. Patients in whom these parameters are normal are likely to be immunocompetent. More importantly, patients in whom either of these parameters is below normal are very likely to be immunocompromised to some extent.

Table 48.2 General principles of vaccination after blood or marrow transplantation

- Avoid all vaccines for at least four months.
  As a result of compromised immune responses, inactive vaccines are unlikely to elicit a response, and live vaccines may be dangerous.

- Avoid live vaccines in immunocompromised patients.
  Live vaccines may cause uncontrolled infection and may be dangerous.

- Avoid spreadable live vaccines such as oral polio in household contacts of immunocompromised patients.
  Spread of live organisms may cause uncontrolled infection in immunocompromised contacts.

- Measure antibody titres after vaccination to ensure efficacy.
  After BMT, in patients who are otherwise normal, immune responses to vaccines are often compromised.

- Multiple doses/courses may be required.
  Response is often inadequate with a single dose or course.

- Bear in mind the possibility of interference with the immune response in patients on intravenous immunoglobulin.
  There is evidence to suggest suboptimal response to vaccines in immunoglobulin recipients.

Table 48.3 shows a recommended reimmunization schedule for transplant recipients excluding those with chronic GvHD, whose schedule is given in Table 48.4. The available data on individual vaccines are discussed separately.

Individual vaccines

Diphtheria toxoid

Diphtheria has recently emerged as a problem in a number of countries where immunization coverage has been high. These outbreaks have been characterized by high fatality rates, a high proportion of cases in adults and an increased incidence of complications [24]. Lum et al. showed that, while antibodies to diphtheria toxoid were present in all patients within the first 100 days after allografting, only two-thirds of normal long-term survivors with immune donors had antibodies. This reduced further to 40% amongst patients with chronic GvHD who were transplanted from immune donors [2].

Chronic GvHD patients have been shown to have an impaired cellular immune response to diphtheria toxoid when vaccinated as early as four months after transplantation [25]. However, immunization with multiple doses of diphtheria toxoid has been reported to result in adequate immune response in paediatric patients autografted using bone marrow depleted of B-lymphocytes 38–54 months after BMT [5], and in allografted thalassaemia patients without chronic GvHD two to six years after BMT [26].

Haemophilus influenzae

Haemophilus influenzae accounts for a significant proportion of pulmonary infections in long-term survivors of BMT [10,27], including those receiving prophylactic penicillin. However, unlike pneumococci,

Table 48.3 Recommended immunization schedule in blood or marrow transplant recipients excluding those with chronic graft-versus-host disease

Vaccine	Schedule	Time post-BMT	Antibody response	Comments
Diphtheria toxoid	Three doses at monthly intervals	1 year	Good	Very immunogenic, so some centres only give one dose
Haemophilus influenzae (Hib)	Two doses 6 months apart	4 months	Good	In UK only used in under 4s as 'herd' immunity good
Influenza	One dose annually	6 months	Good	At least for 2 years, in patients with lung problems; vaccinate household contacts
Measles	One dose	2 years	Good	All children and selected adults
Mumps	One dose	2 years	Good	All children and selected adults
Pneumococcus	One dose	2 years	Variable	Additional drug prophylaxis needed
Poliovirus (inactivated)	Three doses at monthly intervals	1 year	Good	
Rubella	One dose	2 years	Good	Children and potentially fertile female patients
Tetanus toxoid	Three doses at monthly intervals	1 year	Good	In UK, one dose only given as very immunogenic

Table 48.4 Recommended immunization schedule in patients with chronic graft-versus-host disease.

Vaccine	Schedule	Time post-BMT	Antibody response
Diphtheria toxoid	Three doses at monthly intervals	1 year	?
Haemophilus influenzae (Hib)	Three doses at monthly intervals	4 months	Good
Influenza	One dose annually	6 months	?
Pneumococcus	One dose	2 years	Poor
Poliovirus (inactive)	Three doses at monthly intervals	1 year	Good
Tetanus toxoid	Three doses at monthly intervals	1 year	Good

*See contraindications, Table 48.3.

almost all severe disease is related to one capsular serotype (type b) and the Hib vaccine is very effective at preventing infections [1].

The tetanus toxoid-conjugated Hib capsular polysaccharide vaccine is more immunogenic than the unconjugated capsular polysaccharide vaccine and induces protective antibodies in 85% allograft recipients including IgG_2-deficient patients [27]. Between 4 and 18 months after BMT, response to the conjugate vaccine did not correlate with GvHD, immunosuppressive therapy or the time of vaccination. Beyond 18 months from BMT, response correlated with time (increasing efficacy with longer time interval) [27]. Autograft as well allograft recipients receiving a conjugate Hib vaccine at 12 and 24 months or 24 months only developed protective antibodies 80% and 50% of the time [28].

Donor and recipient immunization with the Hib-conjugate vaccine before BMT resulted in higher antibody concentrations in patients as early as three months after BMT compared with immunization of patients after BMT [29]. Higher antibody levels in the early stages post-transplant could potentially decrease the incidence of respiratory-tract infections in patients with lung disease or chronic GvHD.

Hepatitis B

While the risk of hepatitis B infection is not significant in regions with a low prevalence of the virus, the risk and morbidity of the infection in high-prevalence areas are considerable. The risk of infection may be high in the early post-transplant phase due to transfusion requirements.

Pretransplant vaccination of donors can result in adoptive transfer of protective immunity to the recipient [4,30]. Wimperis et al. showed that immunization of the donor alone resulted in transfer of an antibody response to the recipient after T-cell-depleted BMT, whereas immunization of donor as well as recipient resulted in a higher antibody response of a longer duration [4]. Ilan et al. confirmed that pretransplant immunization of donors could result in adoptive transfer of immunity to non-immune marrow recipients [30]. Roughly two-thirds of autograft recipients vaccinated peritransplant developed low-titre antibody responses which could have been protective against hepatitis B-associated complications in the post-transplant phase [31].

Interestingly, it is possible to resolve the hepatitis B carrier state (hepatitis B surface antigen, HBsAg positivity) and chronic hepatitis B through an allograft from an immune (anti-HBs antibody-positive) donor, who could have acquired immunity either through a natural infection [32] or through vaccination [33]. Table 48.5 outlines an approach to hepatitis B immunization in the setting of BMT depending upon the type of graft and the hepatitis B immune status of the patient and the donor.

Influenza

The influenza virus continues to cause annual epidemics of respiratory diseases. Transplant recipients can acquire influenza infections during community epidemics [34,35] and secondary bacterial infections including pneumonia may have serious consequences [35]. Influenza vaccination within the first six months following BMT has been found to be ineffective [36]. However, in patients receiving the vaccine two or more years after BMT, the efficacy was similar to that described in non-immunocompromised hosts [36], with a positive correlation between longer BMT immunization interval and seroconversion. Patients with chronic GvHD responded well to two of the virus strains and poorly to one.

It is also worthwhile vaccinating household contacts of transplant recipients to prevent transmission of influenza through them to patients, especially for patients who are still in the early post-transplant phase.

Measles

A substantial proportion of allograft recipients and some autograft recipients, especially children, lose immunity to measles over a period of time [3,7,37,38]. Measles is an important pathogen in developing countries [39], but apart from occasional outbreaks, it is not a problem elsewhere because of immunization.

Table 48.5 Suggested approach to hepatitis B immunization in BMT, where unspecified recommendations apply to the patient after transplantation

Patient donor	HBs antigen-positive (carrier/hepatitis)	Anti-HBs antibody-positive (immune)	No hepatitis B markers
HBs antigen-positive (carrier/hepatitis)	–	? Multiple-dose boosters immediately after BMT	Vaccinate prior to BMT. Then as indicated on the left
Anti-HBs antibody-positive (immune)	1. Donor leukocyte infusions if patient remains HBs antigen-positive 2. Booster doses if immune, but titres low	Booster doses if titres decline	Booster doses if titres decline
No hepatitis B markers	Immunize donor. Ensure anti-HBs antibody-positive prior to harvest. Then, as above	Revaccinate if antibodies lost. Booster doses if titres decline	Immunize donor pretransplant in areas with high prevalence of hepatitis B. Booster doses after transplant if titres decline.
Autograft	–	Booster doses to ensure titres do not fall	Immunize patient pretransplant in areas with high prevalence of hepatitis B. Booster doses after transplant if titres decline.

Although severe measles can occur in immunocompromised patients, there are no reports of measles following BMT.

The attenuated trivalent measles–mumps–rubella vaccine has been administered to non-immunocompromised allograft recipients beyond two years from transplant with seroconversion [7] and in autografted children [37]. It is not generally recommended for all BMT recipients, but on an individual basis for patients from high-prevalence geographic areas or where the risk for measles is increased [12].

Mumps

As with measles, a large number of allograft and autograft recipients lose immunity to mumps [7,37,38]. Mumps has not been described to be a problem in BMT patients. The attenuated trivalent measles–mumps–rubella vaccine has been administered to non-immunocompromised allograft recipients beyond two years from transplant with seroconversion [7], and in autografted children [37], but is not generally recommended for all BMT recipients [12].

Pneumococcus

Functional hyposplenism is a consequence of total body irradiation and chronic GvHD. Although pneumococcal infections are mainly a problem in patients with chronic GvHD [9] because of their inability to mount an antibody response to the pneumococcal polysaccharide antigen [40], other patients can also be affected. Splenectomized patients and those autografted for Hodgkin's disease and myeloma may be particularly at risk. A number of studies have evaluated pneumococcal vaccination in BMT recipients.

In a study of the 14-valent pneumococcal vaccine in allograft recipients, Winston et al. [41] found that both pre- and post-immunization antibody levels for all serotypes were lower in patients as compared with normal subjects. Antibody responses of patients not on steroids and vaccinated more than seven months after BMT improved with time.

Lortan et al. [42] found that the titres of specific IgG, IgG_1 and IgG_2 pneumococcal antibodies fell significantly after allogeneic BMT compared with pretransplant levels in children. Their response to immunization with a 23-valent vaccine one year or longer after BMT was not significantly different from normal controls except for poorer IgG_2 response. Despite responding, the patients did not achieve a high specific antibody titre after immunization in any immunoglobulin subclass because of the lower pre-immunization levels. Pre-immunization antibody levels and the response to immunization in these patients were not affected by previous splenectomy or chronic GvHD. Immunization of donors before the marrow harvest did not influence the levels of specific antibody a year or more after BMT. Molrine et al. [29] confirmed the observation that pretransplant pneumococcal vaccination of the donor did not affect the recipient's antibody response to post-transplant vaccination.

Avanzini et al. [43] found that all autografted or allografted children vaccinated more than two years after transplantation responded to pneumococcal polysaccharide compared with 20–50% of those vaccinated within two years. Although chronic GvHD influenced the response rate in univariate analysis, only the time between BMT and immunization was significant in multivariate analysis. The improving response to pneumococcal vaccination with increasing time after transplant seems to suggest that B-cell ontogeny follows a sequential programme in which polysaccharide antigens are amongst the last to evoke antibody responses.

Hammarstrom et al. [44] found that over the first year after BMT, pneumococcal antibody levels decreased in most allograft recipients, but not in autograft recipients. None of the patients with chronic GvHD showed normal levels of antibodies at one year. Of the patients who lost immunity after BMT and were vaccinated with a polyvalent pneumococcal vaccine, 34% showed a rise in IgG_2 antibodies, 28% with an increase in IgG_1, and 38% did not respond at all. None of the patients with chronic GvHD showed an increase in IgG_2 antibodies and 75% did not respond at all.

The 23-valent polysaccharide vaccine, apart from being poorly immunogenic, also fails to cover 20% of the commonly encountered pathogenic pneumococcal strains and immunized individuals remain susceptible to them. Life-long prophylactic penicillin V (250 mg twice daily orally) is therefore recommended for all patients who have had total body irradiation prior to an autograft or allograft, patients with chronic GvHD, and splenectomized patients [9,12]. Erythromycin (250 mg twice daily orally) or clarithromycin (250 mg once daily orally) may be used in penicillin-allergic subjects.

The covalent linkage of a polysaccharide antigen to a protein such as tetanus or diphtheria toxoid results in a more immunogenic molecule which evokes a T-cell-dependent immune response which is stronger in an immature immune system and is longer lasting. Conjugated pneumococcal vaccines are being developed.

Poliovirus

Poliomyelitis continues to remain a serious problem in a number of developing countries, and sporadic outbreaks are seen in developed countries in non-immunized individuals [45,46]. Immunity to polio is gradually lost after BMT [47–49].

Engelhard et al. [47] showed that 68–80% of BMT recipients had protective antibodies against the three serotypes of poliovirus 6–96 months after BMT compared with 92–96% before transplant, and titres were significantly lower than before BMT. Immunization with two doses of inactivated polio vaccine 6–96 months after BMT resulted in increased antibody titres in all patients. Presence of GvHD, pre-BMT polio antibody titres, age and the type of graft affected response to the vaccine, but the time from BMT to vaccination did not. Ljungman et al. [48] found that, although almost 70% of allograft recipients were seropositive to all poliovirus types a year after BMT, at least a fourfold decrease in antibody level was seen in roughly half the patients from their pretransplant levels. Half of the patients receiving three inactivated polio vaccine doses responded and the presence of chronic GvHD did not affect the response. Around 20% of autograft recipients were found to have lost antibodies to at least one type of poliovirus a year after autografting [49]. This time-dependent decrease in antibody titres continued in unvaccinated patients in the second and third years. A high proportion of seronegative patients reimmunized with three doses of the inactivated vaccine responded [49].

The inactivated polio vaccine has been successfully administered to paediatric patients autografted using bone-marrow-depleted of B-lymphocytes [5] and in patients allografted for thalassaemia who did not have chronic GvHD [26].

There are no published data on the use of the oral vaccine in transplant recipients or their household contacts. The oral vaccine should certainly be avoided in household contacts of immunocompromised transplant patients.

Rubella

As with measles and mumps, a number of allograft and autograft recipients lose immunity to mumps [7,37,38]. Although rubella has not been reported to be a problem in BMT patients, a number of pregnancies have been reported in transplant recipients [50,51]. The offspring of these women could be at risk of the congenital rubella syndrome, and it would therefore be advisable to revaccinate women with child-bearing potential. The attenuated trivalent measles–mumps–rubella vaccine has been administered to non-immunocompromised allograft recipients beyond two years from the transplant with development of immunity to rubella [7] and in autografted children [37].

Tetanus toxoid

There are data which suggest that tetanus toxoid-specific immunity can be transferred by allografting, and can persist in long-term survivors without immediate pretransplant toxoid administration to donors or to recipients pre- or post-transplant [2,6]. Contrasting observations were made by Ljungman et al. [8] who found that half of the patients who were immune to tetanus before BMT had lost their immunity by one year after BMT, and all the patients who were not reimmunized with tetanus toxoid were seronegative at two years.

Response rates were relatively poor and loss of immunity common in patients immunized with one or two doses of toxoid after BMT [8]. However, primary immunization with three doses of toxoid resulted in 100% response and sustained immunity [8]. Among patients receiving tetanus toxoid 3, 6 and 12 months after T-cell-depleted BMT, only those who had been immunized pretransplant along with their donors responded effectively [52]. Tetanus toxoid administration resulted in adequate immune response in paediatric patients autografted using bone marrow depleted of B-lymphocytes [5] and in thalassaemic patients who did not have chronic GvHD [26].

Gerritsen et al. studied the response to tetanus toxoid in allografted children and autografted or T-depleted allografted adults [53]. In children, who were routinely reimmunized early after BMT, the antibody response was quantitatively superior to that in adults who were not reimmunized early. In the majority of patients, the time required to reach peak antibody level was prolonged and the number of tetanus–toxoid-specific B-cell clones was markedly decreased in comparison with controls. Unlike the controls, production of relatively high concentrations of homogeneous antibodies against a heterogeneous background was seen in BMT recipients. These abnormalities were present up to ten years after BMT, irrespective of the age, the type of transplant or the reimmunization schedule.. Their data indicate that routine reimmunization early after BMT may improve the specific immune response, but because of dysregulated antibody production, long-lasting qualitative defects may be present even after normalization of antibody titres.

Measurement of the immune response to vaccines

Adequacy of the immune response to a vaccine is frequently measured by the serum level of the specific antibody. Although seroconversion does indicate an immune response, it does not necessarily signify protection [1]. Antibody development correlates with clinical protection after some vaccines (e.g. measles and rubella). Antibody development does not indicate immunity after some vaccines but is associated with some protection (e.g. serum vibriocidal antibodies in cholera). In some cases (e.g. tetanus), the antibody titre is crucial and protection is indicated by the level of the circulating antibody.

While routine determination of antibody titres prior to vaccination is not recommended in all transplant recipients [12], post-vaccination determination of antibody levels is useful to monitor antibody response and protection, and assess the need for additional doses of the vaccine.

Adoptive transfer of protective immunity

Although immunity can be transferred adoptively from donor to recipient through an allogeneic blood or marrow graft, the durability of this immune response is uncertain, and most data in clinical practice suggest a fall in antibody titres over a period of time [2–8]. Therefore, adoptive transfer of immunity with allogeneic marrow transplantation probably does not overcome the need for routine reimmunization in the majority of cases.

Shepherd and Noelle [54] showed in a murine model, that while the adoptive transfer of immune splenic B-cells or immune peripheral blood mononuclear cells effectively transferred antigen-specific IgG_1 antibody responses of donor origin to recipients, marrow from immune animals did not transfer a memory response. They suggested that the transfer of immunological memory observed in human BMT may be a consequence of peripheral blood contamination of the harvested donor marrow [54]. The number of B-cells in blood stem-cell harvests from healthy donors is 2.7 to 15.8 times (mean 7.9) higher than marrow [23]. Therefore, it is possible that peripheral blood stem-cell allografts may transfer immunity more effectively and this may be durable.

Serious infections are common in the early phase following allogeneic BMT. Augmentation of immunity to some of the common pathogenic organisms by adoptive transfer could conceivably reduce infection-related mortality and improve outcome. However, adoptive transfer of antibody responses is possible only for recall antigens. Transfer of responses to priming antigens, which would broaden the range of organisms against which patients can be protected, is not successful [55].

Gottlieb et al. [56] immunized marrow donors and/or recipients pretransplant with a polyvalent *Pseudomonas* O-polysaccharide–toxin A conjugate vaccine. When either donor or recipient alone was vaccinated, no increase in specific antibody titres was observed in the recipient post-transplant. However, when both donor and recipient were vaccinated before transplant, antibody titres increased to levels shown to be protective in animal models of Gram-negative sepsis [56]. The requirement for both donor and recipient immunization [55,56] reflects the need for primed donor B-lymphocytes in the marrow inoculum to be transferred into an antigen-containing environment for maximum B-cell proliferation and antibody production.

The adoptive transfer of virus antigen-specific cytotoxic T-lymphocytes from the donor to establish immunity has been shown to be effective for the prevention of cytomegalovirus infections [57], and prevention and treatment of Epstein–Barr virus-induced lymphoproliferation [58] in allograft recipients.

Passive immunization

The indications for passive immunization of BMT recipients using specific immunoglobulin preparations are similar to those in otherwise healthy individuals [1]. Administration of high-dose intravenous immunoglobulin, a form of passive immunization, is commonly employed for up to four months after BMT, especially allogeneic transplantation, for its beneficial effects on infections and GvHD [59]. However, there is evidence that prolonged administration of immunoglobulin (for one year) is associated with delayed immune reconstitution and an increased incidence of infections after discontinuation of immunoglobulin [60]. The role of intravenous immunoglobulin in BMT has been reviewed recently [61].

While reimmunizing BMT recipients, possible interference of immunoglobulin administration with response to vaccination must be borne in mind. Response to the measles–mumps–rubella vaccine in healthy children has been shown to be suboptimal for three months after the administration of 80 mg/kg of immunoglobulin [62]. A similar observation has been made in adult recipients of tetanus–diphtheria vaccine along with tetanus immune globulin [63], but to a much smaller extent.

References

1. Keusch GT and Bart KJ. Immunization principles and vaccine use. In: *Harrison's Principles of Internal Medicine*, 13th edn. KJ Isselbacher, E Braunwald, JD Wilson, JB Martin, AS Fauci and DL Kasper (eds), 1994: 498–511 (New York: McGraw-Hill).
2. Lum LG, Munn NA, Schanfield MS and Storb R. The detection of specific antibody formation to recall antigens after human bone marrow transplantation. *Blood* 1986; **67**: 582–587.
3. Lum LG, Seigneuret MC and Storb R. The transfer of antigen-specific humoral immunity from marrow donors to marrow recipients. *J Clin Immunol* 1986; **6**: 389–396.
4. Wimperis JZ, Brenner MK, Prentice HG et al. Transfer of a functioning humoral immune system in transplantation of T-lymphocyte-depleted bone marrow. *Lancet* 1986; **i**: 339–343.
5. Baumgartner C, Morell A, Hirt A et al. Humoral immune function in pediatric patients treated with autologous bone marrow transplantation for B cell non-Hodgkin's lymphoma. The influence of ex vivo marrow decontamination with anti-Y 29/55 monoclonal antibody and complement. *Blood* 1988; **71**: 1211–1217.
6. Lum LG, Noges JE, Beatty P et al. Transfer of specific immunity in marrow recipients given HLA-mismatched, T cell-depleted, or HLA-identical marrow grafts. *Bone Marrow Transplant* 1988; **3**: 399–406.
7. Ljungman P, Fridell E, Lonnqvist B et al. Efficacy and safety of vaccination of marrow transplant recipients with a live attenuated measles, mumps, and rubella vaccine. *J Infect Dis* 1989; **159**: 610–615.
8. Ljungman P, Wiklund Hammarsten M, Duraj V et al. Response to tetanus toxoid immunization after allogeneic bone marrow transplantation. *J Infect Dis* 1990; **162**: 496–500.
9. Rege K, Mehta J, Treleaven J et al. Fatal pneumococcal infections following allogeneic bone marrow transplantation. *Bone Marrow Transplant* 1994; **14**: 903–906.
10. Aucouturier P, Barra A, Intrator L et al. Long lasting IgG subclass and antibacterial polysaccharide antibody deficiency after allogeneic bone marrow transplantation. *Blood* 1987; **70**: 779–785.
11. Lossos IS, Breuer R, Or R et al. Bacterial pneumonia in recipients of bone marrow transplantation. A five-year prospective study. *Transplantation* 1995; **60**: 672–678.
12. Ljungman P, Cordonnier C, De Bock R et al. Immunisations after bone marrow transplantation: results of a European survey and recommendations from the Infectious Diseases Working Party of the European Group for Blood and Marrow Transplantation. *Bone Marrow Transplant* 1995; **15**: 455–460.
13. Somani J and Larson RA. Reimmunization after allogeneic bone marrow transplantation. *Am J Med* 1995; **98**: 389–398.
14. Lum LG. The kinetics of immune reconstitution after human marrow transplantation. *Blood* 1987; **69**: 369–380.
15. Symann M, Bosly A, Gisselbrecht C, Brice P and Franks C. Immune reconstitution after bone-marrow transplantation. *Cancer Treat Rev* 1989; **16**(Suppl A): 15–19.
16. Atkinson K. Reconstruction of the haemopoietic and immune systems after marrow transplantation. *Bone Marrow Transplant* 1990; **5**: 209–226.
17. Kelsey SM, Lowdell MW and Newland AC. IgG subclass levels and immune reconstitution after T cell-depleted allogeneic bone marrow transplantation. *Clin Exp Immunol* 1990; **80**: 409–412.
18. Storek J and Saxon A. Reconstitution of B cell immunity following bone marrow transplantation. *Bone Marrow Transplant* 1992; **9**: 395–408.
19. Storek J, Ferrara S, Ku N, Giorgi JV, Champlin RE and Saxon A. B-cell reconstitution after human bone marrow transplantation: recapitulation of ontogeny? *Bone Marrow Transplant* 1993; **12**: 387–398.
20. Storek J, Witherspoon RP and Storb R. T cell reconstitution after bone marrow transplantation into adult patients does not resemble T cell development in early life. *Bone Marrow Transplant* 1995; **16**: 413–425.
21. Roberts MM, To LB, Gillis D et al. Immune reconstitution following peripheral blood stem cell transplantation, autologous bone marrow transplantation and allogeneic bone marrow transplantation. *Bone Marrow Transplant* 1993; **12**: 469–475.

22. Ottinger HD, Beelen DW, Scheulen B, Schaefer UW and Grosse-Wilde H. Improved immune reconstitution after allotransplantation of peripheral blood stem cells instead of bone marrow. *Blood* 1996; **88**: 2775–2779.
23. Singhal S, Powles R, Treleaven J, Long S, Rowland A and Mehta J. Comparison of cell yields in a double-blind randomized study of allogeneic marrow versus blood stem cell transplantation. *Br J Haematol* 1996; **93**(Suppl 1): 37.
24. Galazka AM, Robertson SE and Oblapenko GP. Resurgence of diphtheria. *Eur J Epidemiol* 1995; **11**: 95–105.
25. Gratama JW, Verdonck LF, van der Linden JA *et al*. Cellular immunity to vaccinations and herpesvirus infections after bone marrow transplantation. *Transplantation* 1986; **41**: 719–724.
26. Li Volti S, Mauro L, Di Gregorio F *et al*. Immune status and immune response to diphtheria–tetanus and polio vaccines in allogeneic bone marrow-transplanted thalassemic patients. *Bone Marrow Transplant* 1994; **14**: 225–227.
27. Barra A, Cordonnier C, Preziosi MP *et al*. Immunogenicity of *Haemophilus influenzae* type b conjugate vaccine in allogeneic bone marrow recipients. *J Infect Dis* 1992; **166**: 1021–1028.
28. Guinan EC, Molrine DC, Antin JH *et al*. Polysaccharide conjugate vaccine responses in bone marrow transplant patients. *Transplantation* 1994; **57**: 677–684.
29. Molrine DC, Guinan EC, Antin JH *et al*. Donor immunization with *Haemophilus influenzae* type b (HIB)-conjugate vaccine in allogeneic bone marrow transplantation. *Blood* 1996; **87**: 3012–3018.
30. Ilan Y, Nagler A, Adler R *et al*. Adoptive transfer of immunity to hepatitis B virus after T cell-depleted allogeneic bone marrow transplantation. *Hepatology* 1993; **18**: 246–252.
31. Nagler A, Ilan Y, Adler R *et al*. Successful immunization of autologous bone marrow transplantation recipients against hepatitis B virus by active vaccination. *Bone Marrow Transplant* 1995; **15**: 475–478.
32. Ilan Y, Nagler A, Adler R, Tur Kaspa R, Slavin S and Shouval D. Ablation of persistent hepatitis B by bone marrow transplantation from a hepatitis B-immune donor. *Gastroenterology* 1993; **104**: 1818–1821.
33. Ilan Y, Nagler A, Shouval D *et al*. Development of antibodies to hepatitis B virus surface antigen in bone marrow transplant recipient following treatment with peripheral blood lymphocytes from immunized donors. *Clin Exp Immunol* 1994; **97**: 299–302.
34. Potter MN, Foot AB and Oakhill A. Influenza A and the virus associated haemophagocytic syndrome: cluster of three cases in children with acute leukaemia. *J Clin Pathol* 1991; **44**: 297–299.
35. Whimbey E, Elting LS, Couch RB *et al*. Influenza A virus infections among hospitalized adult bone marrow transplant recipients. *Bone Marrow Transplant* 1994; **13**: 437–440.
36. Engelhard D, Nagler A, Hardan I *et al*. Antibody response to a two-dose regimen of influenza vaccine in allogeneic T cell-depleted and autologous BMT recipients. *Bone Marrow Transplant* 1993; **11**: 1–5.
37. Pauksen K, Duraj V, Ljungman P *et al*. Immunity to and immunization against measles, rubella and mumps in patients after autologous bone marrow transplantation. *Bone Marrow Transplant* 1992; **9**: 427–432.
38. Ljungman P, Lewensohn-Fuchs I, Hammarstrom V *et al*. Long-term immunity to measles, mumps, and rubella after allogeneic bone marrow transplantation. *Blood* 1994; **84**: 657–663.
39. de Quadros CA, Olive JM, Hersh BS *et al*. Measles elimination in the Americas. Evolving strategies. *J Am Med Ass* 1996; **275**: 1311–1312.
40. Witherspoon RP, Storb R, Ochs HD *et al*. Recovery of antibody production in human allogeneic marrow graft recipients: influence of time post-transplantation, the presence or absence of chronic graft-versus-host disease, and antithymocyte globulin treatment. *Blood* 1981; **58**: 360–368.
41. Winston DJ, Ho WG, Schiffman G, Champlin RE, Feig SA and Gale RP. Pneumococcal vaccination of recipients of bone marrow transplants. *Arch Intern Med* 1983; **143**: 1735–1737.
42. Lortan JE, Vellodi A, Jurges ES and Hugh-Jones K. Class- and subclass-specific pneumococcal antibody levels and response to immunization after bone marrow transplantation. *Clin Exp Immunol* 1992; **88**: 512–519.
43. Avanzini MA, Carra AM, Maccario R *et al*. Antibody response to pneumococcal vaccine in children receiving bone marrow transplantation. *J Clin Immunol* 1995; **15**: 137–144.
44. Hammarstrom V, Pauksen K, Azinge J, Oberg G and Ljungman P. Pneumococcal immunity and response to immunization with pneumococcal vaccine in bone marrow transplant patients: the influence of graft versus host reaction. *Support Care Cancer* 1993; **1**: 195–199.
45. de Quadros CA, Andrus JK, Olive JM and Carrasco P. Strategies for poliomyelitis eradication in developing countries. *Public Health Rev* 1993–94; **21**: 65–81.
46. Anonymous. Progress towards global poliomyelitis eradication, 1985–1994. *Morb Mortal Wkly Rep* 1995; **44**: 273–275, 281.
47. Engelhard D, Handsher R, Naparstek E *et al*. Immune response to polio vaccination in bone marrow transplant recipients. *Bone Marrow Transplant* 1991; **8**: 295–300.
48. Ljungman P, Duraj V and Magnius L. Response to immunization against polio after allogeneic marrow transplantation. *Bone Marrow Transplant* 1991; **7**: 89–93.
49. Pauksen K, Hammarstrom V, Ljungman P *et al*. Immunity to poliovirus and immunization with inactivated poliovirus vaccine after autologous bone marrow transplantation. *Clin Infect Dis* 1994; **18**: 547–552.
50. Sanders JE, Hawley J, Levy W *et al*. Pregnancies following high-dose cyclophosphamide with or without high-dose busulfan or total-body irradiation and bone marrow transplantation. *Blood* 1996; **87**: 3045–3052.
51. Singhal S, Powles R, Treleaven J, Horton C, Swansburg J, and Mehta J. Melphalan alone prior to allogeneic bone marrow transplantation from HLA-identical sibling donors for hematologic malignancies: alloengraftment with potential preservation of fertility in women. *Bone Marrow Transplant* 1996; 18, **6**: 1049–1057.
52. Wimperis JZ, Brenner MK, Prentice HG, Thompson EJ and Hoffbrand AV. B cell development and regulation after T cell-depleted marrow transplantation. *J Immunol* 1987; **138**: 2445–2450.
53. Gerritsen EJ, van Tol MJ, van't Veer MB *et al*. Clonal dysregulation of the antibody response to tetanus-toxoid after bone marrow transplantation. *Blood* 1994; **84**: 4374–4382.
54. Shepherd DM and Noelle RJ. The lack of memory B cells in immune bone marrow. *Transplantation* 1991; **52**: 97–100.
55. Wimperis JZ, Gottlieb D, Duncombe AS, Heslop HE, Prentice HG and Brenner MK. Requirements for the adoptive transfer

of antibody responses to a priming antigen in man. *J Immunol* 1990; **144**: 541–547.

56. Gottlieb DJ, Cryz SJ Jr, Furer E *et al*. Immunity against *Pseudomonas aeruginosa* adoptively transferred to bone marrow transplant recipients. *Blood* 1990; **76**: 2470–2475.

57. Walter EA, Greenberg PD, Gilbert MJ *et al*. Reconstitution of cellular immunity against cytomegalovirus in recipients of allogeneic bone marrow by transfer of T-cell clones from the donor. *New Engl J Med* 1995; **333**: 1038–1044.

58. Rooney CM, Smith CA, Ng CY *et al*. Use of gene-modified virus-specific T lymphocytes to control Epstein-Barr virus-related lymphoproliferation. *Lancet* 1995; **345**: 9–13.

59. Sullivan KM, Kopecky KJ, Jocom J *et al*. Immunomodulatory and antimicrobial efficacy of intravenous immunoglobulin in bone marrow transplantation. *New Engl J Med* 1990; **323**: 705–712.

60. Sullivan KM, Storek J, Kopecky KJ *et al*. A controlled trial of long-term administration of intravenous immunoglobulin to prevent late infection and chronic graft-vs-host disease after marrow transplantation: clinical outcome and effect on subsequent immune recovery. *Biol Blood Marrow Transplant* 1996; **2**: 44–53.

61. Sullivan KM. Immunomodulation in allogeneic marrow transplantation: use of intravenous immune globulin to suppress acute graft-versus-host disease. *Clin Exp Immunol* 1996; **104**(Suppl 1): 43–48.

62. Siber GR, Werner BG, Halsey NA *et al*. Interference of immune globulin with measles and rubella immunisation. *J Paediatr* 1993; **122**: 204–211.

63. Dal-Re R, Gil A, Gozalez A and Lasheras L. Does tetanus immune globulin interfere with the immune response to simultaneous administration of tetanus–diphtheria vaccine? A comparative clinical trial in adults. *J Clin Pharmacol* 1995; **35**: 420–425.

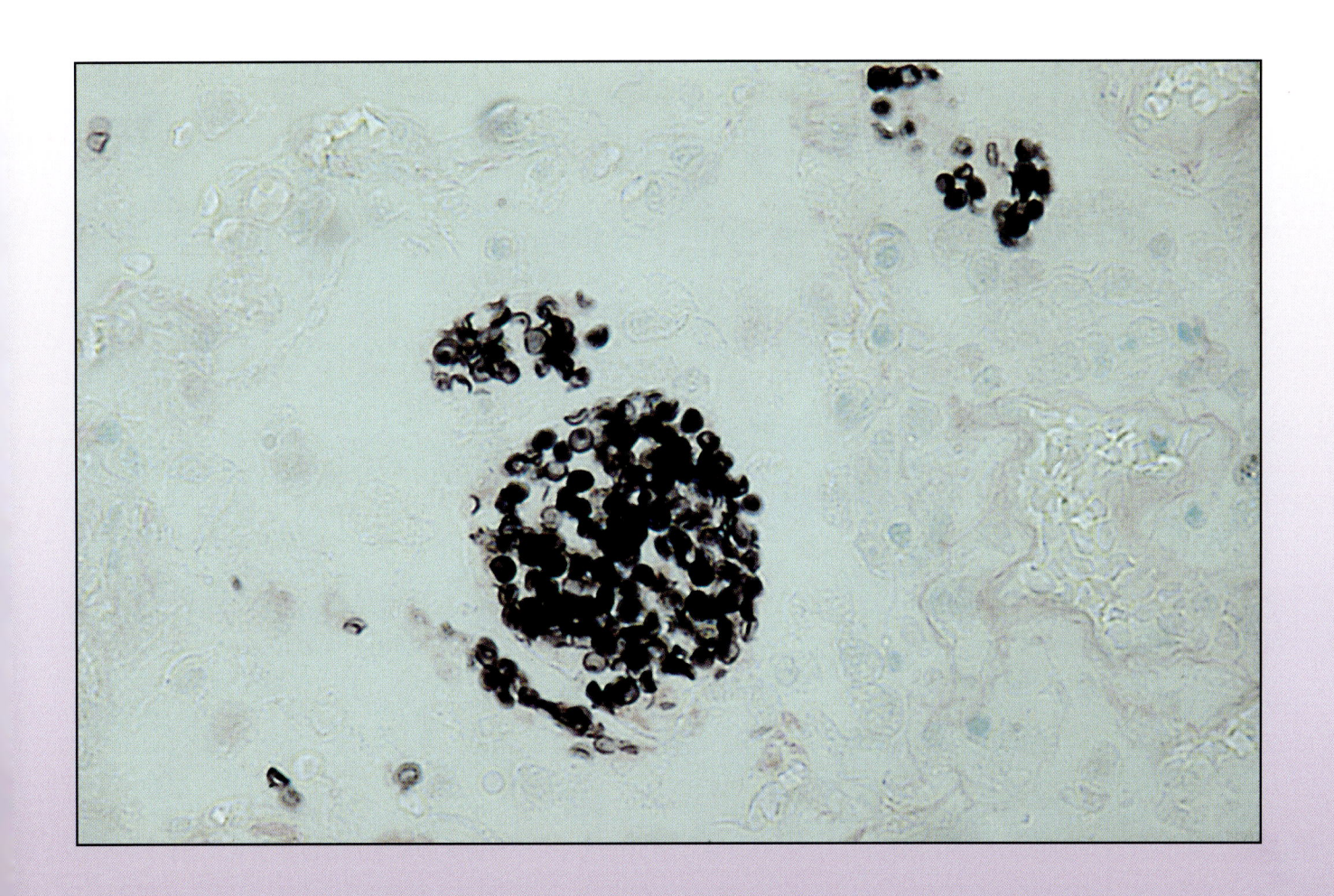

Chapter 49
General infection prophylaxis

Unell Riley

Introduction

Infections during bone marrow transplantation can arise for a number of reasons (Table 49.1) and there are many methods (Table 49.2) of reducing infection risk. The time when these strategies come into operation depends upon where the patient is in the transplant procedure, whether in the immediate neutropenic period, the post engraftment period or late after the transplant.

Table 49.1 Predisposing factors for infection after bone-marrow transplantion

- Neutropenia
- Reduced cell-mediated immunity
- Reduced humoral immunity
- Damage to anatomic barrier
- Hyposplenism
- Medical procedures

Table 49.2 Methods of reducing infection in bone-marrow transplantation patients

- Suppression of endogenous flora
- Reducing acquisition of exogenous flora
- Suppression of latent infection
- Augmentation of host immune function

Suppression of endogenous flora

In the neutropenic phase of the transplant, the combination of neutropenia and damage to the normal anatomic barrier make the patient at particular risk from their own endogenous flora. Therefore, attempts should be made to reduce the microbial load. General measures include proper maintenance of the integument and suppression of microbes on the skin and in the mucosa. Typical regimens include daily chlorhexidine washes or showers to reduce the possible risk of skin colonization by potential pathogens such as *Staphylococcus aureus* and *Corynebacterium jeikeium*. Long-term central venous catheters are a prolonged disruption of the normal anatomic barrier and therefore need particular attention to their care. They should be inserted in sterile conditions in the operating theatre. There is little evidence that the use of a glycopeptide, such as vancomycin, reduces the risk of infection [1]. A sterile occlusive dressing should be kept on the wound for a short period of time, and thereafter the line should be cleaned daily with an antiseptic such as chlorhexidine or povidone-iodine. Manipulation of the line should be kept to a minimum and any procedures involving the line should involve use of an aseptic technique. Shaving should be discouraged since it may cause abrasion to the skin and lead to colonization or infection.

The oropharynx is an important source of infection in a neutropenic patient, and therefore oral hygiene is very important. A dental examination should be carried out well before the bone-marrow transplant and any dental work that is necessary should be performed approximately one month before the transplant to allow proper healing. Brushing the teeth with a soft toothbrush is acceptable if it does not lead to gum damage. Suppression of oropharyngeal flora can be achieved by the use of regular chlorhexidine and nystatin mouthwashes.

Antibiotic prophylaxis/gut decontamination in neutropenia

The gastrointestinal tract is the major source of the aerobic Gram-negative bacilli [2] such as *Escherichia coli* and *Klebsiella pneumoniae* which, after colonization of the gut, can lead to life-threatening Gram-negative sepsis. Disturbance of normal bowel flora, particularly the anaerobic component, may lead to translocation across the bowel wall of aerobic Gram-negative bacilli which may then cause disseminated infection [3]. Therefore, traditionally, gut decontamination regimes have striven to eradicate Gram-negative bacilli from the gut and to maintain the anaerobic flora for colonization resistance. The first of these regimes involved use of non-absorbable antibiotics [4]. Examples included neomycin, colistin and nystatin combinations. Other regimes have used different aminoglycosides or amphotericin B. Evidence for the effectiveness of these selective antimicrobial gut decontamination regimes is conflicting, although most studies show some benefit when they are used in conjunction with protective environments [5]. However, these regimens have the disadvantage that they are expensive, compliance is often poor due to their extreme unpleasantness and their induction of nausea and vomiting, and emergence of resistance, particularly to aminoglycosides, can limit their usefulness. Their early withdrawal can lead to colonization with more resistant hospital organisms which may increase the risk of infection [6,7]. Due to these disadvantages, other more palatable regimens were sought. Trimethoprim-sulphamethoxazole combination (Septrin) has been shown to be more effective than non-absorbable antibiotics in comparative trials [8]. However, it is not effective against *Pseudomonas aeruginosa*. Again, their effectiveness is greatly dependent upon compliance [9] and there are also toxicity problems associated with the regimen. The significant problem of bone-marrow suppression and prolongation of the neutropenic period, particularly in leukaemic patients, has precluded their use in the pre-engraftment phase of the bone-marrow transplant.

The latest development in antibiotic prophylaxis is the use of fluoroquinolones [10]. They have been advocated because of their high activity against aerobic Gram-negative bacilli including *Pseudomonas aeruginosa*, their sparing of the anaerobic gut flora and their higher tolerability. Also, since they achieve high blood levels at the recommended dosage, they have significant systemic prophylactic activity. Use of various quinolones such as ciprofloxacin [11], ofloxacin [12–14], norfloxacin [15,16] and perfloxacin [17] has been shown to be superior in reducing the incidence of Gram-negative sepsis by comparative studies. Most show a significant reduction in duration of fever and also duration of parenteral antimicrobial therapy for infection. The concern about these drugs is their poor activity against Gram-positive organisms such as coagulase-negative staphylococci and viridans streptococci, and these organisms are becoming an increasing cause of sepsis in the neutropenic patient. In one review, quinolone prophylaxis was associated with an increased risk of streptococcal bacteraemia [18]. The mortality rate for streptococcal infection in this review was similar to that of Gram-negative septicaemia.

With the increased importance of streptococcal infections, many have looked at the combination of an antistreptococcal agent with a quinolone for prophylaxis. The addition of roxithromycin to ciprofloxacin has been shown to reduce the incidence of streptococcal infection [19] and the addition of benzylpenicillin has also been suggested [20]. Resistance to ciprofloxacin in coagulase-negative staphylococci and *Staphylococcus aureus* has now been well established [21]. A significant increase in the number of Gram-negative organisms resistant to quinolones has not been universally noticed in units using fluoroquinolone prophylaxis, but isolated cases of increased resistance in a number of units is cause for concern [22–25].

Antibiotic prophylaxis for capsulated bacterial infections

Allogenic bone-marrow transplant patients appear to be at increased risk from bacteraemia with capsulated bacteria after engraftment, particularly in the presence of chronic graft-versus-host disease [26]. This is illustrated by the relatively high incidence of pneumococcal bacteraemia beginning about 100 days post-transplant [27]. This is probably due to two factors:

- the relative deficiency of the IgG_2 subclass in patients who have had a transplant which may last for up to two years. Antibodies to type-specific polysaccharide antigens seem to be restricted to the IgG_2 class [28].
- the presence of chronic graft-versus-host disease which can cause functional and structural hyposplenism [29].

With the considerable risk of overwhelming pneumococcal septicaemia, patients should receive lifelong penicillin prophylaxis starting after engraftment, and they should also receive pneumococcal and *Haemophilus influenza* type b immunization 9–12 months after their bone-marrow transplant [30]. Transplant patients may need reimmunization with pneumococcal vaccine three years after the first dose due to their poor ability to mount an adequate immune response.

Reducing acquisition of exogenous flora

The reduction of exogenous flora is particularly important for a neutropenic bone-marrow patient and can be achieved by a number of methods (Table 49.3).

> **Table 49.3 Reducing acquisition of exogenous flora**
>
> - Protective isolation
>   single-room environment
>   air filtration
>   reverse barrier nursing
>
> - Low-microbial content diet
>
> - Immunotherapy
>   passive immunotherapy
>   active immunization
>   adoptive transfer of antibody response

Environment
Protective isolation
The principle of protective isolation is to reduce the means by which the patient can acquire organisms from external sources and it is at its most effective when combined with decontamination techniques [31]. In its most basic form it would consist of a naturally ventilated room with bathroom facilities. All items brought into the room would be thoroughly cleaned or disinfected and the patient nursed with reverse barrier techniques to reduce all likely routes of a nosocomial infection. There is some evidence suggesting that bone-marrow transplantation can be safely completed without protective isolation [32].

Air filtration
A wide range of organisms can be transmitted as airborne pathogens. These include fungi such as *Aspergillus* species and *Mucor* species, bacteria such as *Legionella* species and protozoan *Pneumocystis carinii*, as well as a number of viruses. Outbreaks have occurred in wards of neutropenic patients nursed in naturally ventilated side-rooms and this has been particularly seen as outbreaks of *Aspergillus* infections, especially when hospital renovation is being carried out or when the ward is near building construction [33–35].

Air-filtration systems are designed to overcome these problems. The most effective and popular system is high-efficiency particulate air filtration (HEPA filtration) [36]. This is thought to remove at least 99.97% of all particles which are $\geq 0.3\,\mu m$ in diameter. Therefore, such a system should remove all bacteria and fungi (and their spores) from the air, but not viruses. They have been used in a number of forms including specially designed laminar air-flow cubicles [37] or plastic tent isolators [38]. Although there is good evidence to suggest that air-flow filtration combined with other methods for reducing exogenous and endogenous microbial exposure does reduce the incidence of infection in bone-marrow transplant patients [39], it does not, however, eliminate fever, and its greatest impact seems to be reducing the incidence of *Aspergillus* infection [40]. Such units are expensive to install and maintain and their cost-effectiveness has been questioned, but they would probably be considered mandatory where hospital construction or renovation is an issue.

Reverse barrier nursing
Contacts from outside should be controlled and kept to a minimum. The hands of healthcare workers and visitors are probably the greatest potential source of nosocomial infection. Therefore, strict attention should be given to hand hygiene. Both staff and visitors should be educated in good hand-washing and aseptic techniques. Hand-washing should be carried out with an antibacterial soap such as chlorhexidine and disposable sterile gloves should be made available. For people spending any length of time in the single room, outer garments (such as white coats) should be removed and a fresh overgown or disposable long-sleeved apron should be worn and changed between patients. Since there is no evidence of nosocomial infection being transmitted by shoes or from the floor, there is no compelling indication for wearing overshoes, and indeed they may lead to unclean shoes contaminating hands. The routine use of masks is also questionable since the spread of infection by nose to hand to patients is more common than by droplets spread, and because the use of masks has a negative psychological effect on patients.

The single-room environment
Walls and floors are not usually thought to be significant sources of nosocomial infection and thus regular cleaning with hot water and detergent of floors and surfaces is all that is usually required. However, there are incidences where the patient may be colonized with a particularly virulent or resistant organism which may contaminate the local

environment and lead to the acquisition of organisms by healthcare workers entering the room. Examples of this are patients who are colonized with vancomycin-resistant enterococci, or patients with *Clostridium difficile* diarrhoea. In these situations, it may be of benefit to perform daily rigorous cleaning of surfaces where healthcare workers have prolonged contact such as door handles and stethoscopes which are kept in the patient's room. Rooms should always be cleaned after they are vacated and before a new patient enters. Taps and sinks can become heavily colonized with environmental pseudomonads and thus should be regularly cleaned. Potted or cut plants should be discouraged since they are a potential source of bacterial or fungal spores and stagnant water can be a potential reservoir for *Pseudomonas* spp.

Low-microbial diet

Since water and food provide a ready source of exogenous microbes, it is essential that a low-microbial diet is provided for patients undergoing gut prophylaxis. Although it is possible to provide totally sterile food by irradiation, this may make food unpalatable. However, with more recent techniques, this problem may be overcome [41]. Since good nutrition is of paramount importance for these patients in their recovery, the aim is to provide the patient with a diet which is as attractive and palatable as possible [42], so as to avoid the significant risks associated with hyperalimentation or parenteral feeding.

As water is a recognized source of environmental pseudomonads and *Acinetobacter* spp., the quality of drinking water should be closely monitored, and sterile or boiled water used whenever possible. Fresh, good-quality food should be brought to the patient for consumption as soon as possible after preparation. Cook–chill or microwave methods of cooking are probably not suitable for the neutropenic patient and dry foods are particularly unsuitable for such preparation [43]. Only pasteurized milk or fruit juices should be used for the neutropenic patient and these should be discarded within 24 hours of opening. Since peppers and spices can be a potential source of bacteria and bacterial and fungal spores, these should also be irradiated [44] or avoided. Nuts, raw vegetables and salads, and raw unpeeled fruit should not be given. Bread should again be as fresh as possible.

Immunotherapy
Passive immunotherapy

This has involved the use of intravenous immunoglobulin to prevent and treat infections in bone-marrow transplant patients. In theory, intravenous immunoglobulin corrects immunoglobulin deficiencies as well as increasing the potential for opisinization and anti-endotoxin and virus neutralization. It may also augment activation of the complement system and immunoregulatory functions which may modify immune thrombocytopenia [45]. Theoretically, it may also be immunosuppressive by its interaction with host cytokines. There are many immunoglobulin preparations available, including standard, hyperimmune or monoclonal products. Most studies show no influence of immunoglobulins on the incidence of bacterial sepsis in bone-marrow transplant patients, but small studies have shown an influence on the number of septicaemia episodes [46] and also suggested a reduced incidence of Gram-negative infections in patients receiving immunoglobulin [47]. However, this does not alter the overall survival of patients. There was great interest in the use of human monoclonal anti-endotoxin antibodies in the treatment of Gram-negative bacteraemia but the effectiveness of this has now been questioned. Since the cost-effectiveness of intravenous immunoglobulin as therapy in chronic lymphocytic leukaemia has not been demonstrated [48], there is no clearly defined role for the use of polyclonal or monoclonal antibacterial antibodies in patients with neutropenia [49].

Active immunization

A number of antibacterial vaccines have been developed. However, the immunocompromised bone-marrow transplant patient does not mount an adequate response to them, which was demonstrated by an unsuccessful vaccine for *Pseudomonas aeruginosa* [50]. Although there is a similar response to the polysaccharide-based vaccines for *Pneumococcus* and *Haemophilus influenza*, limited protection may still be provided [51] and immunization is recommended. Further details are provided in Chapter 48 concerning immunization issues.

Adoptive transfer of antibody responses

This concerns immunity to specific pathogens being achieved by vaccination of the donor prior to transplant. Higher levels of specific antibody can also be achieved by vaccinating both donor and recipient [52]. The effectiveness of this technique has been demonstrated in the production of the IgG$_2$ subclass in bone-marrow transplant patients where both donor and recipient were immunized with carbohydrates from *Pseudomonas aeruginosa* one week before transplant [53]. This allows the potential for immunization protocols against a number of bacteria.

Immunomodulating agents

Recently, there has been much interest in reducing the length and severity of neutropenia in bone-marrow transplant recipients, which would theoretically reduce the severity and incidence of infection in the neutropenic phase of bone-marrow transplantation. The interest has been centred on the recombinant cytokines, granulocyte colony-stimulating factor (G-CSF) [54] and granulocyte–macrophage colony-stimulating factor (GM-CSF) [55]. In separate studies, both agents have been found to reduce the period of neutropenia: G-CSF was shown to decrease the number of documented infections [54] and GM-CSF to reduce the number of febrile days [56]. They act by stimulating granulocyte recovery. Studies have suggested that G-CSF may enhance the activity of neutrophils against bacteria [57] and fungi [58]. Such agents have been shown to be safe and well tolerated, but they do add to the overall cost of care. Further work is currently needed to evaluate the possible use of other cytokines in neutropenic patients.

Special considerations about fungal-infection prophylaxis

Patients with prolonged neutropenia who have received broad-spectrum antibiotics are at particular risk from infection with *Candida* and *Aspergillus* species. For a number of years, oral polyenes such as nystatin and amphotericin lozenges have been used for prophylaxis against *Candida* infections in neutropenic patients. This approach has met with reasonable success. However, these agents are poorly tolerated by patients and this may lead to reduced compliance. In more recent years, the newer triazoles such as fluconazole have been advocated for use in fungal prophylaxis. Studies with fluconazole have shown that it is effective in reducing the incidence of superficial fungal infections such as occur with mucositis [59] and it has been shown to be superior to the oral polyenes [60]. The study conducted by Goodman *et al.* used 400 mg/day fluconazole as prophylaxis and they showed this to be clinically effective in reducing systemic fungal sepsis [61]. A major concern with their use is, however, the theoretical selection of more resistant types of *Candida* such as *Candida krusei*, which are intrinsically resistant to fluconazole. Indeed, studies have shown that there was a higher incidence of *C. krusei* infections in patients who had received fluconazole prophylaxis than those who had not [62,63]. However, with the general reduction in other non-*krusei Candida* species causing infection, the benefits seem to outweigh the disadvantages. Using high-dose fluconazole is expensive and for this reason many units use lower doses of fluconazole for prophylaxis [64]. To date, there is no consensus concerning the ideal, cost-effective dose for use in this situation.

Aspergillus infection is a particular problem in patients with prolonged neutropenia. Since it is acquired by inhalation of *Aspergillus conidia* into the sinuses and lungs, a filtered air supply is essential in units where the risk or incidence of this pathogen is high. However, the use of antifungal prophylaxis for *Aspergillus* is quite contentious. Low-dose amphotericin at 30 mg three times a week does not seem to prevent pulmonary aspergillosis in neutropenic patients [65], although one study showed effectiveness with a higher dose of amphotericin given to patients with a previous history of pulmonary *Aspergillus* infection [66]. However, its routine use should probably be discouraged since amphotericin is associated with significant nephrotoxicity.

The use of topical amphotericin either as a nebulized aerosol [67] or intranasal spray [68] has been investigated, with some studies showing success [69] and others failure [70]. It is often difficult to interpret these studies since most of the time they use historical controls. More definitive studies are needed to determine the efficacy of topical therapy. Further consideration about the use of prophylactic amphotericin is merited in the light of increasing evidence for amphotericin resistance in *Candida* species [71–73]. However, it may be of use in units where air filtration is not available.

The use of itraconozole as prophylaxis against *Aspergillus* if of great interest since this triazole has activity against this fungus, but there are few published data about its prophylactic use [74,75]. Disadvantages for general fungal prophylaxis are its poor activity against *Candida parapsilosis* and *Torulopsis glabrata*, its unpredictable oral bioavailability and possible toxic interactions with cyclosporin. Some of these problems may be overcome by the new oral form which seems to have a greater bioavailability.

References

1. Ranson MR, Oppenheim BA, Jackson A, Kamthon AG and Scarffe JH. Double-blind placebo controlled trial of vancomycin prophylaxis for central venous catheter insertion in cancer patients. *J Hosp Infect* 1990, **15**: 95–102.
2. Schimpff SC, Young VM, Greene WH *et al*. Origin of infection in acute non-lymphocytic leukaemia. Significance of hospital acquisition of potential pathogens. *Ann Intern Med* 1972; **77**: 707–714.
3. Claesner HA, Vollaard EJ and van Saene HK. Long-term prophylaxis of infections by selective decontamination in leucopenia and in mechanical ventilation. *Rev Infect Dis* 1987; **9**: 295–328.
4. Levine AS, Siegel SE, Schreiber AD *et al*. Protected environments and prophylactic antibiotics – a prospective controlled study of their utility in the therapy of acute leukaemia. *New Engl J Med* 1973; **288**: 477–483.
5. Schimpff SC, Greene WH, Young VM, Fortner CL, Jipsen L, Block JB and Wiernek PH. Laminar air flow room reverse isolation with oral non-absorbable antibiotic prophylaxis. *Ann Intern Med* 1975; **82**: 351–358.
6. Pizzo PA, Robichaud KJ, Edward BK, Schumaker C, Kramer BS and Johnson A. Oral antibiotic prophylaxis in patients with cancer: a double-blind, randomised, placebo-controlled study. *J Paed* 1983; **102**: 125–133.
7. Vollaard EJ, Claesner HA and Janssen AJHM. The contribution of Escherichia coli to microbial colonisation resistance. *J Antimicrob Chemother* 1990; **26**: 411–418.
8. EORTC International Antimicrobial Therapy Project Group. Trimethoprim-sulphamethoxazole in the prevention of infection in neutropenic patients. *J Infect Dis* 1984; **150**: 372–379.
9. Watson JG, Jamieson B, Powles RC *et al*. Co-trimoxazole versus non-absorbable antibiotics in acute leukaemia. *Lancet* 1982; **1**: 6–9.
10. Verhoef J, Rosenberg-Arsaka M and Dekker A. Prevention of infection in the neutropenic patient. *Rev Infect Dis* 1989; **11**: S1545–S1550.
11. Arning M, Wolf HH, Aul C, Heyll A, Scharf RE and Schneider WV. Infection prophylaxis in neutropenic patients with acute leukaemia: a randomised, controlled study with ofloxacin, ciprofloxacin and co-trimoxazole/colistin. *J Antimicrob Chemother* 1990; **26**: S137–S142.
12. Winston DJ, Ho WG, Druckner DA, Gale RP and Champlin RE. Ofloxacin versus vancomycin/polymyxin for prevention of infections in granulocytopenic patients. *Am J Med* 1990; **88**: 36–42.
13. Llang RHS, Ying RWH, Chum T-K, Cheu P-Y, Lam WA, So S-Y and Todd D. Ofloxacin versus co-trimoxazole for prevention of infection in neutropenic patients following cytotoxic chemotherapy. *Antimicrob Agents Chemother* 1990; **34**: 215–218.
14. Kern W and Kubble E. Ofloxacin versus trimethoprim-sulphamethoxazole for prevention of infection in patients with acute leukaemia and granulocytopenia. *Infection* 1991; **19**: 73–80.
15. Bow EJ, Rayner E and Louie TJ. Comparison of norfloxacin with co-trimoxazole for infection prophylaxis in acute leukaemia. *Am J Med* 1989; **84**: 847–854.
16. The GIMEMA Infection Programme. Prevention of bacterial infection in neutropenic patients with haematological malignancies. A randomised, multi-centre trial comparing norfloxacin with ciprofloxacin. *Ann Intern Med* 1991; **115**: 7–12.
17. Meunier F. Prevention of infection in neutropenic patients with perfloxacin. *J Antimicrob Chemother* 1990; **26**: S69–S73.
18. Kern W, Kurrle E and Scheiser T. Streptococcal bacteraemia in adult patients with leukemia under-going aggressive chemotherapy: a review of 55 cases. *Infection* 1990; **18**: 138–145.
19. Rosenberg-Arsaka M, Dekker A, Verdonck L and Verhoef J. Prevention of bacteraemia caused by alpha-haemolytic streptococci by roxithromycin (RU-28965) in granulocytopenic patients receiving ciprofloxacin. *Infection* 1989; **17**: 240–244.
20. Guiot HFL, Peters WG, van der Broek PJ, van der Meer JWM, Kramps JA, Willemze R and van Furth R. Respiratory failure elicited by streptococcal septicaemia in patients with cytosine arabinoside, and its prevention by penicillin. *Infect* 1990; **18**: 131–137.
21. Kotilaimen P, Nikoskelainen J and Huovinen P. Emergence of ciprofloxacin-resistant coagulase-negative staphylococcal skin flora in immunocompromised patients receiving ciprofloxacin. *J Infect Dis* 1990; **161**: 41–44.
22. Durand-Gasselin B, Leclereq R, Girard-Pipau F *et al*. Evolution of bacterial susceptibility to antibiotics during a six-year period in a haematology unit. *J Hosp Infect* 1995; **29**: 19–33.
23. Carratala J, Sevilla AF, Tubau F, Callis M and Guidol F. Emergence of quinolone-resistant E. coli bacteraemia in neutropenic patients with cancer who have received prophylactic norfloxacin. *Clin Infect Dis* 1995; **20**: 557–560.
24. Kern W, Andriof E, Oethinger M, Kern P, Hacker J and Marre R. Emergence of quinolone-resistant E. coli at a cancer centre. *Antimicrob Agents Chemother* 1994; **38**: 681–687.
25. Cometta A, Calandra T, Bille J, Galazzo M, Giddey M and Glauser MP. Fluoroquinolone resistant E. coli bacteraemias in neutropenic cancer patients. *Proceedings of the 8th IHS Symposium, Davos, June 23–26 1994* (Abstr 84).
26. Aucouturier P, Barra A, Intrator L *et al*. Long lasting IgG subclass and antibacterial polysaccharide antibody deficiency after allogenic bone marrow transplantation. *Blood* 1987; **70**: 779–795.

27. Winston DJ, Schiffman G, Wang DC et al. Pneumococcal infections after human bone marrow transplantation. *Ann Intern Med* 1979; **91**: 835–841.
28. Barrett DJ and Ayoub EM. IgG$_2$ subclass restriction of antibody to pneumococcal polysaccharides. *Clin Exp Immunol* 1986; **63**: 127–134.
29. Kahls P, Panzer S, Kletter K et al. Functional asplenia after bone marrow transplantation: a late complication related to extensive chronic graft-versus-host disease. *Ann Intern Med* 1988; **109**: 461–464.
30. Working Party of the British Committee for Standards in Haematology Clinical Haematology Task Force. Guidelines for the prevention and treatment of infection in patients with an absent or dysfunctional spleen. *Br Med J* 1996; **312**: 430–434.
31. Neuseef WM and Maki DG. A study of the value of simple protective isolation in patients with granulocytopenia. *New Engl J Med* 1981; **304**: 448–453.
32. Russell JA, Poun M-C, Janes AR, Woodman RC and Ruether BA. Allogenic bone marrow transplantation without protective isolation in adults with malignant disease. *Lancet* 1992; **339**: 38–40.
33. Arnow PM, Anderson RL, Mainos PD and Smith EJ. Pulmonary aspergillosis during hospital renovation. *Am Rev Resp Dis* 1978; **118**: 49–53.
34. Opal SM, Asp AA, Cunnady PB, Morse PL, Burton LJ and Hanmer PG. Efficacy of infection control measures during an outbreak of disseminated aspergillosis associated with hospital construction. *J Infect Dis* 1986; **153**: 634–637.
35. Rogers TR and Barnes RA. Prevention in airborne fungal infections in immunocompromised patients. *J Hosp Infect* 1988; **11**(Suppl A): 515–520.
36. Rhame FS, Streifel AJ, Kersey JH and McGlare PB. Extrinsic risk factors for pneumonia in the patient at high risk of infection. *Am J Med* 1984; **76**: 45–52.
37. Buckner CD, Clift RA, Sanders JE, Meyers JD, Counts GW, Farwell VT and Thomas ED. Protective environment for marrow transplant recipients. *Ann Intern Med* 1978; **89**: 893–901.
38. Watson JG, Rogers TR, Selwyn S and Smith RG. Evaluation of Vickers-Trexlar isolation in children undergoing bone marrow transplantation. *Arch Dis Child* 1997; **52**: 563–568.
39. Petersen FB, Buckner CD, Clift RA, Nelson W, Counts GW, Meyers JD and Thomas ED. Infectious complications in patients undergoing marrow transplantation: a prospective randomised study of the additional effect of decontamination and laminar air flow isolation among patients receiving prophylactic systemic antibiotics. *Scand J Infect Dis* 1987; **19**: 559–567.
40. Barnes RA and Rogers TR. Control of an outbreak of nosocomial aspergillosis by laminar airflow isolation. *J Hosp Infect* 1989; **14**: 89–94.
41. Pryke DC and Taylor PR. The use of irradiated food for immunosuppressed hospital patients in the United Kingdom. *J Human Nutr Diet* 1995; **8**: 411–416.
42. Pattison AJ. Review of current practice in 'clean' diets in the UK. *J Human Nutr Diet* 1993; **6**: 3–11.
43. Vela CR and Wu JF. Mechanism of lethal action of 2450 MHz radiation on micro-organisms. *Appl Environ Microbiol* 1979; **37**: 550–553.
44. MAFF press release 12 June 1991. First Licence Issued to Irradiate Spices and Condiments (London: MAFF).
45. Sullivan KM. Immunoglobulin therapy in bone marrow transplantation. *Am J Med* 1987; **83**(Suppl 4A): S34–45.
46. Peterson FB, Bowden RA, Thornquist M et al. The effect of prophylactic intravenous immune globulin on the incidence of septicaemia in marrow transplant recipients. *Bone Marrow Transplant* 1987; **2**: 141–148.
47. Sullivan K, Kopecky K, Jocom J et al. Immunomodulatory and antimicrobial efficiency of intravenous immunoglobulin in bone marrow transplantation. *New Engl J Med* 1990; **323**: 705–712.
48. Weeks JC, Tierney MR and Weinstein MC. Cost effectiveness of prophylactic intravenous immune globulin in chronic lymphocytic leukaemia. *New Engl J Med* 1991; **325**: 81–86.
49. Dwyer JM. Manipulating the immune system with immune globulin. *New Engl J Med* 1992; **326**: 107–116.
50. Young LS, Meyer RD and Armstrong D. *Pseudomonas aeruginosa* vaccine in cancer patients. *Ann Intern Med* 1973; **79**: 518–527.
51. Winston DJ, Ho WG, Schiffman G, Champlin RE, Feig SA and Gale RP. Pneumococcal vaccination of recipients of bone marrow transplants. *Arch Intern Med* 1983; **143**: 1735–1737.
52. Wimperis JZ, Gottlieb DJ, Duncombe AS, Heslop HE, Prentice HG and Brenner MK. Requirements for the adoptive transfer of antibody responses to a priming antigen in man. *J Immunol* 1990; **144**: 541–547.
53. Gottlieb DJ, Cryz SJ, Furer E, Que JU, Prentice HG, Duncombe AS and Brenner MK. Immunity against *Pseudomonas aeruginosa* adoptively transferred to bone marrow transplant recipients. *Blood* 1990; **76**: 2470–2475.
54. Onno R, Tomonaga M, Kobayashi T et al. Effect of granulocyte colony-stimulating factor and intensive induction therapy in relapsed or refractory acute leukaemia. *New Engl J Med* 1990; **323**: 871–877.
55. Ruff C and Coleman DL. Granulocyte–macrophage colony-stimulating factor pleiotropic cytokine with potential clinical usefulness. *Rev Infect Dis* 1990; **21**: 41–62.
56. Hermann F, Schultz G, Wieser M, Kolbe K, Nicolay U, Noauk M, Lindemann A and Mertelsmann R. Effect of granulocyte–macrophage colony-stimulating factor on neutropenic and related morbidity induced by myelotoxic chemotherapy. *Am J Med* 1990; **86**: 619–624.
57. Roilides E, Walsh TJ, Pizzo PA and Rubin M. Granulocyte colony-stimulating factor enhances the phagocytic and bactericidal activity of normal and defective human neutrophils. *J Infect Dis* 1991; **63**: 579–583.
58. Roilides E, Uhlig K, Venzon D, Pizzo PA and Walsh TJ. Neutrophil oxidative burst in response to blastoconidia and pseudohyphae of *Candida albicans*: augmentation by granulocyte colony-stimulating factor and interferon-gamma. *J Infect Dis* 1992; **166**: 668–673.
59. Samonis G, Ralston K, Karl C, Miller P and Bodey GP. Prophylaxis of oropharyngeal candidiasis with fluconazole. *Rev Infect Dis* 1990; **12**: S369–S373.
60. Walsh TJ, Aoki S, Mechinaud F, Bacher J, Lee J, Rubin M and Pizzo PA. Preventative, early and late anti-fungal chemotherapy with fluconazole in different granulocytopenic models of experimental disseminated candidiasis. *J Infect Dis* 1990; **161**: 755–760.
61. Goodman JL, Winston DJ, Greenfield RA et al. A controlled trial of fluconazole to prevent fungal infections in patients

undergoing bone marrow transplantation. *New Engl J Med* 1992; **326**: 845–851.

62. Wingard JR, Merz WG, Rinaldi MG, Johnson TR, Karp JE and Saral R. Association of *Torulopsis glabrata* infections with fluconazole prophylaxis in neutropenic bone marrow transplant patients. *Antimicrob Agents Chemother* 1993; **37**: 1847–1849.

63. Wingard JR, Merz WG, Rinaldi MG, Johnson TR, Karp JE and Saral R. Increase in *Candida krusei* among patients with bone marrow transplantation and neutropenia treated with fluconazole. *New Engl J Med* 1991; **325**: 1274–1277.

64. Wakerly L, Craig A-M, Malek M *et al*. Fluconazole versus oral polyenes in the prophylaxis of immunocompromised patients: a cost-minimisation analysis. *J Hosp Infect* 1996; **33**: 35–48.

65. Bodey GP and Anaissie EJ. Fluconazole versus intravenous amphotericin B for anti-fungal prophylaxis in leukaemic patients. *Proceedings of the 17th International Congress of Chemotherapy, International Society for Chemotherapy, 1991*.

66. Karp JE, Burch PA and Merz WG. An approach to intensive anti-leukaemia therapy in patients with previous invasive aspergillosis. *Am J Med* 1988; **85**: 203.

67. Connewlly E, Cafferkey MT, Daley PA, Keane CT and McCann SR. Nebulised amphotericin B as prophylaxis against invasive aspergillosis in granulocytopenic patients. *Bone Marrow Transplant* 1990; **5**: 403–406.

68. Meunier-Carpenter F, Schoek R, Guerin G, Muller C and Klastersky J. Amphotericin B nasal spray as prophylaxis against invasive aspergillosis in granulocytopenic patients. *New Engl J Med* 1988; **311**: 1056.

69. Jeffrey GM, Beard MEJ, Ibram RB *et al*. Intranasal amphotericin B reduces the frequency of invasive aspergillosis in neutropenic patients. *Am J Med* 1991; **90**: 85–92.

70. Jorgensen CJ, Dreyfus F, Vaixeler J *et al*. Failure of amphotericin B spray to prevent aspergillosis in neutropenic patients. *Nouv Rev Fr Hematol* 1989; **31**: 327–328.

71. Guinet R, Chanas J, Goullier A, Bonnefoy G and Ambriose-Thomas P. Fatal septicaemia due to amphotericin B-resistant *Candida lusitaniae*. *J Clin Microbiol* 1983; **18**: 443–444.

72. Powderly WG, Kobayashi GS, Herzig GP and Medoff G. Amphotericin B-resistant yeast infection in severely immunocompromised patients. *Am J Med* 1988; **84**: 826–832.

73. Merz WG and Sanford GR. Isolation and characterisation of a polyene-resistant variant of *Candida tropicalis*. *J Clin Microbiol* 1979; **9**: 677–680.

74. Todeschini L. Oral itraconazole plus intranasal amphotericin B in prevention of invasive aspergillosis. *Eur J Clin Microbiol Infect Dis* 1993; **4**: 211.

75. Krcmery Jnr V. Emerging fungal infections in cancer patients. *J Hosp Infect* 1996; **33**: 109–117.

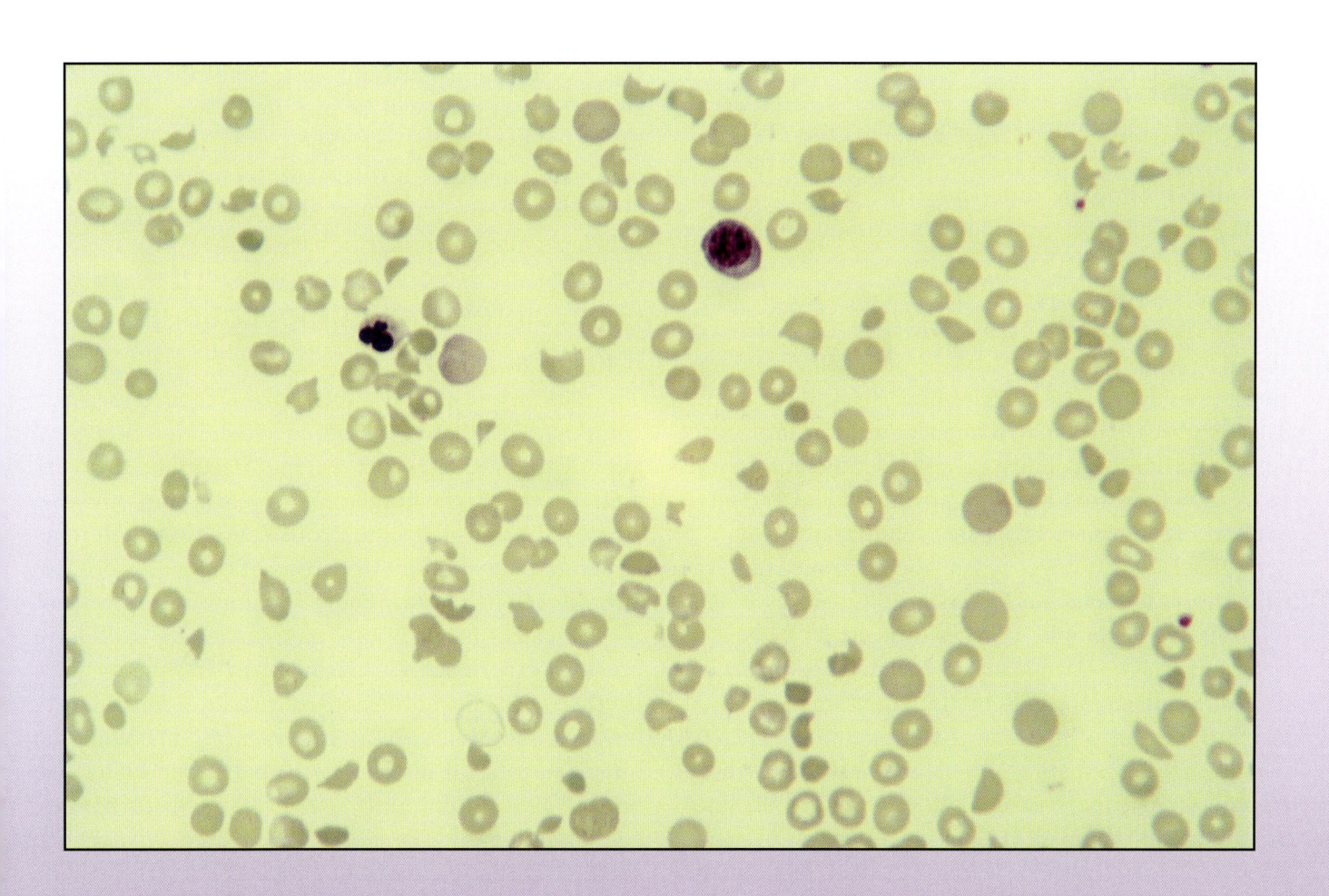

Chapter 50

Complications in the early post-transplant period

Nicola J. Philpott and Edward J. Kanfer

Introduction

A substantial amount of the morbidity and mortality associated with the procedure occurs during the first 100 days following bone-marrow transplantation (BMT), particularly an allograft. Although there is wide variation between centres, due largely to differences in the patient populations studied, most reports estimate an early mortality incidence of 20–30% [1–3] and 1–20% [4–7] after allogeneic and autologous BMT respectively; underlying disease and disease status particularly impact on mortality post-autograft. The possibility of a fatal outcome in the short term following BMT for any individual patient is particularly pertinent given that many transplants are performed at a stage when the average survival expectation without BMT may be considerably longer than this (for example, in cases of acute leukaemia in first remission or chronic myeloid leukaemia in chronic phase). Similarly, BMT is becoming increasingly used in the treatment of non-malignant conditions, such as the haemoglobinopathies, in which survival without transplant may be measured in decades [8,9]. Since outcome following BMT in such cases may be improved if it is performed early in the course of the disorder, prior to the development of significant organ damage, patient selection and pre-BMT counselling are of great importance.

Consideration of the above shapes the practice of BMT in two respects. Firstly, the decision to undertake BMT in a particular case and when best to perform this must be carefully considered. Secondly, during the immediate post-BMT period, the patient will be dependent on a high level of medical and nursing care, akin to management on an intensive care unit. Frequent monitoring in order to detect potential complications and institute appropriate therapy is necessary to limit early morbidity and mortality. BMT should only be performed in centres with the appropriate medical and nursing personnel and investigative facilities [10]. In summary, a high level of commitment is necessary for the patient not to perish from a preventable cause.

This chapter will concentrate on early complications with particular reference to prevention (where possible), diagnostic methods and therapeutic options. Both graft-versus-host disease (GvHD) and specific infections are subjects dealt with in detail elsewhere but they will be mentioned here where they have diagnostic relevance. Generally, such complications are not specific to the underlying disease; where particular diseases bring certain problems, these will be emphasized.

Gastrointestinal complications

Nausea and vomiting

The majority of patients suffer significant nausea and vomiting during the cytoreductive conditioning period [11]. The aetiology may be multifactorial; the very high doses of chemotherapy or chemoradiotherapy employed are usually the major cause, but there may be some contribution from the oral non-absorbable antimicrobials commonly administered prophylactically. In addition, many patients will have previous experience of chemotherapy and the memory of this may be sufficient to produce anticipatory physical symptoms [12]. In practice, this vomiting often causes great distress to the patient and may also result in fluid and electrolyte disturbances, compounding those caused by the cytoreductive regime itself. For these reasons, prophylactic anti-emetic therapy is an absolute requirement before embarking on conditioning therapy. It is good practice to individualize a schedule for each patient as far as is possible; there may be certain medications which have worked well in the past, or conversely, which have produced severe side-effects, for example an oculogyric crisis in a patient given high doses of metoclopramide.

There are many drugs which have been employed for this purpose and each centre will have its particular preferences. Single-agent prophylaxis is often ineffective and it is quite reasonable to choose a schedule comprising two, or sometimes more, drugs. Many centres use a regimen comprising a 5-HT$_3$ antagonist, such as ondansetron or granisetron [13–16], in combination with dexamathasone and/or lorazepam. It is important to note that some agents used in conditioning can cause delayed emesis, for example the platinum drugs used in high-dose therapy for a variety of solid tumours. In these cases, the duration of anti-emetic therapy may need to be increased appropriately.

Mucositis, oesophagitis and gastroduodenitis

A predictable effect of the high-dose conditioning therapy is the occurrence of widespread gastrointestinal mucosal damage. As with many of the other early complications, the severity of this is closely related to intensity of the treatment administered and may, for example, be a particular problem following busulphan, melphalan or total body irradiation (TBI) when used at maximal dosage or in combination. Oropharyngeal mucositis of moderate or greater severity usually begins during the initial 10 days post-conditioning and may last for 14 days before gradually subsiding. It causes substantial discomfort and, in addition, inevitably limits nutritional intake. It should be noted that methotrexate (used for GvHD prophylaxis) may increase the mucositis experienced.

The management of this complication has several aims. Firstly, adequate analgesia is mandatory and this often requires the temporary use of liberal quantities of parenteral opiate drugs. Secondly, the necessity for total parenteral nutrition (TPN) should be assessed early and in most cases will probably be required. Some centres institute TPN prophylactically in all patients and the use of nasogastric feeding for this purpose is being studied in some centres. Thirdly, oral infections should be sought since these may simulate chemoradiotherapy-induced mucositis or at least aggravate this complication. These include candidiasis and particularly herpes simplex virus (HSV), the mucosal ulceration of which may be indistinguishable from that arising secondary to conditioning therapy toxicity. Again, most centres administer prophylactic oral antifungal agents and acyclovir in anticipation of the above. Finally, the use of prophylactic local preparations such as chlorhexidine mouthrinse may modify the severity of mucositis and the propensity towards subsequent systemic infection [17], although this has not been a universal finding [18]. Analgesic/anaesthetic mouthwashes containing benzocaine or cocaine are also frequently used.

As in the case of the oral mucosa, retrosternal and epigastric symptoms, which may include pain, nausea, vomiting and bleeding, during or soon after the conditioning therapy usually reflect mucosal toxicity. H_2-antagonists or proton pump inhibitors are widely used to limit acid production. There are several possible aetiologies for such symptoms occurring later in the post-BMT course which may require specific treatment, including infection (especially candidiasis, HSV and cytomegalovirus (CMV)) and GvHD. Endoscopy is the most useful investigation since this allows direct visualization and biopsy for microbiological and histological diagnosis.

Overt gastrointestinal haemorrhage is uncommon post-BMT. Kaur *et al.* reported an incidence of 7.5%, with a mean onset of eight days post-BMT (range 0–45 days) [19]. The most common cause was widespread oesophagitis and gastritis.

Diarrhoea and typhlitis

Diarrhoea is a common early symptom following conditioning therapy and as such is usually a direct toxic effect of the chemoradiotherapy. Symptomatic preparations are often of benefit and this problem is short-lived in the majority of cases. Much more serious is the development of typhlitis (neutropenic enterocolitis) which occurs, fortunately, in only a very small percentage of patients but carries with it a substantial mortality. It usually occurs within the initial two weeks' post-BMT and presents with fever, abdominal pain and tenderness. Diarrhoea is usual and the patient may become rapidly shocked due to dehydration, intestinal perforation, blood loss and concomitant septicaemia. A plain abdominal X-ray may show a right-sided soft-tissue density due to caecal dilatation. Endoscopy will reveal multiple ulcerated lesions with necrosis and haemorrhage. The exact cause of this complication is unknown but it is thought to be due to a combination of cytotoxic mucosal toxicity, neutropenia and infection. Several infectious agents have been implicated including bacteria, viruses and fungi and it is possible that the simultaneous invasion by a number of organisms is an important factor in this clinical setting. Management should be supportive in the first instance. It is quite common for bacteria to be isolated from blood cultures and this will direct further antibiotic therapy. The patient should be seen initially and then frequently reviewed by a surgeon, since operative intervention may prove life-saving in the event of severe bleeding or intestinal perforation [20].

A very similar clinical picture to the above may be produced by pseudomembranous colitis in association with preceding broad-spectrum antibiotics, although the endoscopic and histological appearances together with

Clostridium difficile isolation and toxin assay will provide the correct diagnosis. Treatment is with oral vancomycin, metronidazole being an effective alternative.

Diarrhoea can be a manifestation of acute GvHD; the appearance of the diarrhoea may be suggestive since it is commonly a green colour, of watery consistency and there may be strands of epithelial cells visible. Contrast radiography may demonstrate several abnormalities but these are not pathognomic [21], and consequently endoscopic examination is the most informative investigation. In addition to providing biopsy material, this may also allow the isolation of infectious organisms, although the coexistence of infection with intestinal GvHD is well recognized.

Pancreatitis and cholecystitis

Pancreatitis is an uncommon complication after BMT, with a reported incidence of less than 5% [22,23]. The aetiology is likely to be multifactorial, including infection, conditioning toxicity, drug toxicity, lipids (in TPN) and perhaps GvHD. Gall-bladder 'sludge' is frequently noted on ultrasound examination in BMT patients [24] and may contribute to the development of pancreatitis and cholecystitis. CMV-induced pancreatitis is rare and generally occurs later in the post-BMT course; other viral causes include adenovirus and varicella-zoster. Pancreatitis should be included in the differential diagnosis of abdominal pain post-transplant. Management is conservative with gut rest, TPN, analgesia, strict fluid balance and glucose monitoring.

Kuttah *et al.* reported cholecystitis in 5 of 35 patients undergoing autologous BMT for acute myeloid leukaemia. All were conditioned with busulphan and cyclophosphamide, and review of patients conditioned with other regimens suggested that a busulphan and cyclophosphamide regimen may predispose to this complication [25].

Hepatic veno-occlusive disease

Hepatic veno-occlusive disease (VOD) is a cause of significant morbidity and mortality following BMT, for which reason it will be considered in detail. VOD produces a clinical syndrome of icterus, tender hepatomegaly and fluid retention. The condition may be fatal and should be considered one of the dose-limiting side-effects of BMT-conditioning regimens.

Clinical features

The classical features of VOD are jaundice, hepatomegaly, weight gain, ascites and right upper quadrant/epigastric pain. Clinical criteria for the diagnosis of VOD have been established by groups from Seattle and Baltimore (see Table 50.1) [26,27].

The signs of more severe disease may include renal failure (hepatorenal syndrome), thrombocytopenia unresponsive to platelet transfusions [28] and hepatic encephalopathy. The timing of these features may be helpful in reaching the diagnosis [29]; although in rare cases VOD can precede the infusion of bone marrow or peripheral blood stem cells, jaundice and weight gain tend to occur within the first 10 days and precede other signs, including clinically apparent ascites, abdominal pain and mental confusion, by several days. The initial rise in hepatic enzymes is often only moderate and evidently out of proportion to the degree of jaundice. It should be noted that the abdominal pain may arise quite suddenly and thus mimic an acute abdominal emergency.

As many as 50% of patients undergoing BMT develop VOD of varying severity; however, there is wide intercentre variation in reported incidence. Some of this disparity may be due to differences in both the intensity of conditioning therapy and the patient populations being transplanted, and in addition it can be assumed that the criteria by which the diagnosis is reached, particularly that of mild VOD, are an

Table 50.1 Diagnostic criteria for hepatic veno-occlusive disease

Seattle

Two of following three within first 20 days post-BMT:
  Jaundice
  Painful hepatomegaly
  Fluid retention

Baltimore

Jaundice (bilirubin >34 mmol/litre) and two of following three:
  Hepatomegaly (usually painful)
  Ascites
  Weight gain >5%.

important variable between centres. However, it is a reasonable generalization that approximately 5% of patients undergoing allogeneic BMT experience life-threatening VOD. The incidence of multi-organ failure increases with the severity of VOD, and adverse prognostic features include the development of renal failure, hepatic encephalopathy and profound jaundice. Only rarely will patients with a serum bilirubin in excess of 400 mmol/litre recover from this complication.

Pathogenesis

An extensive review of the pathogenesis of VOD is beyond the scope of this chapter but the subject has been treated in depth [30]. Briefly, one of the earliest lesions is believed to be endothelial damage related to BMT-conditioning therapy. This results in a local hypercoagulable state due to increased tissue factor production, with activation of the coagulation cascade and downregulation of the natural anticoagulant system via thrombomodulin [31,32]. Immunohistochemical studies have shown deposition of fibrinogen and factor VIII in vessel walls at the interface of the hepatic sinusoids and terminal venules, and levels of antithrombin III and protein C are reduced in VOD [33,34]. Occlusion due to collagen deposition follows [35,36].

While endothelial injury may be an initiating event in VOD, hepatocyte damage is also of importance; hepatocyte necrosis perhaps secondary to glutathione depletion has been reported [37]. Damage to endothelium can also initiate a 'cytokine storm'; the known effects of interleukin-1 (IL-1) and tumour necrosis factor (TNF) suggest a role in the pathogenesis of VOD, and their production by the reticuloendothelial system is known to be increased in response to cytoreductive therapy, irradiation and infection.

Aetiology

Veno-occlusive disease has been described following exposure to pyrrolizidine alkaloids [38,39], hepatic irradiation [36,40] and cytotoxic agents [41–43] and in this context it appears certain that the cause of VOD is the hepatotoxic effects of the very high-dose conditioning therapy for BMT [44,45]. The disease has been observed following single-agent [46–48] or multiple agent therapy [49,50]. In studies utilizing cyclophosphamide alone, busulphan with cyclophosphamide and cyclophosphamide with TBI, the incidence of VOD appeared increased with higher doses of TBI, and with the addition of busulphan to cyclophosphamide versus cyclophosphamide alone [26,51]. Although such data may be difficult to interpret because of the wide variation in incidence of VOD due to the use of different diagnostic criteria, many studies report that the incidence of VOD is increased by the use of the more intensive regimens [26,44,52]. Individual patient characteristics may be of importance; for example, studies have suggested that variation in the pharmacological handling of busulphan results in wide differences in drug exposure ('area under curve', AUC) for patients treated at the same dosage and that this correlates with the incidence of VOD. Dose adjustment on the basis of AUC can reduce the incidence of VOD [53,54].

Other significant predisposing factors include pre-existing biochemical evidence of hepatitis which imparts a threefold increase in the likelihood of VOD development [55], the commencement of conditioning while being treated for bacterial or viral infections [26] and allogeneic versus autologous BMT [26,56]. There is no evidence to suggest that this latter association is due to GvHD and it is more likely a consequence of the use of cyclosporin and/or methotrexate in the allogeneic population [56,57]. Previous irradiation of liver, liver metastases and receipt of second BMT all impart an increased risk of VOD [58–60]. Additional peritransplant factors may include administration of amphotericin B, and prolonged use of broad-spectrum antibiotics [61].

Diagnosis

There are several causes of hepatic dysfunction following BMT, some of which may mimic or coexist with VOD. Table 50.2 lists some of the common differential diagnoses. However, the constellation of symptoms and signs that comprise VOD, together with the timing of their onset, are relatively specific, and in one study these were 89% predictive of a histological confirmation of the clinical diagnosis [55].

The most reliable method of diagnosing of VOD is liver histology; however, the combined problems of platelet refractoriness and coagulopathy make percutaneous liver biopsy too hazardous in most cases. An alternative technique which may avoid this obstacle

Table 50.2 Differential diagnosis of hepatic veno-occlusive disease
Hyperacute hepatic GvHD
Drugs (azoles, co-trimoxazole, cyclosporin, methotrexate)
Viral hepatitis
Fungal infection
Septicaemia
Renal failure
Pericarditis
Heart failure

is a transjugular liver biopsy [62]. Two groups have reported experience of this technique, indicating that adequate specimens can be obtained, that the hepatic venous gradient can be measured (a useful diagnostic parameter in VOD), and that morbidity and mortality associated with the procedure are acceptable [63,64].

Doppler ultrasound examination may show hepatomegaly and reversed or dampened hepatoportal blood flow; experience with this technique suggests that it is relatively specific for the disorder [65]. However, one study failed to identify any ultrasonographic features characteristic of early VOD, when a sensitive and specific diagnostic test would be most valuable [66]. Ultrasound is also, of course, useful for detecting both ascites and intrahepatic abscesses.

Serological and other methods of virus detection should performed, although the clinical diseases they produce are only rarely confused with VOD. The same cannot be said for intrahepatic fungal infection which may be difficult to distinguish from VOD if this occurs soon after conditioning therapy.

Prevention

Patient selection provides little scope for preventing veno-occlusive disease. If circumstances make the decision difficult about whether to transplant a particular patient for other reasons, then the presence of abnormal liver function tests may sway the clinician towards more conservative therapy. Additionally, it may be possible in such cases to be flexible regarding conditioning therapy and avoid agents with a particular hepatotoxic propensity, such as busulphan or TBI. The prophylactic use of heparin to prevent VOD, prompted by a study in patients receiving autologous BMT [67], is employed in some centres. Other (also non-prospective non-randomized) studies have appeared to confirm these findings in allogeneic and autologous BMT recipients [68,69]. However, Bearman *et al.*, using heparin prophylaxis in a group of BMT recipients at high risk of VOD, emphasized the possible hazards of this therapy and also cast some doubt about whether heparin has significant preventative efficacy [70]. Two randomized studies have failed to clarify the issue [71,72].

Other prophylactic treatments which have been reported in VOD include: prostaglandin E_2 [73] which appeared to have some benefit but is toxic; ursodeoxycholic acid, which was well tolerated and produced significant reduction in incidence and death from VOD in a randomized prospective study [74,75]; and pentoxifylline, which proved ineffective [76,77].

Management

Supportive measures will be required with anything other than mild VOD. Special attention should be given to fluid balance, renal function, drug metabolism and coagulation status. Urinary sodium excretion is often impaired and sodium intake should be restricted; the maintenance of intravascular volume may be enhanced by the use of salt-poor albumin infusions. Renal function may be compromised by loop diuretics and it may be more beneficial to use a combination of dopamine (2 µg/kg/min by continuous infusion) with an aldosterone antagonist (e.g. spironolactone 200–400 mg/24 hours). Repeated paracenteses to remove ascites may be necessary to alleviate patient discomfort and also to maintain adequate respiratory function. The development of severe renal and/or hepatic failure require appropriate management which may include haemodialysis and general measures to combat hepatic encephalopathy. These patients are commonly receiving a multitude of drugs and it is important to scrutinize these in the context of renal and hepatic impairment. It should be noted here that cyclosporin A elimination can be delayed through hepatic dysfunction and consequently dosage may require careful adjustment [78]. Severely affected patients will often demonstrate bleeding due both to profound thrombocytopenia and coagulation factor deficiency; these will require replacement therapy although, as noted above, responses to platelet concentrate transfusions may be very poor due either to the VOD itself or coexistent multi-organ failure [27].

Specific therapy for established VOD has been unsatisfactory. There have been reports of the use of prostaglandin E_1 [79]; results are difficult to interpret and have not been confirmed by other investigators. Recombinant tissue plasminogen activator (tPA) has been used with an estimated response rate of 45% [80,81]; however, a randomized prospective study is required to confirm efficacy and to define haemorrhagic risk. Liver transplantation has been carried out successfully [82] but this is unlikely to be a therapeutic option in the majority of cases.

Table 50.3 Causes of pulmonary complications post-BMT

Infection
    Bacterial
    Viral
    Fungal
    Protozoal

Pulmonary oedema
    Fluid overload
    Cardiac dysfunction
    Acute respiratory distress syndrome (ARDS)
        sepsis
        drug toxicity (e.g. cyclosporin A and cytosine arabinoside)

Idiopathic (toxic)

Pulmonary embolism

Pulmonary GvHD

Interstitial pneumonitis

Numerically, pulmonary complications are the single most frequent cause of mortality in the early post-BMT period. Common presentations include dyspnoea and cough, with or without sputum production, hypoxia or fever, associated with localized or diffuse interstitial shadowing on a chest X-ray. A list of possible aetiologies is shown in Table 50.3.

Between 20 and 40% of patients develop interstitial pneumonitis post-BMT [83–85] and of these, up to 50% die of this complication. Infective causes of pneumonitis, which may concern as many as 50% of cases, are discussed in detail elsewhere, and here we will concentrate on the idiopathic variety, which accounts for up to one-third of cases in some series [85].

While the frequency of interstitial pneumonitis *per se* varies according to several factors including the relationship of the donor to patient, that of idiopathic interstitial pneumonitis (IIP) remains fairly constant at 5–10% after allogeneic, syngeneic and autologous BMT [86–89]. This implies that IIP is not related aetiologically to immune mechanisms. There is evidence to show that the incidence of IIP increases with the intensity of conditioning therapy [87] and consequently it appears almost certain that IIP is a result of direct toxicity from the preparative chemotherapy or chemoradiotherapy. There are several conditioning variables which could theoretically influence the frequency of IIP. These include the use, dosage and dose rate of TBI, and whether it is fractionated, whether lung shielding is utilized, the exact nature of the chemotherapy employed in terms of inherent pulmonary toxicity, and the use of methotrexate (and the precise regimen for this) for GvHD prophylaxis. However, there are conflicting reports about the influence of these factors and it is therefore difficult to reach concrete conclusions. Most studies suggest that fractionation of TBI is beneficial although whether complete avoidance of this therapy is the best strategy remains to be determined [89,90]. Patient-specific factors which may increase the risk of developing IIP include the presence of GvHD [91], pre-existing restrictive lung defects and abnormal diffusing capacity [89] and prior exposure to bleomycin [92].

The most common problem is to differentiate IIP from infective causes, pulmonary oedema or haemorrhage. In practice, the decisions relating to further investigations often arise after failure to respond clinically and radiologically to antibiotics and diuretics (if indicated). Bronchoscopy with bronchoalveolar lavage (BAL) has become the first-line investigation [93–95] and the diagnosis of IIP is one of exclusion, for those cases in which there is no evidence of infection, pulmonary oedema or haemorrhage. Late onset IIP in allogeneic BMT must be distinguished from pulmonary GvHD; usually open lung biopsy is required [96], but some centres also employ high-resolution computed tomography scan of the lungs to aid in diagnosis [97].

Therapy for established IIP is supportive in nature. Respiratory failure can be supported mechanically and the use of nitric oxide in this as in other forms of adult respiratory distress syndrome (ARDS) is attracting attention. Steroids are used by several centres although unequivocal evidence of benefit is lacking. The use of heart–lung transplantation in those with chronic pulmonary dysfunction is reported; however, many patients with IIP early after BMT are not suitable candidates for such a procedure.

Renal and urinary-tract complications

Acute renal failure
Incidence
Defining acute renal failure (ARF) as a doubling of the baseline serum creatinine, one study estimated the incidence of this complication post-BMT to be over 60% [98]. In another report, 40% of patients developed renal insufficiency, again defined as a doubling of baseline creatinine, and up to half of these required haemodialysis [99]; however, these data were collected early on in the use of cyclosporin and it is probable that this latter frequency of dialysis requirement does not reflect current experience.

A more recent study of 275 BMT recipients reported an incidence of ARF of 26%, 82% of which occurred within the first month post-BMT [100]. In most of these cases, the aetiology was felt to be multifactorial, but specific causes identified were nephrotoxic drug therapy (29%) and VOD (15%). ARF was significantly more common in allogeneic versus autologous BMT (36% versus 6.5%). There was no proven association with underlying disease, GvHD, sepsis, conditioning regime or sex. Development of ARF had important implications for long-term outcome; patients who developed ARF had a mortality of 45.8%, rising to 88% in those requiring dialysis. Ten-year survival in the ARF group was only 30% versus 53% in those with no renal impairment.

Aetiology
There are a multitude of factors post-BMT which may contribute to renal impairment (Table 50.4), although, as with hepatic VOD, problems with definition criteria result in the wide variation in reported incidence.

Volume depletion
Renal impairment due to actual or relative intravascular volume depletion is usually self-evident in the situations mentioned in Table 50.4; often the cause is multifactorial. Therapy should be designed to correct dehydration, anaemia, hypotension, hypoalbuminaemia, sepsis or shock as dictated by clinical circumstances.

Table 50.4 Causes of post-BMT acute renal failure

Pre-renal*
Vomiting (chemoradiotherapy or acute GvHD)
Diarrhoea (chemoradiotherapy or acute GvHD)
Bleeding, anaemia
Renal
Drugs
aminoglycosides
cyclosporin
amphotericin
cytotoxics, e.g. cisplatinum
Haemolytic uraemic syndrome/thrombotic thrombocytopenic purpura
Sepsis
Hepatorenal syndrome
Radiation nephritis
Post-renal
Haemorrhagic cystitis
Urate nephropathy
*Intravascular volume depletion (actual or relative).

Conditioning therapy
As in many early post-BMT complications, conditioning toxicity may play an important role in renal dysfunction post-BMT. The great majority of patients who undergo BMT do not receive cytotoxic drugs associated with significant renal toxicity, but in those whose therapy includes agents such as platinum compounds, mitomycin C and methotrexate, this complication is a possibility [101]. Acute radiation nephritis following TBI appears to be uncommon although this has been suggested as a cause of microangiopathic renal failure following BMT (see below). However, there is increasing evidence to suggest that radiation is critical in the development of late-onset renal failure. Histologically, renal biopsies from patients with late-onset renal failure are similar to those with a diagnosis of radiation nephritis. Miralbell *et al.* showed a dose-dependent increase in the incidence of late renal dysfunction (at 18 months post-allogeneic BMT) with increasing TBI dosage. There was also a 3.5-fold increase in renal impairment in the presence of GvHD. Based on these findings, renal shielding was recommended to limit the renal radiation dose to 10 Gy, particularly if GvHD risk was high, for example after unrelated donor or mismatched BMT [102]. In general, it may also appear sensible to shield the kidneys to reduce the risk of radiation nephritis if extra-abdominal irradiation is administered, for example, splenic irradiation in chronic myeloid leukaemia. In addition, animal data have suggested that radiation-induced renal damage may be ameliorated by the use of angiotensin-converting enzyme (ACE) inhibitors, such as captopril [103].

Drugs
There are several drugs commonly used in the early post-BMT period which are well-recognized to be associated with renal toxicity. Amphotericin B, aminoglycosides, vancomycin and, less frequently, acyclovir, may all cause renal impairment which usually responds to dose reduction. Unfortunately, it is common for patients to be receiving all of the above drugs in addition to cyclosporin A, which may explain the relative frequency of renal complications. The use of liposomal preparations of amphotericin may reduce the incidence of renal toxicity, but with considerable financial ramifications. Allopurinol is an uncommon cause of progressive renal failure and this seems most frequent in those with pre-existing renal impairment [104].

The renal toxicity of cyclosporin A was noted soon after its introduction into BMT therapy [105,106] and this drug is undoubtedly the most common cause of this complication in this situation. In one study, the use of cyclosporin A resulted in significantly higher serum creatinine in the first 100 days post-BMT, but at one year, there was no significant difference in renal function compared both with pre-BMT values and with a control group treated only with intermittent methotrexate as GvHD prophylaxis [107]. This study also indicated no evidence of renal dysfunction at one year if cyclosporin A was stopped at six months.

A distinct histological appearance of glomerular thromboses with tubular epithelial changes has been reported [108]. There is evidence to suggest that blood levels of cyclosporin A correlate with renal toxicity [109,110] and while many centres attempt to maintain patients within a certain therapeutic range, this can be quite difficult to achieve in the early post-BMT period. For this reason, it may be easier in practice to utilize this renal sensitivity to cyclosporin A by titrating the dose against the serum creatinine, aiming to keep this at or near baseline estimates.

Haemolytic uraemic syndrome
Renal failure due to a thrombotic microangiopathy, termed a 'haemolytic uraemic syndrome' (HUS) or 'thrombotic thrombocytopenic purpura' (TTP), has been increasingly recognized post-BMT; overall incidence has been estimated at between 15 and 20% [99] although severity varies from subclinical to fulminant. The consistent features are a haemolytic anaemia with red-cell fragmentation, thrombocytopenia and renal impairment (acute nephritis). This triad of features is extended to a pentad in TTP with the additional features of fever and neurological impairment, which may be non-specific. It has been variously attributed to cytotoxic chemotherapy, TBI, CMV infection, GvHD and cyclosporin A [105,108,111–115]. However, there is now good evidence to suggest that cytoreductive conditioning, particularly TBI, is the most important aetiological factor in the development of HUS/TTP. Evidence for this includes renal histological similarities with radiation nephritis [116], onset at a similar time point to radiation nephritis in some cases (that is, 6–12

months post-BMT) and reduction in incidence of HUS/TTP in patients treated with non-TBI-containing regimes or renal shielding [117] and in those treated with fractionated TBI [99].

The central histopathological features of BMT-associated HUS are arteriolar and glomerular capillary injury with associated thrombosis [118]. The underlying lesion is thought to be vascular endothelial damage and subsequent stimulation of intravascular coagulation [119].

Although there are exceptions, patients appear to fall into two clinical groups: firstly, those that are relatively mildly affected, who are usually receiving cyclosporin A and often respond to the cessation or reduction in dose of this drug, and secondly, those who are much more severely affected, usually do not respond to any alterations in cyclosporin A regimen and experience a significant morbidity and mortality from this complication. Therapeutic strategies have naturally concentrated on this latter group. Steroids, platelet function inhibitors, prostacyclin, plasma infusions and plasma exchange have all been tried with varying degrees of success or failure. It is notable that the efficacy of plasma exchange in HUS/TTP not associated with BMT has not been mirrored in this subgroup of patients, although currently most centres would nevertheless institute this therapy urgently in severely affected patients. In one report, response rate was only 50% and mortality at three months was more than 85% [120]. Some patients survive with persistent dialysis-dependent renal failure.

Acute tumour lysis syndrome (TLS)

Since the majority of patients undergoing BMT for malignancy have a low tumour load at the time of BMT this complication is rare, with a reported frequency of 1 in 400 cases [99]. Exceptions to this generalization include patients with chronic myeloid leukaemia and high white-cell counts, and those patients with advanced leukaemia or lymphoma undergoing bone-marrow transplant as salvage therapy. Widespread awareness of this potential problem has helped to reduce the incidence of TLS by the use of allopurinol and adequate hydration during cytoreductive therapy. However, on rare occasions, acute renal failure can still occur and such cases may require early dialysis to remove phosphate and purine metabolites.

Haemorrhagic cystitis (HC)

This condition has a bimodal incidence. The symptoms of frequency, dysuria and haematuria may occur acutely in association with the conditioning therapy (early HC), or may arise some weeks later. Haemorrhagic cystitis not only causes great discomfort to the patient and the potential need for multiple red-cell and platelet transfusions, but on occasion may lead to renal failure consequent to obstruction of the outflow tract, requiring insertion of nephrostomy tubes and dialysis support. Late complications of HC include bladder fibrosis with contraction.

The commonest cause of early HC is recognized to be high-dose cyclophosphamide and this toxicity is thought to be due to acrolein (a metabolite of the parent drug) which causes urothelial ulceration and vasculitis [121]. However, several other cytotoxic agents used prior to or during BMT have been associated with HC, although less frequently so, including radiation, busulphan, doxorubicin, cytosine arabinoside and etoposide [122–126]. HC may be worse in patients concurrently receiving busulphan [127]. Viral infection, particularly with adenovirus or BK virus, is the other major cause of HC [128,129]. Electron microscopy and culture of urine is required to exclude such infections; however, these methods may be insensitive in the presence of marked haematuria.

Methods of preventing this complication have included forced alkaline diuresis, bladder irrigation with saline or N-acetylcysteine [130] and the use of 2-mercaptoethanesulphonate sodium (mesna). This agent, which forms an inactive complex with acrolein, has been reported to be of considerable efficacy in the prophylaxis of HC [131,132]. There are several different regimens for mesna in current use; a recommended example is 40% of the cyclophosphamide dose (weight/weight) given as bolus injections at 0, 3, 6 and 9 hours (relative to the cyclophosphamide timing), followed by a further 40% dose infused over 12 hours (totalling 200%). In conjunction with this, intravenous fluids of at least 1.5 litres/m^2 should be administered over the 24 hours. An alternative widely used method is to infuse the total dose (200%) of mesna continuously over 24 hours [133]. Close attention to timing of mesna use is critical for successful prophylaxis of HC. Comparative studies of mesna versus bladder irrigation or forced diuresis have shown that mesna can reduce the incidence of severe HC from 35 to 13% [134]; in a more recent study, mesna and hyperhydration were found to be equally effective [135]. Similarly, Vose et al. reported equal efficacy comparing mesna and continuous bladder irrigation, but mesna-treated patients had less discomfort and fewer urinary-tract infections [136].

Therapy of established HC will depend on severity. While mildly affected patients require nothing in addition to supportive measures (platelet concentrate and blood transfusions as necessary), those with more severe manifestations should be managed in conjunction with a urological surgeon. Continuous bladder irrigation to prevent clot build-up is widely employed. Endoscopic clot removal under general anaesthesia improves patient comfort and can reduce the risk of urinary obstruction. Urinary diversion via nephrostomy tubes may be necessary to preserve renal function. Intravesical therapeutic options include alum [137], prostaglandins [138] and formalin [139]. Many such options are extremely painful for the patient and adequate analgesia is mandatory. Life-threatening haemorrhage will require surgical intervention [140]. In viral HC, antiviral agents have been employed with some success [129,141].

Other causes
Of particular interest has been the evidence that acute renal failure immediately following autologous BMT may be due to the damaging effect of reinfused red-cell stroma on the kidneys, analogous to haemolytic transfusion reactions [142]. The authors subsequently implemented relatively stringent red-cell removal before marrow cryopreservation and their ensuing observations suggested that this procedure had prevented this complication. It is also important to stress that red-cell-depleted cryopreserved infusions can cause intravascular haemolysis and renal failure due to the presence of high concentrations of dimethylsulphoxide (DMSO) used as a cryoprotectant. For this reason the amount of DMSO infused must be carefully controlled, particularly during infusion of multiple peripheral blood stem-cell collections [143].

Cardiovascular complications
Conditioning-related toxicity
Cardiac toxicity due to the conditioning regimen is well described [144] and in most cases this presents with the signs and symptoms of congestive cardiac failure within the initial three weeks post-BMT. It is usually related to the use of high-dose cyclophosphamide [145], although total body irradiation and previous anthracycline exposure may also contribute. Pathologically, the main finding is of myocardial oedema and fibrosis subsequent to endothelial damage. The most important factor dictating the likelihood of cyclophosphamide cardiac toxicity is the amount of drug administered and, in one study, a dose of greater than $1.55 \text{ g/m}^2/\text{day}$ for four days was significantly associated with this complication [146]. In another study of patients receiving 120 mg/kg cyclophosphamide over two days with 10–12 Gy TBI, one-third developed electrocardiographic (ECG) abnormalities in the short term (ST segment, T-wave changes and/or arrhythmias) and 10% had significant cardiac symptoms and signs [147]. In addition, ECG abnormalities of left-ventricular function were common at one month post-BMT but, interestingly, these had reverted to normal at one year [148] confirming the clinical impression that long-term clinically significant cardiac complications are infrequent. However, there is evidence to suggest that late cardiac dysfunction may be relatively common if exercise testing is used for its detection [149].

It would seem sensible from the above that patients with significant cardiac dysfunction pre-BMT should be excluded from this therapy although, perhaps surprisingly, there are few data to support this contention. In practice, the great majority of patients do not have symptoms or signs of cardiac disease prior to BMT and the use of screening procedures to detect minor degrees of dysfunction does not appear to be beneficial [150].

There is no specific therapy currently available which will reverse cyclophosphamide myocardial toxicity and the treatment employed should be as for other patients with congestive cardiac failure. However, this should be aggressively applied since the short-term maximal support of the failing heart usually allows resolution of this clinical problem without significant sequelae. In addition, other coincident complications such as sepsis or pneumonitis are likely to be more difficult to manage successfully in the presence of cardiac failure.

Pericarditis

Pericarditis occurring early after BMT (usually within the first three weeks) presents with chest pain, characteristically retrosternal, radiating to the shoulder tips and ameliorated by sitting forward. Concurrent fever is also common. ECG findings may be minimal or include widespread ST-segment elevation. Echocardiography is required to exclude pericardial effusion; platelet counts should be kept $>50 \times 10^9$/litre to prevent cardiac tamponade due to haemorrhage. This complication appears to be a direct result of conditioning toxicity [151,152].

Hypertension

Hypertension (diastolic blood pressure > 90 mmHg) in the early post-BMT period is common [98]. Cyclosporin A is a direct aetiological factor in many cases [109], but since an estimated 20% of patients not receiving this drug develop hypertension [153], it is clear that other causes should be considered. The most important of these is renal impairment [98] which can also, circuitously, be a toxic effect of cyclosporin A but which may arise for other reasons (see above).

From whatever cause, hypertension requires therapy, particularly since most patients will be thrombocytopenic and at risk of intracerebral bleeding. This can prove surprisingly treatment-resistant and the most useful agents are probably the calcium antagonists (e.g. nifedipine). Cyclosporin A dosage should be adjusted accordingly but, since not all studies have found a correlation between blood levels and hypertension, the best practical guide to this may be the directional trend in serum creatinine.

Endocarditis

Endocarditis, both bacterial and non-bacterial, is probably more frequent post-BMT than generally appreciated. An estimated 7% of allogeneic recipients develop non-bacterial thrombotic (marantic) endocarditis (NBTE) which may lead to multiple emboli involving the brain, kidneys and liver [154]. This complication has also been described following autologous BMT [155]. The pathogenesis remains unclear, but many cases are associated with disseminated intravascular coagulation [156]. An antemortem diagnosis is often difficult because a cardiac murmur is usually not present, and although these lesions may on occasion be detected by echocardiography [157], they are often too small for this to be the case. Clinical evidence of multiple emboli in the absence of fever may suggest the diagnosis and anticoagulant therapy should be instituted, although the benefits of this remain unproven.

Bacterial endocarditis in this setting is often the result of a central venous catheter-related infection and in one study this occurred in 5% of BMT patients [158]; it is clearly important to exclude this complication in those with suggestive clinical features such as persistent or relapsing documented bacteraemia despite appropriate and adequate antibiotic therapy. In contradistinction to NBTE, the valvular lesions of bacterial endocarditis are usually detectable by echocardiography. Therapy should include the removal of any central catheter that remains in situ and a prolonged (four to six weeks) course of antibiotics.

Metabolic complications

In the context of BMT, the syndrome of inappropriate antidiuretic hormone secretion (SIADH) is almost always related to high-dose cyclophosphamide therapy, although it has been reported in association with melphalan [159]. Fluid retention and weight gain during or shortly after the conditioning therapy together with hyponatraemia, hypouricaemia and raised urine osmolality (relative to that of plasma) will suggest the diagnosis. Simple fluid restriction is all that is usually required in this situation which is generally of short duration.

Hypomagnesaemia may be related to therapy with cyclosporin A, aminoglycosides, amphotericin, diuretics and platinum agents. In addition, there may be an associated hypocalcaemia and relative or absolute hypoparathyroidism [160]. Since hypomagnesaemia may be found coincident with hypertension, cyclosporin A toxicity and other symptomatology such as seizures (and may be an aetiological factor in these), plasma magnesium levels should be estimated at intervals and supplementation given as necessary.

Neurological complications

CNS dysfunction is a common occurrence in the early post-BMT period. In a series of autologous BMT and peripheral blood stem cells for Hodgkin's disease, 39%

of patients had early CNS complications including encephalopathy, seizures and CNS haemorrhage [161]. Although the presentation of this may be with focal neurological signs, it is more usual for drowsiness or seizures to dominate the clinical picture. Immediate investigation of CNS symptoms and signs is vital; in the first instance, this should include computed tomography scan of the brain and a lumbar puncture, if this is not contraindicated by signs of raised intracranial pressure. Cerebrospinal fluid microscopy and culture plus newer techniques such as the polymerase chain reaction for herpesviruses or mycobacterial antigens may be useful. Other investigations which can prove helpful in certain clinical settings include magnetic resonance (MRI) imaging and electroencephalography recording. Table 50.5 includes the most frequent causes of neurological dysfunction in approximate order of incidence.

While many cases of neurological dysfunction are secondary to other disorders, neurological symptoms require rapid assessment and investigation since they can be an extremely important sign of serious underlying disease. A recent series of allogeneic BMT reported that neurological events accounted for 26% of all post-BMT deaths [162].

The major causes of respiratory, hepatic and renal failure post-BMT which may lead to neurological signs or symptoms have been discussed above. In almost all cases, the existence of these is conspicuous on clinical grounds and routine laboratory investigations, before CNS complications are evident. However, an exception to this may be the presence of hypoxia which is notoriously easy to overlook from the bedside unless tachypnoea is obvious. For this reason, the initial investigation of the patient with drowsiness or similar symptoms must include arterial blood gas measurement in addition to chest radiography and biochemical tests to detect renal or hepatic impairment.

CNS infection often arises as part of a generalized complication such as septicaemia and, in practice, the investigations and management will not be significantly altered by the CNS involvement. However, there are instances in which CNS symptoms develop in apparent isolation and, in these circumstances, organisms which deserve special consideration are HSV, fungi and *Toxoplasma gondii*. HSV encephalitis appears to be a very rare event now that many centres, as mentioned before, administer prophylactic acyclovir. Varicella-zoster virus (VZV) encephalitis can be devastating post-BMT.

The diagnosis of CNS fungal infection, usually aspergillosis, can be very difficult in the absence of systemic infection since CSF microscopy and cultures are often negative. A computed tomography or MRI brain scan may demonstrate focal lesions. In one series, the majority of cases had evidence of pulmonary fungal infection and spread was presumably haematogenous [163]. The current mainstay of treatment is parenteral amphotericin, now often given in high-dose liposomal form, but the great majority, if not all, of these cases have a fatal outcome despite appropriate therapy.

Toxoplasmosis following BMT was once considered a rarity but this may have been a reflection of the particular patient population being studied. A report from France has suggested that leptomeningeal infection is a reasonably frequent cause of cerebral symptoms post-BMT in those with positive serology

Table 50.5 Neurologic complications post-BMT*

Metabolic disturbance
Respiratory failure
Hepatic failure
Renal failure
Infections
Bacterial
Viral
Fungal
Protozoal
Drug toxicity
Cerebrovascular events
Infarction
Haemorrhage
Thrombotic thrombocytopenic purpura

*CNS leukaemia or lymphoma have not been included since these are uncommon within this time period.

prior to transplant, and a case is made for prophylactic therapy in such patients [164]. A review of the literature has emphasized the pleomorphic presentation of *Toxoplasma* infection and recommended empiric therapy with pyrimethamine and sulphadiazine for BMT patients with neurological dysfunction and no other defined aetiology [165].

Patients with acute or chronic GvHD are at increased risk of CNS infection, particularly due to fungi or viruses. Progressive multifocal leukoencephalopathy due to polyoma virus infection was first reported in AIDS patients. However, it has also been recognized in BMT patients [166].

Several drugs which may have been administered during and after the conditioning therapy may cause or contribute towards CNS dysfunction [167]. These include cytosine arabinoside [168–170], busulphan [171,172], BCNU [173], cisplatinum [174] and intrathecal methotrexate [175]. Cyclosporin A neurotoxicity is also well documented [176] and is probably closely associated with hypomagnesaemia [177]. Other drugs, such as opiates, may produce pronounced effects in the presence of renal or hepatic impairment. Fortunately, many of these drug-related complications are reversible with time. The only relevant prophylactic measures are the use of anticonvulsants during high-dose busulphan therapy (for example, phenytoin 300 mg/24 hours) and the frequent estimation of blood magnesium levels (twice weekly is suggested) in those patients receiving cyclosporin. Post-BMT, both acyclovir and ganciclovir can cause neurological signs. Steroid-induced myopathy and, more rarely, psychosis should also be considered.

CNS haemorrhage is perhaps less frequent than might be anticipated in a group of patients, without exception, experiencing thrombocytopenia but must be excluded in the face of CNS symptoms; computed tomography scanning is probably the most informative investigation. CNS infarction is most commonly associated with endocarditis, bacterial or non-bacterial [178].

Transient or fluctuating neurological symptoms form part of the diagnostic pentad of TTP described earlier; examination of the blood film and assessment of renal function may provide clues to the occurrence of this complication. CSF examination and CNS imaging are generally unhelpful.

References

1. Deeg HJ, Sullivan KM, Buckner CD et al. Marrow transplantation for acute nonlymphoblastic leukemia in first remission – toxicity and long-term follow-up of patients conditioned with single dose or fractionated total-body irradiation. *Bone Marrow Transplant* 1986; **1**: 151–157.
2. McCarthy DM, Barrett AJ, Macdonald D et al. Bone marrow transplantation for adults and children with poor risk acute lymphoblastic leukaemia in first complete remission. *Bone Marrow Transplant* 1988; **3**: 315–322.
3. Geller RB, Saral R, Piantadosi S et al. Allogeneic bone marrow transplantation after high-dose busulfan and cyclophosphamide in patients with acute nonlymphocytic leukemia. *Blood* 1989; **73**: 2209–2218.
4. Gorin NC, Herve P, Aegerter P et al. Autologous bone marrow transplantation for acute leukaemia in remission. *Br J Haematol* 1986; **64**: 385–395.
5. Armitage JO. Bone marrow transplantation in the treatment of patients with lymphoma. *Blood* 1989; **73**: 1749–1758.
6. Holland HK, Dix SP, Geller RB et al. Minimal toxicity and mortality in high-risk breast cancer patients receiving high-dose cyclophosphamide, thiotepa, and carboplatin plus autologous marrow/stem-cell transplantation and comprehensive supportive care. *J Clin Oncol* 1996; **14**: 1156–1164.
7. Beyer J, Kramar A, Mandanas R et al. High-dose chemotherapy as salvage treatment in germ cell tumors: a multivariate analysis of prognostic variables. *J Clin Oncol* 1996; **14**: 2638–2645.
8. Olivieri NF, Nathan DG, MacMillan JH et al. Survival in medically treated patients with homozygous beta-thalassemia. *New Engl J Med* 1994; **331**: 574–578.
9. Davies SC. Bone marrow transplant for sickle cell disease – the dilemma. *Blood Rev* 1993; **7**: 4–9.
10. British Committee for Standards in Haematology Clinical Haematology Task Force. Guidelines on the provision of facilities for the care of adult patients with haematological malignancies (including leukaemia and lymphoma and severe bone marrow failure). *Clin Lab Haematol* 1995; **17**: 3–10.
11. Chapko MK, Syrjala KL, Schilter L, Cummings C and Sullivan KM. Chemoradiotherapy toxicity during bone marrow transplantation: time course and variation in pain and nausea. *Bone Marrow Transplant* 1989; **4**: 181–186.
12. Divgi AB. Oncologist-induced vomiting: the Igvid syndrome. *New Engl J Med* 1989; **320**: 189–190.
13. Tyers MB, Bunce KT and Humphrey PP. Pharmacological and anti-emetic properties of ondansetron. *Eur J Cancer Clin Oncol* 1989; **25**(Suppl 1): 5–9.
14. Viner CV, Selby PJ, Zulian GB et al. Ondansetron – a new safe and effective antiemetic in patients receiving high-dose melphalan. *Cancer Chemother Pharmacol* 1990; **25**: 449–453.
15. Lazarus HM, Bryson JC, Lemon E, Pritchard JF and Blumer J. Antiemetic efficacy and pharmacokinetic analyses of the serotonin antagonist ondansetron (GR 38032F) during multiple-day chemotherapy with cisplatin prior to autologous bone marrow transplantation. *J Nat Cancer Inst* 1990; **82**: 1776–1778.
16. Prentice HG, Cunningham S, Gandhi L, Cunningham J, Collis C and Hamon MD. Granisetron in the prevention of

irradiation-induced emesis. *Bone Marrow Transplant* 1995; **15**: 445–448.
17. Ferretti GA, Ash RC, Brown AT, Parr MD, Romond EH and Lillich TT. Control of oral mucositis and candidiasis in marrow transplantation: a prospective, double-blind trial of chlorhexidine digluconate oral rinse. *Bone Marrow Transplant* 1988; **3**: 483–493.
18. Weisdorf DJ, Bostrom B, Raether D *et al.* Oropharyngeal mucositis complicating bone marrow transplantation: prognostic factors and the effect of chlorhexidine mouth rinse. *Bone Marrow Transplant* 1989; **4**: 89–95.
19. Kaur S, Cooper G, Fakult S and Lazarus HM. Incidence and outcome of overt gastrointestinal bleeding in patients undergoing bone marrow transplantation. *Dig Dis Sci* 1996; **41**: 598–603.
20. Shamberger RC, Weinstein HJ, Delorey MJ and Levey RH. The medical and surgical management of typhlitis in children with acute nonlymphocytic (myelogenous) leukemia. *Cancer* 1986; **57**: 603–609.
21. Fisk JD, Shulman HM, Greening RR, McDonald GB, Sale GE and Thomas ED. Gastrointestinal radiographic features of human graft-versus-host disease. *Am J Roentgenol* 1981; **136**: 329–336.
22. Werlin SL, Casper J, Antonson D and Calabro C. Pancreatitis associated with bone marrow transplantation in children. *Bone Marrow Transplant* 1992; **10**: 65–69.
23. Shore T, Bow E, Greenberg H *et al.* Pancreatitis post-bone marrow transplantation. *Bone Marrow Transplant* 1996; **17**: 1181–1184.
24. Teefey SA, Hollister MS, Lee SP *et al.* Gallbladder sludge formation after bone marrow transplant: sonographic observations. *Abdominal Imaging* 1994; **19**: 57–60.
25. Kuttah L, Weber F, Creger RJ *et al.* Acute cholecystitis after autologous bone marrow transplantation for acute myeloid leukemia. *Ann Oncol* 1995; **6**: 302–304.
26. McDonald GB, Hinds MS, Fisher LD *et al.* Veno-occlusive disease of the liver and multiorgan failure after bone marrow transplantation: a cohort study of 355 patients. *Ann Intern Med* 1994; **118**: 255–267.
27. Jones RJ, Lee KSK, Beschorner WE *et al.* Veno-occlusive disease of the liver following bone marrow transplantation. *Transplantation* 1987; **44**: 778–783.
28. Rio B, Andreu G, Nicod A *et al.* Thrombocytopenia in veno-occlusive disease after bone marrow transplantation or chemotherapy. *Blood* 1986; **67**: 1773–1776.
29. McDonald GB, Sharma P, Matthews DE, Shulman HM and Thomas ED. The clinical course of 53 patients with veno-occlusive disease of the liver after marrow transplantation. *Transplantation* 1985; **36**: 603–608.
30. Bearman SI. The syndrome of hepatic veno-occlusive disease after marrow transplantation. *Blood* 1995; **85**: 3005–3020.
31. Gertler JP and Abbott WM. Prothrombotic and fibrinolytic function of normal and perturbed endothelium. *J Surg Res* 1992; **52**: 89–95.
32. Shulman HM, Gown AM and Nugent DJ. Hepatic veno-occlusive disease after bone marrow transplantation. Immunohistochemical identification of the material within occluded central venules. *Am J Pathol* 1987; **127**: 549–558.
33. Gordon B, Haire W, Kessinger A, Duggan M and Armitage J. High frequency of antithrombin-III and protein C deficiency following autologous bone marrow transplantation for lymphoma. *Bone Marrow Transplant* 1991; **8**: 497–502.
34. Faioni EM, Krachmalnicoff A, Bearman SI *et al.* Naturally occurring anticoagulants and bone marrow transplantation: plasma protein C predicts the development of veno-occlusive disease of the liver. *Blood* 1993; **81**: 3458–3462.
35. Shulman HM and McDonald GB. Liver disease after marrow transplantation. In: *The Pathology of Bone Marrow Transplantation*. GE Sale and HM Shulman (eds), 1984: 104–135 (New York: Masson).
36. Fajardo LF and Colby TV. Pathogenesis of veno-occlusive liver disease after radiation. *Arch Pathol Lab Med* 1980; **104**: 584–588.
37. Deleve LD. Dacarbazine toxicity in murine liver cells: a model of hepatic endothelial injury and glutathione defense. *J Pharmacol Exp Ther* 1994; **268**: 1261–1270.
38. Selzer G and Parker RGF. Senecio poisoning exhibiting as Chiari's syndrome: a report on 12 cases. *Am J Pathol* 1951; **27**: 885–907.
39. Bras G, Jelliffe DB and Stuart KL. Veno-occlusive disease of liver with nonportal type of cirrhosis, occurring in Jamaica. *Arch Pathol* 1954; **57**: 285–300.
40. Reed GB Jr and Cox AJ Jr. The human liver after radiation injury. A form of veno-occlusive disease. *Am J Pathol* 1966; **48**: 597–611.
41. McLean E, Bras G and McLean AE. Venous occlusions in the liver following dimethylnitrosamine. *Br J Exp Pathol* 1965; **46**: 367–369.
42. Griner PF, Elbadawi A and Packman CH. Veno-occlusive disease of the liver after chemotherapy of acute leukemia. Report of two cases. *Ann Intern Med* 1976; **85**: 578–582.
43. Gill RA, Onstad GR, Cardamone JM, Maneval DC and Sumner HW. Hepatic veno-occlusive disease caused by 6-thioguanine. *Ann Intern Med* 1982; **96**: 58–60.
44. Shulman HM, McDonald GB, Matthews D *et al.* An analysis of hepatic veno-occlusive disease and centrilobular hepatic degeneration following bone marrow transplantation. *Gastroenterology* 1980; **79**: 1178–1191.
45. Beschorner WE, Pino J, Boitnott JK, Tutschka PJ and Santos GW. Pathology of the liver with bone marrow transplantation. Effects of busulfan, carmustine, acute graft-versus-host disease, and cytomegalovirus infection. *Am J Pathol* 1980; **99**: 369–385.
46. McIntyre RE, Magidson JG, Austin GE and Gale RP. Fatal veno-occlusive disease of the liver following high-dose 1,3-bis(2-chloroethyl)-1-nitrosourea (BCNU) and autologous bone marrow transplantation. *Am J Clin Pathol* 1981; **75**: 614–617.
47. Lazarus HM, Gottfried MR, Herzig RH *et al.* Veno-occlusive disease of the liver after high-dose mitomycin C therapy and autologous bone marrow transplantation. *Cancer* 1982; **49**: 1789–1795.
48. Kanfer EJ, Peterson FB, Buckner CD *et al.* A phase I study of high dose dimethylbusulfan followed by autologous bone marrow transplantation in patients with advanced malignancy. *Cancer Treat Rep* 1987; **71**: 101–102.
49. Jacobs P, Miller JL, Uys CJ and Dietrich BE. Fatal veno-occlusive disease of the liver after chemotherapy, whole-body irradiation and bone marrow transplantation for refractory acute leukaemia. *South African Med J* 1979; **55**: 5–10.
50. Woods WG, Dehner LP, Nesbit ME *et al.* Fatal veno-occlusive disease of the liver following high dose chemotherapy,

irradiation and bone marrow transplantation. *Am J Med* 1980; **68**: 285–290.
51. Ringden O, Ruutu T, Remberger M *et al*. A randomized trial comparing busulfan with total body irradiation as conditioning in allogeneic marrow transplant recipients with leukemia: a report from the Nordic Bone Marrow Transplantation Group. *Blood* 1994; **83**: 2723–2730.
52. Kanfer EJ, Buckner CD, Fefer A *et al*. Allogeneic and syngeneic marrow transplantation following high dose dimethylbusulfan, cyclophosphamide and total body irradiation. *Bone Marrow Transplant* 1987; **1**: 339–346.
53. Grochow LB, Piantadosi S, Santos G and Jones R. Busulfan dose adjustment decreases the risk of hepatic veno-occlusive disease in patients undergoing bone marrow transplantation. *Proc Am Ass Cancer Res* 1992; **33**: 200.
54. Grochow LB. Busulfan disposition: the role of therapeutic monitoring in bone marrow transplantation induction regimens. *Semin Oncol* 1993; **20**: 18–25.
55. McDonald GB, Sharma P, Matthews DE, Shulman HM and Thomas ED. Veno-occlusive disease of the liver after bone marrow transplantation: diagnosis, incidence and predisposing factors. *Hepatology* 1984; **4**: 116–122.
56. Dulley FL, Kanfer EJ, Appelbaum FR *et al*. Veno-occlusive disease of the liver after chemoradiotherapy and autologous bone marrow transplantation. *Transplantation* 1987; **43**: 870–873.
57. Deeg HJ, Shulman HM, Schmidt E, Yee GC, Thomas ED and Storb R. Marrow graft rejection and veno-occlusive disease of the liver in patients with aplastic anemia conditioned with cyclophosphamide and cyclosporine. *Transplantation* 1986; **42**: 497–501.
58. Ayash LJ, Hunt M, Antman K *et al*. Hepatic veno-occlusive disease in autologous bone marrow transplantation of solid tumors and lymphomas. *J Clin Oncol* 1990; **8**: 1699–1706.
59. Sanders JE, Buckner CD, Clift RA *et al*. Second marrow transplants in patients with leukemia who relapse after allogeneic marrow transplantation. *Bone Marrow Transplant* 1988; **3**: 11–19.
60. Radich JP, Sanders JE, Buckner CD *et al*. Second allogeneic marrow transplantation for patients with recurrent leukemia after initial transplant with total-body-irradiation-containing regimens. *J Clin Oncol* 1993; **11**: 304–313.
61. Nevill TJ, Barnett MJ, Klingemann HG, Reece DE, Shepherd JD and Phillips GL. Regimen-related toxicity of a busulfan–cyclophosphamide conditioning regimen in 70 patients undergoing allogeneic bone marrow transplantation. *J Clin Oncol* 1991; **9**: 1224–1232.
62. Carreras E, Granena A, Rozman C *et al*. Transvenous liver study as a diagnostic approach to veno-occlusive disease after bone marrow transplantation. *Bone Marrow Transplant* 1988; **3**(Suppl 1): 255–256.
63. Shulman HM, Gooley T, Dudley MD *et al*. Utility of transvenous liver biopsies and wedged hepatic venous pressure measurements in sixty marrow transplant recipients. *Transplantation* 1995; **59**: 1015–1022.
64. Carreras E, Granena A, Navasa M *et al*. Transjugular liver biopsy in BMT. *Bone Marrow Transplant* 1993; **11**: 21–26.
65. Morris CL, Babcock DS, Pietryga DW and Neudorf SM. Doppler ultrasonography for evaluation of venoocclusive disease (VOD) of the liver. *J Cell Biochem* 1990; Suppl 14A: C519.
66. Hommeyer SC, Teefey SA, Jacobson AF *et al*. Veno-occlusive disease of the liver: prospective study of US evaluation. *Radiology* 1992; **184**: 683–686.
67. Cahn JY, Flesch M, Plouvier E, Herve P and Rozenbaum A. Venous occlusive disease of the liver and autologous bone marrow transplantation. Preventive role for heparin? *Nouv Rev Fr Hematol* 1985; **27**: 27–28.
68. Rio B, Lamy T and Zittoun R. Preventive role of heparin for liver veno-occlusive disease (VOD). *Bone Marrow Transplant* 1988; **3**: 266.
69. Mozzana R, Lambertenghi DG, Della Volpe A, Fossati V and Selva S. Use of minidoses of heparin and liver venoocclusive disease (VOD) in patients treated with autologous and allogeneic BMT. *Bone Marrow Transplant* 1990; **5**(Suppl 2): 86.
70. Bearman SI, Hinds MS, Wolford JL *et al*. A pilot study of continuous infusion heparin for the prevention of hepatic veno-occlusive disease after bone marrow transplantation. *Bone Marrow Transplant* 1990; **5**: 407–411.
71. Marsa Vila L, Gorin NC, Laporte JP *et al*. Prophylactic heparin does not prevent liver veno-occlusive disease following autologous bone marrow transplantation. *Eur J Haematol* 1991; **47**: 346–354.
72. Attal M, Huguet F, Rubie H *et al*. Prevention of hepatic veno-occlusive disease after bone marrow transplantationation by continuous infuson of low-dose heparin: a prospective randomized trial. *Blood* 1992; **79**: 2834–2840.
73. Gluckman E, Jolivet I, Scrobohaci ML *et al*. Use of prostaglandin E1 for prevention of liver veno-occlusive disease in leukaemic patients treated by allogeneic bone marrow transplantation. *Br J Haematol* 1990; **74**: 277–281.
74. Essell JH, Thompson JM, Harman GS *et al*. Pilot trial of prophylactic ursodiol to decrease the incidence of veno-occlusive disease of the liver in allogeneic bone marrow transplant patients. *Bone Marrow Transplant* 1992; **10**: 367–372.
75. Essell J, Schroeder M, Thompson J, Harman G, Halvorson R and Callander N. A randomized double-blind trial of prophylactic ursodeoxycholic acid (UDCA) versus placebo to prevent veno-occlusive disease (VOD) of the liver in patients undergoing allogeneic bone-marrow transplantation (BMT). *Blood* 1994; **84**: A250.
76. Attal M, Huguet F, Rubie H *et al*. Prevention of regimen-related toxicities after bone marrow transplantation by pentoxifylline: a prospective, randomized trial. *Blood* 1993; **82**: 732–736.
77. Clift RA, Bianco JA, Appelbaum FR *et al*. A randomized controlled trial of pentoxifylline for the prevention of regimen-related toxicities in patients undergoing allogeneic marrow transplantation. *Blood* 1993; **82**: 2025–2030.
78. Yee GC, Kennedy MS, Storb R and Thomas ED. Effect of hepatic dysfunction on oral cyclosporin pharmacokinetics in marrow transplant patients. *Blood* 1984; **64**: 1277–1279.
79. Ibrahim A, Pico JL, Ostronoff M *et al*. Use of prostaglandin E1 for the treatment of veno-occlusive disease of the liver following autologous bone marrow transplantation. *Bone Marrow Transplant* 1990; **5**(Suppl 2): 82.
80. Baglin TP, Harper P and Marcus RE. Veno-occlusive disease of the liver complicating ABMT successfully treated with recombinant tissue plasminogen activator (rt-PA). *Bone Marrow Transplant* 1990; **5**: 439–441.

81. Patton DF, Harper JL, Wooldridge TN, Gordon BG, Coccia P and Haire WD. Treatment of veno-occlusive disease of the liver with bolus tissue plasminogen activator and continuous infusion antithrombin III concentrate. *Bone Marrow Transplant* 1996; **17**: 443–447.
82. Nimer SD, Milewicz AL, Champlin RE and Busuttil RW. Successful treatment of hepatic veno-occlusive disease in a bone marrow transplant patient with orthotopic liver transplantation. *Transplantation* 1990; **49**: 819–821.
83. Weiner RS, Bortin MM, Gale RP *et al*. Risk factors associated with interstitial pneumonitis following allogeneic bone marrow transplantation for leukemia. *Transplant Proc* 1985; **17**: 470–474.
84. Piedbois P, Cordonnier C, Levy C *et al*. Diffuse interstitial pneumonitis following BMT – incidence and relationship with parameters of single fraction TBI. *Bone Marrow Transplant* 1988; **3**: 273.
85. Granena A, Carreras E, Rozman C *et al*. Interstitial pneumonitis after BMT: 15 years experience in a single institution. *Bone Marrow Transplant* 1993; **11**: 453–458.
86. Meyers JD, Flournoy N and Thomas ED. Non-bacterial pneumonitis after allogeneic bone marrow transplantation: a review of ten years' experience. *Rev Infect Dis* 1982; **4**: 1119–1132.
87. Appelbaum FR, Meyers JD, Fefer A *et al*. Nonbacterial nonfungal pneumonia following marrow transplantation in 100 identical twins. *Transplantation* 1982; **33**: 265–268.
88. Pecego R, Hill R, Appelbaum FR *et al*. Interstitial pneumonitis following autologous bone marrow transplantation. *Transplantation* 1986; **42**: 515–517.
89. Carlson K, Backlund L, Smedmyr B, Oberg G and Simonsson B. Pulmonary function and complications subsequent to autologous bone marrow transplantation. *Bone Marrow Transplant* 1994; **14**: 805–811.
90. Kanfer EJ and McCarthy DM. Cytoreductive preparation for bone marrow transplantation in leukaemia: to irradiate or not? *Br J Haematol* 1989; **71**: 447–450.
91. Crawford SW, Longton G and Storb R. Acute graft-versus-host disease and the risks for idiopathic pneumonia after marrow transplantation for severe aplastic anemia. *Bone Marrow Transplant* 1994; **12**: 225–231.
92. Hartsell WF, Czyzewski EA, Ghalie R and Kaizer H. Pulmonary complications of bone marrow transplantation: a comparison of total body irradiation and cyclophosphamide to busulfan and cyclophosphamide. *Int J Radiat Oncol Biol Phys* 1995; **32**: 69–73.
93. Crawford SW, Bowden RA, Hackman RC, Gleaves CA, Meyers JD and Clark JG. Rapid detection of cytomegalovirus pulmonary infection by bronchoalveolar lavage and centrifugation culture. *Ann Intern Med* 1988; **108**: 180–185.
94. Robbins RA, Linder J, Stahl MG *et al*. Diffuse alveolar hemorrhage in autologous bone marrow transplant recipients. *Am J Med* 1989; **87**: 511–518.
95. Leskinen R, Taskinen E, Volin L, Tukiainen P, Ruutu T and Häyry P. Use of bronchoalveolar lavage cytology and determination of protein contents in pulmonary complications of bone marrow transplant recipients. *Bone Marrow Transplant* 1990; **5**: 241–245.
96. Gondo H, Harada M, Hara N *et al*. Idiopathic interstitial pneumonitis possibly associated with chronic graft-versus-host disease. *Rinsho Ketsueki* 1993; **34**: 183–189.
97. Graham NJ, Muller NL, Miller RR and Shepherd JD. Intrathoracic complications following allogeneic bone marrow transplantation: CT findings. *Radiology* 1991; **181**: 153–156.
98. Kone BC, Whelton A, Santos G, Saral R and Watson AJ. Hypertension and renal dysfunction in bone marrow transplant recipients. *Q J Med* 1988; **69**: 985–995.
99. Zager RA. Acute renal failure in the setting of bone marrow transplantation. *Kidney Int* 1994; **46**: 1443–1458.
100. Gruss E, Bernis C, Tomas JF *et al*. Acute renal failure in patients following bone marrow transplantation: prevalence, risk factors and outcome. *Am J Nephrol* 1995; **15**: 473–479.
101. Wadler S and Dutcher JP. Renal failure related to drugs and disease. In: *Handbook of Hematologic and Oncologic Emergencies*. JP Dutcher and PH Wiernik (eds), 1987 (New York: Plenum).
102. Mirabell R, Bieri S, Mermillod B *et al*. Renal toxicity after allogeneic bone marrow transplantation: the combined effects of total-body irradiation and graft-versus-host disease. *J Clin Oncol* 1996; **14**: 579–585.
103. Moulder JE, Cohen EP, Fish BL and Hill P. Prophylaxis of bone marrow transplant nephropathy with captopril, an inhibitor of angiotensin-converting enzyme. *Radiat Res* 1993; **136**: 404–407.
104. Hande KR, Noone RM and Stone WJ. Severe allopurinol toxicity: description and guidelines for prevention in patients with renal insufficiency. *Am J Med* 1984; **76**: 47–56.
105. Powles RL, Clink HM, Spence D *et al*. Cyclosporin A to prevent graft-versus-host disease in man after allogeneic bone marrow transplantation. *Lancet* 1980; **i**: 327–329.
106. Hows JM, Palmer S, Want S, Dearden C and Gordon Smith EC. Serum levels of cyclosporin A and nephrotoxicity in bone marrow transplant patients. *Lancet* 1981; **ii**: 145–146.
107. Yee GC, McGuire TR, St Pierre BA *et al*. Minimal risk of chronic renal dysfunction in marrow transplant recipients treated with cyclosporine for 6 months. *Bone Marrow Transplant* 1989; **4**: 691–694.
108. Shulman HM, Striker G, Deeg HJ, Kennedy M, Storb R and Thomas ED. Nephrotoxicity of cyclosporin A after allogeneic marrow transplantation: glomerular thromboses and tubular injury. *New Engl J Med* 1981; **305**: 1392–1395.
109. Barrett AJ, Kendra JR, Lucas CF *et al*. Cyclosporin A as prophylaxis against graft-versus-host disease in 36 patients. *Br Med J* 1982; **285**: 162–166.
110. Hows JM, Chipping PM, Fairhead S, Smith J, Baughan A and Gordon-Smith EC. Nephrotoxicity in bone marrow transplant recipients treated with cyclosporin A. *Br J Haematol* 1983; **54**: 69–78.
111. Atkinson K, Biggs JC, Hayes J *et al*. Cyclosporin A associated nephrotoxicity in the first 100 days after allogeneic bone marrow transplantation: three distinct syndromes. *Br J Haematol* 1983; **54**: 59–67.
112. Marshall RJ and Sweny P. Haemolytic–uraemic syndrome in recipients of bone marrow transplants not treated with cyclosporin A. *Histopathology* 1986; **10**: 953–962.
113. Holler E, Kolb HJ, Hiller E *et al*. Microangiopathy in patients on cyclosporine prophylaxis who developed acute graft-versus-host disease after HLA-identical bone marrow transplantation. *Blood* 1989; **73**: 2018–2024.
114. Chappell ME, Keeling DM, Prentice HG and Sweny P. Haemolytic-uraemic syndrome after bone marrow

transplantation: an adverse effect of total body irradiation? *Bone Marrow Transplant* 1988; **3**: 339–347.
115. Tschuchnigg M, Bradstock KF, Koutts J, Stewart J, Enno A and Seldon M. A case of thrombotic thrombocytopenic purpura following allogeneic bone marrow transplantation. *Bone Marrow Transplant* 1990; **5**: 61–63.
116. Down JD, Berman AJ, Warhol M, Yeap B and Mauch P. Late complications following total-body irradiation and bone marrow rescue in mice: predominance of glomerular nephropathy and hemolytic anemia. *Int J Radiat Biol* 1990; **57**: 551–565.
117. Lawton CA, Barber Derus SW, Murray KJ, Cohen EP, Ash RC and Moulder JE. Influence of renal shielding on the incidence of late renal dysfunction associated with T-lymphocyte deplete bone marrow transplantation in adult patients. *Int J Radiat Oncol Biol Phys* 1992; **23**: 681–686.
118. Antignac C, Gubler MC, Leverger G, Broyer M and Habib R. Delayed renal failure with extensive mesangiolysis following bone marrow transplantation. *Kidney Int* 1989; **35**: 1336–1344.
119. Cohen H, Bull HA, Seddon A *et al*. Vascular endothelial cell function and ultrastructure in thrombotic microangiopathy following allogeneic bone marrow transplantation. *Eur J Haematol* 1989; **43**: 207–214.
120. Silva VA, Frei Lahr D, Brown RA and Herzig GP. Plasma exchange and vincristine in the treatment of hemolytic uremic syndrome/thrombotic thrombocytopenic purpura associated with bone marrow transplantation. *J Clin Apheresis* 1991; **6**: 16–20.
121. Cox PJ. Cyclophosphamide cystitis: identification of acrolein as the causative agent. *Biochem Pharmacol* 1979; **28**: 2045–2049.
122. Goldstein AG, D'Escrivan JC and Allen SD. Haemorrhagic radiation cystitis. *Br J Urol* 1968; **40**: 475–478.
123. Millard RJ. Busulphan-induced hemorrhagic cystitis. *Urology* 1981; **18**: 143–144.
124. Ershler WB, Gilchrist KW and Citrin DL. Adriamycin enhancement of cyclophosphamide-induced bladder injury. *J Urol* 1980; **123**: 121–122.
125. Renert WA, Berdon WE and Baker DH. Haemorrhagic cystitis and vesicoureteric reflux secondary to cytotoxic therapy for childhood malignancies. *Am J Roentgenal* 1973; **117**: 664–669.
126. Blume KG, Forman SJ, O'Donnell MR *et al*. Total body irradiation and high-dose etoposide: a new preparatory regimen for bone marrow transplantation in patients with advanced hematologic malignancies. *Blood* 1987; **69**: 1015–1020.
127. Morgan M, Dodds A, Atkinson K, Szer J, Downs K and Biggs J. The toxicity of busulphan and cyclophosphamide as the preparative regimen for bone marrow transplantation. *Br J Haematol* 1991; **77**: 529–534.
128. Rice SJ, Bishop JA, Apperley J and Gardner SD. BK virus as cause of haemorrhagic cystitis after bone marrow transplantation. *Lancet* 1985; **ii**: 844–845.
129. Jurado M, Navarro JM, Hernandez J, Molina MA and DePablos JM. Adenovirus-associated haemorrhagic cystitis after bone marrow transplantation successfully treated with intravenous ribavirin. *Bone Marrow Transplant* 1995; **15**: 651–652.
130. Tolley DA. The effect of N-acetylcysteine on cyclophosphamide cystitis. *Br J Urol* 1977; **49**: 659–661.
131. Link H, Neef V, Niethammer D and Wilms K. Prophylaxis of haemorrhagic cystitis due to cyclophosphamide-conditioning for bone marrow transplantation. [Letter] *Blut* 1981; **43**: 329–330.
132. Blacklock H, Ball L, Knight C, Schey S and Prentice G. Experience with mesna in patients receiving allogeneic bone marrow transplants for poor prognostic leukaemia. *Cancer Treat Rev* 1983; **10**(Suppl A): 45–52.
133. Brugieres L, Hartmann O, Travagli JP *et al*. Hemorrhagic cystitis following high-dose chemotherapy and bone marrow transplantation in children with malignancies: incidence, clinical course, and outcome. *J Clin Oncol* 1989; **7**: 194–199.
134. Hows JM, Mehta A, Ward L *et al*. Comparison of mesna with forced diuresis to prevent cyclophosphamide induced haemorrhagic cystitis in marrow transplantation: a prospective randomised study. *Br J Cancer* 1984; **50**: 753–756.
135. Shepherd JD, Pringle LE, Barnett MJ, Klingemann HG, Reece DE and Phillips GL. Mesna versus hyperhydration for the prevention of cyclophosphamide-induced hemorrhagic cystitis in bone marrow transplantation. *J Clin Oncol* 1991; **9**: 2016–2020.
136. Vose JM, Reed EC, Pippert GC *et al*. Mesna compared with continuous bladder irrigation as uroprotection during high-dose chemotherapy and transplantation: a randomized trial. *J Clin Oncol* 1993; **11**: 1306–1310.
137. Kennedy C, Snell ME and Witherow RO. Use of alum to control intractable vesical haemorrhage. *Br J Urol* 1984; **56**: 673–675.
138. Mohiuddin J, Prentice HG, Schey S, Blacklock H and Dandona P. Treatment of cyclophosphamide-induced cystitis with prostaglandin E_2. *Ann Intern Med* 1984; **101**: 142.
139. Shrom SH, Donaldson MH, Duckett JW and Wein AJ. Formalin treatment for intractable hemorrhagic cystitis: a review of the literature with 16 additional cases. *Cancer* 1976; **38**: 1785–1789.
140. Andriole GL, Yuan JJ and Catalona WJ. Cystotomy, temporary urinary diversion and bladder packing in the management of severe cyclophosphamide-induced hemorrhagic cystitis. *J Urol* 1990; **143**: 1006–1007.
141. Chapman C, Flower AJ and Durrant ST. The use of vidarabine in the treatment of human polyomavirus associated acute haemorrhagic cystitis. *Bone Marrow Transplant* 1991; **7**: 481–483.
142. Smith DM, Weisenburger DD, Bierman P, Kessinger A, Vaughan WP and Armitage JO. Acute renal failure associated with autologous bone marrow transplantation. *Bone Marrow Transplant* 1987; **2**: 195–201.
143. Yellowlees P, Greenfield C and McIntyre N. Dimethylsulphoxide-induced toxicity. *Lancet* 1980; **ii**: 1004–1006.
144. Cazin B, Gorin NC, Laporte JP *et al*. Cardiac complications after bone marrow transplantation – a report on a series of 63 consecutive transplantations. *Cancer* 1986; **57**: 2061–2069.
145. Gottdeiner JS, Appelbaum FR, Ferrans VJ, Deisseroth A and Zeigler J. Cardiotoxicity associated with high-dose cyclophosphamide therapy. *Arch Intern Med* 1981; **141**: 758–763.
146. Goldberg MA, Antin JH, Guinan EC and Rappeport JM. Cyclophosphamide cardiotoxicity: an analysis of dosing as a risk factor. *Blood* 1986; **68**: 1114–1118.

147. Kupari M, Volin L, Suokas A, Timonen T, Hekali P and Ruutu T. Cardiac involvement in bone marrow transplantation: electrocardiographic changes, arrhythmias, heart failure and autopsy findings. *Bone Marrow Transplant* 1990; **5**: 91–98.

148. Kupari M, Volin L, Suokas A, Hekali P and Ruutu T. Cardiac involvement in bone marrow transplantation: serial changes in left ventricular size, mass and performance. *J Int Med* 1990; **227**: 259–266.

149. Larsen RL, Barber G, Heise CT and August CS. Exercise assessment of cardiac function in children and young adults before and after bone marrow transplantation. *Paediatrics* 1992; **89**: 722–729.

150. Bearman SI, Petersen FB, Schor RA et al. Radionuclide ejection fractions in the evaluation of patients being considered for bone marrow transplantation: risk for cardiac toxicity. *Bone Marrow Transplant* 1990; **5**: 173–177.

151. Appelbaum F, Strauchen JA, Graw RG Jr et al. Acute lethal carditis caused by high-dose combination chemotherapy. A unique clinical and pathological entity. *Lancet* 1976; **i**: 58–62.

152. Reykdal S, Sham R and Kouides P. Cytarabine-induced pericarditis: a case report and review of the literature of the cardio-pulmonary complications of cytarabine therapy. *Leuk Res* 1995; **19**: 141–144.

153. Loughran TP, Deeg HJ, Dahlberg S, Kennedy MS, Storb R and Thomas ED. Incidence of hypertension after marrow transplantation among 112 patients randomized to either cyclosporine or methotrexate as graft-versus-host disease prophylaxis. *Br J Haematol* 1985; **59**: 547–553.

154. Patchell RA, White CL, Clark AW, Beschorner WE and Santos GW. Nonbacterial thrombotic endocarditis in bone marrow transplant patients. *Cancer* 1985; **55**: 631–635.

155. Diez Martin JL, Habermann TM, Gastineau DA, Solberg LA Jr and Letendre L. Nonbacterial thrombotic endocarditis in autologous bone marrow transplantation. *Am J Med* 1988; **85**: 742–744.

156. Kim H-S, Suzuki M, Lie JT and Titus JL. Nonbacterial thrombotic endocarditis and disseminated intravascular coagulation. *Arch Pathol Lab Med* 1977; **101**: 65–68.

157. Siegel RJ, Ginzton LE, Flanagan K and Criley JM. Marantic endocarditis: diagnosis by 2-D echocardiography. *Chest* 1981; **80**: 118–119.

158. Martino P, Micozzi A, Venditti M et al. Catheter-related right-sided endocarditis in bone marrow transplant recipients. *Rev Infect Dis* 1990; **12**: 250–257.

159. Greenbaum Lefkoe B, Rosenstock JG, Belasco JB, Rohrbaugh TM and Meadows AT. Syndrome of inappropriate antidiuretic hormone secretion. A complication of high-dose intravenous melphalan. *Cancer* 1985; **55**: 44–46.

160. Freedman DB, Shannon M, Dandona P, Prentice HG and Hoffbrand AV. Hypoparathyroidism and hypocalcaemia during treatment for acute leukaemia. *Br Med J* 1982; **284**: 700–702.

161. Snider S, Bashir R and Bierman P. Neurologic complications after high-dose chemotherapy and autologous bone marrow transplantation for Hodgkin's disease. *Neurology* 1994; **44**: 681–684.

162. Gallardo D, Ferra C, Berlanga JJ et al. Neurologic complications after allogeneic bone marrow transplantation. *Bone Marrow Transplant* 1996; **18**: 1135–1139.

163. Boes B, Bashir R, Boes C, Hahn F, McConnell JR and McComb R. Central nervous system aspergillosis. Analysis of 26 patients. *J Neuroimaging* 1994; **4**: 123–129.

164. Derouin F, Gluckman E, Beauvais B et al. Toxoplasma infection after human bone marrow transplantation: clinical and serological study of 80 patients. *Bone Marrow Transplant* 1986; **1**: 67–73.

165. Seong DC, Przepiorka D, Bruner JM, Van Tassel P, Lo WK and Champlin RE. Leptomeningeal toxoplasmosis after allogeneic marrow transplantation. Case report and review of the literature. *Am J Clin Oncol* 1993; **16**: 105–108.

166. Bogdanovic G, Grandien M, Brytting M and Fridell E. BK and JC viruses – two polyomaviruses causing disease in immunosuppressed patients. *Läkartidningen* 1992; **89**: 3925–3926.

167. Kaplan RS and Wiernik PH. Neurotoxicity of antineoplastic drugs. *Semin Oncol* 1982; **9**: 103–130.

168. Lazarus HM, Herzig RH, Herzig GP, Phillips GL, Roessmann U and Fishman DJ. Central nervous system toxicity of high-dose systemic cytosine arabinoside. *Cancer* 1981; **48**: 2577–2582.

169. Dunton SF, Nitschke R, Spruce WE, Bodensteiner J and Krous HF. Progressive ascending paralysis following administration of intrathecal and intravenous cytosine arabinoside. *Cancer* 1986; **57**: 1083–1088.

170. Johnson NT, Crawford SW and Sargur M. Acute acquired demyelinating polyneuropathy with respiratory failure following high-dose systemic cytosine arabinoside and marrow transplantation. *Bone Marrow Transplant* 1987; **2**: 203–207.

171. Marcus RE and Goldman JM. Convulsions due to high-dose busulphan. *Lancet* 1984; **ii**: 1463.

172. Sureda A, Perez de Oteyza J, Garcia Larana J and Odriozola J. High-dose busulfan and seizures. *Ann Intern Med* 1989; **111**: 543–544.

173. Ramirez G, Wilson W, Grage T and Hill G. Phase II evaluation of 1,3-bis(2-chloroethyl)-1-nitrosourea (BCNU; NSC-409962) in patients with solid tumors. *Cancer Chemother Rep* 1972; **56**: 787–790.

174. Daugaard GK, Petrera J and Trojaborg W. Electrophysiological study of the peripheral and central neurotoxic effect of cisplatin. *Acta Neurol Scand* 1987; **76**: 86–93.

175. Geiser CF, Bishop Y, Jaffe N, Furman L, Traggis D and Frei E III. Adverse effects of intrathecal methotrexate in children with acute leukemia in remission. *Blood* 1975; **45**: 189–195.

176. Joss DV, Barrett AJ, Kendra JR, Lucas CF and Desai S. Hypertension and convulsions in children receiving cyclosporin A. *Lancet* 1982; **i**: 906.

177. Thompson CB, June CH, Sullivan KM and Thomas ED. Association between cyclosporin neurotoxicity and hypomagnesaemia. *Lancet* 1984; **ii**: 1116–1120.

178. Patchell RA, White CL, Clark AW, Beschorner WE and Santos GW. Neurologic complications of bone marrow transplantation. *Neurology* 1985; **35**: 300–306.

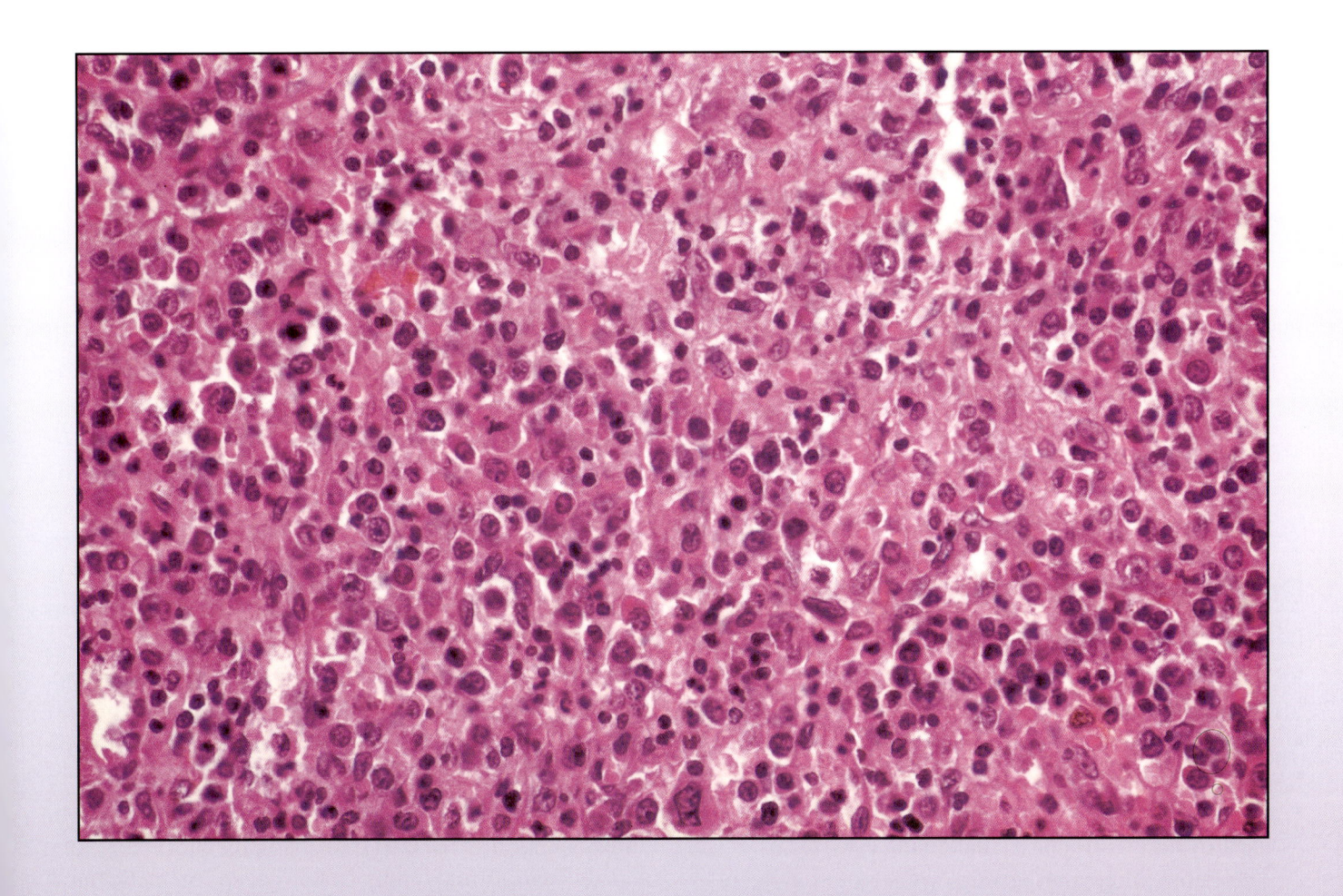

Chapter 51

Neurological aspects of stem-cell transplantation

Paul V. Marks

Introduction

Problems affecting either the central nervous system (CNS) or peripheral nervous system can occur in patients undergoing stem-cell transplantation. It is convenient to discuss and classify these problems in the following manner:
1. drug related neurological problems;
2. problems associated with suppressed or recovering marrow;
3. distinguishing original disease recurrence from complications of transplantation, as well as investigating neurological problems that may be associated with malignant disease such as paraneoplastic phenomena.

Drug-related neurological problems

Drugs used in the treatment of malignant disease and for immunosuppression can be classified under the following headings:
- cytotoxic agents;
- drugs which affect the immune response;
- sex hormones and hormone antagonists which are used in the treatment of malignant disease.

The most important group are cytotoxic agents, many of which have recognized neurotoxicity, the most notable of which are the vinca alkaloids. It should, of course, be appreciated that neurological problems can develop indirectly through the myelosuppression which these agents can produce, and this may result in an increased likelihood of intracranial haemorrhage or infection due to thrombocytopenia and neutropenia, respectively. These problems are discussed in greater detail in the next section.

Cytotoxic drugs can be divided into the following categories:
- alkylating agents;
- cytotoxic antibiotics;
- anti-metabolites;
- vinca alkaloids and etoposide; and
- others

Extensive experience has been gained with the use of alkylating agents such as cyclophosphamide, chlorambucil, carmustine and melphalan. However, neurological side-effects are extremely rare. Cytotoxic antibiotics such as doxorubicin, bleomycin and daunorubicin are also remarkably free of central or peripheral nervous system toxicity. Antimetabolites may be associated with CNS toxicity. Fluorouracil can be associated with a cerebellar syndrome and fludarabine can cause idiosyncratic CNS toxicity which is unpredictable.

Vinca alkaloids are undoubtedly the most neurotoxic of all cytotoxic drugs [1]. Vincristine commonly causes peripheral and autonomic neuropathy. Vinblastine, although more toxic to the bone marrow, tends to cause less neurological problems. The neurological side-effects of vincristine are manifest as sensory disturbance and paraesthesae associated with loss of deep tendon reflexes or difficulty with phonation due to involvement of the recurrent laryngeal nerves. The onset of weakness is an absolute contraindication to the further use of vinca alkaloids. Recovery does occur but can be slow, and is slowest in older patients who also tend to develop symptoms at an earlier stage in the use of the agent.

A variety of other cytotoxic drugs are neurotoxic. Cisplatin and carboplatin may cause peripheral neuropathy and high-tone hearing loss. Such complications tend to be more common and severe with cisplatin compared with carboplatin. Paclitaxel, which is a taxane used to treat patients with refractory ovarian carcinoma, may also cause in peripheral neuropathy.

Patients who have undergone bone-marrow transplantation may also be given to a variety of agents which affect the immune response. The various side-effects of corticosteroid therapy are well known, but it should not be forgotten that mental disturbances such as euphoria or depression can occur and weakness due to proximal myopathy may be observed, even in patients who have been taking steroids for comparatively short periods of time. Cyclosporin can cause peripheral neuropathy, paraesthesiae and burning sensations in the hands and feet. Cyclosporin may also be associated with confusion and an increased tendency to seizure.

Tacrolimus, a macrolide immuno-suppressant, has a similar mode of action to cyclosporin, but the incidence of neurotoxicity tends to be greater. Neuropsychiatric symptoms such as agitation, depression, anxiety and nightmares may be observed. It is also ototoxic and vestibulotoxic and can cause migrainous headaches as well as photophobia.

The interferons can cause in neuropsychiatric complications and should be avoided in those with a history of depression or epilepsy which is inadequately controlled. Depression of the level of consciousness may also be seen, particularly when higher doses of interferon α are used, and especially in elderly subjects.

It should not be overlooked that many patients who are to undergo a stem-cell transplantation procedure will already have been exposed to some of the above-mentioned agents when they underwent their initial chemotherapy designed to treat the presenting disease, and they may therefore embark upon the procedure with neurological problems which can be exacerbated by the drugs used for the transplant.

Problems associated with suppressed or recovering marrow

Platelets

Thrombocytopenia may predispose patients to spontaneous intracranial or intraspinal haemorrhage. Spontaneous haemorrhage is uncommon when the platelet count is above $50\,000 \times 10^9$/litre but becomes a matter of concern when the count is less than $20\,000 \times 10^9$/litre. Haemorrhage may occur into the subdural space (Figure 51.1) or into the parenchyma of the brain itself, resulting in an intracerebral haematoma.

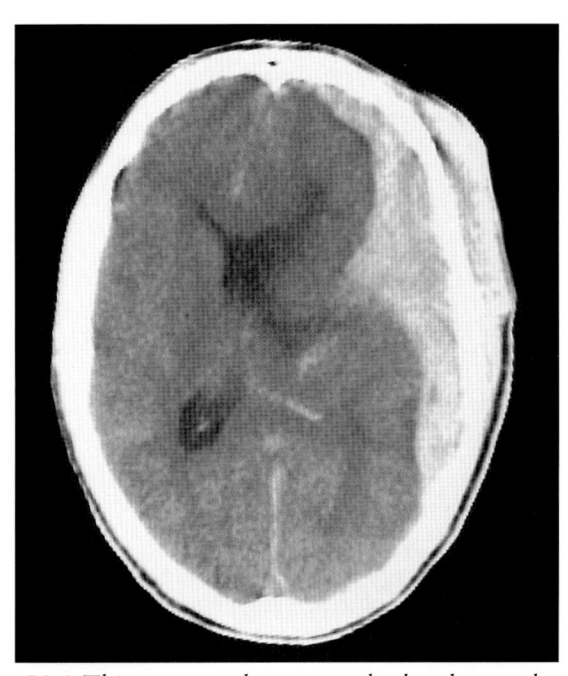

Figure 51.1 This computed tomography head scan shows an acute subdural haematoma which is producing shift of midline structures. This patient was markedly thrombocytopenic.

Spontaneous haemorrhage into the extradural space is extremely uncommon. Acute haemorrhage may present as an expanding intracranial lesion, with decreasing level of consciousness which may or may not be associated with focal neurological deficit. An intracerebral haematoma, which ruptures through the pia mater into the subarachnoid space, may be associated with signs of meningeal irritation and a picture indistinguishable from that of subarachnoid haemorrhage. Urgent investigation and neurosurgical referral is essential. A full blood count and clotting screen should be obtained and arrangements made for the patient to have a computed tomography scan of the head. Lesions exerting a significant mass effect associated with a depressed level of consciousness require immediate neurosurgical intervention. The principles of management involve pre-operative correction of the platelet count and evacuation of the haematoma by craniotomy. For chronic subdural collections, evacuation through burr holes is usually sufficient.

Spontaneous spinal haemorrhage from thrombocytopenia is extremely rare. The condition is usually associated with spinal pain of sudden onset, often with radicular radiation. This is followed by signs of spinal dysfunction ranging from sensory disturbance to complete paraplegia. Urgent investigation is mandatory and magnetic resonance imaging scanning is the imaging modality of choice. Rapid neurosurgical referral and intervention is required to prevent complete loss of spinal cord function.

Leukopenia

Upper respiratory-tract infections and intrathoracic sepsis can render the transplant patient vulnerable to intracranial abscess (Figure 51.2), subdural empyema or meningitis. Frontal sinusitis with suppuration can result in thrombophlebitis of emissary veins with spread of infection into the frontal lobe of the brain. Middle-ear sepsis can result in temporal lobe or cerebellar abscess, but it should not be overlooked that dental sepsis, particularly when associated with periodontal disease, can also cause brain abscess. Intrathoracic sepsis spreads via the bloodstream to the brain producing single or multiple abscesses typically in the distribution of the middle cerebral artery. Brain abscess may present with symptoms and signs of raised intracranial pressure, focal neurological deficit or epilepsy.

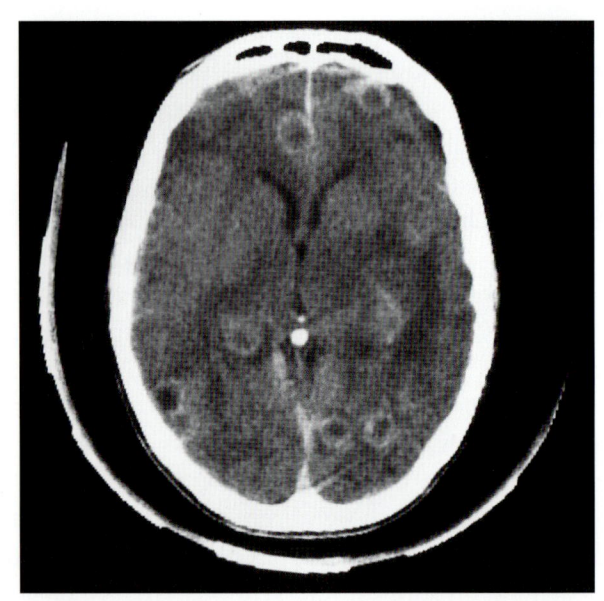

Figure 51.2 This computed tomography scan shows multiple ring-enhancing lesions which were cerebral abscesses. The patient was immunocompromised and had severe dental sepsis and periodontal disease.

Subdural empyema is a serious condition with a high mortality even in normal individuals, but in the post transplant patient the situation is far more serious. Typically, the patient presents with a toxic state with epilepsy, often status epilepticus and dysfunction affecting an entire cerebral hemisphere.

A patient suspected of intracranial sepsis should have a computed tomography head scan with and without contrast and, assuming no mass lesion is identified and there is a high index of suspicion that meningitis is present, a lumbar puncture should be carried out. Measurements of cerebrospinal fluid (CSF) pressure as well as the cellular and glucose content of the CSF should be made. If an intracranial abscess or subdural empyema are shown on the scan, urgent neurosurgical referral is required. The principles of management are drainage of the pus, and high-dose triple antibiotic therapy until the identity and sensitivities of the organism are established, whereupon the antibiotic regime is tailored to the organism or organisms that have been isolated. Sometimes, in the presence of small multiple abscesses, it is difficult to obtain material for microbiological evaluation, in which case the abscesses are treated conservatively with high-dose antibiotic therapy and sequential scanning to assess the effectiveness of the treatment. In some circumstances, if a small deep-seated abscess is present, it can be aspirated stereotactically and material can be retrieved for microbiological assay.

Subdural empyema is treated by craniotomy and thorough irrigation of the subdural space so that all pus and necrotic material are washed out. The patient is given triple antibiotic therapy, usually consisting of benzylpenicillin, metronidazole and chloramphenicol or ciprofloxacin until the sensitivities of the organism are known.

Although patients undergoing stem-cell transplantation are vulnerable to pyogenic infections, one of the main concerns when neurological deterioration develops is whether they are developing an exotic opportunistic infection. A considerable degree of expertise has been gained in the management of these conditions, chiefly due to experience with the acquired immune deficiency syndrome (AIDS) [2]. It should be appreciated that not only can infective problems occur in immunocompromised patients which may be viral, bacterial, fungal or protozoal, but also malignant lymphoma enters into the differential diagnosis of those presenting with mass lesions. It is useful to categorize lesions into diffuse and focal pathology.

Focal lesions

Toxoplasmosis may be seen in immunocompromised patients after stem-cell transplantation. Toxoplasmosis is due to infestation with the parasite *Toxoplasma gondii*. Lesions in the brain are usually multiple, though occasionally they may be solitary (Figure 51.3).

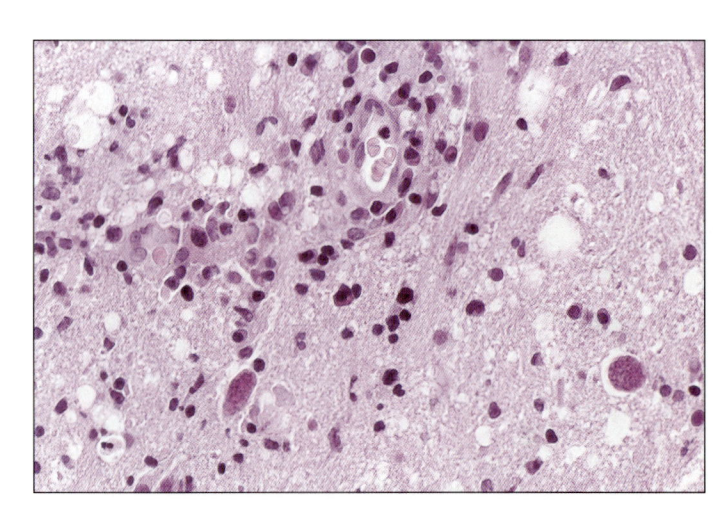

Figure 51.3 Toxoplasmosis. This section shows a mixed, predominantly chronic, inflammatory infiltrate around small vessels with two cysts filled with cystozoites. (Haematoxylin & Eosin, original magnification × 130.)

Patients classically present with headache, confusion, seizures, fever and focal neurological deficit.

Lymphoma may be responsible for between 10 and 25% of mass lesions in patients who are immunocompromised or who have undergone stem-cell transplantation. It may be primary in origin or secondary to systemic lymphoma which may have developed as a second tumour or be part of the original disease process [3]. The most common lymphoma seen intracranially is a high-grade B-cell non-Hodgkin's type (Figure 51.4). Again, patients tend to present with confusion, focal deficit and epilepsy.

Progressive multifocal leukoencephalopathy is probably the third most common condition seen in patients who are immunocompromised. The disease is caused by the JC virus which is a double-stranded DNA papovavirus. The virus causes focal areas of demyelination (Figure 51.5) and this usually becomes clinically apparent with dementia, blindness and focal neurological deficit.

Infection with *Cryptococcus neoformans* is another possibility to be borne in mind in immunocompromised patients. This argyrophilic capsulated yeast can cause a meningitis and cases of cerebral abscess have been described.

Other mass lesions seen in immunocompromised patients include tuberculomas (Figure 51.6) and atypical mycobacterial infections. It should also be appreciated that areas of focal cerebral infarction can be seen following attacks of meningitis which may lead to endarteritis obliterans of small perforating arteries. Metastatic disease from the original pathology or leukaemic relapse for which the stem-cell transplantation was carried out must also enter into the differential diagnosis.

The management of focal lesions in immunocompromised patients is difficult and challenging. Experience both from human

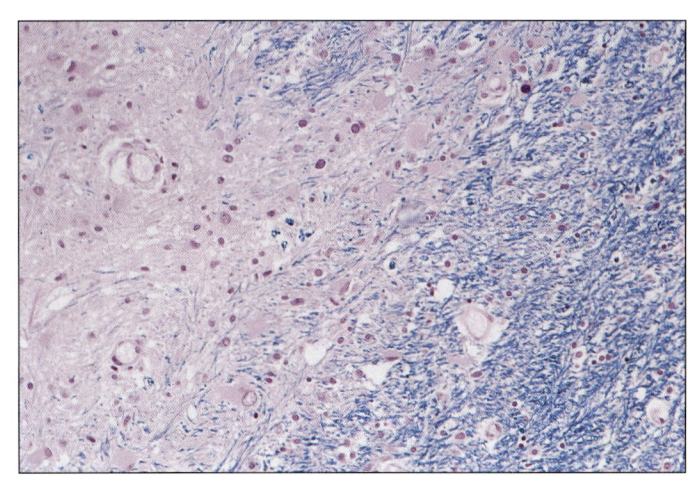

Figure 51.5 Progressive multifocal leukoencephalopathy. This section shows an area of demyelination which is associated with large atypical astrocytes and (top right) oligodendroglial basophilic inclusions which obliterate the normal nuclear pattern. (Haematoxylin & Eosin, counter-stained with Luxol Fast Blue, original magnification × 52.)

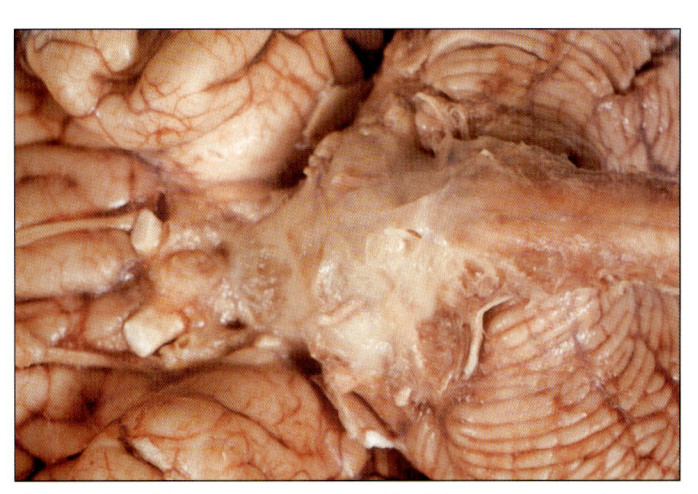

Figure 51.6 Tuberculous meningitis. This specimen shows a predominantly basal exudate which fills the subarachnoid space and encases the basal vessels.

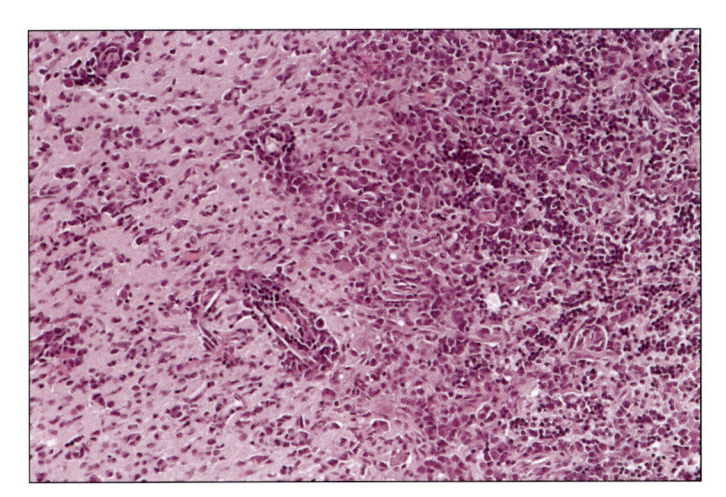

Figure 51.4 High-grade malignant lymphoma of the CNS. This section shows malignant lymphoid cells which are infiltrating the adjacent brain with a perivascular and interstitial pattern. The large malignant cells contrast with the associated (reactive) infiltrate of small lymphocytes. (Haematoxylin & Eosin, original magnification × 52.)

immunodeficiency virus (HIV) and transplant patients has shown that the outcome is unfavourable, irrespective of pathology in patients in poor clinical and immunological condition at presentation. Experience has shown that if computed tomography scanning reveals an enhancing lesion it is appropriate to administer a seven- to ten-day course of antitoxoplasmal therapy. The computed tomography scan is then repeated and if partial resolution has not occurred, stereotactic biopsy is undertaken if at all feasible. Non-enhancing focal lesions generally do not require biopsy. Cerebral toxoplasmosis can be treated medically with sulphadiazine and pyrimethamine, with the possible addition of clindamycin. Steroids such as dexamethasone can be employed if there is marked surrounding oedema associated with such a focal lesion, but they are not recommended as a first line of therapy. Stereotactic biopsy is not recommended when lesions fail to resolve with antitoxoplasmal therapy and a diagnosis of cerebral lymphoma is suspected.

In skilled neuropathological hands, the diagnostic yield from stereotactic biopsy specimens is high (Figures 51.7a,b) and the differentiation of infective from non-infective pathologies is usually possible. Primary cerebral lymphoma is associated with a poor prognosis and the mean survival without treatment ranges from six weeks to six months. Factors which adversely affect the prognosis include multicentric origin, meningeal or periventricular location and histological features indicative of high-grade malignancy. Tumours of low grade such as centroblastic/centrocytic lymphomas have a better prognosis than the higher-grade lesions. Lymphoma is very responsive to radiotherapy, but full doses of treatment may not be possible following intensive preparative regimens. Whole brain radiotherapy is recommended in view of the frequency of multicentric origin, and this can be combined with cytotoxic chemotherapy [4,5].

Diffuse lesions

Cerebral atrophy may be seen in patients who have undergone stem-cell transplantation. Infection with cytomegalovirus (CMV) can produce diffuse cerebral atrophy. Atrophy may also be seen with non-viral infections such as chronic cryptococcal meningitis. The presence of diffuse, poorly defined areas of low attenuation on computed or high signal T2-weighted magnetic resonance imaging are usually attributable to viral infection.

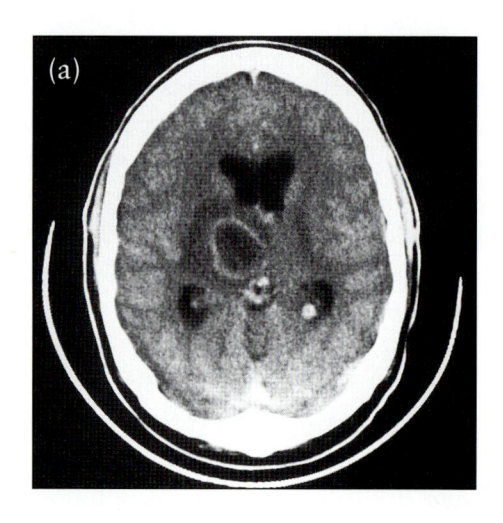

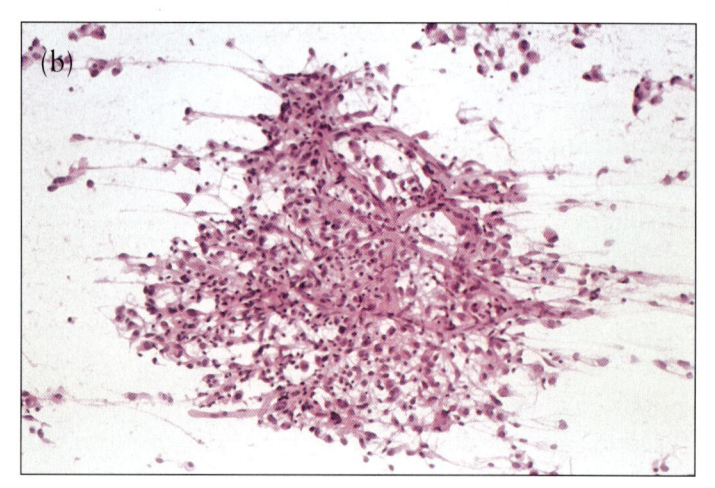

Figure 51.7 (a) This contrast-enhanced computed tomography scan shows a lesion in the thalamus which was thought to represent an abscess. A stereotactic biopsy was performed. (b) A smear was made of the biopsy specimen which proved diagnostic and shows a gemistiocytic astrocytoma rather than an abscess in this immunosuppressed patient. (Haematoxylin & Eosin, original magnification × 250.)

Distinguishing original disease recurrence from complications of transplantation

Many aspects of this complex problem have been discussed in the section above and it will have been appreciated that stereotactic biopsy of mass lesions may provide not only a safe but also an accurate diagnostic tool to help in such situations. Despite this, many neurological problems may arise in transplant patients of which clarification proves to be extremely difficult and challenging. A structured approach to the analysis of the problem coupled with a sound knowledge of the mechanisms by which malignant diseases and their treatment may affect the central and peripheral nervous systems is essential. Close cooperation with neurological and neurosurgical colleagues is essential as it is difficult for the stem-cell transplant physician to be conversant with all the nuances of neurological disorders.

It should be remembered that paraneoplastic phenomena may result in neurological disorders in such patients. Paraneoplastic cerebellar degeneration is recognized in Hodgkin's disease and a paraneoplastic neuropathy can occur as a complication of bronchogenic carcinoma as well as with ovarian cancer [6,7].

Guillain–Barré syndrome with its acute sensory and motor neuropathy can occur with Hodgkin's disease, certain solid tumours, chronic lymphocytic leukaemia [8] and after stem-cell transplantation [9].

In conditions where there may be a paraproteinaemia such as in multiple myeloma and Waldenstrom's macroglobulinaemia, a peripheral neuropathy may occur [10]. It has been shown that the paraprotein will usually have antibody activity against carbohydrate epitopes shared by the peripheral nerve myelin glycolipid sulphated glucuronyl paragloboside and the CNS and peripheral nerve glycoprotein myelin-associated glycoprotein [11].

It should not be forgotten that peripheral nerve and plexus problems that may be seen in this group of patients may be attributable to the effects of radiation which was used in the management of the original disease [12]. It is unusual for such problems to develop until at least six months after radiotherapy, and it can be very difficult to distinguish problems of this nature from neoplastic infiltration of the involved nerves. The symptoms of radiation-induced damage tend to be insidious and hence the appearance of a rapidly progressive problem usually portends a neoplastic aetiology [13].

Unfortunately, despite sophisticated imaging techniques and methods of assay such as the polymerase chain reaction (PCR), neurological problems in patients who have undergone stem-cell transplantation may remain undiagnosed during life. In such circumstances, if a fatal outcome ensues, a careful neuropathological autopsy can provide important information which may facilitate diagnosis during life in similar cases (Figure 51.8).

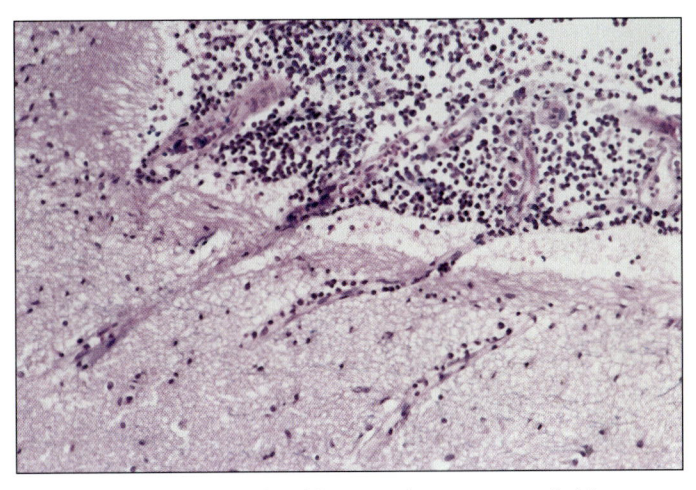

Figure 51.8 Meningeal infiltration by acute myeloblastic leukaemia. Abnormal myeloid cells fill the subarachnoid space and extend for varying distances around penetrating pial vessels. It was thought that this patient, who had undergone marrow transplantation, was disease-free but he was suffering from progressive cranial nerve palsies. (Haematoxylin & Eosin/Luxol Fast Blue.)

References

1. Donaghy MJ. Selected side-effects: 18. Vincristine and neuropathies. *Prescribers' J* 1996; **36**: 116–119.
2. Viswanathan R, Ironside J, Bell JE, Brettle RP and Whittle IR. Stereotaxic brain biopsy in AIDS patients: does it contribute to patient management? *Br J Neurosurg* 1994; **8**: 307–311.
3. Parekh HC, Sharma RR, Lynch PG, Keogh AJ and Prabhu SS. Primary cerebral lymphoma: report of 24 patients and review of the literature. *Br J Neurosurg* 1992; **6**: 563–573.
4. Hochberg FH and Miller DC. Primary central nervous system lymphoma. *J Neurosurg* 1988; **68**: 835–853.
5. Neuwelt EA, Balaban E, Diehl J *et al*. Successful treatment of primary central nervous system lymphomas with chemotherapy after osmotic blood–brain barrier opening. *Neurosurgery* 1983; **12**: 662–671.
6. Horwich MS, Cho L, Porro RS and Posner JB. Subacute sensory neuropathy: a remote effect of carcinoma. *Ann Neurol* 1977; **19**: 2–7.
7. Hammack J, Kotanides H, Rosenblum MK and Posner JB. Paraneoplastic cerebellar degeneration. II. Clinical and immunologic findings in 21 patients with Hodgkin's disease. *Neurology* 1992; **42**: 1938–1943.
8. Currie S, Henson RA, Morgan HG and Poole AJ. The incidence of non-metastatic neurological syndromes of obscure origin in the reticuloses. *Brain* 1970; **93**: 629–641.
9. Perry A, Mehta J, Iverson T, Treleaven J and Powles R. Guillain-Barré syndrome after bone marrow transplantation. *Bone Marrow Transplant* 1994; **14**(1): 165–169.

10. Kyle RA and Dyck PJ. Neuropathy associated with the monoclonal gammopathies. In: *Peripheral Neuropathy*. PJ Dyck and PK Thomas (eds), 1993: 1275–1287 (Philadelphia: WB Saunders).
11. Willison HJ, Trapp BD, Bacher JD, Dalakas MC, Griffin JW and Quarles RH. Demyelination induced by intraneural injection of human anti-MAG antibodies. *Muscle Nerve* 1988; **11**: 1169–1176.
12. Thomas PK and Holdorff B. Neuropathy due to physical agents. In: *Peripheral Neuropathy*. PJ Dyck and PK Thomas (eds), 1993: 990–1013 (Philadelphia: WB Saunders).
13. Hughes RAC, Britton T and Richards M. Effects of lymphoma on the peripheral nervous system. *J Roy Soc Med* 1994; **87**: 526–530.

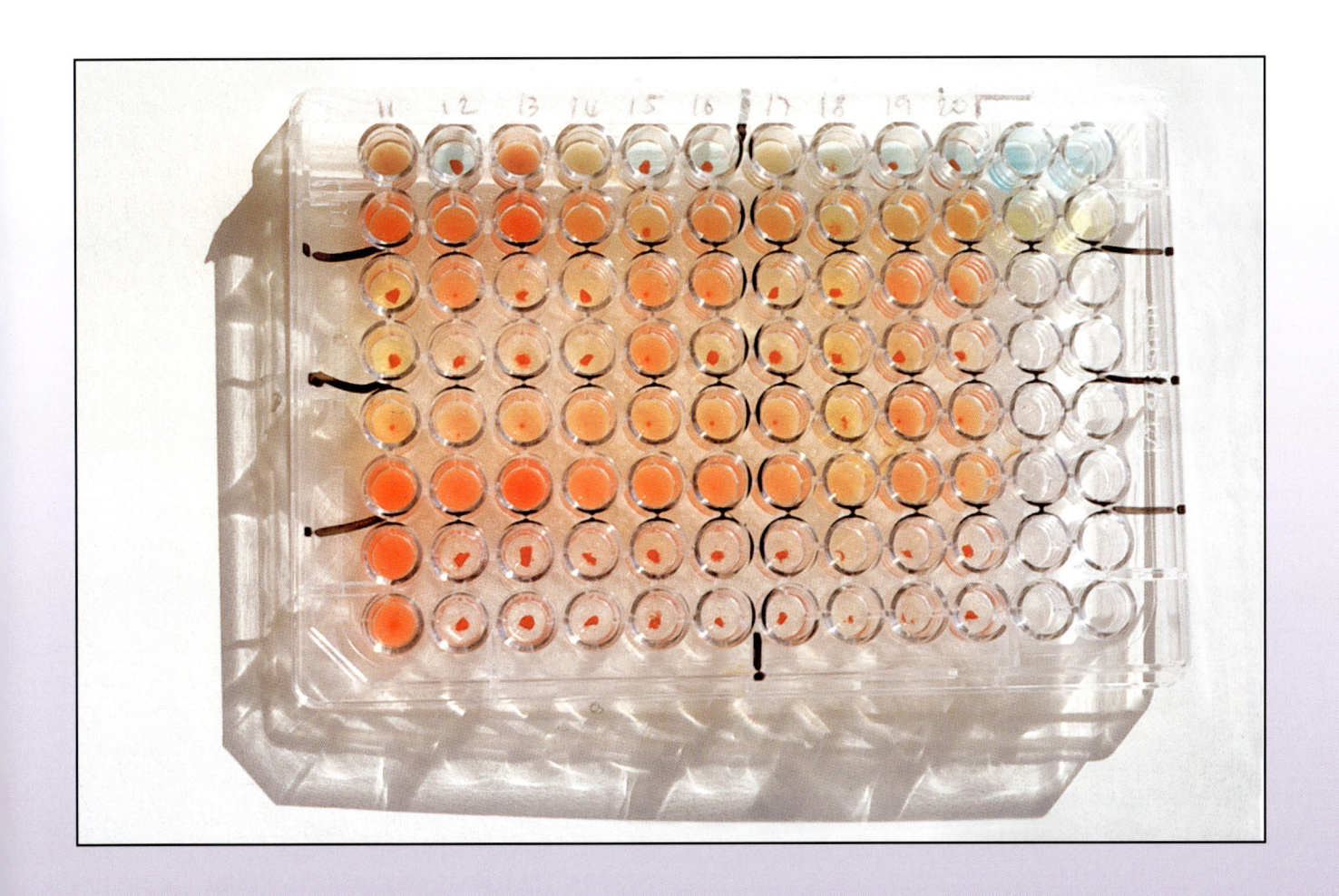

Chapter 52
Blood transfusion support

Mahes de Silva, Marcela Contreras and Ruth Warwick

Introduction

The increasing indications for bone-marrow transplantation (BMT) [1] are having an impact on the higher volume of blood transfusion support required for such patients during the early stages of engraftment. Ensuring the supply of safe products of the highest quality involves the entire process from the recruitment and selection of blood donors, the collection, testing, processing and storage of blood donations, to the final issue of components to hospitals. The concept of total quality management, when applied appropriately in blood transfusion centres, requires that each of these processes, compliant with standards and regulatory affairs, is involved in the delivery of safe products of optimum performance to the bedside. It includes ensuring that patient needs, as determined by clinicians, are prioritized [2].

Despite the fact that blood supplies has never been safer, blood components should only be prescribed when the benefits outweigh the risks, and transfusion policies should constantly be reviewed in the light of new developments which might decrease transfusion requirements. Blood transfusion still carries the following risks:
- infectious complications from those agents for which we routinely screen, such as hepatitis B virus (HBV), hepatitis C virus (HCV), human immunodeficiency virus (HIV), etc. (due to, for example, failure of tests, window period of infectivity), and for those for which we do not test;
- alloimmunization to blood cells with its immunological consequences;
- errors of identification leading to haemolytic transfusion reactions;
- bacterial contamination, especially of platelet concentrates; and
- immune modulation by transfusion.

Blood transfusion support for bone-marrow transplantation has been well reviewed by several authors [3–7].

Red cell transfusions

The greatest need for red blood cell transfusions is during the first four weeks post-BMT with a peak at week 2 and a gradual levelling off thereafter. Generally, red blood cell transfusions are given to maintain a haematocrit of approximately 30% [8].

Wulff *et al.* (1983) [9] showed that the average number of red blood cell units required per adult patient to keep the haematocrit above 25–30% was 9, with a range of 1–82. Factors such as the primary diagnosis, clinical complications and treatment given, influence the red cell support required by each patient. For example, patients with relapsed leukaemia require greater support compared with patients with aplastic anaemia or leukaemia in remission [4]. Delayed or slow engraftment usually increase the period during which red blood cell support is required, and complications such as graft failure, bleeding gastrointestinal ulcers and infections may increase the number of red-blood cell transfusions required. Drug therapy may also have an influence, and patients given cyclosporin A for graft-versus-host disease (GvHD) prophylaxis have been noted to have increased red-blood cell requirements compared to patients given methotrexate [10]. It has been shown that both red-blood cell and platelet requirements increase with the age of the patient. Up to the age of 16 years, body weight is closely related to age, and both platelet and red-blood cell requirements increase with the age of the patient. However, beyond the age of 16 years, patient body weight has a lower predictive value for red blood cell transfusion needs than the age of the BMT recipient [11].

ABO compatibility between donor and recipient

Bone-marrow transplants between human leukocyte antigen (HLA)-matched, ABO incompatible donor–recipient pairs may be undertaken successfully and mixed haematopoietic chimaerism is consistent with long-term graft survival [12]. Donor stem-cell proliferation does not appear to be inhibited by circulating ABO antibodies in the recipient.

ABO blood groups of the donor–recipient pair affect both the selection of the ABO group of blood components for transfusion, and the extent of red blood cell support required. In the Caucasian population, 15–20% of HLA-compatible pairs are ABO-identical and the provision of red blood cell transfusion is straightforward (Table 52.1).

In major ABO incompatibility, anti-A and anti-B of recipient origin may persist in the plasma for some months and the direct antiglobulin test (DAT) may

> **Table 52.1 Red cell transfusion**
>
> - In the Caucasian population 15–20% of HLA-compatible pairs are ABO identical.
> - The lifespan of residual recipient-derived red-blood cells following allogeneic BMT is about 40 days.
> - Circulating recipient-type IgG and IgM have an intrinsic half-life of about 20 days and 6 days, respectively.

become positive after engraftment, when donor-derived incompatible red cells enter the circulation. On the other hand, in minor ABO incompatibility, donor lymphocytes may produce ABO antibodies [13]. In one study, 3 of 5 recipients of minor ABO-incompatible BMT developed ABO haemagglutinins against their inherited red-cell ABO group after an interval of 10–27 months post-BMT.

The lifespan of residual recipient-derived red blood cells following allogeneic BMT is about 40 days [14] and circulating recipient-type IgG and IgM have an intrinsic half-life similar to that of healthy individuals, i.e. about 20 days and 6 days, respectively [15,16]. However, recipient-derived immunoglobulins may persist long beyond their intrinsic half-lives, due to continued synthesis by recipient lymphocytes/plasma cells which survive the conditioning regimen [12]. Thus, two separate immune systems and two separate haematopoietic systems may co-exist in a single host simultaneously and it is not surprising that mismatches mainly in the ABO but also in other blood group systems may lead to adverse interactions.

Major ABO incompatibility

Major ABO incompatibility consists of the presence of ABO antibodies in the BMT recipient directed against ABO antigens on the marrow donor red cells. This combination is seen in 15–20% of HLA-compatible donor–recipient pairs in European Caucasians. There is a risk of haemolysis occurring either at the time of marrow infusion or in the ensuing weeks when engraftment takes place.

Haemolysis at the time of marrow infusion has largely been eliminated as a clinically significant problem by depleting red cells from the bone-marrow harvest [17]. A disadvantage of this type of manipulation is the possible loss of mononuclear cells, including progenitor cells. Another option available, particularly if the recipient ABO antibody titre is very high, is to lower the antibody concentration by either conventional plasma exchange or by the use of an immuno-absorbent column prior to BMT, permitting the marrow to be infused safely without adverse effects.

While immediate haemolysis is not often a problem, delayed haemolytic transfusion reactions may be an important cause of morbidity following ABO-mismatched transplantation and the risk of clinically significant haemolysis has been estimated to be about 10% [12]. Haemolysis may begin either as early as three days' post-BMT or several weeks later when donor-derived red blood cells begin to appear in the circulation. No correlation has been found between the pretransfusion ABO haemagglutinin titre in the recipient and the number of days that ABO antibodies are detected post-transplantation [18].

When immune haemolysis occurs as a result of major ABO incompatibility, additional requirements are only for red cells. In one study, patients who had a major ABO-mismatched BMT and suffered immune haemolysis required a mean of 20 units red blood cells each in the post-transplantation period, compared with a mean of 6 units in patients with compatible BMT [12]. When the ABO haemagglutinin titres are high, there is a slight delay in production of red cells by the graft, although white cell and platelet production appear to be uninhibited. This may be explained by the finding of ABO antigens in 49.5% of BFU-E and 83.5% of CFU-E, as defined by erythroid colony assays [19]. With time, the ABO antibody concentration in the recipient falls, and larger numbers of red cells of donor origin enter and survive in the peripheral circulation. Eventually, the recipient ABO haemagglutinins become undetectable.

Red-cell aplasia following BMT

Rarely, red-cell aplasia may develop following ABO-incompatible BMT. In one study [20], pure red-cell aplasia lasting five to eight months was observed in 3 of 15 consecutive patients receiving HLA-identical but major ABO-incompatible grafts. The recipient's anti-A titre before infusion of the red blood cell depleted bone-marrow harvest was very high in one case, but within the normal range in the two other patients. The decline in haemagglutinin titre which usually occurs during the first four weeks' post-BMT did not occur and the titres rose and remained elevated for 19–28 weeks. Red blood cell engraftment and reticulocyte recovery ultimately occurred spontaneously and coincided with the decrease of haemagglutinin titres to <16. In these patients, the mean red blood cell requirement was 21 units while the mean red blood cell transfusion requirement of patients given ABO-matched grafts was 5.4 units. This phenomenon probably reflects the persistence of functional B-lymphocytes in the recipient, but may also reflect a delay of erythroid engraftment. It appears that cyclosporin A therapy has a potential role in the pathogenesis of pure red blood cell aplasia following ABO-incompatible BMT.

Minor ABO incompatibility

Minor ABO incompatibility is defined as the presence of ABO antigens on the recipient's red cells which are lacking in the donor, who consequently has antibodies against recipient's red cells, i.e. group O donor and group A, B or AB recipient. In general, group O subjects have the strongest ABO antibodies. Minor ABO incompatibility occurs with a frequency of approximately 10–15% of HLA matched donor recipient pairs. In these cases, it is the donor-derived antibodies that influence the outcome and may result in a slightly higher red blood cell requirement as a result of the shortening of the lifespan of recipient red cells. This may happen when engraftment occurs and donor lymphocytes, usually group O, produce ABO antibodies incompatible with the recipient's red blood cells. Usually there is no significant shortening of red blood cell lifespan and when engraftment is successful, recipient red blood cells disappear from the circulation. In these cases, there is no significant delay in marrow engraftment and mortality directly attributable to immunohaematological problems arising from minor ABO incompatibility has not been reported (Table 52.2).

Rh blood groups

Mismatches involving the Rh blood group system do not appear to be associated with impaired engraftment, reduction in overall patient survival or

Table 52.2 Minor ABO incompatibility

- Presence of ABO antigens on *recipient* red cells which are lacking in the donor.
- Thus, *donor* has antibodies against *recipient* red cells (group O *donor* into group A, B or AB *recipient*, or AB *recipient* and group A or B *donor*).
- Group O subjects usually have the strongest ABO antibodies.
- Minor ABO incompatibility occurs in approximately 10–15% of HLA-matched *donor–recipient* pairs.
- When engraftment occurs, *donor* lymphocytes, usually group O, produce ABO antibodies incompatible with the *recipient* red cells.
- There is usually no significant shortening of red-cell lifespan, and no significant delay in marrow engraftment.
- Mortality directly attributable to immunohaematological problems arising from minor ABO incompatibility has not been reported.

increased risk of GvHD [13,14,21]. However, in one report [14] of 4 Rh-positive recipients who received grafts from Rh-negative donors, 2 patients developed anti-D at 12 and 15 weeks following BMT. It is not known whether the Rh-negative donors were previously immunized and whether anti-Rh developed from previously sensitized passenger lymphocytes. Also, both patients received at least four Rh-positive platelet concentrates during the first month post-BMT, which, if red cell contaminated, may have been responsible for the alloimmunization.

Blood grouping and red-blood cell antibody testing

Prior to bone-marrow harvest, the donor's ABO and Rh blood groups should be established and the presence of atypical red cell antibodies excluded. This is important both in case the donor requires red cell transfusions during or after bone-marrow harvesting and also because it influences the selection of blood products for the BMT recipient. (In the UK, about

0.3% of random blood donors and 3% of multiparous women have atypical red-cell alloantibodies in their plasma.)

No compatibility testing is required prior to the transfusion of blood products that contain either no red-blood cells or are only minimally contaminated with such cells. However, when transfusing products such as fresh frozen plasma, platelets and cryoprecipitate, which contain ABO haemagglutinins, selection of the appropriate ABO group is important in order to prevent haemolysis.

Following transplantation, close attention should be paid to the selection of blood components of the most appropriate blood group.

Selection of blood groups of red cells and products for transfusion

Major ABO incompatibility

The potential for haemolysis is greatest when there is major ABO incompatibility. ABO antibodies in the recipient will either destroy or coat donor-derived red blood cells when the DAT may become positive. Following a major ABO-mismatched BMT, the DAT is positive in about 40% of cases [22] but only a minority will experience clinically significant haemolysis. In these cases, red cells compatible with the recipient's ABO group should be given until the recipient-derived ABO antibodies disappear and the DAT becomes negative. This usually takes three to six weeks, following which red cells of the marrow donor type should be transfused. In view of the possibility of ABO antibodies being IgG, pretransfusion compatibility testing of BMT recipients should include an indirect antiglobulin test (IAT).

Plasma-containing blood products should be of the recipient's inherited ABO type until conditioning commences prior to BMT; thereafter plasma components compatible with the donor's ABO type should be selected for transfusion (see Figure 52.1 and Table 52.3).

ABO minor incompatibility

In these cases, either the donor is group O with the recipient being of another ABO group or the recipient is group AB and the donor is either group A or B. Red cells given should be of the donor's ABO type from the time of conditioning prior to transplantation, especially if the donor is group O.

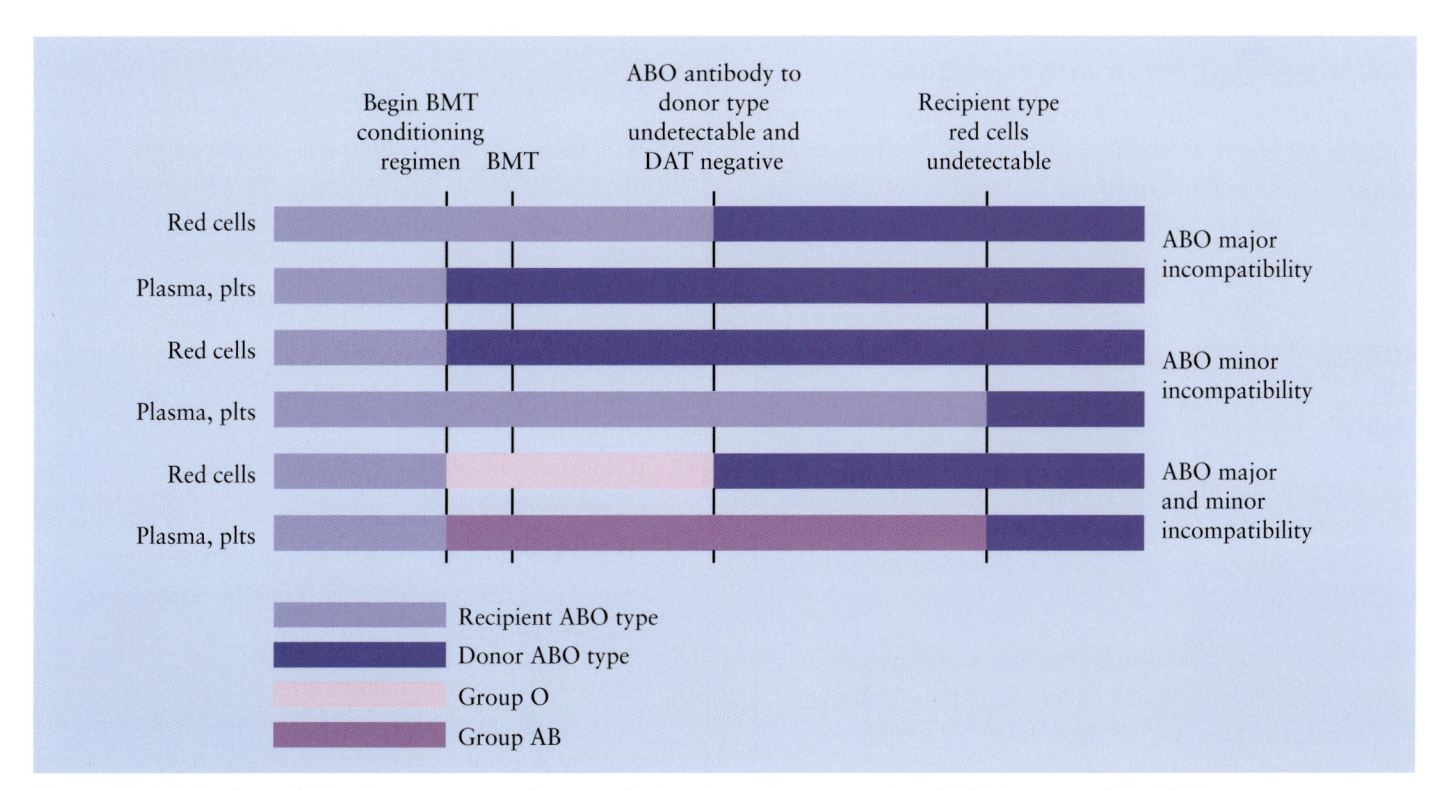

Figure 52.1 Selection of blood components for transfusion in patients receiving ABO-incompatible BMT.

> **Table 52.3 Major ABO incompatibility**
>
> - ABO antibodies in *recipient* either destroy or coat *donor*-derived red cells.
> - Following a major ABO-mismatched BMT, the DAT is positive in about 40% of cases.
> - Only a minority of patients experience significant haemolysis.
> - May take 3–6 weeks, after which red cells of the marrow *donor* type should be transfused.
> - Because ABO antibodies may be IgG, pretransfusion compatibility testing of BMT *recipients* should include an indirect antiglobulin test.
> - Red cells compatible with *recipient* ABO group should be given until the *recipient-derived* ABO antibodies disappear and DAT becomes negative.

Plasma-containing products should be of the recipient's inherited ABO type until engraftment has occurred and recipient red cells are no longer detectable (Table 52.4).

ABO major and minor incompatibility

This occurs when the bone-marrow donor is group A and the recipient group B or vice versa. In these cases, group O red cells should be selected for transfusion from the time of conditioning prior to transplantation until donor ABO antibodies are undetectable and the DAT is negative. Red cells of the donor ABO type should be selected thereafter (Table 52.5).

These patients should receive plasma-containing products of group AB from conditioning up to the time when recipient type red cells are no longer detectable in the circulation. Thereafter, products of the donor ABO type are safe for transfusion.

Selection of Rh blood group

Where there is RhD incompatibility between donor and recipient, Rh-negative blood products should be used to avoid delayed haemolytic transfusion reactions as a result of either the recipient's lymphocytes or donor's grafted lymphocytes producing anti-D (Table 52.6).

The red cells of the donor's group may be detected before the relevant antibody disappears. The recorded hereditary blood group of the recipient should only be

> **Table 52.5 Major and minor ABO incompatiblity**
>
> - Group A *donor* and group B *recipient*, or vice versa.
> - O red cells should be transfused from conditioning until *donor* ABO antibodies undetectable and DAT negative. Red cells of *donor* ABO type should be selected thereafter.
> - AB plasma-containing products should be used from conditioning until *recipient* red cells no longer detectable. Then, products of *donor* ABO type are safe.

> **Table 52.4 Selection of blood products after BMT with major ABO incompatibility**
>
> - Appropriate ABO group of fresh frozen plasma, platelets and cryoprecipitate (which contain ABO haemagglutinins) should be selected to prevent haemolysis.
> - These should be of the *recipient's* inherited ABO type until conditioning commences prior to BMT; then plasma components compatible with *donor* ABO type should be used.

> **Table 52.6 Selection of Rh blood group**
>
> - Differences in donor and recipient unlikely to be clinically significant.
> - Occasional development of anti-D reported in D-negative recipients, but they had also received D-positive platelets.
> - Where RhD incompatibility exists, Rh-negative blood products should be used to avoid possible delayed haemolytic transfusion reactions.

changed when the relevant ABO antibody can no longer be detected in the recipient's serum by an indirect antiglobulin test (IAT) and the DAT is negative.

Platelet transfusion support

The quality of platelet concentrates for transfusion has improved significantly in recent years. Processing methods are designed to reduce or deplete the white-cell content, thus reducing metabolic activity, avoiding the consequent deleterious decrease in pH, which is damaging to platelet viability. A lower white cell content also leads to a reduction in the release of proteolytic enzymes and cytokines from leukocytes. An additional benefit of leukoreduction and leukodepletion is the decrease in transmission and reactivation of viruses with strong affinity for leukocytes, such as cytomegalovirus (CMV), Epstein–Barr virus (EBV), human T-cell lymphotrophic virus (HTLV) and HIV. Moreover, allogeneic leukocytes lead to an *in vivo* mixed leukocyte reaction which might trigger the activation of latent viruses in host leukocytes (Table 52.7). Current plastic containers for platelet concentrates have high permeability, increasing oxygen availability, thus maintaining the oxidative phosphorylation of platelets during storage and avoiding a drop in pH. Well temperature-controlled (20–22°C) agitating incubators allow optimal storage of platelet concentrates for five days (Table 52.8).

The outcome of platelet transfusions should be monitored routinely in BMT patients. As a minimum, platelet counts 1 hour or 24 hours post-transfusion should be examined. Several formulas are used, which take into consideration the number of platelets administered as a dose, and the body surface area or blood volume of the recipient. The outcome is expressed as a percentage of platelets recovered in the circulation or as an increment per 10^{11} platelets transfused. The post-transfusion platelet increment used in calculating the percentage platelet recovery or corrected count increment (CCI) is determined by subtracting the pretransfusion platelet count from the platelet count 10 minutes, 1 hour or 24 hours post-transfusion. A CCI at 1 hour of <7.5, a platelet recovery <20% at 1 hour or a CCI at 24 hours of <4.5 are considered failures of platelet transfusion therapy.

In the 1980s, it was not unusual for the recipient of an HLA-identical or a one-antigen mismatched marrow transplant to receive a mean of 44 or 80 doses of platelet concentrates, depending upon the centre [9,10]. Patients with aplastic anaemia or acute lymphoblastic leukaemia particularly required support in the first month after transplantation and this increased with the age of the patient. In addition, the GvHD prophylaxis regimen, acute GvHD itself, HLA matching, the rate of engraftment and high-risk malignancies, all influenced the degree of platelet transfusion support needed [7]. The impact of granulocyte colony-stimulating factor (G-CSF) mobilized peripheral blood stem cells (PBSC) has diminished the requirements for platelet support in the autograft [23] and sibling allogeneic setting [24] and may impinge upon the unrelated PBSC setting if the use of G-CSF becomes permitted by unrelated donor

---

Table 52.7 Reduction of white cells from platelets

- Reduces metabolic activity, avoiding the decrease in pH, which is damaging to platelet viability.
- Lower white-cell content reduces release of proteolytic enzymes and cytokines from leukocytes.
- Decreases transmission and reactivation of viruses with affinity for leukocytes (CMV, EBV, HTLV, HIV).
- Allogeneic leukocytes lead to an *in vivo* mixed leukocyte reaction which might trigger activation of latent viruses in host leukocytes.

Table 52.8 Platelet storage

- Plastic containers have high permeability, increasing oxygen availability and thus maintaining oxidative phosphorylation of platelets during storage and avoiding a drop in pH.
- Temperature-controlled (20–22°C) agitating incubators allow optimal storage of platelet concentrates for 5 days.

registries. The benefits extend to reduced donor exposure and systems savings [25]. However, there are also concerns regarding long-term safety of G-CSF administration and the need for central lines for effective apheresis of PBSC in a number of donors [26].

It is likely that thrombopoietin will further reduce, although not abolish, the need for platelet support in the future [27].

Platelet transfusion trigger

The prophylactic support of patients with bone-marrow failure prevents lethal haemorrhage but sometimes results in unnecessary transfusion with the concomitant infectious and immunological risks, in addition to cost implications. As early as 1962, it was demonstrated that there was a relationship between the platelet count and risk of haemorrhage, but no threshold was determined [28]. The threshold at which platelet support is traditionally given is based upon historical practice rather than evidence. In the 1980s, most BMT centres in the UK and in USA used platelet counts of 20 or 30×10^9/litre as the platelet transfusion trigger. In 1987, a US National Institutes of Health (NIH) consensus conference suggested that factors other than the platelet count were relevant to platelet transfusion [29]. A study in 1992 suggested 5×10^9/litre as a safe transfusion trigger for induction in acute myeloid leukaemia [20], but a subsequent study discriminated between stable patients in whom a trigger of 10×10^9/litre was used and those with a consumptive state due to factors such as fever, disseminated intravascular coagulopathy (DIC), and drug-induced antibodies, in whom a trigger of 20×10^9/litre was maintained [30]. Using these triggers, fewer platelet concentrates were used overall and there was no significant difference between the study group and a retrospective control group.

The issue of prophylactic platelet transfusions versus platelet transfusions on demonstrable clinical need has been discussed [31] with the conclusion, by some, that production-related thrombocytopenia should be treated with transfusion at platelet levels below 5×10^9/litre; clinical judgement should be used to assess the bleeding for counts between 5 and 10×10^9/litre. When dysfunction of platelets leads to bleeding, then the cause, such as drug-induced thrombocytopenia, should be addressed. Platelet transfusions should be administered until the underlying cause of the platelet dysfunction can be eliminated.

HLA immunization

Traditional platelet concentrate production technology from whole blood donations involved the preparation of platelet-rich plasma (PRP) by centrifugation. This method is still used in several countries, including the USA. New, more efficient techniques for the preparation of platelet concentrates, particularly those which use pooled buffy coat layers as a source of platelet concentrates, are now available. With these new techniques, the number of donations required for a pool with an adult dose of $2.5-3 \times 10^{11}$ platelets has decreased from a standard six or eight to just four, with resultant reduction in the donor exposure rate. Another advantage of this technology is reduced levels of contaminating white cells to about 0.08×10^9 per pooled platelet concentrate compared with about 0.24×10^9 per pool of six concentrates obtained by the original PRP method.

Alloimmunization to major histocompatibility complex (MHC) antigens is not uncommon; it is due to the presence in blood components of antigen-presenting cells carrying class II HLA antigens [32]. Hence, significant reduction in the numbers of white cells in cellular blood components has led to a lower incidence of HLA immunization, and consequently, less refractoriness to platelet transfusions. HLA immunization is considerably more frequent than immunological refractoriness; for example, 30–35% of patients in BMT centres supplied by the North London Blood Centre have HLA antibodies, yet only 6–8% become immunologically refractory to platelet transfusions. This low figure is attributed to the low white-cell content of the platelet pools obtained by the buffy-coat or 'top and bottom' methodology. It is known that significant leukodepletion of red-blood cell and platelet concentrates can delay, and possibly prevent, alloimmunization [33,34]. Platelets themselves do not carry HLA class II antigens and are therefore unable to induce primary HLA immunization. White-cell contamination can be reduced to less than 5×10^6 per unit by leukodepletion with third-generation filters or by collecting platelets by apheresis with the new COBE – LRS (leukoreduction system) system. It has been stated that prevention of alloimmunization by leukodepletion improves the post-transfusion platelet increment when concomitant clinical factors known to reduce the platelet increment are absent [35]. In one prospective randomized study, the difference in HLA alloimmunization was considerable between patients who received routine versus leukodepleted random platelet and red-cell concentrates, with a rate of 46% compared with 11%, respectively [36]. In another prospective study, alloimmunization was shown to be dramatically reduced to 3%, by prestorage leukodepletion of red-cell and platelet concentrates for multitransfused patients with bone-marrow failure without a prior history of sensitization, and to 31% in patients with previous sensitizing events [37]. Leukodepletion did not prevent secondary HLA alloimmunization or refractoriness in another study of patients who had received previous blood transfusions or who had been pregnant [38].

No clear clinical benefit was obtained when filtration was undertaken at the bedside [39] because in this setting little control of the filtration process can be exerted and the age of the products to be filtered is uncontrolled. Quality assurance of the entire process of filtration is required, including counting of residual white cells in all filtered components during the validation process, or alternatively, by using statistical process control methods; neither technique can be applied to bedside filtration. In animal studies, it seems that delayed filtration increases the likelihood of inducing refractoriness, perhaps as a result of releasing soluble antigens or microparticles into the plasma [40]. However, it is unlikely that this mechanism operates in humans, as soluble HLA antigens cannot induce primary immunization.

Another benefit of prestorage filtration lies in the prompt removal of white cells which would otherwise release cytokines and may result in febrile transfusion reactions [41,42]. Indeed, the supernatants of stored platelet concentrates have been shown to lead to reactions in recipients and this was related to the level of white-cell contamination of the concentrates [43]. Alternative techniques to prevent HLA alloimmunization have been attempted, such as ultraviolet (UVB) irradiation of platelet concentrates but, so far, have been found to be impractical or ineffective [44].

In acute myeloid leukaemia, it has been suggested that leukocyte depletion of blood components has favourable effects on the recovery of haematopoiesis, on the requirement for the transfusion of blood components, on the occurrence of serious infections and on relapse-free survival [45]. These claims require further investigation.

Immunological refractoriness to platelet transfusions

Platelet transfusion refractoriness is the failure to achieve adequate response to platelet transfusion on at least two consecutive occasions. It is not uncommon and it may be due to: (i) poor quality of platelet concentrates (insufficient numbers, non viable platelets due to poor storage conditions, etc.); (ii) non-alloimmune mechanisms (splenomegaly, DIC, fever/infection, drug-induced antibodies, platelet autoantibodies, circulating immune complexes) and alloimmune mechanisms (mostly HLA class I antibodies, but occasionally antibodies to human platelet antigens (HPA) and ABO antibodies). In one series, refractoriness to platelet transfusions was present in 44% consecutive patients with haematological malignancies, and 88% of these occurred in the presence of non-immune causes but were present in combination with immune causes in 21%. Alloimmune causes alone were present in 25% of unsuccessful platelet transfusions [46]. It is unusual for HLA alloantibodies to develop before 10–14 days after the first alloantigen exposure and it is more common for alloimmunization to develop in patients with aplastic anaemia than in those with acute leukaemia [2]; the difference is perhaps related to the presence or absence of immunosuppressive therapy.

Demonstration of an alloimmune aetiology for platelet transfusion refractoriness revolves around the detection by lymphocytotoxicity of HLA antibodies in the context of clinical refractoriness. In general, such antibodies have a broad HLA specificity, although usually more potent antibodies with an underlying, narrower specificity can be found. However, some weaker, non-complement-fixing HLA antibodies have been associated with refractoriness; they may only be demonstrable by antiglobulin-based methods such as enzyme-linked immunoassays [47], or by lymphocyte immunofluorescence. Immunological refractoriness may occasionally be related to platelet-specific antibodies such as anti-HPA-1a [49] and ABO antibodies may also play a role [50]. Patients receiving only ABO-matched platelets have a lower incidence of refractoriness [51] and it has been suggested that circulating immune complexes may be associated with ABO-incompatible platelet transfusions, which would lead to the destruction of platelets as innocent bystanders [52]. Antibodies to plasma proteins have also been associated with platelet refractoriness [53].

If patients have clinical bleeding, or very low platelet counts unresponsive to random platelet transfusions on at least two occasions, in the presence of HLA antibodies, it is likely that they will benefit from the provision of HLA-matched platelets. Patients on prophylactic platelet transfusion regimes who are confirmed to be immunologically refractory will also require HLA-matched platelet transfusions. This requires the use of an extensive HLA-typed apheresis donor panel where HLA class I homozygous donors are particularly useful. In London, a panel of over 3000 HLA-typed regular apheresis donors is used, and in The Netherlands a national panel of nearly 20 000 HLA-typed donors is available for this purpose. HLA-C and -DR are irrelevant since they are not expressed or are only weakly expressed on platelets. In any case, a large number of HLA-typed donors is needed and the judicious use of intelligently mismatched platelets utilizing cross-reactive class I antigens to find matches may widen the pool of available donors. Knowledge of the degree of expression of different HLA class I antigens on platelets is also useful. However, even with good HLA matches, increments may not be seen, either because of the concomitant presence of non-immune refractoriness or because of platelet-specific antibodies [54] or cross-reacting HLA antibodies to public HLA determinants. Cross-matching by a variety of techniques, such as a solid-phase platelet adherence method, against a panel of random platelet concentrates may enable compatible units to be identified when no HLA-typed apheresis donor panel is available, or for patients in whom either the HLA type cannot be identified or who have such unusual HLA types that matches cannot be found [55].

It is essential to monitor the effectiveness of such specialist support with platelet increment studies. These identify donors whose platelet transfusions give rise to optimal increments, or conversely, those where no beneficial effect can be seen. Some patients may bleed even with matched platelet transfusions and in these circumstances very large doses of platelets may be necessary [56]. In addition, the immune status of the patient may change with time, with up to 42% of patients losing their HLA antibodies over time and having no further need for matched platelets. This may be the result of the development of anti-idiotypic antibodies which downregulate the HLA alloimmune response [57]. It is therefore recommended that HLA antibodies in refractory patients are monitored on a monthly basis.

Apheresis platelets (single donor platelet; SDP)

Platelets from single donors have certain advantages, mainly in reducing allogeneic donor exposure and probability of bacterial contamination (only one venepuncture required). Some apheresis systems, such as the COBE-Spectra fitted with the LRS meet the criteria for leukodepletion without the need to use leukodepletion filters. If available in stock, single-donor platelet units can be used to screen for cross-match-compatible units for refractory patients and also to screen for HLA-matched units for selected patients. However, SDP are expensive to collect compared with platelets prepared from buffy coats. Both types of preparation, i.e. SDP and buffy coat-derived platelets, contain fewer leukocytes and hence lower cytokine levels, with a lower incidence of febrile transfusion reactions.

Prevention of transfusion-associated cytomegalovirus (CMV) infection

Cytomegalovirus infection is a major cause of morbidity and mortality in bone-marrow transplant patients. Cytomegalovirus does not reside in the plasma in appreciable amounts and infection by transfusion only occurs following transmission by cellular blood components. The virus is presumed to reside in the mononuclear cell fraction but also in granulocytes, and risk of infection is probably related to the number and white cell content of CMV-seropositive products administered. Red cells, platelets and granulocyte concentrates have all been implicated in transfusion-transmitted CMV, while fresh frozen plasma, cryoprecipitate and deglycerolized red cells have not. Transfusion of unscreened cellular components leads to transfusion-transmitted CMV infection in approximately 30% of seronegative BMT recipients [58]. When CMV safe blood products are transfused, the rate of seroconversion drops to approximately 1–3% [59,60] Therefore, it is now standard practice to administer 'CMV-safe' cellular blood products to CMV seronegative bone-marrow transplant recipients of CMV-seronegative BMT.

In the UK, 45–50% of blood donors are CMV seronegative and it is generally possible to satisfy the requirements of patients who need CMV-seronegative cellular blood components. However, elsewhere, where the rate of seropositivity is higher or when the only HLA-matched platelet concentrate required by a refractory CMV-seronegative patient is from a CMV-seropositive donor, other measures should be taken. It has been determined that leukodepletion by filtration is an effective alternative to the use of seronegative blood products for prevention of transfusion-associated CMV infection in BMT recipients [61], and leukodepleted platelet concentrates, with $<1 \times 10^7$ white cells/adult dose should be used in such situations. Leukodepleted platelet concentrates would have the additional benefit of reducing alloimmunization to HLA antigens, thereby postponing or eliminating immunological platelet transfusion refractoriness, as well as preventing febrile reactions. However, white-cell depletion by filtration is very expensive and it is more cost-effective to test routine donors for CMV antibodies. This has the added benefit of the ability to maintain routine stocks of CMV-seronegative red cells. To be safe, filtration procedures must be undertaken in a carefully controlled and validated manner to ensure that $<5 \times 10^6$ leukocytes are present in each dose of platelets. To be effective, this should be undertaken in the laboratory, 6–8 hours after, but within 48–72 hours of donation (prestorage leukodepletion). As stated above, some cell separators provide leukodepleted platelet concentrates, without the need for filtration. White-cell depletion is very expensive; it was estimated in 1993 that the cost of white-blood cell depletion of all cellular blood products by filtration in the UK would be £12 million [62].

Treatment of the febrile neutropenic post-transplant patient

Granulocyte transfusions are used infrequently, partly because of improved antibiotic therapy and alternative therapies involving the administration of intravenous immunoglobulin and the use of recombinant growth factors, but also because of the risks associated with such transfusions. They may induce alloimmunization [63], transmit infection, such as CMV, or result in pulmonary infiltrates, particularly if the recipient has anti-HLA or granulocyte-specific antibodies or if the patient is receiving amphotericin B [64]. If non-irradiated, they may result in transfusion-associated GvHD. However, patients with persistent neutropenia and concomitant infection, unresponsive to therapy, may require granulocyte transfusion support from unrelated donors. Controlled studies of therapeutic granulocyte transfusions in neutropenia have shown that benefit to patients is dependent upon the administration of an adequate dose of white cells [65]. However, the results of such trials have been complicated by antibiotic responses in the control groups. Adequate dosage has been estimated at $2–3 \times 10^{10}$ polymorphonuclear cells per day, with treatment continued until the patient's white-cell count is above 0.5×10^9/litre. These numbers of granulocytes would be present in about 15 units of donated blood. It has therefore been suggested that G-CSF stimulation of donors prior to leukapheresis may be required to provide adequate numbers of cells [66], but this raises ethical issues for those involved in the care of volunteer donors. Strauss surveyed 30 reports in the literature of the use of G-CSF in a variety of different infections. The largest number of evaluable patients were those with bacterial septicaemia, in whom there was an overall 62% treatment success rate. The number of controlled trials using granulocyte transfusions comprised only seven. Among these, three reported success in treatment, two partial success and two reported no success [65]. It has also been suggested, in the context of chronic granulomatous disease, that alloimmunization to HLA or granulocyte-specific antigens may reduce the effectiveness of granulocyte transfusions and that these transfusions should not be used in such circumstances unless matched donors can be found [67].

There are two sources of granulocytes:
- buffy coats from routine donations; and
- leukapheresis of stimulated or unstimulated donors.

The ethics of using G-CSF in normal donors are contentious. Both types of product require irradiation because of the high content of viable lymphocytes and should be transfused as soon as possible after collection. Buffy coats obtained for the production of platelet concentrates, by the semi-automated 'top-and-bottom' system, are rich in granulocytes and platelets. The buffy coats contain 10–20% of red cells present in a single donation and their presence requires cross-matching prior to use. In adults, transfusion of 5 units of buffy coats will increase the patient's haemoglobin by 1 g/litre, thus limiting the usefulness of such components in addition to providing relatively low numbers of white cells and increasing donor exposure and risk of transfusion-transmitted infection. Hence, if therapeutic granulocyte transfusions are needed, these should be supplied as apheresis concentrates and in adequate doses for the appropriate length of time [68].

Immunotherapy of malignancy

It is anticipated that there will be a significant increase in the need for a new component for cancer therapy in the form of white cells for passive immune therapy to enhance the antileukaemic effect of the graft [69,70]. There have now been more than 250 transplant recipients who have relapsed and who have been treated with donor white-cell transfusions [71]. The highest response rates have been seen in chronic myeloid leukaemia, and lymphocyte infusions might even benefit recipients who have not undergone a previous transplant procedure [69]. In addition, infusions of donor leukocytes have been used to treat EBV virus-associated lymphoproliferative disease after bone-marrow transplantation [72], raising the ethical issues of approaching unrelated bone-marrow volunteer donors for a second donation. This also requires a new view of what constitutes a 'blood component'. However, it remains to be shown whether use of these new components results in a balance between GvHD and graft-versus-leukaemia effect which is beneficial.

Transfusion-associated GvHD

Quite apart from the graft-versus-host disease (GvHD) associated with bone-marrow or PBSC transplants, there is the possibility that the immunosuppressed recipient, having undergone total body irradiation and chemotherapy, may develop transfusion-associated GvHD. This disease is a devastating sequel to engraftment of donor lymphocytes contained in blood or blood components and may result in catastrophic bone-marrow hypoplasia with death from infection. It is entirely preventable by gamma-irradiation, which results in chromosomal damage to transfused lymphocytes, thus preventing their proliferation: 25 Gy is the recommended minimum dose for blood components [73]. Ultraviolet irradiation with UVB has been investigated as an alternative to gamma-irradiation, but has not been clinically assessed [74].

Certainly, all patients who have undergone allogeneic or autologous bone-marrow transplantation should receive irradiated cellular components, both in the period prior to stem-cell transplantation and in the post-transplant period. This should be continued at least until immunosuppressive therapy is withdrawn, usually about six months after transplantation, but should be extended if chronic post-transplant GvHD persists. This applies to both the autograft and allograft settings [75]. The effect of 25-Gy gamma-irradiation on platelet viability and function is negligible, but there is a slight reduction in the viability of irradiated red-cell components. The Food and Drug Administration in the USA has recommended that irradiation may be performed at any time following collection, but that the red-cell units should only be used up to a maximum of 28 days from the time of irradiation, or to the end of the unit's normal expiry date, whichever is the shorter. Gamma-irradiation also increases potassium-ion egress from red cells into the supernatant. The level of potassium ions in the red-cell supernatant is approximately double that at any given time for a non-irradiated counterpart. However, the potassium-ion levels are still very tolerable and, except in clinical situations with particular sensitivity to high concentrations of potassium ions, such as renal failure, use of irradiated blood is inconsequential upon recipient potassium-ion load.

Summary

The Blood Transfusion Service has a role to play in the support of patients undergoing bone-marrow transplantation. This includes provision of high-quality, safe blood components, which may be buffy coat or leukocyte depleted, to prevent HLA sensitization, platelet refractoriness or febrile transfusion reactions. Special donor panels are required to provide specific components matched for HLA or platelet antigens. Volume of blood component support for individual patients may diminish with the use of PBSC and recombinant growth factors, especially when the clinical use of thrombopoietin commences. The resultant reduction in donor exposure is to be welcomed. On the other hand, the transfusion service may need to broaden its activities to include procurement of allogeneic lymphocytes or granulocytes for passive immunological treatment of leukaemias and to treat infectious complications of chemotherapy in BMT and PBSC recipients. Testing of blood and stem-cell donors for CMV, or the provision of filtered equivalent 'CMV safe' products is a requirement in the BMT setting. Centralized gamma-irradiation, carefully quality controlled with thermoluminescent dosimetry, documentation and tracking will prevent third-party transfusion-associated GvHD in a cost-effective manner.

References

1. Gratwohl A, Hermans J, Baldomero H, Tichelli A, Goldman JM and Gahrton G. Indications for haemopoietic precursor cell transplants in Europe. *Br J Haematol* 1996; **92**: 35–43.
2. Moss F and Garside P. The importance of quality: sharing responsibility for improving patient care. *Br Med J* 1995; **310**: 996–999.
3. Slichter SJ. Transfusion and bone marrow transplantation. *Transfus Med Rev* 1988; **2**(1): 1–17.
4. Klumpp TR. Immunohematologic complications of bone marrow transplantation. *Bone Marrow Transplant* 1991; **8**: 159–170.
5. McCullough J. The role of the blood bank in transplantation. *Arch Pathol Lab Med* 1991; **115**: 1195–1200.
6. Petz LD. Immunohematologic problems associated with bone marrow transplantation. *Transfus Med Rev* 1987; **1**(2): 85–100.
7. Pihlstedt P, Paulin T, Sundberg B, Nilsson B and Ringdèn O. Blood transfusion in marrow graft recipients. *Ann Haematol* 1992; **65**: 66–70.
8. Bensinger WI. Transfusion support in bone marrow transplantation. Bone marrow transplantation. *Prog Transfusion Med* 1988; **3**: 159–163.
9. Wulff JC, Santner TJ, Storb R et al. Transfusion requirements after HLA-identical marrow transplantation in 82 patients with aplastic anemia. *Vox Sang* 1983; **44**: 366–374.
10. Bensinger W, Petersen FB, Banaji M et al. Engraftment and transfusion requirements after allogeneic marrow transplantation for patients with acute non-lymphocytic leukemia in first complete remission. *Bone Marrow Transplant* 1989; **4**: 409–414.
11. Mehta J, Powles R, Horton C, Milan S, Singhal S and Treleaven J. Relationship between donor–recipient blood group incompatibility and serum bilirubin after allogeneic bone marrow transplantation from HLA-identical siblings. *Bone Marrow Transplant* 1995; **15**: 853–858.
12. Sniecinski IJ, Oien L, Petz LD and Blume KG. Immuno-hematological consequences of major ABO-mismatched bone marrow transplantation. *Transplantation* 1988; **45**(3): 530–534.
13. Hows J, Beddow K, Gordon-Smith E et al. Donor-derived red blood cell antibodies and immune hemolysis after allogeneic bone marrow transplantation. *Blood* 1986; **67**(1): 177–181.
14. Lasky LC, Warkentin PI, Kersey JH, Ramsay NKC, McGlave PB and McCullough J. Hemotherapy in patients undergoing blood group incompatible bone marrow transplantation. *Transfusion* 1983; **23**(4): 277–285.
15. Wells JV and Fridenberg HH. Metabolism of radio-ionated IgG in patients with abnormal serum IgG levels. 1. Hyper-gammaglobulinaemia. *Clin Exp Immunol* 1971; **9**: 761–760.
16. Ho WG, Champlin RE, Feig SA and Gale RP. Transplantation of ABH incompatible bone marrow: gravity sedimentation of donor marrow. *Br J Haematol* 1984; **57**: 155–162.
17. Blacklock HA, Gilmore MJML, Prentice HG et al. ABO-incompatible bone-marrow transplantation: removal of red blood cells from donor marrow avoiding recipient antibody depletion. *Lancet* 1982; **11**: 1061–1064.
18. Gmür JP, Burger J, Schaffner A et al. Pure red cell aplasia of long duration complicating major ABO-incompatible bone marrow transplantation. *Blood* 1990; **75**(1): 290–295.
19. Blacklock HA, Katz F, Michalevicz R et al. A and B blood group antigen expression on mixed colony cells and erythroid precursors: relevance for human allogeneic bone marrow transplantation. *Br J Haematol* 1984; **58**: 267–276.
20. Gmur J, Burger J, Shcanz U, Fehr J and Schaffner A. Safety of stringent prophylactic platelet transfusion policy for patients with acute leukaemia. *Lancet* 1991; **338**: 1223–1226.
21. Berkman EM and Caplan SN. Engraftment of Rh-positive marrow in a recipient with Rh antibody. *Transplant Proc* 1977; **8**(1) (Suppl 1): 215–218.
22. Buckner CD, Clift RA, Sanders JE et al. ABO-incompatible marrow transplants. *Transplantation* 1978; **26**: 233–238.
23. Kessinger A and Armitage JO. The evolving role of autologous peripheral stem cell transplants following high dose therapy for malignancy. *Blood* 1991; **77**: 211–213.
24. Bensinger WI, Weaver CH, Appelbaum FR et al. Transplantation of allogeneic peripheral blood stem cells mobilised by recombinant human granulocyte colony stimulating factor. *Blood* 1995; **85**(6): 1655–1658.
25. Holyoake T and Franklin IM. Bone marrow transplants from peripheral blood. Set to transform medical oncology. *Br Med J* 1994; **309**: 4–5.
26. Anderlini P, Przepiorka D, Seong D et al. Clinical toxicity and laboratory effects of granulocyte colony-stimulating factor (filgrastim) mobilisation and blood stem cell apheresis from normal donors, and analysis of charges for the procedures. *Transfusion* 1996; **36**: 590–595.
27. Kaushansky K. Thrombopoietin: the primary regulator of platelet production. *Blood* 1995; **86**(2): 419–431.
28. Gaydos LA, Freireich EJ and Mantel N. The quantitative relationship between platelet count and hemorrhage in patients with acute leukaemia. *New Engl J Med* 1962; **266**(18): 905–909.
29. Platelet Transfusion Therapy. Consensus Conference. *J Am Med Ass* 1987; **257**: 1777–1780.

30. Gil-Fernandez JJ, Alegre A, Fernandez-Villalta MJ et al. Clinical results of a stringent policy on prophylactic platelet transfusion: non-randomised comparative analysis in 190 bone marrow transplant patients from a single institution. *Bone Marrow Transplant* 1996; **18**: 931–935.
31. Shlicter SJ. Platelet transfusions a constantly evolving therapy. *Thrombosis Haemostasis* 1991; **66**(1): 178–188.
32. Claas FHJ, Smeenk RJT, Schmidt R, van Steenbrugge GJ and Eernisse JG. Alloimmunisation against the MHC antigens etc. *Exp Haematol* 1981; **9**(1): 84–89.
33. Consensus Conference: Leucocyte Depletion of Blood and Blood Components (1993) held at the Royal College of Physicians, Edinburgh, 18–19 March.
34. Heddle NM and Blajchman MA. The leukodepletion of cellular blood products in the prevention of HLA-alloimmunisation and refractoriness to allogeneic platelet transfusions. *Blood* 1995; **85**(3): 603–606.
35. Heddle NM. The efficacy of leukodepletion to improve platelet transfusion response: a critical appraisal of clinical studies. *Transfus Med Rev* 1994; **8**(1): 15–28.
36. van Marjwik Kody M, van Prooijen HC, Moes M, Bosma-Stants I and Akkerman JWN. Use of leukodepleted platelet concentrates for the prevention of refractoriness and primary HLA alloimmunization: a prospective, randomized trial. *Blood* 1991; **77**(1): 201–295.
37. Novotny VMJ, van Doorn R, Witvliet MD, Claas FHJ and Brand A. Occurrence of allogeneic HLA and non-HLA antibodies after transfusion of prestorage filtered platelets and red blood cells. *Blood* 1995; **85**(7): 1736–1741.
38. Sintnicolaas K, van Marwijk Kooij M, van Prooijen HC et al. Leukocyte depletion of random single-donor platelet transfusions does not prevent secondary human leukocyte antigen-alloimmunization and refractoriness: a randomized prospective study. *Blood* 1995; **85**(3): 824–828.
39. Williamson LM, Wimpersis JZ, Williamson P et al. Bedside filtration of blood products in the prevention of HLA alloimmunisation – a prospective randomised study. *Blood* 1994; **83**: 3028–3035.
40. Blajchman MA, Bardossy L, Carmen RA, Goldman M, Heddle NM and Singal DP. An animal model of allogeneic donor platelet refractoriness: the effect of the time of leucodepletion. *Blood* 1992; **79**(5): 1371–1375.
41. Muylle L. The role of cytokines in blood transfusion reactions. *Blood Rev* 1985; **9**: 77–83.
42. Wadhwa M, Seghatchian MJ, Lubenko A et al. Cytokine levels in platelet concentrates: quantitation by bioassays and immunoassays. *Br J Haematol* 1996; **93**: 225–234.
43. Heddle NM, Klama L, Singer J et al. The role of the plasma from platelet concentrates in transfusion reactions. *New Engl J Med* 1994; **331**(10): 625–628.
44. Grijzenhout MA, Aarts-Riemens MI, de Gruijl FR, van Weelden H and van Prooijen HC. UVB irradiation of human platelet concentrates does not prevent HLA alloimmunization in recipients. *Blood* 1994; **84**(10): 3524–3531.
45. Oksanen K and Elonen E. Impact of leucocyte-depleted blood components on the haematological recovery and prognosis of patients with acute myeloid leukaemia. *Br J Haematol* 1993; **84**: 639–647.
46. Doughty HA, Murphy MF, Metcalfe P, Rohatiner AZS, Lister TA and Waters AH. Relative importance of immune and non-immune causes of platelet refractoriness. *Vox Sang* 1994; **66**: 200–205.
47. Brubaker DB and Romine M. Relationship of HLA and platelet reactive antibodies in alloimmunised patients refractory to platelet therapy. *Am J Hematol* 1987; **26**: 341–352.
48. Kickler T, Kennedy SD and Braine HG. Alloimmunisation to platelet specific antigens on glycoproteins IIb–IIIa and Ib/IX in multiply transfused thrombocytopenic patients. *Transfusion* 1990; **30**: 622–625.
49. Ogaswara K, Ueki J, Takenaka M and Furihata K. Study on the expression of ABH antigens on platelets. *Blood* 1993; **82**: 993–999.
50. Heal JM, Rowe JM, McMican A, Masel D, Finke C and Blumberg N. The role of ABO matching in platelet transfusion. *Eur J Haematol* 1993; **50**: 110–117.
51. Heal JM, Masel D, Rowe JM and Blumberg N. Circulating immune complexes involving the ABO system after platelet transfusion. *Br J Haematol* 1993; **85**: 566–572.
52. Heal JM, Cowles J, Masel D, Rowe JM and Blumberg N. Antibodies to plasma proteins. *Br J Haematol* 1992; **80**: 83–90.
53. Evenson DA, Stroncek DF, Pulkrabek EH, Perry J, Radford J, Miller JS and Verfaille C. Post transfusion purpura following bone marrow transplantation. *Transfusion* 1995; **35**: 688–693.
54. O'Connell BA, Lee EJ, Rothko K, Hussein MA and Schiffer A. Selection of histocompatible apheresis platelet donors by crossmatching random donor platelet concentrates. *Blood* 1992; **79**: 527–531.
55. Guidelines for platelet transfusions. British Committee for Standards in Haematology, Working Party of the Blood Transfusion Task Force. *Transfusion Med* 1992; **2**: 311–318.
56. Atlas E, Freedman J, Blanchette V, Kazatchkine MD and Semple JW. Downregulation of the anti-HLA alloimmune response by variable region reactive (anti-idiotypic) antibodies in leukaemic patients transfused with platelet concentrates. *Blood* 1993; **81**(2): 538–542.
57. Hillyer CD, Emmens RK, Zago-Novaretti M and Berkman EM. Methods for the reduction of transfusion-transmitted cytomegalovirus infection: filtration versus the use of seronegative donor units. *Transfusion* 1994; **34**(10): 929–934.
58. Logan S, Barbara K and Kovar I. Cytomegalovirus screened blood for neonatal intensive care units. *Arch Dis Child* 1988; **63**: 753–755.
59. Miller WJ, McCullough J, Balfour HH et al. Prevention of cytomegalovirus infection following bone marrow transplantation: a randomized trial of blood product screening. *Bone Marrow Transplant* 1991; **7**: 227–234.
60. Bowden RA, Slichter SJ, Sayers M et al. A comparison of filtered leukocyte-reduced and cytomegalovirus (CMV) seronegative blood products for the prevention of transfusion-associated CMV infection after marrow transplant. *Blood* 1995; **86**(9): 3598–3603.
61. Smith R. Filtering white cells from blood for transfusion. *Br Med J* 1993; **306**: 810.
62. Applebaum FR, Trapani RJ and Graw RG Jr. Consequences of prior alloimmunisation during granulocyte transfusion. *Transfusion* 1977; **17**(5): 460–464.
63. Wright DG, Robichaud KJ, Pizzo PA and Deisseroth AB. Lethal pulmonary reactions associated with the combined use

of amphotericin B and leukocyte transfusions. *New Engl J Med* 1981; **304**: 1185–1189.

64. Strauss RG. Therapeutic granulocyte transfusion in 1993. *Blood* 1993; **81**(7): 1675–1678.
65. Bensinger WI, Price TH, Dale DC *et al*. The effects of daily recombinant human granulocyte colony-stimulating factor administration on normal granulocyte donors undergoing leukapheresis. *Blood* 1993; **81**: 1883–1888.
66. Stroncek DF, Leonard K, Eiber G, Malek HL, Gallin JI and Leitman SF. Alloimmunisation after granulocyte transfusions. *Transfusion* 1996; **36**: 1009–1015.
67. Kalmin ND and Grindon AJ. Pheresis with the IBM 2997. *Transfusion* 1981; **21**(3): 325–329.
68. Horowitz MM, Gale RP, Sondel PM *et al*. Graft-versus-leukemia reactions after bone marrow transplantation. *Blood* 1990; **75**: 555–562.
69. Kolb JH, Schattenberg A, Goldman JM *et al*. Graft-versus-leukemia effect of donor lymphocyte transfusions in marrow grafted patients. European Group for Blood and Marrow Transplantation Working Party on Chronic Leukemia. *Blood* 1995; **86**: 2041–2050.
70. Gale RP and Butturini A. Cancer treatment in the blood bank: a growth industry? *Transfusion* 1995; **35**: 889–890.
71. Papadopoulos EB, Ladanyi M, Emanuel D *et al*. Infusions of donor leucocytes to treat Epstein–Barr virus associated lymphoproliferative disorders after allogeneic bone marrow transplantation. *New Engl J Med* 1994; **330**: 1185–1191.
72. BCSH Blood Transfusion Task Force: Guidelines on gamma irradiation of blood components for the prevention of transfusion-associated graft-versus-host disease. *Transfusion Medicine* 1996: **6**: 261–271.
73. Oluwole S, Engelstad K and James T. Prevention of graft-versus-host disease and bone marrow rejection: kinetics of induction of tolerance by UVB modulation of accessory cells and T cells in the bone marrow inoculum. *Blood* 1993; **81**: 1658–1665.
74. Williamson LM and Warwick RM. Transfusion-associated graft-versus-host disease and its prevention. *Blood Rev* 1995; **9**: 251–261.

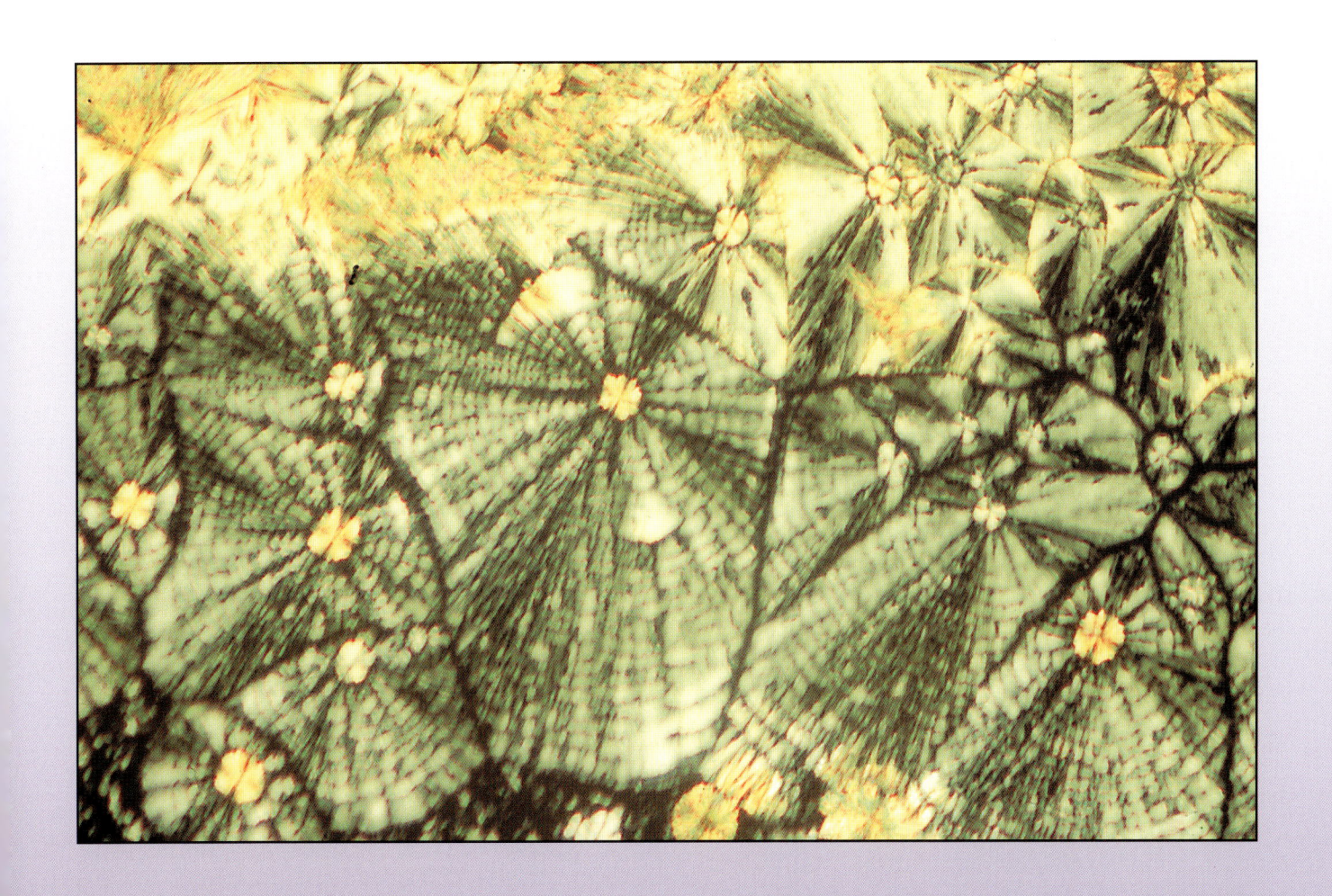

Chapter 53

Nutritional support

Louise Henry and Virginia Souchon

Introduction

Nutrition support is an important part of the care of the patient undergoing bone-marrow transplantation. Deeg et al. [1], in a retrospective review of patient outcomes in relation to body weight, found that underweight patients had a higher mortality in the early post-transplant period. It has also been suggested that weight loss is correlated with protein loss, and weight loss in excess of 15% was associated with objective impairment of several physiological parameters including muscle strength and respiratory function [2]. It is therefore likely that underweight patients would benefit from nutrition intervention prior to transplant and also during the post-transplant period. While most units involved in the treatment of such patients have developed modified low microbial diets and frequently use parenteral nutrition there is little research to support their use [3,4]. Perhaps the most important development in nutrition support for these patients would be the instigation of large, well-designed trials investigating the use of low microbial diets, parenteral nutrition and enteral nutrition.

Nutritional requirements are increased in all patients following conditioning therapy, and the very complications provoking an increased nutritional requirement decrease the patient's desire and ability to eat and drink, i.e. treatment side-effects which include mucositis, anorexia, nausea, vomiting, diarrhoea, malabsorption, infection and graft-versus-host disease (GvHD) [5–7] (see Table 53.1). Active nutritional support is necessary to prevent weight loss and muscle wasting, and to aid full recovery of the haematopoietic and immune systems [8]. Artificial nutrition support such as enteral and parenteral nutrition plays an important role if patients are unable to ingest sufficient fluid and nutrients.

Nutritional assessment and support should be carried out before bone-marrow transplantation (BMT) and continued throughout hospitalization and at subsequent outpatient visits. This ensures the early identification of nutritional problems and hopefully instigation of measures to prevent deterioration in nutritional status.

Issues relating to BMT which may potentially affect nutritional status

Underlying disease

The underlying disease state which has led to the patient undergoing transplantation may influence nutritional requirements. A recent study emphasizes that patients with advanced chronic myeloid leukaemia (CML) can present with anorexia and weight loss [9]. This appears to be in contrast to patients suffering from other haematological malignancies. For such patients, previous chemotherapy regimens leading up to transplantation are likely to have influenced nutritional status. Side-effects of treatment can include prolonged anorexia, diarrhoea, malabsorption, nausea and vomiting, dysgeusia and weight loss. If possible, patients should be given the opportunity to regain nutritional status and physical strength before transplant (Table 53.1).

Cytoreductive treatment and type of transplant

The type of chemotherapy regimen and the use of total body irradiation (TBI) will influence the nature and severity of post-transplant complications and hence may induce adverse effects on nutritional status.

Table 53.1 Issues relating to BMT which may potentially affect nutritional status

Underlying disease/previous treatment
Cytoreductive conditioning
Type of transplant

Gastrointestinal problems
    oral mucositis and oesophagitits
    xerostomia
    altered saliva
    dysgeusia
    nausea and vomiting
    diarrhoea

Graft-versus-host disease
Infection
Psychosocial issues, e.g. depression

Generally, patients receiving TBI experience worse mucositis, more diarrhoea and are at greater risk of developing thickened secretions, all of which can greatly compromise nutritional status [10]. Papadopoulou et al. [11] found that children who received TBI required parenteral nutrition for longer periods and also experienced more significant weight loss than those children receiving chemotherapy only. Patients undergoing allogeneic transplant are also at risk of developing GvHD, which can have very adverse effects on nutritional status [5,6,12,13].

Patients undergoing stem-cell transplants are likely to experience less profound effects on nutritional status because of the shorter recovery period.

Gastrointestinal problems

Gastrointestinal problems occurring as a result of conditioning therapy may be aggravated by the onset of GvHD. Mucositis, xerostomia, altered salivary secretion, oral infections, oesophagitis, dysgeusia, nausea, vomiting and diarrhoea all contribute to morbidity following BMT [13] causing problems with nutrition.

Oral mucositis and oesophagitis

Oral mucositis generally occurs 4–10 days after conditioning therapy [6] and may persist for three to four weeks. Palliative measures such as topical anaesthesia, intravenous narcotic analgesics and meticulous mouth care are used for symptomatic relief. Healing begins with marrow engraftment, complete recovery commonly occurring within 20 days [14]. However, if acute GvHD is present, it may take longer, especially if local infections with bacteria, fungi or viruses occur [13]. Regular mouth care is vital to attenuate these problems [14,15]. Bland, cool, soft foods are best tolerated, and glucose polymers such as Polycose and Maxijul can added to increase the energy density of soft foods. Patients should also be encouraged to take sip feeds such as Ensure Plus, Entera, and Fortisip.

The use of artificial nutrition support should be considered if the patient is likely to have mucositis for more than seven days.

Xerostomia

Decreased salivation occurs after TBI and with the use of anti-emetics. The rate of improvement is very variable. For the majority of patients, saliva production returns to near normal levels within two to three months. However, for some, especially those who have undergone TBI or who have chronic GvHD, it may persist indefinitely [15]. Good oral hygiene is important because the normal cleansing function of saliva is absent. Management of xerostomia includes frequent normal saline rinses and careful tooth brushing using a soft-bristled brush to avoid gum trauma and local infection [13]. Methylcellulose solutions, artificial saliva (e.g. Glandosane), and salivary stimulants in the form of citric acid beverages, sugar-free chewing gum, slices of citrus fruit and boiled sweets may be beneficial [15]. Patients should be encouraged to eat soft, moist foods and to drink with food to avoid 'gagging' while eating. Foods such as bread, cakes and meat seem to be particularly difficult to swallow.

Long-term xerostomia requires regular dental treatment and topical fluoride to prevent or reduce dental decay [13]. Xerostomia often leads to dysgeusia, which can further reduce food intake. For persistently thickened secretions it may be necessary to consider nasogastric or gastrostomy tube feeding.

Total body irradiation can contribute to production of thickened saliva and oral mucous [10]. The condition may be so extreme that intubation is necessary to maintain the airway, particularly in the presence of GvHD. Swallowing such saliva may contribute to nausea and vomiting. Extremely thick saliva usually only persists for two to three weeks after TBI, and resolves with healing of the oral mucosa and marrow engraftment. It may, however, recur with dehydration and certain medications. Early mouth care can help to reduce the severity of this condition. Clear fluids, tea, ice lollies and jellies are best tolerated. Saline rinses before eating and drinking may help. Mouthwashes containing alcohol should be avoided, since they tend to dry and irritate the mucosa [13].

Dysgeusia

A loss or alteration in the sense of taste can severely reduce desire for food [16]. Patients often complain of an unpleasant taste pervading all foods, especially savoury foods. Common causes include TBI, cyclophosphamide, morphine and antibiotics [6,15]. Taste normally recovers within 30–50 days of BMT. Management involves experimenting with spicy, highly flavoured foods (in the absence of mucositis) and emphasizing the other aspects of food including presentation, texture, aroma and colour. Good mouth care is essential.

Oral infections

There is an increased risk of bacterial, fungal and viral infections secondary to neutropenia, mucositis and xerostomia. Oral candidiasis is common. Herpetic lesions may occur and can be difficult to differentiate from chemoradiotherapy mucositis. Pain from these infections may limit oral intake. Topical or systemic antibiotics, antiviral and antifungal agents can be administered, and some centres use prophylactic agents such as acyclovir.

Nausea and vomiting

This is multifactorial in aetiology, causes ranging from the side-effect of cytoreductive therapy to nausea related to taking antibiotics. Management should always include the prescription of anti-emetics. When severe vomiting occurs, oral intake should be discouraged to prevent aspiration. Diet should include clear liquids, dry salty foods, fruit and chilled or iced foods. It is important to avoid foods that are very sweet, greasy or have a strong odour. Patients are also discouraged from drinking or eating too fast. High-energy drinks served frozen as iced lollies or taken through a straw can be helpful. For prolonged vomiting, parenteral nutrition should be considered.

Diarrhoea

The incidence and severity of diarrhoea are variable. Diarrhoea is a common side-effect of chemotherapy and TBI. It is often exacerbated by the use of antibiotics, especially the oral non-absorbable antibiotics used to sterilize the gastrointestinal tract. Graft-versus-host disease and gastrointestinal infections are other potential causes of diarrhoea. Patients with diarrhoea experience a significant decrease in nutritional status and well-being [11].

Management of diarrhoea should always be through drug intervention; dietary manipulation will not be enough. Where profuse diarrhoea is in evidence, the patient will be absorbing very little and may require parenteral nutrition. Some patients, particularly those with chronic GvHD affecting the gut, may benefit from a low lactose, gluten-free diet.

Infection

It is suggested that patients can be vulnerable to food-borne infections and endogenous infections from normally non-pathogenic bacteria. Consequently, the majority of BMT units operate some level of food restrictions and some continue to use gut sterilization. The issues surrounding this area are discussed below.

Graft-versus-host disease

Very little data exist concerning the effects of acute or chronic GvHD on nutritional status or the appropriate dietary management. Corticosteroid therapy often causes fluid gain which may mask muscle wastage and general deterioration in nutritional status. In high doses, it can also lead to non-insulin-dependent diabetes which can further compromise intake through the restriction of high-calorie foods. From our own clinical practice, acute and chronic GvHD affecting the skin lead to increased nutritional requirements and muscle wasting. Such patients should be encouraged to use nutritional supplements and may benefit from overnight supplementary nasogastric feeding.

Acute GvHD affecting the gut may cause profuse diarrhoea. In such circumstances, parenteral nutrition should be given. In the past, particular GvHD diets have been suggested [17]. However, their efficacy has not been well researched. Diet should be reintroduced gradually, with some patients benefiting from a low allergen diet, i.e. low in lactose, milk-free, gluten-free and egg-free. These diets are, however, very limiting and it can be difficult to meet nutritional requirements. For some patients where malabsorption is a problem, a peptide feed and low allergen diet may be beneficial.

For chronic GvHD affecting the gut, patients may require short-term enteral feeding, particularly if mucositis is a problem.

When GvHD affects the liver it can be difficult to maintain nutritional status. Patients often experience anorexia (frequently accompanied by early satiety). Parenteral nutrition is likely to adversely affect liver function [18]. It is therefore advisable to encourage nutritional supplements and consider nasogastric feeding. There is no research to support the use of a low fat diet. Patients with veno-occlusive disease often experience similar side-effects and may also benefit from nasogastric feeding. Parenteral nutrition is not indicated because of fluid balance problems and the likelihood of it causing further liver-function abnormalities.

Dietary restrictions for immunocompromised patients

The restrictions recommended for immunocompromised patients are controversial, with no clear national guidelines. No empirical research exists concerning the efficacy of low microbial diets, the most recent studies tending to concentrate on auditing current practice in UK centres [19–21]. Unfortunately, such audits can only highlight common practice and are not indicative of the best practice regarding patient care. Research considering the benefits of gut sterilization, protective isolation and sterile or low microbial diets is limited and contradictory [22,23].

The dietary restrictions recommended can be costly to implement, confusing and inconsistent. They should reflect the overall philosophy of the centre towards isolation procedures. The regimen is often dependent upon the cooking facilities available, funds, and the number of patients requiring such a diet at any one time.

Foodborne infections

Foodborne infections are on the increase in the UK, particularly in the home [24]. The role of food as a source of infection has long been recognized. The microorganisms most commonly responsible are *Salmonella*, *Clostridium perfringes*, *Staphylococcus aureus* and *Bacillus* spp. The incidence of *Campylobacter* spp. and *Escherichia* coli O157-related infections is also increasing [23].

Since food-related pathogens require conditions of moisture and warmth, a source of nutrition (usually protein) and an appropriate atmosphere in order to thrive, the most common causes of food poisoning [26] are secondary to:

- using contaminated food;
- storing food at the incorrect temperature (i.e. ambient temperature);
- cross-contamination between raw and cooked food;
- undercooking meat, meat products, eggs and poultry;
- not thawing adequately frozen meat and poultry before cooking;
- incorrect reheating of foods; and
- infected food-handlers.

The risk of food poisoning can be reduced by good food hygiene practice in the hospital and home. Staff and patients should be given food hygiene advice and, if possible, basic training in the subject [26].

General research concerning food poisoning and the knowledge that immunocompromised patients are more vulnerable to such infections has led to the use of dietary restriction. The level of restriction required is unknown. In fact, three recent audits of practice have suggested a move towards liberalization of the diet. At present, there are three levels of food restrictions in the UK [19–21] (see Table 53.2).

Sterile diets Sterile diets were exclusively used for the first BMT patients and are now largely out of favour, with only one or two UK centres using such diets [19–21]. Foods are sterilized by autoclaving, prolonged baking, gamma-irradiation or canning, with the aim of producing food that has no bacterial or fungal growth [3,27–29]. Although this diet carries a minimal risk of foodborne infection, it does have the drawback that only a limited number of foods can be fully sterilized and remain palatable (dairy products are said to acquire a 'wet dog' flavour after gamma-irradiation!) [30].

Most systems of sterilization use expensive equipment and require specially trained nursing or catering staff for their use. The cost considerations of such a diet mean that a sterile diet is not appropriate for smaller BMT units.

Low microbial diets 'Low microbial diet' is a term which covers a wide variety of dietary restrictions. Generally, the diet involves using well-cooked foods prepared in hygienic conditions and aims to provide a nutritionally adequate, palatable diet. The low microbial diet is more widely used than the sterile diet and was developed to offset the limitations of the sterile diet [19–21,31]. Several authors suggest that food preparation and cooking is carried out at ward level and that there should be a ward kitchen,

Table 53.2 Types of food restrictions used with patients undergoing bone-marrow transplantation

Sterile diets
Low microbial diets
Modified hospital (ward) diets

preferably with a 'dirty kitchen' for cleaning crockery, etc. This type of food service requires specially trained nursing or catering staff. The foods permitted vary considerably, although raw fruit and salad are invariably prohibited. Packaged, individual portions of foods such as breakfast cereals tend to be used [21,31,32]. Some centres use disposable crockery, or crockery stored under ultraviolet light [32].

The rationale of such dietary restrictions is to decrease total bacterial count and eliminate pathogens, while at the same time providing greater flexibility and palatability than is the case with sterile diets.

The advantage is that a low microbial diet allows greater food choice than a sterile diet. Ward-based catering staff allows greater flexibility and may better meet the catering needs of patients from ethnic minorities, and children. It is also cheaper than a sterile diet system.

The disadvantage is that such a diet is more expensive than a modified hospital diet. The diet also restricts food choice for the patient to a great extent. As no national guidelines exist, the restrictions might be confusing and inconsistent, thus leading to problems with patient anxiety and non-compliance [33].

Modified ward diets A modified ward diet is a diet where food is prepared in the hospital kitchen and served as normal. The exact nature of any restrictions within this are variable. Most units exclude salad, unpeeled fruits and uncooked vegetables. Reviews of practice in the UK suggest that this is the most common type of food service for neutropenic patients [19–21].

The rationale for a modified ward diet is that patients are not being nursed in strict protective isolation and therefore do not require particular restrictions other than good food hygiene practices. Gut sterilization is not normally being used. This diet is most useful for units where patients are not nursed in isolation. It is also the cheapest option. No additional facilities are required. The patient has greater food choice. However, there is an increased risk of food poisoning with this diet and less control over the food eaten by vulnerable patients. Safety of the diet may be increased by ensuring that food is freshly prepared and served immediately, that patients, staff and carers receive food-handling training and that the food brought in by friends and family for the patient is closely monitored. The use of microwave ovens should also be restricted and ward storage facilities such as refrigerators and freezers regularly checked [32].

Controversial areas
Water The use of tap water is frequently debated in the literature [3,31,34]. Sterile and boiled cooled water are advocated by those centres employing sterile or clean food diets. Unfortunately, while there may be minimal risk of contamination of such water, it is also unpalatable and may lead to the patient drinking less [19]. Mineral waters are not as safe from contamination by pathogens. They are not subject to the same levels of microbiological stringency as tap water and higher levels of contamination may therefore be present [35]. Several centres allow patients to drink specific brands of mineral water; however, it is difficult to guarantee safety [19–21]. Bibbington *et al.* [19] found 40% of centres permitted tap water.

A related area is the use of the ice machines. Bacteria such as *Mycobacteria*, *Legionella*, *Pneumophila*, *Cryptosporidium* and *Pseudomonas* have been isolated from such machines. The contamination is likely to be due to poor design of machines, the presence of 'still' water and poor maintenance. Several authors suggest the use of sterile water to make ice-cubes in ice-cube trays or bags [13,31,34].

Fruit and vegetables Several pathogenic agents have been isolated from fresh, raw fruit and vegetables. These include hepatitis A in watercress, *Escherichia coli*, *Staphylococcus aureus*, *Klebsiella* species in salads and *Pseudomonas* in bananas [3,31,36–40], and it has been demonstrated that enteric viruses cannot be removed from the surface of vegetables by washing alone [41]. Cooked and canned fruit and vegetables are usually acceptable to patients as part of the food restrictions. Peeled fruits are permitted in several centres [19–21]. Salads are permitted in 5% of units sampled by Bibbington *et al.* [19].

Dairy products and eggs Since the *Salmonella* scare of the 1980s, hospitals are no longer permitted to serve soft-cooked eggs. All neutropenic or potentially neutropenic patients should only eat well-cooked eggs.

Consequently, foods made with raw egg such as home-made mayonnaise and eggnog should be avoided. Most BMT units allow well-cooked eggs. Milk is sometimes restricted to only ultra-high temperature (UHT) or sterilized. As the flavour of the milk is altered by heat treatment, patients may be discouraged from drinking such milk. Yoghurt is not allowed on over half the BMT units sampled [19].

Slow-ripened soft cheeses such as Brie, Camembert, blue-veined cheese and goats' cheeses should be avoided as they are associated with *Listeria monocytogenes*, *Salmonella paratyphoid* and *Brucella militarises*, etc. [42]. However Bibbington et al. [19] indicates that, controversially, this is not always enforced. Cream cheese, hard cheese and processed cheese such as cheese spreads are considered to be less hazardous.

Seasonings Herbs and spices may carry fungal spores, and are therefore only used in most centres if cooked. Pepper is associated with *Aspergillus* and several centres permit pepper only if it is included in cooked or irradiated food [3,19,21,43].

Cooking with microwave ovens Microwave cooking does not sterilize food. Research has shown that foods cooked in a microwave oven consistently yield more Gram-positive bacteria than do foods cooked in conventional ovens [44]. Page and Martin [45] also found that bacteria could survive on the inner surfaces of the microwave oven. Microwave heating is uneven and less effective than conventional cooking and its use should be limited. Review of UK centres dealing with immunocompromised patients revealed that the majority of centres discourage the use of microwave ovens. However, one centre did use microwave ovens [21]. Gibbon [20] found that the very unsafe practice of reheating cook–chill foods in the microwave oven was used in some centres.

Cook–chill foods Cook–chill foods are not ideal for neutropenic patients as there are many opportunities for bacterial contamination of such foods [26,32]. They have been associated with the growth of several pathogenic bacteria including *Listeria monocytogenes* and *E. coli* O157 [26], but if they are to be used (and Gibbons [20] suggests that this is the case in sixteen UK centres), then the catering department must ensure very high standards of food hygiene, with frequent testing of food samples to guarantee patient safety [26].

Nutritional assessment

Pretransplant assessment

The purpose of a pretransplant nutritional assessment is to ascertain overall nutritional status and to identify potential risk factors and nutritional requirements. It also offers the opportunity of obtaining baseline anthropometric measurements such as mid upper-arm circumference and triceps skinfold thickness. Information concerning past medical history, biochemical data, medications and dietary history are of assistance [46,47]. Specific food requirements, likes and dislikes, food allergies or intolerances, and the presence of therapeutic or alternative diets potentially restricting food intake may be discussed [47]. Patients and relatives should be alerted to the possibility of eating difficulties during the BMT period. They will also need to be informed of the clean/sterile food policy of the particular BMT unit. Patients who have lost 10–20% of their body weight should endeavour to regain this prior to BMT. Nutritional intervention is aimed at increasing protein and calorie intake, by administering commercial enteral supplements or initiating artificial nutrition support early.

Severe weight loss is common following BMT. Anorexia and eating difficulties can last for months, with the TBI-associated somnolence period aggravating the problem. For this reason, even 'ideal weight' patients are advised to try to gain extra weight in the two to four weeks prior to BMT.

Post-transplant assessment

Assessment of nutritional status is very problematic, particularly in the early post-transplant period [6]. Several methods are used in the research literature concerning nutrition and BMT. However, many are unreliable and inaccurate and therefore the validity of claims made by researchers should be questioned.

Weight

Body weight is an unreliable indicator of nutritional status during the early post-transplant period because of fluid and electrolyte changes. Weight may increase or remain stable despite loss of lean body tissue.

Sequential measures after discharge home may be useful as an indicator of nutritional status [6].

Anthropometry is useful if measurements can be made over a long period of time. This allows the estimation of muscle and fat mass. However, skinfold measurements are not very sensitive to change and are open to intra-observer error. They are also affected by fluid and electrolyte imbalance, and their use may result in severe bruising in patients with low platelet levels [5,6,18].

Biochemical measures such as serum albumin are not reliable indicators of nutritional status [48–50]. They tend to reflect the severity of illness in patients and are affected by a number of factors including acute phase responses secondary to febrile episodes and GvHD [49]. The regular use of blood products in BMT patients also renders them unreliable as nutrition markers [6]. Haematological and immunological measures are also wholly unsuitable measures of nutritional status in such a patient population [6].

Nitrogen balance

This method of assessing the nutritional adequacy of nutrition support is problematic from a practical point of view. The presence of diarrhoea or urinary incontinence makes collection very inaccurate, and the insensitivity of the measure (impaired renal or hepatic function and immobility) greatly influences results. It is futile to aim for a positive nitrogen balance in critically ill patients as they are unlikely to be able to utilize high protein intakes [18].

Bioelectrical impedance

This is an inaccurate way of estimating fat and muscle mass in such patients as it is greatly influenced by fluid imbalance [18]

Development of a prognostic nutritional index for BMT patients would greatly assist in identifying patients at risk and in monitoring the efficacy of nutrition support.

Nutrient requirements

Energy

Requirements are increased secondary to chemotherapy, TBI, infection, and the rapid cell turnover associated with GvHD during the first 30–50 days after BMT [5,46]. Energy requirements are undoubtedly increased (despite a reduction in activity levels for most patients), although quantifying the increase is difficult. A small study looking at energy expenditure suggests that patients can require between 30 and 50 kcal/kg body weight (dependent on sex and presence of sepsis or GvHD) [51]. Geibig et al. [52] suggest 30–35 kcal/kg body weight. It is advisable to avoid overfeeding particularly when commencing parenteral nutrition, as this can cause additional physical stress and may led to fluid and electrolyte abnormalities as well as changes in liver function. It is therefore advisable to start feeding at 30 kcal/kg body weight and review this depending upon changes in clinical condition and nutritional status. Energy needs may have to be adjusted according to activity when patients are discharged from hospital.

Nitrogen

Keller et al. [53] have established that patients experience marked protein catabolism due to increased protein turnover and leucine oxidation. Protein requirements are related to age, body size, organ function and catabolic corticosteroid treatment. They are calculated at approximately twice the recommended daily allowance, although adults may require 0.17–0.25 grams of nitrogen per kilogram of body weight, particularly during septic episodes [5,46,54]. Excessively high nitrogen intakes are not advisable as it is unlikely that the nitrogen will be assimilated, particularly during sepsis and critical illness. In addition, it is also essential to ensure that energy requirements are met if nitrogen is to be utilized properly. Research also suggests that maintaining some level of activity is essential in the preservation of lean body mass [15].

Fluid

Fluid requirements are calculated according to body surface area or weight [46]:

Greater than 20 kg:	1500 ml/m^2
Less than 20 kg:	100 ml/kg/day for first 10 kg, plus 50 ml/kg/day for each kilogram between 10–20 kg

Fluids must be increased during episodes of fever, diarrhoea and other gastrointestinal fluid losses, and may require restriction during episodes of hepatic, cardiac or renal dysfunction [46].

Vitamin and mineral requirements

There is little information concerning vitamin requirements in patients undergoing BMT. It is recommended that amounts of vitamins A, D, E, K, folic acid, ascorbic acid, B complex and biotin are increased [55]. Antila *et al.* [56] have suggested that zinc requirements may be slightly increased. Medication such as cyclosporin may also increase requirements for some minerals such as magnesium [11].

Methods of nutritional support

During the first few weeks following BMT, anorexia, nausea and vomiting reduce voluntary food intake, while mucositis and enteritis contribute towards malabsorption. Catabolism, fever, infection and organ failure further increase nutritional stress.

Early nutritional support is important in BMT because patients are known to lose body tissue, especially during the first few weeks. Bone-marrow transplantation constitutes a nitrogen-depleting stress factor, and studies have revealed losses of body cell mass >2kg in the first four weeks [55]. The aim of nutrition support is normally maintenance rather than repletion of body cell mass, as for the majority of patients nutritional status is fairly good at the onset of treatment. Before instigating artificial nutritional support, it should be estimated that this is likely to be required for at least one week.

The two forms of nutritional support available to BMT patients are enteral (i.e. via the gastrointestinal tract) feeding and total parenteral nutrition (see Table 53.3).

Oral nutrition

The first method of enteral feeding to be tried should be the provision of food itself. The 'healthy eating' guidelines for the general public are not applicable to this patient population. Generally, patients require foods with a high-energy and protein density. Strict food restrictions can further compound the problem of poor food intake. For example, many transplant centres exclude yoghurt and ice-cream, foods which generally appeal to patients with dry or sore mouths [17,31]. Oral nutritional intake is very poor during the first four weeks post-transplant and patients may consume as little as 150–424 kcal/day. The reasons for this include psychological factors such as those relating to hospitalization and protective isolation. Patients may become afraid to eat, anticipating nausea, vomiting or pain [13]. Others may refuse to eat, since eating is the one function over which they still have control. Dietary intake should be encouraged but never forced. Nutritional counselling can be helpful. Enteral nutritional support is made easier if the food service is flexible enough to provide food and drink when patients want it. Research has shown that patients request 40% of their food between 5 pm and midnight [13]. Some BMT centres have a family kitchen which is open at all hours, allowing relatives and friends to prepare foods familiar to the patient [57]. This is particularly helpful in centres treating overseas patients. Providing foods that are tempting as well as nutritious is a challenging task for the dietitian, nurse and catering staff.

Appetite generally improves by three to four weeks following BMT [54] but it may be months before

Table 53.3 Methods of nutrition support used in bone-marrow transplantation

Nasogastric feeding
Patients unable to achieve an adequate oral nutritional intake, including those with severe weight loss, mucositits, nausea and xerostomia
Patients requiring short-term feeds
Gastrostomy feeding
Patients requiring long-term enteral nutrition support
Jejunostomy feeding
Patients requiring nutrition support and who have poor gastric emptying
Parenteral feeding
Non-functioning gastrointestinal tract
Severe mucositis
Severe vomiting
Profuse diarrhoea
Severe hepatic abnormalities

patients eat sufficient 'normal' food to meet their requirements. This can result in continuing weight loss and the need for constant nutritional support and assessment.

Nutritionally complete supplements

These are available on prescription. They are nutritionally complete (in 1500 ml), clinically lactose-free, gluten-free and UHT/sterile until opened. They are milk-like in taste, appearance and texture. There are a wide range of flavours, including 'neutral', fruit flavours and soup flavours. They can be served hot or cold. Despite a wide range of flavours, patients are often reluctant to take such supplements and can very rarely drink adequate volumes to meet their nutritional requirements The main hurdles to supplement consumption are taste fatigue, poor palatability and texture.

Nasogastric feeding

Historically, parenteral nutrition has been the method of choice when providing nutrition support for transplant patients [58]. However, recent research findings from the field of critical care medicine have suggested that early instigation of enteral feeding and prolonged enteral feeding during illness helps to maintain gut function and reduce the risk of passage of bacteria across the intestinal mucosa. Nasogastric feeding is also considerably cheaper than parenteral nutrition. Research is limited in the BMT setting. However, it is likely that the same will be true for patients undergoing BMT. There are currently studies under way looking at the question of the efficacy and feasibility of nasogastric feeding in this patient population [59].

Historically, there are several objections to nasogastric feeding including gastric erosion by feeding tubes, body image issues and the risk of bleeding [58]. These issues can be addressed by using fine-bore polyurethane nasogastric tubes and giving platelet cover in thrombocytopenic patients. If patients are prepared for the possibility of needing a nasogastric tube, and if the practice is commonplace, then body image issues should be easily overcome. Infection via the tube should be minimized if nasogastric tubes are kept patent and flushed regularly.

For patients with diarrhoea or malabsorption there are a wide range of specialist feeds that can be used which cater for patients with different nutritional needs, e.g. peptide feeds for patients with malabsorption.

Tube feeding also has a role to play in the pretransplant period, however, and in the later post-transplant period, particularly for patients needing supplementary feeding in the home environment.

Gastrostomy tubes

These are useful for patients requiring prolonged enteral feeding, particularly if they are at home. They overcome the problem of altered body image by virtue of the fact that the tube is concealed. Gastrostomy tubes can be inserted endoscopically or surgically and are relatively easy to remove. They are a potential site for infection and therefore great care should be taken in cleaning the insertion site, and antibiotics should be given prophylactically on insertion. Gastrostomy tubes should not be used in patients with acute or chronic GvHD affecting the gut, as wound healing is likely to be poor [60].

Jejunostomy tubes

These can be used to provide prolonged nutritional support in patients with impaired gastric emptying. They require surgical insertion. As with gastrostomy tubes, they should not be used in patients with poor wound healing.

Parenteral nutrition

The widespread use of right atrial catheters in the BMT setting allows parenteral nutrition to be part of standard supportive care [61]. It is not always required, however. Parenteral nutrition is expensive and is associated with a higher patient risk than is enteral nutrition. Individual nutritional support programmes can make it possible to use the enteral route to support BMT [61].

One study, comparing parenteral nutrition to an individualized enteral feeding programme during BMT, showed that enteral feeding was not as effective in maintaining weight. Important clinical outcomes such as rate of haematopoietic recovery, length of hospitalization and survival were, however, not affected. Enteral feeding was also associated with lower risks and costs, suggesting that parenteral nutrition is not necessarily superior and should be reserved for patients in whom enteral feeding has failed [61].

Parenteral nutrition is beneficial in the support of poorly nourished patients undergoing BMT and is especially recommended for the under 10 age groups. In some BMT units, it is started before transplant as a prophylactic measure [4]. Weisdorf et al. [4,8] suggest that prophylactic parenteral nutrition in well-nourished patients leads to a slight improvement in survival. However, time to engraftment did not differ, and neither did the incidence of GvHD.

The overall goal of parenteral nutrition is to provide sufficient protein and energy to preserve body stores, and in well-nourished individuals, to maintain rather than increase body cell mass [61,62]. It should not be started if it is anticipated that such nutrition will be required for less than one week. It should be continued until the patient is managing to eat 50% of his or her requirements. Cyclic administration of parenteral nutrition is advisable (i.e. feeding for ≤ 18 hours) as it provides a period free from infusion to allow physiotherapy and a shower [63]. Fat-free parenteral nutrition is not recommended.

Several recent studies considered the use of glutamine-supplemented parenteral nutrition in patients undergoing BMT [64–66]. Several studies have found that the addition of glutamine improved nitrogen balance, shortened hospital stay and lowered incidence of infection [64,66,67]. Young [59] found that glutamine improved mood.

Complications of parenteral nutrition during BMT

Infection
Parenteral nutrition-related infections can be reduced if a dedicated line is used. Breaking the line for drug administration or blood sampling may lead to contamination of nutrient solutions [68].

Fluid overload
Since BMT patients receive large volumes of fluid in the form of blood products and antibiotics, the volume of parenteral nutrition may require adjustment in order to prevent fluid overload. More concentrated dextrose and lipid solutions may be used, and sodium may be eliminated or reduced from parenteral nutrition [5,48,54].

Problems associated with excessive carbohydrate administration
Large amounts of parenteral glucose solutions are associated with hepatomegaly and fatty liver [15]. Hyperglycaemia may occur with excessive carbohydrate use, requiring administration of insulin. Providing fat as 30–40% of total calories can help obviate this.

Muscle wasting
Despite adequate parenteral protein and energy, muscle wasting and negative nitrogen balance are common during BMT. Patients lose muscle protein and gain body fat. Physiotherapy plays an important role in preserving muscle stores during BMT [15].

Specific nutritional requirements
The formulae for calculating protein and energy requirements have been mentioned earlier in this chapter. Parenteral protein solutions containing essential and non-essential amino acids are available in varying concentrations designed to meet protein requirements within volume restrictions. The most recent trend has been towards developing glutamine containing solutions. The same applies to dextrose and lipid solutions. Both water-soluble and fat-soluble parenteral vitamin solutions are available. All patients require the addition of electrolytes, although requirements vary between individuals [55]. Hypokalaemia and hypomagnesaemia may occur during hospitalization due to antibiotic use and increased gastrointestinal losses, and require careful supplementation.

Parenteral nutrition tolerance should be monitored daily using serum turbidity and glucose levels. Lipid clearance tests are carried out weekly if the patient is receiving 50% or more of his calories as lipid, if serum triglyceride levels are elevated or in the presence of pancreatitis or liver disease [5].

Parenteral nutrition should be continued until patients are able to consume 50% of their required calories [69]. Outpatient programmes have been started in the USA in order to facilitate discharge and avoid re-admission to hospital for nutritional support. This is currently not feasible in the UK due to funding and organizational difficulties.

Discharge planning
The importance of good nutrition should be emphasized to patients prior to discharge. The two most important points to discuss are dietary

requirements and food hygiene. Dietary advice may involve practical advice on increasing protein and calorie intake at home, and the prescription of nutritional supplements if necessary. Patients should be reminded that nutritional requirements remain high, despite relative inactivity. Patients may also need advice on coping with eating difficulties such as nausea, xerostomia and taste changes.

Lenssen *et al.* [7] conducted a retrospective review of the nutrition-related problems experienced following allogeneic transplant, and found that oral sensitivity, xerostomia, dysgeusia, diarrhoea and limited capacity for exercise were commonplace amongst this transplant group. Weight loss was recorded in 28% of the sample 3–12 months after transplant. Her study highlights the importance of ongoing nutrition support and monitoring nutritional status in transplant patients.

Body weight is a more reliable indicator of nutritional status in BMT outpatients than in inpatients [5]. Patients should therefore be weighed regularly in order that weight changes can be noticed and addressed before they become too severe. In our experience, short-term supplementary feeding via a fine-bore nasogastric feeding tube in the home setting is often well tolerated by patients and is relatively easily arranged. It is also worthwhile considering the use of appetite stimulants such as megestrol acetate where there is no obvious cause for anorexia [70].

Dietary advice for home

The majority of patients are discharged home when they are reasonably fit and have an adequate white blood cell count. At this point the hospital environment is likely to present a greater infection risk than home [3]. Several studies have highlighted the risk of foodborne pathogens as mentioned earlier. It is essential that patients are advised to avoid 'high-risk' foods, as there have been reported cases of Listeria meningitis after bone-marrow transplantation [71,72]. Advice regarding food hygiene (e.g. checking the temperature of the refrigerator, checking 'use by' dates, etc.), and the avoidance of 'high-risk' foods as defined by the Ministry of Agriculture, Fisheries and Foods (MAFF) (see Table 53.4) should be given as a basic minimum. Some centres extend this to a very strict regimen of no poultry, shellfish or tap water for three months [21]. There is no research to support this level of restriction, and it may lead to a reduction in food intake and a consequently adverse effect on nutritional status.

There should not be an assumption that the patient and his or her carers are knowledgeable in the area of food hygiene. Written and verbal advice should be given to all patients on discharge from hospital. Patients should remain on the basic food restriction for a minimum of three months or for as long as they are taking immunosuppressive drugs such as cyclosporin.

Table 53.4 Foods to be avoided by immunocompromised patients*

Unpasteurized milk and milk products
Soft mould-ripened cheese, e.g. Brie, Camembert and blue-veined cheeses
Soft whip ice-cream from machines
Raw or lightly cooked eggs
Pâté

*Source: Department of Health and Ministry of Agriculture, Fisheries and Foods.

Appendix

Increasing protein and calorie intake
- Fortified milk (1 pint of whole milk + 2oz skimmed milk powder) may be used in place of ordinary milk in soups, milk puddings, drinks.
- Extra butter or margarine may be added to vegetables, sauces and soups.
- Cream may be added to soups, sauces and desserts.
- Milk may be used in jellies, soups and porridge.
- Glucose polymer may be added to drinks, soups, porridge, jellies, milk puddings, and drinking water (approximately four teaspoons per serving or 70 g per 750 ml water).
- Small frequent meals should be encouraged.

Taste changes
Metallic taste
Sharp or acidic flavours may help, such as fruit juices, fresh/tinned fruit, lemon juice, vinegar, salad cream or mayonnaise. Red meat often tastes metallic, and may improve with marinating in fruit juice, wine or sweet-and-sour sauce. Some people find it best to replace red meat for the better tolerated flavours of chicken, fish, eggs and cheese.

Sweet taste
Adding salt may help to soften a sweet taste. It may also be helpful to replace sugar with a glucose polymer (e.g. Maxijul or Polycose).

Salty taste
Adding sugar may help to soften a salty taste.

Mouth blindness
Here it may be necessary to enhance the flavour of foods using herbs, spices, lemon juice, garlic, chutney, tomato and other sauces.

Xerostomia
- Provide regular drinks to moisten the mouth throughout the day, especially at meal times.
- Serve foods with plenty of sauce or gravy.
- Ice-cubes and ice lollies may stimulate salivation, and can soothe a dry mouth.
- Fruit drops or pineapple chunks can stimulate saliva production.
- Chewing gum can stimulate saliva production, although some people find it makes the mouth even drier. Dental health gum or sugar-free gum is preferable.

Mucositis
- Soft, bland foods are often easiest to eat, e.g. soups, minced meat, fish in sauce, milk puddings.
- Food should not be served too hot; cold and chilled foods are best tolerated.
- Sharp, spicy or salty foods should be avoided, as should rough or dry foods.
- Encourage nourishing drinks to replace or supplement (Build-up, Fresubin, Fortisip, or home-made milkshakes made with fortified milk).
- Offer drinks with a straw. This may help the patient to avoid sensitive areas of the mouth.
- Try freezing juices or milk drinks into ice lollies which can be soothing to a sore mouth.

Nausea and vomiting
- Cold foods do not have such a strong aroma and may be better tolerated.
- Milkshakes and cool drinks drunk from a carton with a straw are virtually odourless.
- Serve small meals frequently.
- Avoid highly flavoured or spiced foods.
- Offer foods that are high in carbohydrates but low in fat (clear jellies, clear soups, dry crackers, toast, tinned fruit, instant whips made with skimmed milk).
- Offer drinks between meals.
- Ice lollies made from fruit juices or high-protein milk drinks (fortified with glucose polymers) are easily tolerated.

Diarrhoea
- Reduce dietary fibre intake by avoiding whole-grain cereals, wholemeal bread, fruit, vegetables and nuts, and encourage foods low in fibre such as white bread, refined cereals (cornflakes, rice krispies) potatoes (without skins) pasta and white rice. Meat, fish, eggs, milk and cheese can be eaten in normal quantities.
- Avoid highly spiced foods.
- Encourage plenty of fluid.
- Some patients may benefit from reducing dietary intake of lactose and fat.

References

1. Deeg HJ, Seidel K, Bruemmer B, Pepe MS and Appelbaum FR. Impact of patient weight on non-relapse mortality after marrow transplantation. *Bone Marrow Transplant* 1995; **15**: 461–468.
2. Hill GL. Body composition research: implications for the practice of clinical nutrition. *J Parenteral Enteral Nutrition* 1992; **16**: 197–218.
3. Aker SN and Cheney CL. The use of sterile and low microbial diets in ultraisolation environments. *J Parenteral Enteral Nutrition* 1983; **7**: 390–397.
4. Weisdorf S, Lysne J, Wind D et al Positive effect of prophylactic total parenteral nutrition on long term outcome of bone marrow transplantation. *Transplantation* 1987; **43**(6): 833–838.
5. Aker SN, Lenssen P, Darbinian J, Cheney CL and Cunningham B. Nutritional assessment in the marrow transplant patient. *Nutritional Support Serv* 1983; **3**: 22–27.
6. Keenan AM. Nutritional support of the bone marrow transplant patient. *Nursing Clin North Am* 1989; **24**: 383–392.
7. Lenssen P, Sherry ME, Cheney CL et al. Prevalence of nutrition-related problems among long-term survivors of allogeneic marrow transplantation. *J Am Dietetic Ass* 1990; **90**: 835–842.
8. Weisdorf S, Hofland C, Sharp HL, Teasley K, Schissel K and McGlave P. Total parenteral nutrition in bone marrow transplantation: a clinical evaluation. *J Paediatr Gastroenterol Nutrition* 1984; **3**(1): 95–100.
9. Savage DG, Szydlo RM and Goldman JM. Clinical features in 430 patients with chronic myeloid leukaemia seen at a referral centre over a 16 year period. *Br J Haematol* 1997; **96**(1): 111–116.
10. Zerbe MB, Parkerson SG, Ortlieb ML and Spitzer T. Relationship between oral mucositis and treatment variables in bone marrow transplant patients. *Cancer Nursing* 1992; **15**(3): 196–205.
11. Papadopoulou A, Nathavitharana KA, Williams MD, Darbyshire PJ and Booth IW. Diarrhoea and weight loss after bone marrow transplantation in children. *Paed Haem Oncol* 1994; **11**(6): 601–611.
12. Stern JM and Lenssen P. Food and nutrition services for the BMT patient. In: *Bone Marrow Transplantation. Administrative and Clinical Strategies.* PC Buchsel and MB Whedon (eds), 1995 (London: Jones and Bartlett).
13. Moe G, Aker SN and Schubert MM. Enteral management. In: *Nutritional Assessment and Management During Marrow Transplantation. A resource manual.* P Lenssen and SN Aker (eds), 1985: 31–44 (Seattle: Murray).
14. Ford R and Ballard B. Acute complications after bone marrow transplantation. *Semin Oncol Nursing* 1988; **4**: 15–24.
15. Cunningham BA, Morris G, Cheney CL, Buergel N, Aker SN and Lenssen P. Effects of resistive exercise on skeletal muscle in marrow transplant recipients receiving total parenteral nutrition. *J Parenteral Enteral Nutrition* 1986; **10** (6): 558–563.
16. Boock CA and Reddick JE. Taste alterations in bone marrow transplant patients. *J Am Dietetic Ass* 1991; **91** (9): 1121–1122.
17. Gauvreau JM, Lenssen P, Cheney CL, Aker SN, Hutchinson ML and Barale KV. Nutritional management of patients with intestinal graft-versus-host disease. *J Am Dietetic Ass* 1981; **79**: 673–675.
18. Payne-James J, Grimble G and Silk D (eds). *Artificial Nutrition Support in Clinical Practice*, 1995 (London: Edward Arnold).
19. Bibbington A, Wilson P and Jones M. Audit of nutritional advice given to bone marrow transplant patients in the United Kingdom. *Clin Nutrition* 1993; **12**: 233–235.
20. Gibbon J. A review of current dietary practices. In: *Bone Marrow Transplant Units Throughout the UK.* BSc Dissertation, University of Cardiff, 1996.
21. Pattison AJ. Review of current practice in clean diets in the UK. *J Human Nutr Diet* 1993; **6**: 3–11.
22. Levine AS, Siegel S, Schneiber AD, Hauser J, Preisler H, Goldstein IM et al. Protected environments and prophylactic antibiotics. *New Engl J Med* 1973; **288**(10): 477–483.
23. Yates JW and Holland JF. A controlled study of isolation and endogenous microbial suppression in acute myeloid leukaemia patients. *Cancer* 1973; **32**: 1490–1498.
24. Sheard JB. Food poisoning cases are nearly double the level of 1970. *Environmental Health* 1987; **85**: 10–15.
25. Communicable Disease Report. Foodborne Disease Surveillance in England and Wales: 1989–1991. *CDR Review* 1993; **12**(3) (London: Public Health Laboratory Service).
26. Barrie D. The provision of food and catering services in hospital. *J Hosp Infect* 1996; **33**: 13–33.
27. Reimer AO and Tillotson JL. Food science procedures for reverse isolation. *J Am Dietetic Ass* 1966; **48**: 381–384.
28. Swain JF and Hargleroad MJ. Minimal bacteria diets: an assessment for implementation. *J Am Dietetic Ass* 1976; **69**: 258–261.
29. Dong FM, Hashisaka AE, Rasco BA, Einstein MA, Mar DR and Aker SA. Irradiated or aseptically prepared frozen dairy desserts: acceptability to bone marrow transplant patients. *J Am Dietetic Ass* 1992; **92**: 719–723.
30. Watson P and Bodey GP. Sterile food service for patients in protected environments. *J Am Dietetic Ass* 1970; **56**: 515–520.
31. Pizzo PA, Purvis DS and Waters C. Microbiological evaluation of food items. *J Am Dietetic Ass* 1982; **81**: 272–279.
32. Thomas B (ed.) *Manual of Dietetic Practice*, 2nd edn., (Oxford 1994) Blackwell Scientific Publications).
33. Henry CL. Case Study Dossier: Food Restrictions on a Bone Marrow Transplant Unit. MSc Thesis (Cancer Care), 1995 (Sutton: Centre for Cancer and Palliative Care Studies).
34. Oniboni AC. Infection in the neutropenic patient. *Semin Oncol Nursing* 1990; **6**(1): 50–60.
35. Bischofberger T, Chas SK, Schmitt R, Konig B and Schmidt-Lorenz W. The bacterial flora of non-carbonated, natural mineral water from the springs to reservoir and glass and plastic bottle. *Int J Food Microbiol* 1990; **11**: 51–72.
36. Fowler JL and Foster JF. A microbiological survey of three fresh green salads – can guidelines be recommended for these foods? *J Milk Food Technol* 1976; **39**(2): 111–113.
37. Groisak B. Introduction of Pseudomonas aeruginosa into a hospital via vegetables. *Appl Environ Microbiol* 1972; **24**: 567–570.
38. Remington JS and Schimpff SC. Please don't eat the salads. *New Engl J Med* 1981; **304**: 433–435.
39. Shooter RA, Faiers MC, Cooke EM, Brenden AL and Farrell SM. Isolation of *Escherichia coli, Pseudomonas aeruginosa*

40. Wright C, Kominos SD and Yee RB. Enterobacteriacae and *Pseudomonas aeruginosa* recovered for vegetable salads. *Appl Environ Microbiol* 1976; **31**(3): 435–454.
41. Konowalchuk J and Speirs JI. Survival of enteric viruses on fresh vegetables. *J Milk Food Technol* 1975; **38**(8): 469–472.
42. Rampling A. Raw milk cheese and *Salmonella*. *Br Med J* 1996; **312**: 67–68.
43. Eccles NK and Scott GM. *Aspergillus* in pepper. *Lancet* 1992; **339**: 618.
44. Fruin J and Guthertz L. Survival of bacteria cooked by microwave oven, conventional oven and slow cookers. *J Food Protection* 1982; **45**: 695–698.
45. Page WJ and Martin WG. Survival of microbial films in a microwave oven. *Canadian J Microbiol* 1978; **24**: 460–465.
46. Dickson B and Barale KV. Nutritional assessment. In: *Nutritional Assessment and Management During Marrow Transplantation. A Resource Manual*. P Lenssen and SN Aker (eds), 1995: 5–15 (Seattle: Murray).
47. Buchsel PC and Whedon MB. *Bone Marrow Transplantation. Administrative and Clinical Strategies*, 1995 (London: Jones and Bartlett).
48. Barzaghi A, Rovelli A, Piroddi A, Balduzzi A, Pirovano L, Colombini A and Uderzo C. Six years experience of total parenteral nutrition in children with haematological malignancies at a single centre: management; efficacy and complications. *Paed Haem Oncol* 1996; **13**(40): 349–358.
49. Muscaritoli M, Conversano L, Cangiano C, Capri S, Laviano A, Arcese W and Fanelli FR. Biochemical indices may not accurately reflect changes in nutritional status after allogeneic bone marrow transplantation. *Nutrition* 1995; **11**(5): 433–436.
50. Taveroff A, McArdle AH and Rybka WB. Reducing parenteral energy and protein intake improves metabolic homeostasis after bone marrow transplantation. *Am J Clin Nutr* 1991; **54**(6): 1087–1092.
51. Szeluga DJ, Stuart RK, Brookmeyer R, Utermohlen V and Santos GW. Energy requirements of parenterally fed bone marrow transplant recipients. *J Parenteral Enteral Nutrition* 1985; **9**: 139–143.
52. Geibig CB, Owens JP, Mirtallo JM, Bowers D, Nahikian-Nelms M and Tutshka P. Parenteral nutrition for marrow transplant recipients: evaluation of increased nitrogen dose. *J Parenteral Enteral Nutrition* 1991; **15**(2): 184–188.
53. Keller U, Kraenzlin E, Gratwohl A *et al*. Protein metabolism assessed by 1-^{13}C-leucine infusions in patients undergoing bone marrow transplantation. *J Parenteral Enteral Nutrition* 1990; **14**(5): 480–484.
54. Driedger L and Burstall CD. Bone marrow transplantation: dietitian's experience and perspective. *J Am Dietetic Ass* 1987; **87**: 1387–1388.
55. Cunningham BA. Parenteral management. In: *Nutritional Assessment and Management During Marrow Transplantation. A Resource Manual*. P Lenssen and SN Aker (eds), 1985: 45–63 (Seattle: Murray).
56. Antila HM, Salo MS, Kirvela O, Nanto V, Rajamaki A and Toivanen A. Serum trace element concentrations and iron metabolism in allogeneic bone marrow transplant recipients. *Ann Med* 1992; **24**: 55–59.
57. Cunningham BA, Lenssen P, Aker SN, Gittere K, Cheney CL and Hutchinson MM. Nutritional considerations during marrow transplantation. *Nursing Clin North Am* 1983; **18**: 585–596.
58. Hermann VM and Petruska PJ. Nutrition support in bone marrow transplant recipients. *Nutr Clin Practice* 1993; **8**: 19–27.
59. Young M. Senior Dietitian, Hammersmith Hospital, 1997. Personal communication.
60. Ringwald-Smith K, Krance R and Stricklin L. Enteral nutrition support in a child after bone marrow transplant. *Nutr Clin Practice* 1995; **10**: 140–143.
61. Szeluga DJ, Stuart RK, Brookmeyer R, Utermohlen V and Santos GW. Nutritional support of bone marrow transplant recipients: a prospective, randomized clinical trial comparing total parenteral nutrition to an enteral feeding program. *Cancer Res* 1987; **47**: 3309–3316.
62. Cheney CL, Gittere K, Abson K *et al*. Body composition changes in marrow transplantation. *Cancer* 1987; **59**: 1515–1519.
63. Reed MD, Lazarus HM, Herzig RH, Halpin TC, Gross S, Husak MP and Blumer JL. Cyclic parenteral nutrition during bone marrow transplantation in children. *Cancer* 1983; **51**: 1563–1570.
64. MacBurney M, Young LS, Ziegler TR and Wilmore DW. A cost-evaluation of glutamine-supplemented parenteral nutrition in adult bone marrow transplant patients. *J Am Dietetic Ass* 1994; **94**: 1263–1266.
65. Young LS, Bye R, Scheltinga M, Ziegler TR, Jacobs DO and Wlimore DW. Patients receiving glutamine-supplemented intravenous feedings report an improvement in mood. *J Parenteral Enteral Nutrition* 1993; **17**: 422–427.
66. Scloerb PR and Amare M. Total parenteral nutrition with glutamine in bone marrow transplantation and other clinical applications (a randomised, double blind study). *J Parenteral Enteral Nutrition* 1993; **17**: 407–413.
67. Zeigler TR, Young LS, Benfell K *et al*. Clinical and metabolic efficacy of glutamine supplemented parenteral nutrition after bone marrow transplantation. *Ann Intern Med* 1992; **116**: 821–828.
68. Baughen R. Nutrition for leukaemia patients. *Nursing Standard* 1988; 6: 22–23.
69. Lenssen P, Moe GL, Cheney CL, Aker SN and Deeg HJ. Parenteral nutrition in marrow transplant recipients after discharge from the hospital. *Exp Haematol* 1983; **11**: 974–981.
70. Tchekmedyian NS, Hickman M and Heber D. Treatment of anorexia and weight loss with megestrol acetate in patients with cancer or acquired immunodeficiency syndrome. *Semin Oncol* 1991; **18** (Suppl 2): 35–42.
71. Long SG, Leyland MJ and Milligan DW. Listeria meningitis after bone marrow transplantation. *Bone Marrow Transplant* 1993; **12**: 537–539.
72. Want SV, Lacey SL, Ward L and Buckingham S. An epidemiological study of listeriosis complicating a bone marrow transplant. *J Hosp Infect* 1993; **1223**: 299–304.

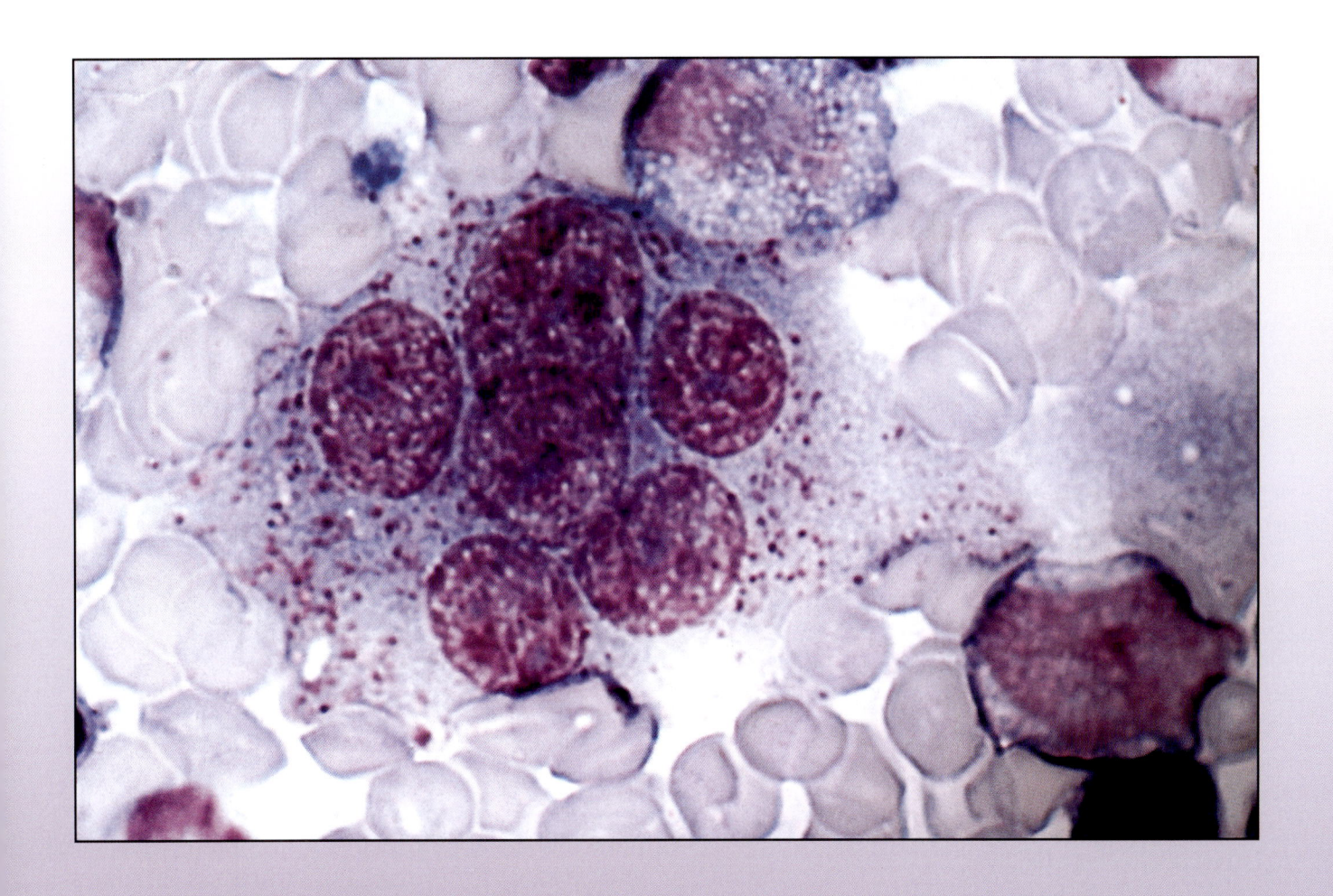

Chapter 54

Re-adaptation to normal life

Michael A. Andrykowski and Richard P. McQuellon

Introduction

Bone-marrow transplantation (BMT) is a physically and psychologically demanding procedure requiring major life adjustments for most patients. Both patient and family members are likely to experience stressful changes in their normal daily activities and functioning as a consequence of BMT. Even under the best of circumstances, patients face the challenge of adaptation to their illness and post-BMT treatment sequelae, as well as re-integration into social, family and work life after BMT. The extent to which patients successfully readapt to normal life after BMT varies as a function of a variety of factors including the demands of prior treatment, demographic and psychological characteristics of the patient, clinical status of the disease and available social support resources (Table 54.1). Here we describe issues related to both patient adaptation to illness as well as re-adaptation to normal life, review the existing literature pertinent to the post-BMT functioning of adult BMT recipients, and discuss psychosocial or behaviourally-oriented interventions that could facilitate readaptation to normal life following BMT.

Adaptation to illness

The BMT experience leaves few recipients completely unchanged. Ample research has demonstrated that BMT is often associated with a number of longstanding physical and psychosocial sequelae [1–8]. Even when such sequelae or 'late effects' are limited in number or extent, BMT recipients must live with the continual threat of disease recurrence. Thus, adaptation following BMT shares many similarities to adaptation to any chronic physical illness [9–13].

Adaptation to chronic physical illness requires that a defined set of tasks be managed [9]. Successful performance of these tasks requires that the sick individual assume the patient role, in other words, behave like a patient, at least temporarily. For example, rehabilitation following accidental trauma, intensive treatment regimens for cancer, kidney transplantation, or cardiac surgery all require a prolonged period of hospitalization and convalescence. The business executive accustomed to independent functioning may find it difficult to assume a role where he or she must comply with prescribed activities, take numerous medications, and rely on others for managing even the simplest of tasks, such as toileting. In the family context, assuming the patient role may mean relinquishing other more valued roles such as active parent, provider or recreational companion. However, for successful adaptation to illness to occur, an individual must adopt the role of the patient, at least on a temporary basis (see Table 54.2).

Assuming the role of the patient is similar to adoption of the 'sick role' first described by sociologist Talcott Parsons [14,15]. According to Parsons, the sick role includes privileges as well as obligations. Privileges accorded the sick role include exception from normal duties and freedom from blame for illness. Obligations associated with the sick role include recognizing the illness status as undesirable and taking steps to get

Table 54.1 Factors affecting adaptation to normal life after BMT
Demands of prior treatment
Demographic and psychological aspects of patient
Clinical status of disease
Available social support resources

Table 54.2 Adaptive tasks in chronic illness (adapted from Moos and Schaefer [9])
Illness-related
Dealing with pain and incapacitation
Dealing with the hospital environment and special treatment procedures
Developing adequate relationships with professional staff
General
Preserving a reasonable emotional balance
Preserving a satisfactory self-image
Preserving relationships with family and friends
Preparing for an uncertain future

well. In other words, one of the obligations of the sick role is to work towards eliminating its necessity. Thus, the sick role includes those actions taken by patients which are designed to restore health or to facilitate a return to 'normal life'. While the concept of the 'sick role' is perhaps best suited to understanding patient behaviour associated with more time-limited, acute illness episodes, it is also useful in settings where a prolonged convalescence is required. In particular, the concept of the sick role can be useful in the BMT setting since it provides a means of understanding the reactions of medical staff or family members to the patient who is evidencing slow functional recovery. While the BMT patient is not necessarily culpable for failing to recover and readapt to normal life *per se*, they may be held responsible for the failure to exert efforts to do so. For example, if a BMT patient fails to make efforts to sit up in a chair, walk or otherwise exercise during BMT hospitalization, or is inactive at home following BMT discharge, the patient will quickly hear directives to change this behaviour. From the viewpoint of medical staff and family, it is the patient's obligation to work to get well, and thus ultimately abandon the sick role. The prolonged period of convalescence that may be necessary following BMT may clash with family or staff's expectations of how long the patient is comfortably allowed to maintain the sick role.

The potential for conflict between BMT recipients and both family or medical staff is great, particularly when disabilities that limit post-BMT functioning are relatively invisible, for example, fatigue. Family and coworkers, who are programmed by their understanding of the sick role to expect a full return to normal, may be exasperated and frustrated by the limitations imposed by the patient's fatigue. The potential for disappointment and conflict is exacerbated since the patient may 'look normal', yet be incapable of even simple tasks, such as climbing stairs, without immediate rest.

Successful adaptation to changes in daily functioning brought on by illness and its treatment, and re-integration into normal roles and activities are important tasks for patients during and following intensive medical care. Even when medical treatment can be viewed as 'successful' by most criteria, re-adaptation to normal life is not assured. In fact, various maladaptive responses to illness characterized by a failure to 'return to normal' despite objectively successful treatment have been identified. Most notable perhaps, is the cluster of psychological and behavioral responses known as 'cardiac invalidism' [16–18]. In the early years of cardiac rehabilitation, it was assumed that the patient would need a period of bed rest and minimal exertion following a myocardial infarction, a type of medically imposed invalidism [16]. Cardiac invalidism, however, has come to mean a self-imposed inactive or invalid-like lifestyle following a myocardial infarction, even though exercise and a return to an active life are viewed as medically possible and recommended.

A distinct parallel to this syndrome is evident at times in the BMT setting. It is common for BMT patients to view themselves as damaged and fragile and their medical condition as dangerously volatile even if this view may not appear to be medically justified. This 'post-BMT invalidism' can limit re-adaptation following BMT by causing some patients to unnecessarily restrict the normal activities of daily living. A more subtle, but much less typical, form of maladaptive response observed clinically occurs when a patient identifies so strongly with the sick role that he is unwilling to relinquish it following treatment. Such patients may have adjusted to utilizing so-called 'secondary gains', such as reduced responsibilities at home and in the work setting. Full recovery may be less desirable for this unusual patient, since recovery requires assuming additional responsibility.

Many serious, chronic conditions that require intensive medical treatment share elements in common with BMT. The cardiac patient may require high-risk surgery followed by intensive inpatient and outpatient rehabilitation efforts and lifestyle changes. The renal transplant recipient will need immunosuppressive drugs and prolonged medical surveillance and follow-up after a period of intense treatment. Both of these conditions may be life-threatening, a source of chronic worry, interrupt social and family life, physical and emotional well-being, and functional status. Indeed, most solid-organ transplants involve high-risk medical procedures, and all solid-organ transplant recipients require long-term medical follow-up. However, while BMT shares many elements in common with other conditions that require intensive medical treatment, BMT has its own unique set of demands that require initial adaptation followed by readaptation to some degree of normal life.

Adaptation to bone-marrow transplantation

The specific adaptational challenges posed by BMT can vary considerably from patient to patient. For some patients, BMT is simply another challenge in an already long series of adaptational necessities they may have faced. These patients have undergone prior conventional treatment for their underlying disease before eventually becoming BMT candidates. Such patients may have already had anything from several months to many years to adapt to the initial diagnosis and treatment of their disease. For other patients, such as women with breast cancer with a high risk of relapse following conventional therapy, BMT is used as a first-line therapy. The breast cancer patient treated with autologous BMT for high-risk disease may have had little time to adapt to the initial diagnosis. Consequently, the tasks of adapting to both the initial diagnosis and the patient role are superimposed upon the task of adapting to the physical and psychological rigours posed by the BMT treatment itself. Furthermore, the nature and quality of the adaptive demands placed upon an individual by BMT may also vary greatly as a function of the family life cycle or developmental stage of the recipient. For example, the patient with a spouse and young children is likely to feel an extraordinary burden during the inpatient and convalescence phase of treatment. Conversely, the young adult without a spouse or partner is likely to be challenged by the need to surrender recently gained independence in the light of the need for his or her parents to reassume a primary care-giving role.

In general, BMT can be considered as a moderate-to-severe stressor for most people given that it requires lengthy hospitalization, life-threatening treatment, interruption of social relations, disruption of work, the potential for financial burden and physical sequelae. Each step or stage of the BMT process, from the decision to undergo treatment to the post-BMT convalescence, has its own stressors and quality of life challenges [19,20]. While general models of coping and adaptation to stress [21–23], as well as more specific models addressing adaptation to chronic illness [10,11,24] have been described elsewhere, there is little information regarding specific adaptational strategies utilized by patients following BMT. Hence, there is a clear need for study in this area [4].

Returning to normal following BMT: a review of the literature

The general question of whether or not an individual has returned to 'normal' has wide intuitive appeal. The simplest route to this information is to ask the BMT patient directly: 'Do you believe that you have "returned to normal"?' Yet, in practice, this question is difficult to answer. First, the BMT patient's disease course and treatment are superimposed upon a larger process of growth, development and life change. In other words, while BMT can profoundly alter the life course and circumstances of some patients, some changes would have occurred even in the absence of BMT. For example, compared to their pre-BMT status, many patients report subtle difficulties in memory or recall and/or a reduced capacity to engage in vigorous physical exercise.

These changes may simply reflect the normal functional changes due to the process of ageing, particularly when a considerable period of time has elapsed between initial diagnosis and treatment and recovery following BMT. Normal physical and psychological functioning for any person at any particular point in time is a subtly changing standard. This makes it difficult to assess the degree to which observed physical or psychological changes are true sequelae of BMT or are part of the normal growth and development process. Furthermore, a BMT recipient's definition of 'normal' may subtly change as a consequence of their disease and treatment. What was once viewed as normal physical and psychological functioning may now be unattainable, and what was once thought of as disability may now be viewed as normal.

Additionally, in judging the degree to which one has returned to normal following BMT, an individual may place more or less emphasis on certain aspects of physical or psychological functioning. Areas of deficit or change may be downplayed in significance, while areas of strength or status may be given greater weight in making global judgments of whether or not one has returned to normal. This unequal weighting of areas of functioning is a vexing problem for researchers and underscores the subjectivity of normality for the individual patient. [25] As a result, some BMT recipients may view themselves as 'normal' despite the objective existence of BMT-induced physical or psychological changes.

Only a single study has directly assessed BMT recipients' perceptions of whether they had 'returned to normal' following their transplant [26]. The 172 respondents ranged from 12 to 124 months post-transplant (autologous or allogeneic) for a malignant condition. All respondents were in disease remission at time of study. While 48% of the sample reported that they viewed themselves as 'back to normal' following BMT, 32% stated that they did not view themselves as such. The remaining 20%, while stating that they had indeed returned to normal, nevertheless qualified this assertion by indicating one or more specific areas of deficit. Respondents were also questioned regarding eight specific areas of functioning and asked to indicate whether their current status was 'normal' 'almost normal' or 'not normal' (see Table 54.3). For only three of the eight areas did 50% or more of respondents indicate that their current status was 'normal': socializing with friends (62%), personal appearance (54%) and ability to think clearly and remember (50%). In contrast, over 25% of BMT recipients reported that their current status was explicitly 'not normal' with regard to engaging in vigorous physical exercise (43%), engaging in sexual activity (32%) and working outside the home (28%). In general, areas involving physical activity or exertion were most likely to be viewed as having not returned to normal following BMT. On the other hand, patient status in areas not involving physical activity was most likely to be viewed as having returned to normal.

In addition to examining BMT recipients' perceptions of whether or not they had returned to normal, information regarding recipients' expectations for their post-BMT recovery were also obtained [26]. About half of the study sample (47%) indicated that they had, indeed, expected that they would have returned to normal by the time of their study participation (a mean of over three years post-BMT). An additional 25% maintained that they recalled no particular expectations for their recovery, typically recalling instead that at the time of their BMT they were concentrating solely on survival and not the quality of their survival. Only 19% of BMT recipients indicated that they had not expected to return to normal following BMT. In general, even when a period of convalescence and recovery was anticipated, its length was often underestimated. Many respondents indicated that they had anticipated a period of only weeks or a few months at most before a return to normal was achieved.

The large and growing literature on post-BMT quality of life (QoL) also furnishes some insight into the issue of returning to normal after BMT. Studies involving QoL assessments both before and after BMT, while distinctly uncommon, provide a means for examining the impact of BMT upon various functional

Table 54.3 Percentage of BMT respondents (n = 172) reporting current status was 'not normal', 'almost normal' or 'normal' for various domains (from Andrykowski et al. [26])

Domain	Not normal	Almost normal	Normal
Work outside the home	28	23	49
Doing hobbies/recreation	21	35	44
Socializing with friends	12	26	62
Engaging in sexual activity	32	32	36
Engaging in vigorous physical activity	43	36	21
Work around home/garden	22	29	49
Personal appearance	9	37	54
Ability to think clearly/remember	13	37	50

domains. In a study of 67 allogeneic recipients ($n = 31$ at 12 months follow-up), the authors found physical function was most impaired 90 days post-BMT with a return to pre-BMT functioning in most areas by 12 months post-BMT [27]. The investigators concluded that while the majority of study participants had returned to full-time employment with normal physical and psychosocial functioning by one year, recovery required longer than one year for approximately 40% of study participants. In general, poorer one-year emotional status was associated with greater pre-BMT family conflict and unmarried status. Poorer physical status was associated with more severe chronic graft-versus-host disease (GvHD) and greater pre-BMT physical impairment and family conflict.

In a second study of 28 allogeneic BMT recipients, little difference was found in mean scores for the group as a whole on various measures of physical and psychosocial status obtained both pre-BMT and 12–16 months post-BMT [28]. However, analysis of scores for individual patients indicated that physical and psychosocial status improved markedly following BMT for some patients while that of others declined. Females and younger patients were most likely to evidence improvements in physical and psychological functioning following BMT. In a study of 52 recipients ($n = 24$ patients at follow-up) 3–24 months post-autologous BMT for breast cancer, significant improvement in mean scores on functional well-being, overall QoL and mood was recorded between pre-BMT and post-BMT assessments [29]. No differences were found in group mean scores obtained at the pre- and post-BMT assessments with regard to physical, social/family and emotional well-being, and perceived social support. Twelve of 24 patients reported normal activity at the time of the post-BMT assessment with the remaining patients reporting some symptoms with regard to patient-rated performance status. However, at the post-BMT assessment, approximately one-third of respondents reported problems with depression, sexuality or fatigue. Some of these patients had reported 'normal' activity, thus illustrating again that patients may view their functioning as essentially normal while nevertheless acknowledging areas of significant deficit. Overall QoL and mood improved at the post-BMT assessment and QoL compares favourably with that reported by breast cancer patients treated with conventional therapies [30].

Finally, in a study of 54 autologous BMT recipients ($n = 34$ patients who completed assessments at each time point), psychological and neuropsychological status was assessed pre-BMT, 1–3 days post-BMT and 1–2 days prehospital discharge (mean of 36 days post-BMT) [31]. A general decline in neuropsychological performance was evident between the pre-BMT and pre-discharge assessments. Whereas distress generally declined over the course of the study in patients with haematological malignancies, patients with breast cancer evidenced similar distress levels at the pre-BMT and predischarge assessments.

In summary, the prospective, longitudinal studies described above suggest that physical and psychological recovery are well underway by the first year post-BMT, with many patients reporting similar or superior post-BMT functional status relative to their pre-BMT baseline. However, these studies are limited by both a short duration of follow-up and relatively small sample sizes. As a result, it is not known whether physical or functional deficits evident at assessments 12–24 months post-BMT represent relatively permanent areas of deficit or simply a slower temporal course of recovery. Additionally, the small sample sizes raise the question of representativeness of study findings. However, even given adequate sample sizes and longer follow-up, prospective studies of post-BMT physical and functional recovery pose some interpretive difficulties. Specifically, it is unclear whether QoL assessments conducted immediately prior to pre-BMT conditioning provide a true baseline for gauging normal functioning. Many patients undergo BMT following one or more courses of conventional (i.e. low-dose) cytotoxic therapy. Thus, patients' functional status may already be markedly different from normal even as they prepare to undergo BMT. Comparison of pre- and post-BMT QoL assessments may thus be misleading. If pre-BMT QoL measures exceed identical post-BMT QoL measures, one might conclude that some QoL deficits exist and patients' QoL has not returned to normal. On the other hand, however, if pre-BMT QoL measures are equal or are inferior to post-BMT QoL measures, the conclusion that QoL is unaffected or that normal functioning is regained is warranted only to the degree that the pre-BMT assessment constitutes a true baseline of 'normal' functioning and status. Of course, this true baseline problem is present whenever disease status is assessed following diagnosis, since the diagnosis itself can affect emotional well-being and other QoL domains immediately. It becomes a greater problem when the question involves assessing the patient's subjective sense of returning to normal. The only way to resolve this issue would be to collect QoL data prior to diagnosis or to compare BMT recipients to matched controls on general QoL measures.

Information regarding recovery of normal functioning following BMT is also potentially available from retrospective studies of post-BMT QoL and functioning. Fortunately, many fairly large-scale retrospective studies (i.e. sample sizes > 100) currently exist [28,32–39]. Furthermore, most of these studies include BMT recipients several years or more post-BMT, thus shedding more light upon long-term functional recovery than is possible in the presently available prospective studies. In general, these studies suggest that many, perhaps most, BMT recipients report an essentially 'normal' QoL. However, even the patients who appear to adapt most successfully following BMT may experience what have been called 'islands' of significant life disruption [40]. The remaining group of BMT recipients tend to report a range of problems or deficits including low self-esteem, depression, psychological distress, fatigue and lack of energy, occupational disability, impaired social relationships, sexual dysfunction, sleep difficulties, cognitive impairment, and limitations upon performance of household tasks and typical recreational activities [3–5]. (Table 54.4). Unfortunately, none of these studies collected identical data from a comparison group of generally healthy individuals without a history of cancer or BMT. Such comparison data would provide an invaluable normative standard, allowing inferences regarding the extent to which BMT recipients have recovered normal QoL and functional status. While it is tempting to speculate that results from retrospective, cross-sectional studies suggest that a significant number of BMT recipients fail to return to normal following BMT, the absence of comparison data from age- and gender-matched healthy individuals makes such an interpretation tenuous. An additional problem with the available retrospective, cross-sectional studies of post-BMT QoL is that they do not report on relapsed patients who might arguably report worse overall QoL when compared to disease-free BMT recipients. Thus,

Table 54.4 Problems reported after BMT

Low self-esteem

Depression

Psychological stress

Fatigue and lack of energy

Occupational disability

Impaired social relationships

Sexual dysfunction

Sleep difficulties

Cognitive impairment

Limitations upon performance of household tasks and recreational activities

the statement that post-BMT QoL is generally good and that most recipients report a return to normal clearly needs to be qualified by noting that many BMT recipients have relapsed or expired along the way.

In making global judgements regarding whether or not they have 'returned to normal' following BMT, patients typically use their pre-illness status or the perceived status of an age and gender similar other as benchmarks. Therefore, in lieu of a true prediagnosis baseline or a suitably matched healthy comparison group, one useful strategy is to ask BMT recipients to compare their current status to their prediagnosis status or to the status of a typical person their own age. Several studies have asked BMT recipients to provide global ratings of current physical health and QoL [29,32,37]. By themselves, these ratings are difficult to interpret. Asking patients to provide additional ratings of their own health and QoL 'prior to your diagnosis' as well as the health and QoL of a 'typical person your age' provides some context within which ratings of current health and QoL can be judged [27]. Using this approach, it was found that BMT patients as a group rated their current health and QoL as significantly poorer than both their own prediagnosis health and QoL as well as that of a typical person their age [27]. Relative to two different baseline standards, therefore, BMT recipients reported that, on the whole, their current status had not returned to normal. While this strategy does not negate the desirability of a true prediagnosis baseline or normative comparison group, it is a strategy worth considering by those conducting cross-sectional, retrospective research.

Finally, in considering whether or not an individual has 'returned to normal' following BMT, emphasis has typically been placed upon the extent to which recipients have recovered from the well-known negative physical and psychosocial sequelae potentially associated with BMT. However, the experience of life-threatening disease and treatment can also trigger a range of salutary psychosocial reactions. These can include increased self-esteem, greater appreciation for life, enhanced interpersonal relationships, or heightened spirituality [41–44]. Not surprisingly, reports of such positive responses have been documented in BMT recipients [41,42,44]. Interestingly, such positive sequelae are often juxtaposed with a variety of negative, often severe, physical and psychosocial sequelae. Most significantly, this research has suggested that positive psychosocial reactions can continue to exert an impact upon the lives of BMT recipients many years following BMT. Thus, the experience of a life-threatening disease and BMT can be associated with temporary or relatively permanent deviations from normal in both positive as well as negative directions. Even if an individual has fully recovered from any negative physical or functional sequelae of BMT, they may nevertheless still not have returned to normal. In fact, it is common for BMT recipients to indicate that while they believe they have fully recovered from the physical rigours of their disease and transplant, they also believe that their illness experience has left them irrevocably altered in some deeper psychological or spiritual sense.

Interventions to facilitate re-adaptation to normal life

Since BMT recipients are at risk of experiencing a variety of negative physical and psychosocial problems, efforts to minimize the negative impact of such sequelae and to facilitate re-adaptation to normal life are of obvious importance. While some rehabilitation efforts are no doubt incorporated into routine clinical follow-up on an informal basis, little attempt has been made to systematically develop, implement and evaluate clinical interventions to maximize QoL and to facilitate re-adaptation following BMT. In fact, only a single, preliminary pilot study addressing this issue could be identified. Decker and colleagues investigated the effects of participation in a cardiopulmonary exercise program in 12 allogeneic BMT recipients [45]. The exercise programme consisted of three weekly exercise sessions using a stationary bicycle for a minimum of 30 minutes each session at 85% of maximum heart rate. While the authors suggested that poor performance status might make the intervention difficult to implement during the first few months post-BMT, the intervention was well accepted and easy to perform at approximately four months post-BMT. Results at follow-up testing eight months post-BMT, however, were equivocal due to the limited numbers of patients available for study.

Some useful strategies for rehabilitative interventions for BMT recipients can be appropriated from successful interventions utilized in other clinically similar populations. Specifically, there is a growing literature documenting the ability of various interventions to enhance psychosocial functioning and adaptation in cancer patients following conventional cytotoxic therapy [46–55]. A variety of different psychosocially oriented intervention approaches can be identified, including cognitive–behavioural interventions, provision of information and education, non-behavioural counselling or psychotherapy, and provision of social support [46]. Often, these distinct approaches can be effectively combined as components of a larger multi-factorial intervention. For example, Fawzy and colleagues randomly assigned 66 post-surgical malignant melanoma patients to either a structured psychoeducational group intervention ($n = 38$) or a no-intervention control group ($n = 28$) [55]. The intervention groups consisted of 7 to 10 patients who met for 90 minutes weekly for six consecutive weeks. The intervention included four components: health education, enhancement of illness-related problem-solving skills, training in stress management and psychological support. Results of a six-month follow-up indicated that participation in the intervention reduced psychological distress and enhanced effective coping in the long term. Interestingly, the intervention also appeared to enhance the likelihood of survival in a six-year follow-up [54], a finding which has also been reported following participation in a supportive group intervention for women with metastatic breast cancer [51].

Group-oriented interventions have the obvious advantages of both being able to capitalize on the provision of social support and maximize the number of patients able to participate at a given time. However, individually oriented interventions have also been utilized with success [56,57]. For example, Greer and colleagues randomly assigned cancer patients to an adjuvant psychological therapy condition or a no-intervention control condition [57]. The adjuvant psychological therapy intervention consisted of a minimum of six weekly one-hour therapy sessions with the patient, accompanied by their spouse, if appropriate. A cognitive–behavioural approach was utilized emphasizing the personal meaning of cancer to the patient as well as coping with specifically identified stressors and problems. Results of a four-month follow-up indicated that participants in the intervention condition evidenced significantly less physical and psychological distress relative to their counterparts in the control condition.

While both of the basic intervention strategies described above would appear to be translatable into the post-BMT setting, some caution is warranted. First, psychological distress and/or self-reported coping behaviours have been the primary outcome indices evaluated. Furthermore, length of follow-up for these indices has often been limited. As a result, the long-term impact of psychosocial interventions on overall functional recovery has been less extensively studied. Second, the ability to implement group intervention in the BMT setting might be limited given that BMT patients at a particular transplant centre are often relatively few in number and drawn from a wide geographical area. While the alternative is a more individualized intervention approach, this, of course, has the disadvantage of increased expense. This expense can be reduced by focussing upon intervening only with those BMT recipients who are most at risk for poor functional outcomes following BMT. Potential risk factors for greater post-BMT psychosocial morbidity can be gleaned from the general cancer [58], as well as the BMT literature [59]. These include poor social support, increased physical co-morbidity, more extensive treatment and disease, lower socioeconomic status, a history of substance abuse or psychiatric problems and a limited or rigid repertoire of coping skills (Table 54.5).

Table 54.5 Risk factors for psychosocial morbidity

Poor social support
Increased physical co-morbidity
More extensive treatment and disease
Lower socioeconomic status
History of substance abuse or psychiatric problems
Limited or rigid repertoire of social skills

Summary

For most individuals electing to undergo BMT, the BMT procedure offers the strongest possibility of a cure for their underlying disease. The term 'cure', however, can have several different meanings. To the oncologist or BMT clinical staff, 'cure' most likely refers to a condition where the individual is alive with no evidence of disease for some specified period of time. To the BMT patient, however, disease cure is likely to imply far more. Specifically, the lay definition of 'cure' incorporates not only the eradication of the underlying disease that necessitated BMT but also a full restoration of health with its implied recovery of normal functioning [26]. It is not surprising, therefore, that many BMT recipients and family members link the attainment of a cure for their disease with a full 'return to normal'.

Even when BMT is followed by a biological cure as well as an apparent complete recovery of normal functioning, a complete 'return to normal' may still not be evident. Re-adaptation following BMT requires not only a biological cure, but a psychological and social cure as well [60]. A 'psychological cure' is attained when the BMT recipient is able to acknowledge and accept his illness as a past event with little current interference in normal activities. A 'social cure' is attained when the BMT patient functions socially without consideration of his history of cancer and treatment. In both cases, a 'cure' is attained to the degree that status as a BMT recipient becomes a less and less salient aspect of an individual's personal or social identity. One clear impediment to attaining either a psychological or social cure is the ever present threat of disease recurrence that exists following BMT.

In fact, the threat of recurrence carries even more ominous implications in the BMT setting relative to that experienced by cancer patients who have undergone conventional therapy [61,62]. Since BMT patients are being treated with the 'last line of defence', so to speak, palliative care or a second transplant remain the only viable option in the event of disease recurrence. In light of the continual threat of recurrence and the serious implications of such, it is not surprising to hear even long-term BMT survivors remark that 'it will never be the same again'.

The diagnosis and treatment of cancer, and especially the bone-marrow transplantation experience, exact a heavy toll on recipients and family members. For the fortunate patient, the diagnosis, treatment and recovery process become but a small portion of the patient's larger 'life story' [63]. This usually occurs with the passage of time and the gradual resumption of valued roles and activities, and the recovery of psychological, social and physical functioning. While many BMT patients may indeed 'never be the same' following their transplant, to the extent that they and others are able to view their disease and its treatment as a subplot rather than their entire life story, they can usually be considered to have accomplished a successful re-adaptation to normal life.

References

1. Winer EP and Sutton LM. Quality of life after bone marrow transplantation. *Oncology* 1994; **8**: 19–27.
2. Patenaude AF. Psychological impact of bone marrow transplantation: current perspectives. *Yale J Biol Med* 1990; **63**: 515–519.
3. Hjermstad MJ and Kaasa S. Quality of life in adult cancer patients treated with bone marrow transplantation – a review of the literature. *Eur J Cancer* 1995; **31A**: 163–173.
4. Andrykowski MA. Psychosocial factors in bone marrow transplantation: a review and recommendations for research. *Bone Marrow Transplant* 1994; **13**: 357–375.
5. Andrykowski MA. Psychiatric and psychosocial aspects of bone marrow transplantation. *Psychosomatics* 1994; **35**: 13–24.
6. Hurd DD. Bone Marrow transplantation: an overview. In: *Recent Results in Cancer Research, Volume 132. Infectious Complications in Bone Marrow Transplantation*. SC Schimpf (ed.), (New York: Springer-Verlag).
7. Dicke KA. Late effects after allogeneic bone marrow transplantation. *Bone Marrow Transplant* 1994; **14**(Suppl 4): S11–3.
8. Giri N, Davis EA and Vowels MR. Long-term complications following bone marrow transplantation in children. *J Paediatr Child Health* 1993; **29**: 201–205.
9. Moos RH and Schaefer JA. The crisis of physical illness: an overview and conceptual approach. In: *Coping with Physical Illness: New perspectives*. RH Moos (ed.), 1984: 3–25 (New York: Plenum).
10. Rowland JH. Psychological factors and adaptation. In: *Handbook of Psycho-oncology: Psychological Care of the Patient with Cancer*. JC Hollland and JH Rowland (eds), 1989: 23–71 (New York: Oxford University Press).
11. Andersen BL, Kiecolt-Glaser JK and Glaser R. A biobehavioral model of cancer stress and disease course. *Am Psychol* 1994; **49**: 389–404.
12. Thompson SC. In sickness and in health: chronic illness, marriage, and spousal caregiving. In: *Helping and Being Helped: Naturalistic Studies*. The Claremont Symposium on Applied Psychology. S Spacapan and S Oskamp (eds), 1992: 115–151 (Newbury Park CA: Sage Publications).
13. Cole RE. *How Do Families Cope with Chronic Illness?* 1993 (Hillsdale NJ: Lawrence Erlbaum).
14. Parsons T. *The Social System*. 1951 (New York: Free Press).
15. Parsons T. The sick role and the role of the physician reconsidered. *Milbank Mem Fund Quart* 1975; **53**: 257–278.
16. Burch GE and DePasquale NP. There is such an entity as a cardiac invalid. *Am Heart J* 1969; **78**: 426.
17. Crumlish CM. Coping and emotional response in cardiac surgery patients. *Western J Nursing Res* 1994; **16**: 57–68.
18. Brown JS and Rawlinson M. Relinquishing the sick role following open-heart surgery. *J Health Social Behavior* 1975; **16**: 12–27.
19. Brown HN and Kelly MJ. Stages of bone marrow transplantation: a psychiatric perspective. *Psychosomatic Med* 1976; **38**: 439–446.
20. Andrykowski MA and McQuellon RP. Bone marrow transplantation. In: *Handbook of Psycho-oncology*. J Holland, PB Jacobsen, M Lederberg and R McCorkle (eds) (New York: Oxford University Press). In press for early 1998.
21. Lazarus RS. Coping theory and research: past, present, and future. *Psychosomatic Med* 1993; **55**: 234–247.
22. Lazarus RS. From psychological stress to the emotions: a history of changing outlooks. *Ann Rev Psychol* 1993; **44**: 1–21.
23. Lazarus RS and Folkman S. *Stress, Appraisal, and Coping*. 1984 (New York: Springer).
24. Mullan F. Seasons of survival: reflections of a physician with cancer. *New Engl J Med* 1985; **313**: 270–273.
25. Cella DF. Quality of life: concepts and definition. *J Pain Symptom Management* 1994; **9**: 186–192.
26. Andrykowski MA, Brady MJ, Greiner CB et al. 'Returning to normal' following bone marrow transplantation: outcomes, expectations and informed consent. *Bone Marrow Transplant* 1995; **15**: 573–581.
27. Syrjala KL, Chapko MK, Vitaliano PP, Cummings C and Sullivan KM. Recovery after allogeneic marrow transplantation: prospective study of predictors of long-term physical and psychosocial functioning. *Bone Marrow Transplant* 1993; **11**: 319–327.
28. Andrykowski MA, Bruehl S, Brady MJ and Henslee-Downey PJ. Physical and psychosocial status of adults one-year after bone marrow transplantation: a prospective study. *Bone Marrow Transplant* 1995; **15**: 837–844.
29. McQuellon RP, Craven B, Russell GB et al. Quality of life in breast cancer patients before and after autologous bone marrow transplantation. *Bone Marrow Transplant* 1996; **18**: 579–584.

30. McQuellon RP, Muss HB, Hoffman SL, Russell G, Craven B and Yellen SB. Patient preferences for treatment of metastatic breast cancer: a study of women with early-stage breast cancer. *J Clin Oncol* 1995; **13**: 858–868.
31. Ahles TA, Tope DM, Furstenberg C, Hann D and Mills L. Psychologic and neuropsychologic impact of autologous bone marrow transplantation. *J Clin Oncol* 1996; **14**: 1457–1462.
32. Andrykowski MA, Greiner CB, Altmaier EM *et al.* Quality of life following bone marrow transplantation: findings from a multicentre study. *Br J Cancer* 1995; **71**: 1322–1329.
33. Baker F, Wingard JR, Curbow B *et al.* Quality of life of bone marrow transplant long-term survivors. *Bone Marrow Transplant* 1994; **13**: 589–596.
34. Baker F, Curbow B and Wingard JR. Role retention and quality of life of bone marrow transplant survivors. *Social Sci Med* 1991; **32**: 697–704.
35. Bush NE, Haberman M, Donaldson G and Sullivan KM. Quality of life of 125 adults surviving 6–18 years after bone marrow transplantation. *Social Sci Med* 1995; **40**: 479–490.
36. Schmidt GM, Niland JC, Forman SJ *et al.* Extended follow-up in 212 long-term allogeneic bone marrow transplant survivors. Issues of quality of life. *Transplantation* 1993; **55**: 551–557.
37. Chao NJ, Tierney DK, Bloom JR *et al.* Dynamic assessment of quality of life after autologous bone marrow transplantation. *Blood* 1992; **80**: 825–830.
38. Wingard JR. Functional ability and quality of life of patients after allogeneic bone marrow transplantation. *Bone Marrow Transplant* 1994; **14**(Suppl 4): S29–33.
39. Wingard JR, Curbow B, Baker F and Piantadosi S. Health, functional status, and employment of adult survivors of bone marrow transplantation. *Ann Intern Med* 1991; **114**: 113–118.
40. Andersen BL, Anderson B and deProsse C. Controlled prospective longitudinal study of women with cancer: II. Psychological outcomes. *J Consulting Clin Psychol* 1989; **57**: 692–697.
41. Curbow B, Somerfield MR, Baker F, Wingard JR and Legro MW. Personal changes, dispositional optimism, and psychological adjustment to bone marrow transplantation. *J Behavioral Med* 1993; **16**: 423–443.
42. McLaurin T. *Keeper of the Moon: A Southern Boyhood*. 1991 (New York: WW Norton).
43. Andrykowski MA, Brady MJ and Hunt JW. Positive psychosocial adjustment in potential bone marrow transplant recipients: Cancer as a psychosocial transition. *Psycho-Oncology* 1993; **2**: 201–276.
44. Fromm K, Andrykowski MA and Hunt J. Positive and negative psychosocial sequelae of bone marow transplantation: Implications for quality of life assessment. *J Behavioral Med* 1996; **19**: 221–240.
45. Decker WA, Turner-McGlade J and Fehir KM. Psychosocial aspects and the physiological effects of a cardiopulmonary exercise program in patients undergoing bone marrow transplantation (BMT) for acute leukemia (AL). *Transplant Proc* 1989; **21**: 3068–3069.
46. Meyer TJ and Mark MM. Effects of psychosocial interventions with adult cancer patients: a meta-analysis of randomized experiments. *Health Psychol* 1995; **14**: 101–108.
47. Andersen BL. Psychological interventions for cancer patients to enhance the quality of life. *J Consulting Clin Psychol* 1992; **60**: 552–568.
48. Spiegel D. Health caring. Psychosocial support for patients with cancer. *Cancer* 1994; **74**: 1453–1457.
49. Spiegel D. Psychosocial intervention in cancer. *J Nat Cancer Inst* 1993; **85**: 1198–1205.
50. Spiegel D. Can psychotherapy prolong cancer survival? *Psychosomatics* 1990; **31**: 361–366.
51. Spiegel D, Bloom JR, Kraemer HC and Gottheil E. Effect of psychosocial treatment on survival of patients with metastatic breast cancer. *Lancet* 1989; **ii**: 888–891.
52. Fawzy FI, Fawzy NW, Arndt LA and Pasnau RO. Critical review of psychosocial interventions in cancer care. *Arch Gen Psychiatry* 1995; **52**: 100–113.
53. Fawzy FI and Fawzy NW. A structured psychoeducational intervention for cancer patients. *Gen Hosp Psychiatry* 1994; **16**: 149–192.
54. Fawzy FI, Fawzy NW, Hyun CS *et al.* Malignant melanoma. Effects of an early structured psychiatric intervention, coping, and affective state on recurrence and survival 6 years later. *Arch Gen Psychiatry* 1993; **50**: 681–689.
55. Fawzy FI, Kemeny FI, Fawzy NW *et al.* A structured psychiatric intervention for cancer patients: I. Changes over time in methods of coping and affective disturbance. *Arch Gen Psychiatry* 1990; **47**: 720–725.
56. Gordon WA, Freidenbergs I, Diller L *et al.* Efficacy of psychosocial intervention with cancer patients. *J Consulting Clin Psychol* 1980; **48**: 743–759.
57. Greer S, Moorey S, Baruch JD *et al.* Adjuvant psychological therapy for patients with cancer: a prospective randomised trial. *Br Med J* 1992; **304**: 675–680.
58. Andersen BL. Surviving cancer. *Cancer* 1994; **74**: 1484–1495.
59. Futterman AD, Wellisch DK, Bond G and Carr CR. The Psychosocial Levels System. A new rating scale to identify and assess emotional difficulties during bone marrow transplantation. *Psychosomatics* 1991; **32**: 177–186.
60. Van Eys J. Living beyond cure. Transcending survival. *Am J Pediatr Hematol Oncol* 1987; **9**: 114–118.
61. Mahon SM. Managing the psychosocial consequences of cancer recurrence: implications for nurses. *Oncol Nursing Forum* 1991; **18**: 577–583.
62. Cella DF, Mahon SM and Donovan MI. Cancer recurrence as a traumatic event. *Behavioral Med* 1990; **16**: 15–22.
63. McQuellon RP and Hurt GJ. The healing power of cancer stories. *J Psychosocial Oncol* 1993; **11**: 95–108

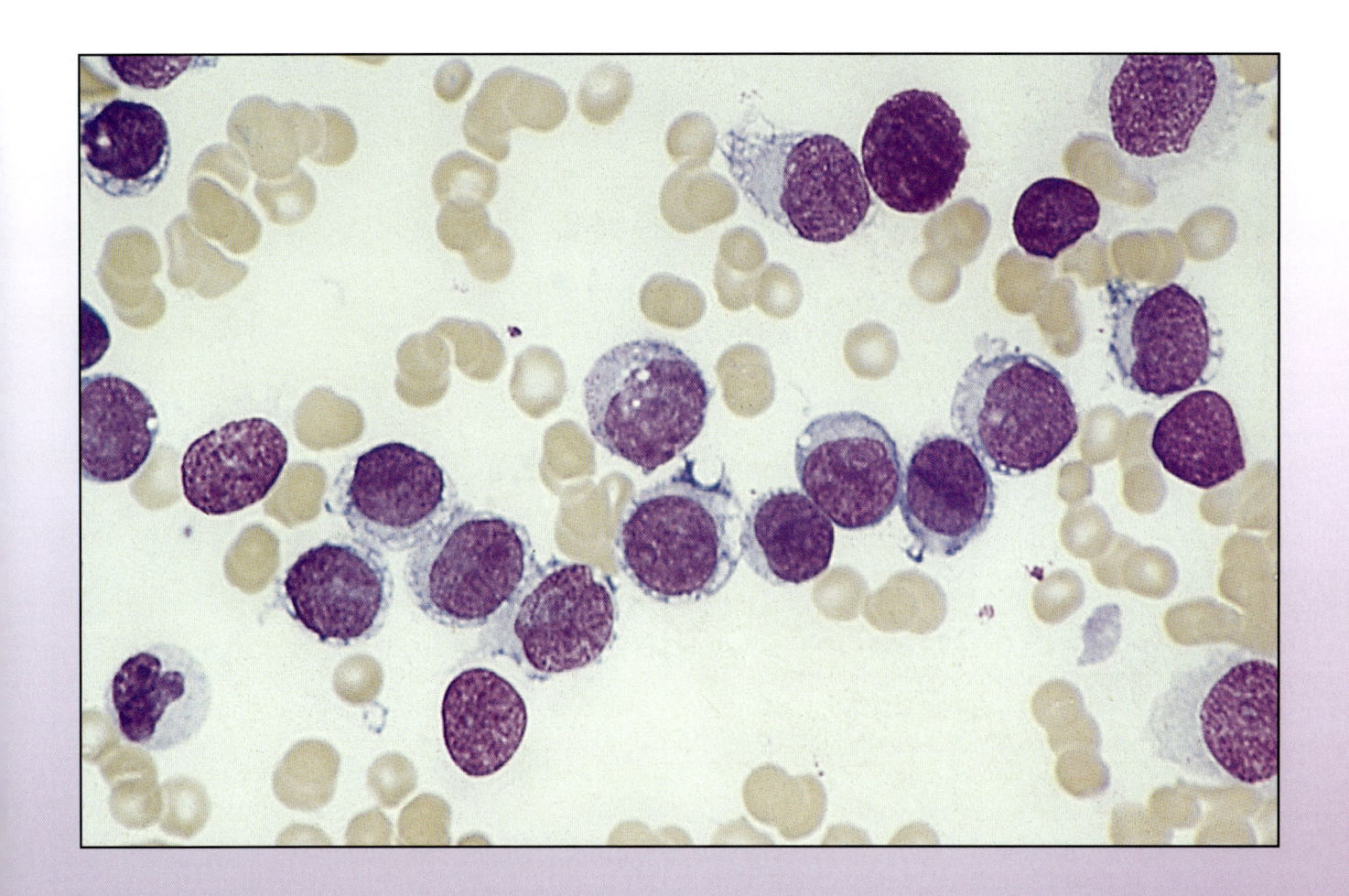

Chapter 55

Paediatric problems

Sally E. Kinsey

Introduction

The most common indication for bone-marrow transplantation (BMT) in children is acute lymphoblastic leukaemia (ALL), usually in second remission. As a result, most patients come to BMT having received significant amounts of previous chemotherapy. The long-term effects of BMT are therefore cumulative with previous therapy received and cannot be considered in isolation. Here, the late effects of chemotherapy and radiotherapy given in childhood will be considered and, although BMT issues take priority for purposes of discussion, they are not restricted solely to BMT-associated effects, as the principles of cumulative toxicity are similar. Long-term effects unique to the post-BMT situation will be highlighted.

Children tolerate acute toxicities much better than adults but the growing child is more vulnerable to delayed adverse sequelae – many of which may not be apparent for many years following the BMT procedure. Sixty per cent of children with malignant disease can now expect to be cured having been treated with intensive chemotherapy and radiotherapy schedules. The continuing improvement in long-term outlook for children comes on the back of increasing intensity of therapy which thereby potentially increases the development of late sequelae. Many of the late effects of therapy are expected in both adults and children. However, as the child is still growing and developing, there is potential for more serious late effects being apparent in the future.

The continuing improvement in survival following malignant disease in childhood is due primarily to the increasing intensity of therapy. With cure rates as they currently stand, it has been predicted that by the year 2000, 1 in 2000 adults will be survivors of ALL in childhood [1]. It may not be for many years that the full extent of long-term problems following BMT in childhood are manifest.

Organ toxicity is dependent upon individual cell susceptibility. Organs with high cell turnover such as bone marrow, gastrointestinal mucosa and testis are much more susceptible to the effects of chemotherapy and radiotherapy compared with tissues with very slow, or no, replication, including neurones and muscle cells (Table 55.1). Unfortunately, when damage does occur to tissues with low susceptibility and hence with

Table 55.1 Susceptibility of organs to treatment-related damage

High susceptibility	Low susceptibility
Bone marrow	Neurones
Gastrointestinal tract	Muscle cells
Testis	Connective tissue
Epidermis	
Liver	

Table 55.2 Late effects of bone-marrow transplantation in childhood

Growth
    Severe growth failure
    Growth hormone deficiency
    Early-onset puberty
    Chronic malabsorption and weight loss
    Obesity (secondary to radiation and steroids)

Endocrine system
    Hypothyroidism
    Gonadal failure
        Males
            reduced sperm production
            reduced gonadal endocrine function
        Females
            primary amenorrhoea
            absent secondary sexual characteristics
            secondary ovarian failure

Cardiovascular system
    Myocarditis/pericarditis
    Cardiomyopathy

Pulmonary system
    Fibrosis
    Pneumonitis
        GvHD
        Chemotherapy
        Radiotherapy
Interstitial pneumonitis
Restrictive lung damage
Obstructive lung disease
Obliterative bronchiolitis

Paediatric problems

Table 55.2 Continued

Neurological/neuropsychological
    Reduced IQ
    Learning difficulties
    Leukoencephalopathy
    Radionecrosis
    Intracranial calcification

Gastrointestinal system
    Malabsorption, diarrhoea and weight loss
    Sicca syndrome – dry mouth
    Mucosal lichenoid change

Renal system
    Hypertension and fluid retention
    Impaired glomerular function
    Haemorrhagic cystitis
    Haemolytic uraemic syndrome/thrombotic thrombocytopenic purpura

Musculoskeletal system
    Contracture formation
    Extravasation injuries
    Arthritis

Bone
    Osteopenia/osteoporosis
    Avascular necrosis

Skin
    Hyperpigmentation
    Depigmentation, sclerosis
    Subcutaneous thinning
    Poor hair and nail growth

Second malignancies
    Brain tumours
    Epstein–Barr virus-associated lymphoma
    Secondary leukaemia
    Glioma
    Melanoma
    Squamous-cell carcinoma
    Thyroid carcinoma

Other
    Dental abnormalities
    Cataract formation
    Hearing loss (antibiotic related)
    Immunological abnormalities
        hyposplenia/asplenia
        decreased humoral immunity
        decreased cell-mediated immunity
    Infection

slow repair potential, any damage is likely to result in a long-term or permanent deficit (Table 55.2).

Effects of BMT on growth

The effects of intensive chemotherapy and BMT conditioning regimes on growth are multifactorial and include growth hormone deficiency following cranial irradiation or busulphan [2], hypothyroidism, early onset of puberty (resulting in the early closure of epiphyses and shortened final height) [3] and inhibition of vertebral growth resulting in short spinal length (Figure 55.1). At puberty, growth is dependent on the interaction between growth hormone and sex

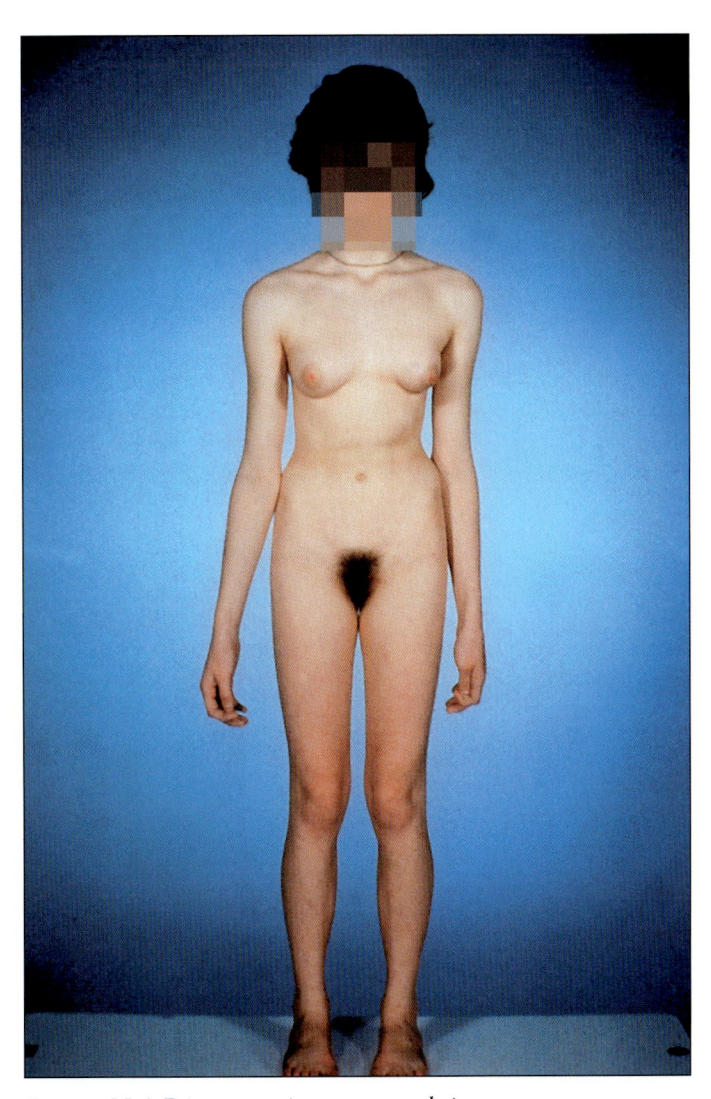

Figure 55.1 Disproportionate growth in a young woman, showing shortening of the spine and normal growth of limbs. Her arms appear too long, because of spinal shortening.

hormones. Abnormalities of hormone secretion and their treatment are covered in Chapter 56.

Severe growth failure (less than the fifth centile) is seen in 10–15% of children following antileukaemia treatment regimes [4], with a worsening of growth dependent upon associated central nervous system (CNS)-directed therapy and/or total body irradiation (TBI). Long-term effects are related to age (with most severe growth impairment in children treated under the age of three years), dose of irradiation given (greatest morbidity seen following ≥ 30 Gy, with much milder effects seen following 18–24 Gy), and fractionation of radiation dose, with lesser morbidity associated with multiple fractionation regimes [5] (Figures 55.2 and 55.3; Table 55.3).

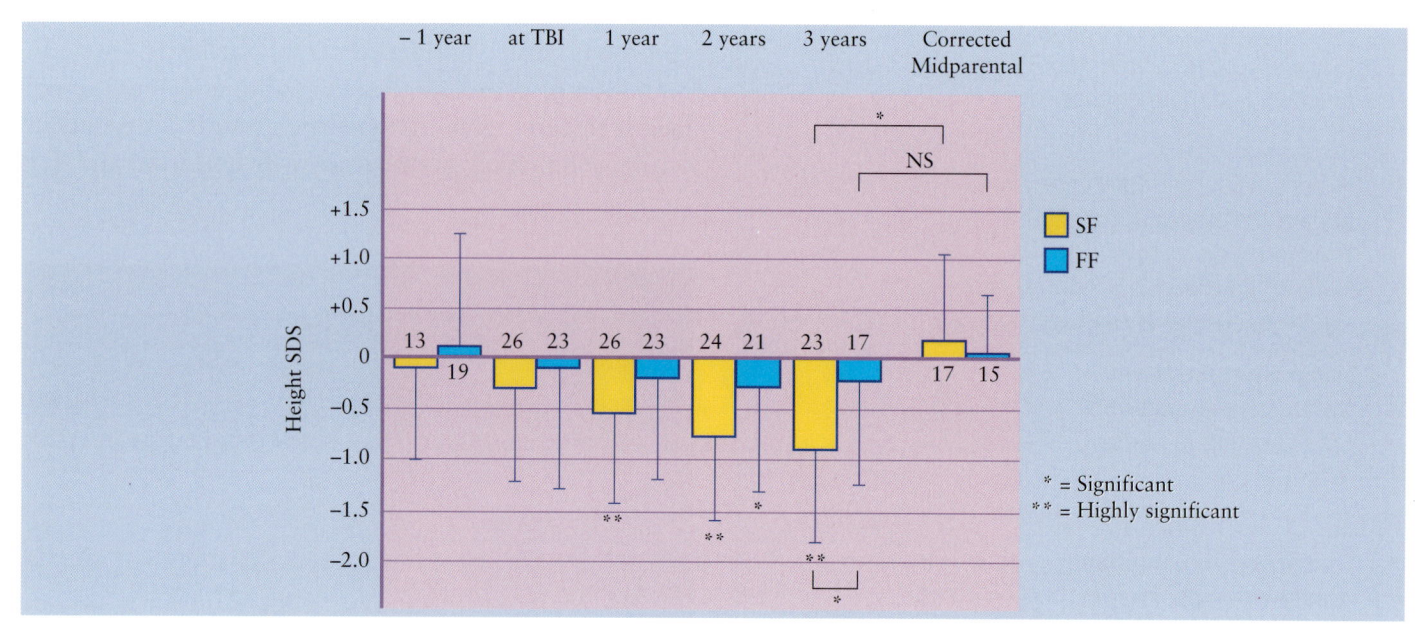

Figure 55.2 The effects on growth of total body irradiation (TBI) on 49 patients after TBI for BMT. Height standard deviation scores following single fraction (SF) and fractionated (FF) TBI. Numbers refer to the number of patients, of the 49, with measurements at the different time points with respect to TBI.

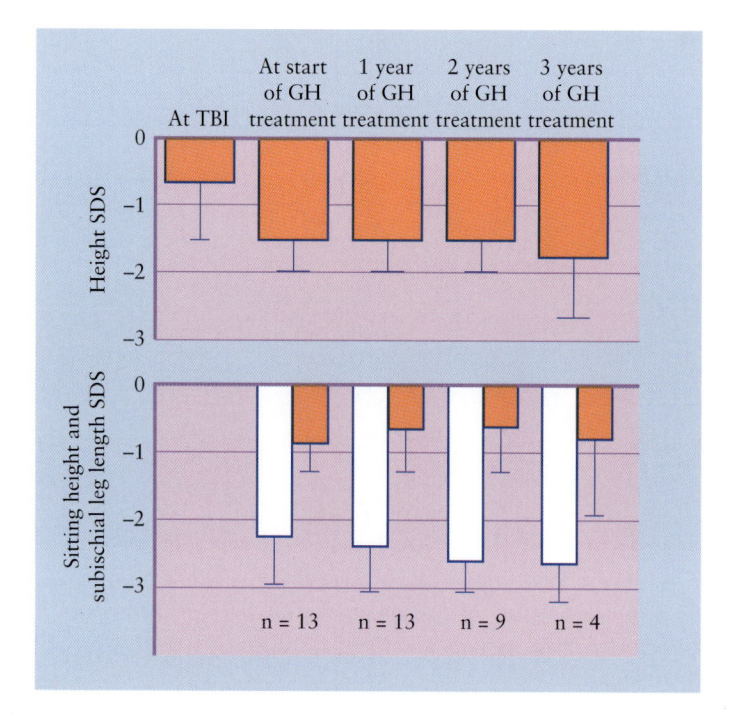

Figure 55.3 The effects of growth hormone administration on growth after TBI, showing no catch up. First year: 13 U/m²/week; second year: 18 U/m²/week. Progressive loss of sitting height, but maintenance of growth in subischial leg length.

> **Table 55.3** Factors worsening long-term effects of BMT
>
> - Young age (most impairment in children treated under the age of three years)
> - Dose of irradiation (greatest morbidity seen after > 30 Gy: much milder effects seen following 18–24 Gy).
> - Single-fraction radiation. Fractionation of radiation dose precipitates fewer sequelae.

Effects of BMT on the cardiovascular system

It is well recognized that cardiac toxicity is seen in a dose-related way following anthracycline therapy in both adults and children [6,7]. Additional mediastinal radiation contributes to the development of long-term problems [8]. Cardiac damage induced by anthracyclines is thought to be due to free-radical generation [9] causing damage to mitochondrial membranes and subsequent myofibrillar lysis. This causes degeneration of myocytes, interstitial fibrosis and hypertrophy of remaining myocytes (as lost myocytes are not replaced), resulting in an inadequate left-ventricular mass. The initial myocyte loss may be asymptomatic or be manifest as a myocarditis/pericarditis syndrome immediately associated with anthracycline administration [10]. The left-ventricular wall becomes relatively thin and may fail to maintain adequate function at times of increased cardiovascular stress, e.g. with the pubertal growth spurt, strenuous exercise or the demands of pregnancy leading to cardiac embarrassment. Both TBI and cyclophosphamide as BMT conditioning modalities may add to previous cardiotoxicity.

Although the ideal parameter for monitoring cardiac function is not clear, 6–12 monthly assessment by echocardiography, to measure left-ventricular ejection fraction and electrocardiography (ECG) is recommended [7].

Myocyte loss and myocardial fibrosis are likely to be associated with much earlier cardiac morbidity in those treated as children than in a previously untreated adult patient group. It seems likely that in 10–20 years time, we may see early onset of coronary artery disease and ischaemic heart disease in the individuals who have received TBI and cyclophosphamide at an early age.

Effects of BMT on the respiratory system

Pulmonary sequelae of BMT are multifactorial, with radiation, chemotherapeutic agents, graft-versus-host disease (GvHD), interstitial pneumonitis and infection being contributory.

Restrictive pulmonary defects are common after BMT. In one reported series [11], 20% of patients were found to have a reduced vital capacity, total lung capacity and impaired diffusion capacity one year following BMT. Restrictive defects may improve with time. Obstructive defects [12], however, may be permanent and may continue to worsen, particularly in those with GvHD. GvHD may be manifest as obliterative bronchiolitis and severe obstructive airways disease. Idiopathic interstitial pneumonitis developing within 100 days from BMT is associated with worse pulmonary effects.

Monitoring of pulmonary function is recommended, with an annual chest radiograph and formal pulmonary function tests.

Effects of BMT on the renal system

Long-term renal complications are most likely to be secondary to nephrotoxic agents required during the transplant period, i.e. cyclosporin, aminoglycoside antibiotics and amphotericin. With the antimicrobial agents, this tends to be manifest as glomerular tubular abnormalities with Fanconi syndrome and chronic electrolyte loss. The consequences of sepsis during neutropenia resulting in hypotension and reduced renal perfusion (including acute tubular necrosis) may lead to chronic renal impairment. Late-onset renal dysfunction may be seen as a consequence of radiation nephritis following TBI [13].

Neurological and neuropsychological complications of BMT

Total body irradiation as conditioning for BMT usually follows previous CNS-directed therapy, either intrathecal methotrexate, high-dose intravenous methotrexate or cranial irradiation. This combination of treatment is likely to lead to long-term problems which include reduction in IQ score and subtle learning difficulties [14,15] at one end of the spectrum, to leukoencephalopathy with severe progressive neurological deterioration at the other [16]. Educational performance may be impaired with a more noticeable deficit seen in girls [17]. Impairment tends to be manifest as a decrease in verbal IQ and reduced attention and concentration. The younger the age of the patient at time of therapy, the greater the effects appear to be. This is associated with a number of changes on computed tomography imaging of the brain [14]. These changes include attenuation of white matter, ventricular dilatation, intracerebral calcification and cerebral atrophy [18].

Cranial irradiation doses of either 24 Gy or 18 Gy do not differ in their effect on cognitive function. However, more severe neurological deficit is seen with increasing cumulative radiotherapy doses, particularly with short time intervals between two radiation exposures [19,20].

Readjusting to normal life following BMT may be difficult, not only as intellectual capacity may be altered, but also because of the desire to equal peers. Behavioural problems, impaired attainment of social skills and lower levels of satisfaction may cause further problems [21].

Effects of BMT on the gastrointestinal system

Chronic GvHD may result in sclerodermatous change of the gut associated with dysphagia and stricture formation, or a chronic malabsorption syndrome and weight loss. Intermittent abdominal pain and spasmodic diarrhoea may occur concurrently with chronic GvHD, and it is often difficult to distinguish whether infection is also present.

Hepatic complications after BMT are most frequently due to chronic GvHD or chronic hepatitis C infection [22].

Ophthalmological effects of BMT

Cataracts are induced by irradiation in a dose-related fashion, as has been known for some time (Figure

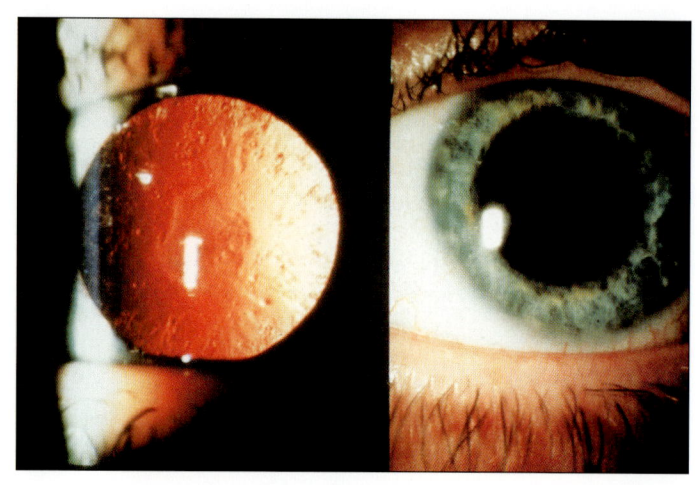

Figure 55.4 Cataract formation after total body irradiation.

55.4). Their development may be hastened by the use of steroids which are also cataractogenic [19], but a protective effect may be derived from the use of heparin, perhaps to treat veno-occlusive disease, although the mode of action is unclear.

Deeg and colleagues [23] reported an 80% risk of developing cataracts at six years following single-fraction TBI which is reduced to an 18% risk with fractionated regimes. The risk is also reduced with single-fraction regimes using low-dose rates [24]. Antineoplastic agents may also be implicated in cataract formation [25]. In a recent study of children with acute myeloid leukaemia (AML) treated with either high-dose chemotherapy alone or with an additional BMT with TBI conditioning, only those receiving BMT developed cataracts, but this was seen in 6 of 7 patients by three years following BMT [26]. Most patients require surgery for removal of cataracts, which is well tolerated and successful [23].

Other ophthalmic complications of BMT include dry eyes as a component of keratoconjunctivitis sicca seen with chronic GvHD or as a direct radiotherapy effect and may also be complicated by obstruction of the nasolacrimal duct [27].

Dental effects of BMT

Dental abnormalities and problems may be seen following TBI, cranial irradiation and chemotherapy and may result in poor root development with reduced life expectancy of dentition, grooves, pits and discolouration of the enamel, poor enamel and dentine development and poor saliva production either as a direct effect of radiotherapy or as a component of chronic GvHD-associated sicca syndrome.

Hypoplasia of the mandible and maxilla and increased bone resorption following radiotherapy contribute to dental loss. Tooth decay is a common feature particularly with poor saliva production and frequently is seen on unusual dental surfaces [28]. Careful and thorough dental hygiene and regular dental review must be encouraged.

Effects of BMT on bone

Osteoporosis and osteopenia are common following BMT (Figure 55.5) and may be related to radiotherapy, prolonged steroid therapy, chronic GvHD or premature menopause. Osteoporosis is difficult to detect as 30% bone mineral loss has to occur before it is apparent radiologically. More sensitive analysis and monitoring is possible by quantitative computed tomography scanning or dual-exposure X-ray absorptiometry (DEXA) scanning, the latter involving less radiation exposure.

Osteoporosis and avascular necrosis may both result in pathological fractures with poor subsequent bone healing.

Second malignancies

Individuals treated for malignant disease in childhood have an increased risk of developing second malignancies [29] to which initial diagnosis, type of chemotherapy (particularly alkylating agents), radiotherapy and BMT are contributory [30]. Epipodophyllotoxins are recognized to have an oncogenic potential [31], being associated with the development of secondary AML with specific cytogenetic abnormalities of 11q23 [32].

The long-term risk of second malignancy following therapy for ALL is 2.5–8% at 15 years [33] and a 2–3% incidence of brain tumours within 10 years of treatment has been reported [29,33]. All except one, were in individuals who had received 24 Gy cranial irradiation or TBI. Cranial irradiation for ALL is also associated with an increased incidence of thyroid malignancy and adenoma formation. The thyroid receives as much as 7.5% of the total irradiation dose within the radiation field [34].

The Seattle group have reported a series of BMT recipients in whom the incidence of second malignancy was 6.69 times that of primary cancer in the general population [35] from which TBI was a predictor for second malignancy. The types of second malignancy described include: B-cell non-Hodgkin's lymphoma, basal-cell carcinoma, squamous-cell carcinoma, leukaemia, glioma, melanoma and sarcoma.

An increased incidence of pigmented naevi is commonly found in association with TBI and chemotherapy [36] (Figure 55.6). With the additional risks of development of malignant change on exposure to ultraviolet radiation, care should be taken to prevent excessive sun exposure.

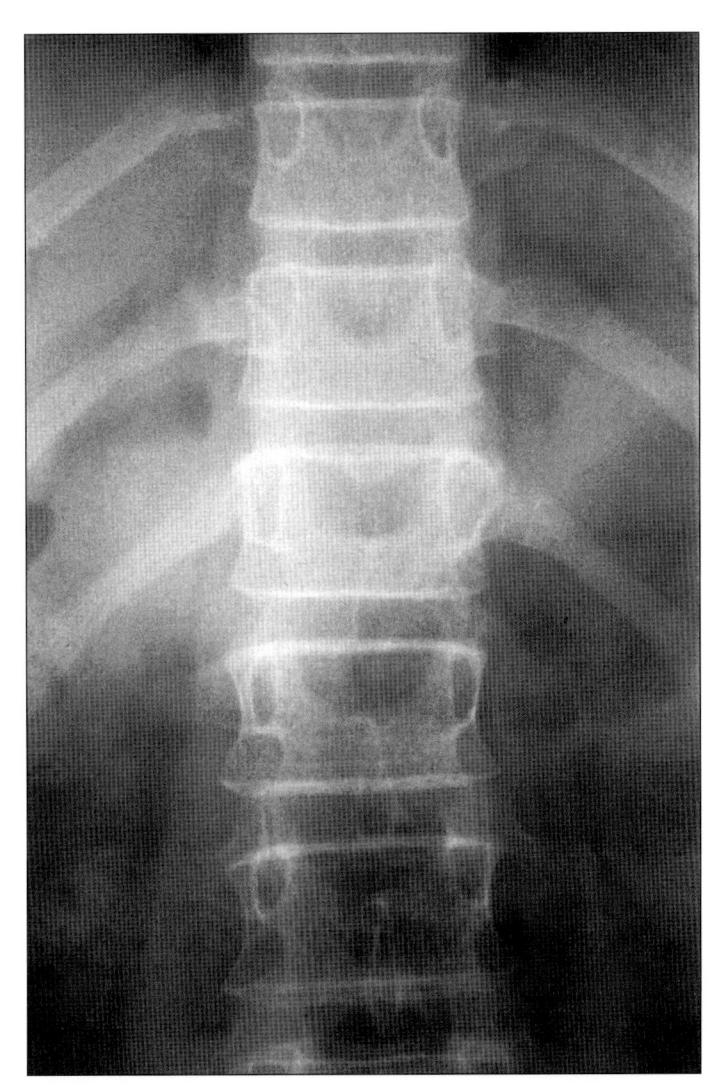

Figure 55.5 Severe osteoporosis of the spine secondary to growth hormone deficiency and radiation.

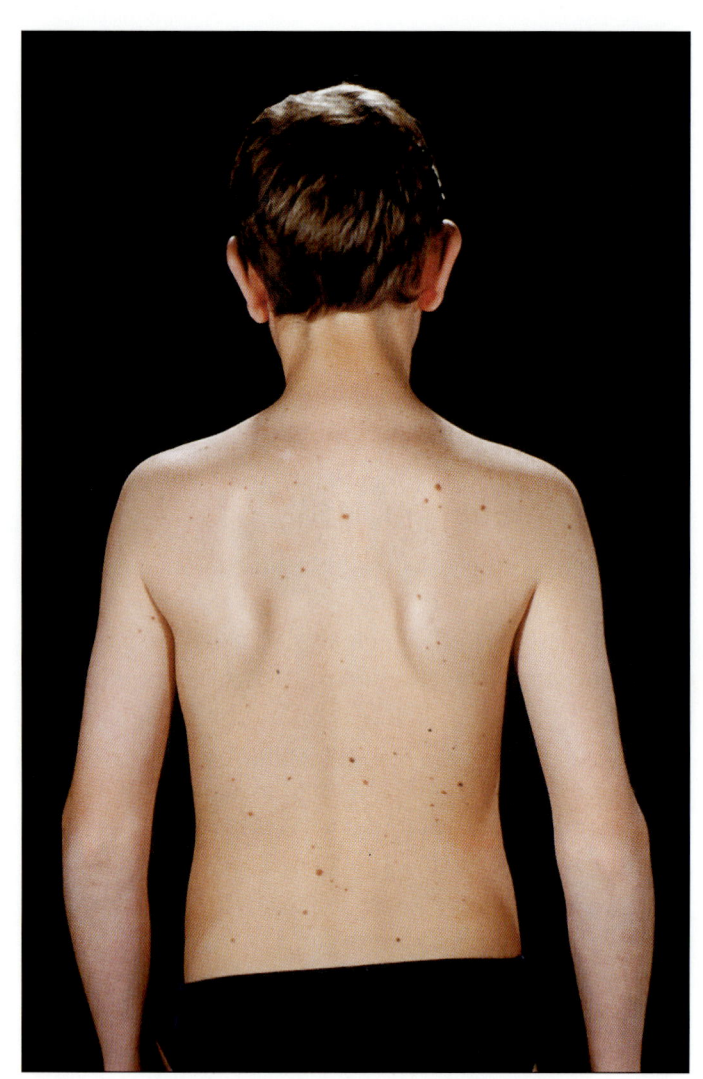

Figure 55.6 Multiple moles following chemoradiotherapy.

Table 55.4 Follow-up investigations post-BMT

General examination
    height (including sitting height) and weight, skin, mouth, teeth, eyes, joints

Full blood count and differential biochemical profile
    liver function
    renal function
    electrolytes

Chest X-ray

Echocardiogram and ECG (yearly)

Pulmonary function tests (yearly)

Bone age (yearly)

Thyroid function tests (yearly)

Endocrine assessment (yearly)

Immunoglobulins (yearly)

Vaccination titres (18 months and 2 years)

Audiology assessment (1 year, followed-up if necessary)

Ophthalmological review (yearly)

Conclusions

Improved survival is undoubted for those successfully undergoing BMT. However, there are many insidious and delayed effects of TBI and chemotherapy regimes. It is essential not only to monitor those effects which are already recognized in order that signs, symptoms and pathogenesis may be ameliorated but also to remain alert to any newly emerging problems (Table 55.4).

Identification of long-term risks and quality of survival must be weighed against striving for survival at any cost. In the future, we should be aiming to deliver therapy on a risk-related basis, thus intensifying therapy to those with high-risk disease and even decreasing therapy for those with good prognosis.

References

1. Meadows AT, Kreimas NL and Belasco JB. The medical cost of cure: sequelae in survivors of childhood cancer. In: *Status of the Curability of Childhood Cancers*. MP Sullivan and J van Eys (eds), 1980: 263–276 (New York: Raven Press).
2. Wingard JR, Plotnick LP, Freemer CS et al. Growth in children after bone marrow transplantation: busulphan plus cyclophosphamide versus cyclophosphamide plus total body irradiation. *Blood* 1992; **79**: 1068–1073.
3. Davies HA, Didcock E, Didi M, Ogilvy-Stuart A, Wales JKH and Shalet SM. Disproportionate short stature after cranial irradiation and combination chemotherapy for leukaemia. *Arch Dis Child* 1994; **70**: 472–475.
4. Robison LL, Nesbit ME, Sather HN et al. Height of children successfully treated for acute lymphoblastic leukaemia: a report from the Late Effects Study Committee of Children's Cancer Study Group. *Med Paediatr Oncol* 1985; **13**: 14.
5. Thomas BC, Plowman PN, Leiper AD et al. Growth following single fraction and fractionated total body irradiation for bone marrow transplantation. *Eur J Paediatr* 1993; **152**: 888–892.

6. Bistow MR, Billingham ME, Mason JW et al. Clinical spectrum of anthracycline antibiotic cardiotoxicity. *Cancer Treat Rep* 1978; **62**: 873–879.
7. Hale JP and Lewis IJ. Anthracyclines: cardiotoxicity and its prevention. *Arch Dis Child* 1994; **71**: 457–462.
8. Hancock SL, Donaldson S and Hoppe R. Cardiac disease following treatment of Hodgkin's disease in children and adolescents. *J Clin Oncol* 1993; **11**: 1208–1215.
9. Bristow MR, Mason JW, Billingham ME et al. Doxorubicin cardiomyopathy; evaluation by phonocardiography, endomyocardial biopsy and cardiac catheterisation. *Ann Intern Med* 1978; **88**: 168–175.
10. Lipshultz SE and Sallan SE. Cardiovascular abnormalities in long-term survivors of childhood malignancy. *J Clin Oncol* 1993; **11**: 1199–1203.
11. Springmeyer SC, Flournoy N, Sullivan KM et al. Pulmonary function changes in long term survivors of allogeneic bone marrow transplantation. In: *Recent Advances in Bone Marrow Transplantation*. RP Gale (ed.) 1983: 343–353 (New York: Alan R Liss).
12. Tait DC, Burnett AK, Robertson AG et al. Subclinical pulmonary function defects following autologous and allogeneic bone marrow transplantation. *Int J Radiat Oncol Biol Phys* 1991; **20**: 1219–1227.
13. Tarbell NJ, Guinan EC, Niemeyer C et al. Late onset of renal dysfunction in survivors of bone marrow transplantation. *Int J Radiat Oncol Biol Phys* 1988; **15**: 99–104.
14. Jannoun L and Chessells JM. Long-term psychological effects of childhood leukaemia and it treatment. *Paediatr Haematol Oncol* 1987; **4**: 293–308.
15. Eiser C. Intellectual abilities among survivors of childhood leukaemia as a function of CNS irradiation. *Arch Dis Child* 1978; **53**: 391–395.
16. Bleyer A. Neurological sequelae of methotrexate and ionising radiation: a new classification. *Cancer Treat Rev* 1981; **65**: 89–98.
17. Waber DP, Tarbell NJ, Kahn CM et al. The relationship of sex and treatment modality to neuropsychologic outcome in childhood acute lymphoblastic leukaemia. *J Clin Oncol* 1992; **10**: 810–817.
18. Peylan-Ramu N, Poplack DG, Pizzo PA et al. Abnormal CT scans of the brain in asymptomatic children with acute lymphoblastic leukaemia after prophylactic treatment of the central nervous system with radiation and intrathecal chemotherapy. *New Engl J Med* 1978; **298**: 815–819.
19. Leiper AD. Late effects of total body irradiation. *Arch Dis Child* 1995; 72: 382–385.
20. Ochs J and Mulhern RK. Late effects of antileukaemic treatment. *Ped Clin North Am* 1988; **35**: 815–833.
21. Sawyer M, Crettenden A and Toogood I. Psychological adjustment of families of children and adolescents treated for leukaemia. *Am J Paediatr Hematol Oncol* 1986; **8**: 200–207.
22. Shuhart MC and McDonald GB. Gastrointestinal and hepatic compications. In: *Bone Marrow Transplantation*. SJ Forman, KG Blume and ED Thomas (eds), 1994: 454–481 (Oxford: Blackwell Scientific Publications).
23. Deeg H J, Flourney N, Sullivan KM et al. Cataracts after total body irradiation and marrow transplantation: a sparing effect of dose fractionation. *Int J Radiat Oncol Biol Phys* 1984; **10**: 957–964.
24. Barrett A, Nicholls J and Gibson B. Late effects of total body irradiation. *Radiother Oncol* 1987; **9**: 131–135.
25. Fraunfelder FT and Meyer SM. Ocular toxicity of anti-neoplastic agents. *Ophthalmology* 1983; **90**: 1–3.
26. Leisner R, Leiper AD, Hann IM et al. Late effects of intensive treatment for acute myeloid leukaemia and myelodysplasia in children. *J Clin Oncol* 1994; **12**: 916–924.
27. Hanada R and Ueoka Y. Obstruction of nasolacrimal ducts closely related to GvHD after bone marrow transplantation. *Bone Marrow Transplant* 1989; **4**: 125–126.
28. Dahloff G, Barr M, Bolme P et al. Disturbances in dental development after TBI in BMT recipients. *Oral Surg Oral Med Oral Pathol* 1988; **65**: 41–44.
29. Mike V, Meadows AT and D'Angio GJ. Incidence of second malignant neoplasms in children: results of an international study. *Lancet* 1982; **ii**: 1326–1331.
30. Hawkins MM, Draper GJ and Kingston JE. Incidence of second primary tumours among children cancer survivors. *Br J Cancer* 1987; **56**: 339–347.
31. Hawkins MM, Kinnier Wilson LM, Stovall MA et al. Epipodophyllotoxins, alkylating agents and radiation and risks of secondary leukaemia after childhood cancer. *Br Med J* 1992; **304**: 951–958.
32. Pedersen-Pjergaard J, Pedersen M, Roulston D and Philip P. Different genetic pathways in leukemogenesis for patients presenting with therapy-related myelodysplasia and therapy-related acute myeloid leukaemia. *Blood* 1995; **86**: 3542–3552.
33. Neglia JP, Meadows AT, Robison LL et al. Second neoplasms after acute lymphoblastic leukaemia in childhood. *New Engl J Med* 1991; **325**: 1330.
34. Rogers PC, Fryer CJ and Hussein S. Radiation dose to the thyroid in treatment of acute lymphoblastic leukaemia (ALL). *Med Paediatr Oncol* 1982; **10**: 385.
35. Witherspoon RP, Fisher LD, Schoch G et al. Secondary cancers after bone marrow transplantation for leukaemia or aplastic anaemia. *New Engl J Med* 1989; **321**: 784–789.
36. Hughes BR, Cunliffe WJ and Bailey CC. The development of excess numbers of benign melanotic naevi in children after chemotherapy for malignancy. *Br Med J* 1989; **299**: 88–91.

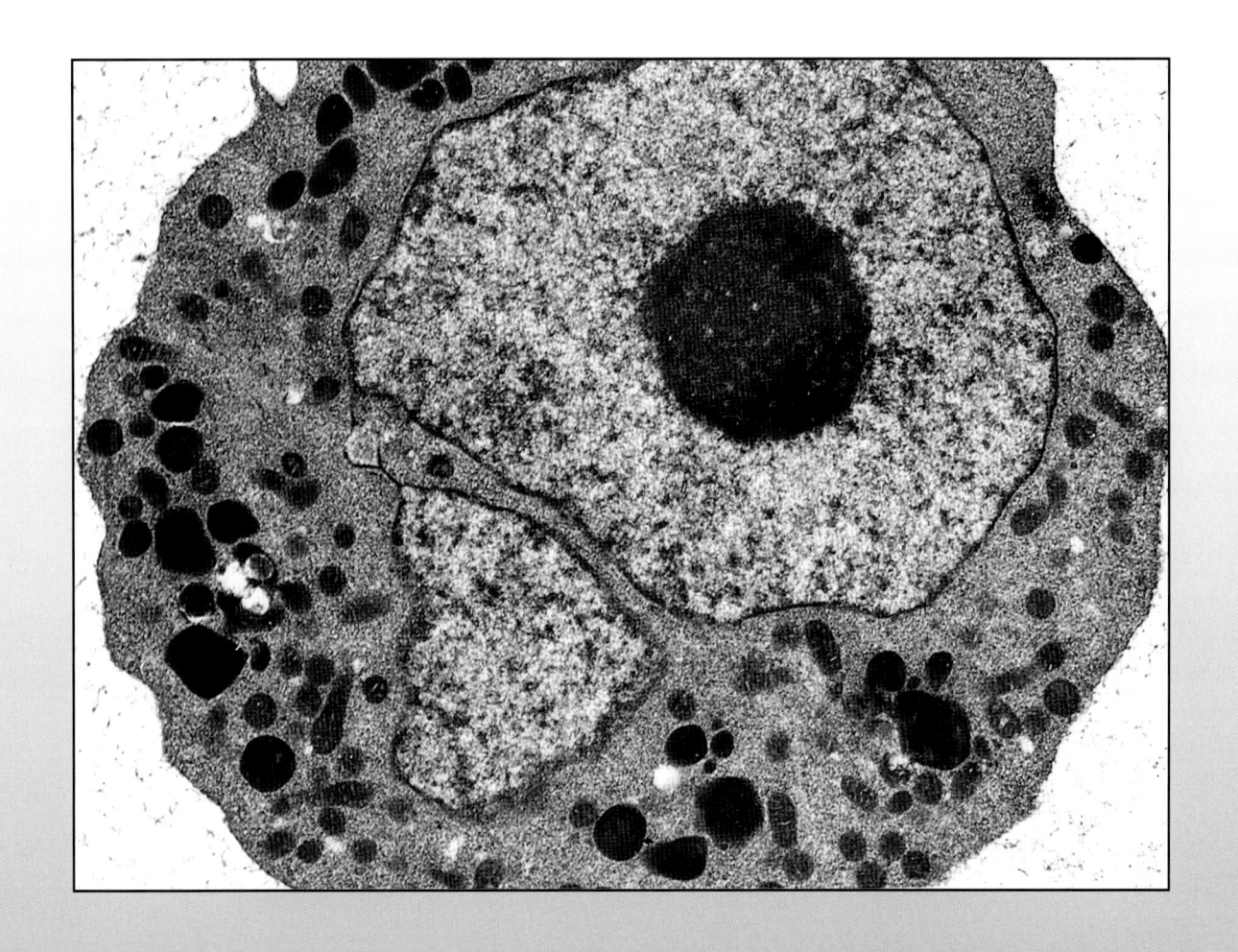

Chapter 56
Endocrine and reproductive dysfunction in adults

Stephen M. Shalet

Introduction

Commonly used marrow-transplant preparative regimens have included either total body irradiation (TBI), high-dose chemotherapy or both. In the survivors there is a high risk of endocrine and reproductive dysfunction. The relative risk of these adverse events is influenced by the underlying pathological condition, previous treatment for that condition, the use of TBI and the irradiation schedule, and the nature and quantity of the cytotoxic drugs used in the bone-marrow transplantation (BMT) preparative regimen.

Pituitary gland

The most sensitive indication of damage to the hypothalamic–pituitary axis, particularly following irradiation, is biochemical evidence of growth hormone (GH) deficiency. In contrast with most of the paediatric studies, GH secretion appears uninfluenced by TBI administered in adult life. Littley et al. [1] studied 18 adults who had received TBI (10–13.2 Gy over three days) and a BMT between 17 and 55 months earlier. The mean peak GH response to an Insulin Tolerance Test (ITT) was 64 mU/litre and all 18 patients achieved a peak growth hormone response of 20 mU/litre or greater (range 21–146 mU/litre). These results support the belief that the hypothalamic–pituitary axis of adults compared with that of children is less vulnerable to irradiation damage. The data also indicate that such patients will not be candidates for GH replacement therapy in adult life.

Confirmation of normal pituitary function is provided by the high gonadotrophin levels, normal prolactin, absence of biochemical evidence of adrenocorticotrophic hormone (ACTH) and thyroid-stimulating hormone (TSH) deficiency or clinical evidence of diabetes insipidus [1]. The only contradictory data relate to two patients reported by Mills et al. [2] who showed an inadequate cortisol and GH response to an insulin tolerance test within eight months of chemotherapy, single fraction TBI (10.5 Gy) and autologous BMT for T-cell lymphoblastic lymphoma.

The raised gonadotrophin levels indicate that the hypothalamic–pituitary axis is capable of responding normally to the loss of negative feedback associated with primary gonadal damage. Thus the dysfunction of the pituitary–gonadal axis is entirely a consequence of damage to the gonadal component.

In-depth studies of the impact of high-dose chemotherapy on pituitary function in adults have not been carried out. In children, however, there is much less evidence that chemotherapy can induce hypothalamic–pituitary dysfunction [3] compared with the numerous studies citing radiation-induced GH deficiency [4–8]. Thus, we would expect normal pituitary function in those adults receiving high-dose chemotherapy as their preparative regimen for a BMT. The findings which reflect normal pituitary function are summarized in Table 56.1.

Table 56.1 Confirmation of normal pituitary function

High gonadotrophin levels
Normal prolactin
Absence of biochemical evidence of GH, ACTH and TSH deficiency
Absence of clinical evidence of diabetes insipidus

Thyroid gland

It has been recognized for many years that external irradiation to the neck may lead to thyroid dysfunction and predispose to thyroid tumours. After a TBI dose of 10–12 Gy, the typical biochemical finding is a mildly elevated basal TSH level and a normal serum thyroxine concentration [7,9–11]. Frank biochemical hypothyroidism with a more elevated TSH level and low thyroxine concentration is less common. The thyroid dysfunction occurs in both children [7,9–10] and adults [1] following TBI and may be transient [9].

It is known from studies of children receiving craniospinal irradiation for brain tumours [12,13] that the addition of chemotherapy significantly increases the risk of thyroid dysfunction. The contribution of chemotherapy to the thyroid dysfunction occurring after TBI and BMT has not yet been clarified.

The incidence of thyroid dysfunction following fractionated TBI (15–16%) [7,11] appears significantly less than that following single-dose TBI (46–48%)

[10,11,14]. However, the long-term natural history of irradiation-induced thyroid dysfunction is unknown, and thus the timing of the peak incidence of biochemical thyroid abnormalities has not been established for different TBI schedules.

It has been suggested that hyperfractionated radiation might lower the incidence of thyroid dysfunction but a retrospective study did not support this hypothesis. Boulad et al. [15] studied thyroid function in 150 patients (100 paediatric and 50 adult) who received BMT and underwent radiation-based preparative regimens; 129 patients received hyperfractionated TBI to a total dose of 13.75 Gy or 15 Gy and 10 patients received total lymphoid irradiation to a total dose of 6 Gy. Twenty-one of the 139 patients (15.1%) who received hyperfractionated radiation were found to have developed hypothyroidism, 11–88 months after transplant (median 49 months). Analysis revealed no significant difference in the incidence of thyroid dysfunction at six years after transplant for any of the following risk factors: age, sex, diagnosis, dose of TBI, type of BMT or the presence or absence of chronic graft-versus-host-disease (GvHD). Thus the incidence of thyroid dysfunction following hyperfractionated radiation (15.1%) is lower than that reported after a single dose but comparable with that associated with fractionated irradiation.

Up to now there have been reports of thyroid papillary carcinoma in children but not adults following TBI and BMT [4,16].

The majority of endocrinologists treat all children with an elevated TSH level with thyroxine replacement, irrespective of whether or not the thyroxine concentration is normal or low. In this way, the increase in theoretical risk of thyroid cancer, associated with a raised TSH level in a child who has undergone irradiation to the thyroid, is normalized. The situation is less clear in adults with an isolated elevation of TSH, although clearly, if symptomatic, the patient should be offered thyroxine replacement. There are no data to suggest, however, that the potential risk for thyroid malignancy would be lowered even further if the TSH level were to be suppressed into the undetectable range of a highly sensitive TSH assay; furthermore, such a policy would probably lead to a great number of patients being overtreated with thyroxine.

Adrenal gland

Littley et al. [1] did not find any evidence of impaired hypothalamic–pituitary–adrenal function in 18 adult patients, who underwent a BMT and received TBI (10–13.2 Gy over three days) up to 55 months before they were studied endocrinologically. In all 18 subjects the basal (0900 hours) cortisol level was normal (> 250 nmol/litre) ranging from 262 to 615 nmol/litre and the peak cortisol response to insulin hypoglycaemia (626–1105 nmol/litre) exceeded the minimum normal response (500 nmol/litre).

The adrenal gland itself appears to be resistant to the effects of irradiation and the secretion of ACTH from the pituitary gland is only affected by doses of irradiation substantially in excess of the typical TBI dose (10–13 Gy).

Ovaries

The LD_{50} (the radiation dose causing the death of 50 per cent of cells) for the human oocyte has been estimated to be less than 4 Gy [17]. Therefore it is not surprising that a high prevalence of primary ovarian failure is found after TBI. Sanders et al. [18] studied 144 women transplanted for leukaemia following 120 mg/kg cyclophosphamide and 9.2–15.75 Gy TBI. Amenorrhoea, decreased oestradiol levels and elevated gonadotrophin levels were present for the first three years after BMT in all 144 women. Nine showed evidence of recovery of ovarian function with restoration of menses, normal gonadotrophin and oestradiol levels between three and seven years after BMT. The age of the patient and schedule of TBI are significantly associated with the potential for recovery of ovarian function [18,19].

With increasing age at transplant, the probability of restoration of ovarian function decreases by a factor of 0.8 per year of age [18]. Patients who received 12 Gy fractionated TBI were 4.8 times more likely to recover ovarian function than those receiving 10 Gy single-dose or 15.75 Gy fractionated TBI [18]. After TBI, ovarian failure occurs quickly, usually within three months [1] and the majority of women are symptomatic within six months [20].

In women receiving cytotoxic drug therapy but not TBI before BMT, the potential for recovery of ovarian function is dependent on the chemotherapy regimen. All 43 women studied by Sanders et al. [18] following

200 mg/kg cyclophosphamide and a BMT for aplastic anaemia developed amenorrhoea. Thirty-six had a return of normal menstrual cycles between 3 and 42 months following BMT. All 27 women under 26 years of age but only five of 16 women over 26 years of age recovered normal ovarian function. In contrast, after a BMT preparation regimen with busulphan plus cyclophosphamide, none of 50 women evaluated one to two years after BMT demonstrated recovery of ovarian function. All showed elevated gonadotrophin levels and a low oestradiol concentration [21].

Chatterjee et al. [22] studied the acute effects of high-dose chemotherapy or TBI or both on ovarian function. All women showed subtle evidence of ovarian dysfunction before BMT, with lower basal and human menopausal gonadotrophin (HMG)-stimulated oestradiol levels, higher basal follicle-stimulating hormone (FSH) levels and exaggerated FSH responses to an acute bolus of gonadotrophin-releasing hormone (GnRH) than seen in controls. The conditioning regimens employed before BMT caused further ovarian damage; gonadotrophin levels rose further into the menopausal range, basal oestradiol levels fell and became unresponsive to HMG stimulation three to four months after BMT. Contrary to expectation, the hormonal changes occurring acutely were similar in patients undergoing radiation-based regimens and those conditioned with high-dose chemotherapy alone. In the women studied by Chatterjee et al. [22], it is not yet known if the prospects for recovery of ovarian function are better following their chemotherapy regimens. If this is the case, however, then their results would imply that the severity of ovarian dysfunction occurring acutely after BMT cannot be used to predict the long-term prospects of recovery of ovarian function.

In recent years, there have been several reports of post-BMT pregnancies [23]. A total of over thirty pregnancies in women with aplastic anaemia resulting predominantly in live births have been reported and summarized by Lipton et al. [23] and Sanders [21]. In all cases, conditioning regimens involved cyclophosphamide at various doses but no TBI.

More recently, Salooja et al. [24] reported recovery of ovarian function in six out of 10 women following treatment for acute myeloid leukaemia (AML) with a high-dose chemotherapy regimen (cyclophosphamide, daunorubicin, carmustine, cytosine arabinoside (Ara-C) and 6-thioguanine) with autologous BMT. Five of the six menstruating women became pregnant between 4 and 40 months following BMT. Three pregnancies went to term and each resulted in the delivery of a full-term normal infant.

The prognostic implication is clear. Chemotherapy regimens which use cyclophosphamide are associated with a high chance of restoration of ovarian function; ovulatory cycles are restored and pregnancy is possible, unlike the situation following high-dose busulphan/cyclophosphamide. Patients should be counselled accordingly.

Following TBI, the incidence of reported pregnancy is less common. A total of 12 pregnancies in nine women resulting in 6 live births, 4 spontaneous and 1 therapeutic abortion and 1 pending are now reported [23] in women conditioned with cyclophosphamide and TBI before BMT for acute leukaemia. Only 3 of the 12 pregnancies occurred in women aged over 25 years at the time of BMT.

The expected findings for hormonal function in women after BMT are summarized in Table 56.2.

Table 56.2 Post-BMT findings in females

Amenorrhoea
Decreased oestradiol levels
Elevated gonadotrophin levels

Testis

There is evidence to show that the germinal epithelium of the testis is more vulnerable to the effects of both cytotoxic chemotherapy and irradiation than either the ovary or the Leydig cell [25]. Therefore, the universal finding of damage to the germinal epithelium would be anticipated following both gonadotoxic chemotherapy and irradiation. Occasionally, germ-cell dysfunction induced by high-dose chemotherapy and TBI administered as a single fraction at a dose of 7.5 Gy appears to be amenable to recovery as demonstrated by a return to normal of the previously elevated FSH level with time [26]. Animal evidence suggests that irradiation administered as a fractionated schedule is

Table 56.3 Post-BMT findings in males
Azoospermic
Small testes
Normal testosterone level
Normal or mildly elevated LH level
Grossly raised FSH level
Androgen replacement therapy rarely required

more deleterious to spermatogenesis than the same total irradiation dose in a single fraction.

In a very large review [21] of 417 men evaluated between one and twelve years after BMT with TBI-containing regimens, 323 submitted semen for analysis but only 5 demonstrated a normal sperm count and the other 318 subjects remained azoospermic. These 5 men fathered 9 normal children; all received 10 Gy single exposure TBI [21]. None of those receiving fractionated TBI demonstrated recovery of spermatogenesis.

Rarely, however, has recovery of spermatogenesis been described in adults even after fractionated TBI [1]. Recovery of spermatogenesis is more likely in those receiving conditioning for BMT with high-dose chemotherapy only. The potential for recovery is influenced by the nature and quantity of the cytotoxic drugs administered [25].

The basal testosterone level is within the normal range in the vast majority of men studied one to four years after high-dose chemotherapy and fractionated TBI for a BMT [1]. Chatterjee et al. [27] however, have shown that in men transplanted for lymphoma, there is evidence of reduced Leydig cell reserve even before BMT. Furthermore, the basal testosterone and the human chorionic gonadotrophin (HCG)-stimulated testosterone levels are lowered further within two to three months after BMT irrespective of conditioning with either TBI or high-dose chemotherapy [27].

Thus, the typical patient will be azoospermic and have small testes; characteristic biochemical findings include a normal testosterone level, normal or mildly elevated luteinizing hormone (LH) level and a grossly raised FSH level. Androgen replacement therapy is required rarely. The usual findings for hormonal function in men after BMT are summarised in Table 56.3. Fertility issues in general are discussed more fully in Chapter 57.

Conclusions

In the adult patient, the risk of hypothyroidism requires regular monitoring. However, the major endocrine needs of the patient are in the field of reproductive medicine. The reproductive endocrinologist/gynaecologist will need to consider fertility counselling, including the possibility of donor oocyte and in vitro fertilization. Young women with ovarian failure require hormone-replacement therapy for relief of menopausal symptoms, to avoid osteoporosis, and to reduce the risk of ischaemic heart disease. All of these adult survivors deserve regular endocrine input into their long-term management.

References

1. Littley MD, Shalet SM, Morganstern GR and Deakin DP. Endocrine and reproductive dysfunction following fractionated total body irradiation in adults. *Q J Med* 1991; **287**: 265–274.
2. Mills W, Chatterjee R, McGarrigle HHG, Linch DC and Goldstone AH. Partial hypopituitarism following total body irradiation in adult patients with haematological malignancy. *Bone Marrow Transplant* 1994; **14**: 471–473.
3. Roman J, Villaizan CJ, Garcia-Foncillas J, Azcona C, Salvador J and Sierrasesumaga L. Chemotherapy-induced growth hormone deficiency in children with cancer. *Med Paediatr Oncol* 1995; **25**: 90–95.
4. Sanders JE, Buckner CD, Sullivan KM et al. Growth and development in children after bone marrow transplantation. *Horm Res* 1988; **30**: 92–97.
5. Papadimitriou A, Uruena M, Hamill G, Stanhope R and Leiper AD. Growth hormone treatment of growth failure secondary to total body irradiation and bone marrow transplantation. *Arch Dis Child* 1991; **66**: 689–692.
6. Borgstrom B. and Bolme P. Growth and growth hormone in children after bone marrow transplantation. *Horm Res* 1988; **30**: 98–100.
7. Ogilvy-Stuart AL, Clark DJ, Wallace WHB, Gibson BE, Stevens RF, Shalet SM and Donaldson MDC. Endocrine deficit after fractionated total body irradiation. *Arch Dis Child* 1992; **67**: 1107–1110.
8. Olshan JS, Willi SM, Gruccio D and Moshang T. Growth hormone function and treatment following bone marrow transplant for neuroblastoma. *Bone Marrow Transplant* 1993; **12**: 381–385.
9. Katsanis E, Shapiro RS, Robison LL, Haake RJ, Kim T, Pescovitz O and Ramsay NKC. Thyroid dysfunction following bone marrow transplantation: long-term follow-up of 80 pediatric patients. *Bone Marrow Transplant* 1990; **5**: 335–340.

10. Borgstrom B and Bolme P. Thyroid function in children after allogenic bone marrow transplantation. *Bone Marrow Transplant* 1994; **13**: 59–64.
11. Sanders JE and The Seattle Bone Marrow Transplant Team. The impact of marrow transplant preparative regimens on subsequent growth and development. *Semin Hematol* 1991; **28**: 244–249.
12. Livesey EA and Brook CGD. Thyroid dysfunction after radiotherapy and chemotherapy of brain tumours. *Arch Dis Child* 1989; **64**: 593–595.
13. Ogilvy-Stuart AL, Shalet SM and Gattamaneni HRG. Thyroid function following the treatment of brain tumours in children. *J Paediatr* 1991; **119**: 733–737.
14. Thomas BC, Stanhope R, Plowman PN and Leiper AD. Endocrine function following single fraction and fractionated total body irradiation for bone marrow transplantation in childhood. *Acta Endocrinologica* 1993; **128**: 508–512.
15. Boulad F, Bromley M, Black P, Heller G, Sarafoglou K, Gillio A and Papadopoulos E. Thyroid dysfunction following bone marrow transplantation using hyperfractionated radiation. *Bone Marrow Transplant* 1995; **15**: 71–76.
16. Uderzo C, Van Lint MT, Rovelli A *et al*. Papillary thyroid carcinoma after total body irradiation. *Arch Dis Child* 1994; **71**: 256–258.
17. Wallace WHB, Shalet SM, Hendry JH, Morris-Jones PH and Gattamaneni HR. Ovarian failure following total abdominal irradiation in childhood: the radiosensitivity of the human oocyte. *Br J Radiol* 1989; **62**: 995–998.
18. Sanders JE, Buckner CD, Amos D *et al*. Ovarian function following marrow transplantation for aplastic anaemia or leukaemia. *J Clin Oncol* 1988; **6**: 813–818.
19. Spinelli S, Chiodi S, Bacigalupo A *et al*. Ovarian recovery after total body irradiation and allogenic bone marrow transplantation: long-term follow up of 79 females. *Bone Marrow Transplant* 1994; **14**: 373–380.
20. Cust MP, Whitehead MI, Powles R, Hunter M and Milliken S. Consequences and treatment of ovarian failure after total body irradiation for leukaemia. *Br Med J* 1989; **299**: 1494–1497.
21. Sanders JE. Growth and development after bone marrow transplantation. In: *Bone Marrow Transplantation*. SJ Forman, KG Blume and ED Thomas (eds), 1994: 527–537 (London: Blackwell Scientific Publications).
22. Chatterjee R, Mills W, Katz M, McGarrigle HH and Goldstone AH. Prospective study of pituitary–gonadal function to evaluate short-term effects of ablative chemotherapy or total body irradiation with autologous or allogenic marrow transplantation in post-menarchial female patients. *Bone Marrow Transplant* 1994; **13**: 511–517.
23. Lipton JH, Derzko C, Fyles G, Meharchand J and Messner HA. Pregnancy after BMT: three case reports. *Bone Marrow Transplant* 1993; **11**: 415–418.
24. Salooja N, Chatterjee R, McMillan AK *et al*. Successful pregnancies in women following single autotransplant for acute myeloid leukaemia with a chemotherapy ablation protocol. *Bone Marrow Transplant* 1994; **13**: 431–435.
25. Shalet SM. Cancer therapy and gonadal dysfunction. In: *Clinical Endocrine Oncology*. R Sheaves, P Jenkins and JH Wass (eds), 1997 (Oxford: Blackwell Scientific Publications).
26. Sklar CA, Kim TH and Ramsay NKC. Testicular function following bone marrow transplantation performed during or after puberty. *Cancer* 1984; **53**: 1498–1501.
27. Chatterjee R, Mills W, Katz M, McGarrigle HH and Goldstone AH. Germ cell failure and Leydig cell insufficiency in post-pubertal males after autologous bone marrow transplantation with BEAM for lymphoma. *Bone Marrow Transplant* 1994; **13**: 519–522.

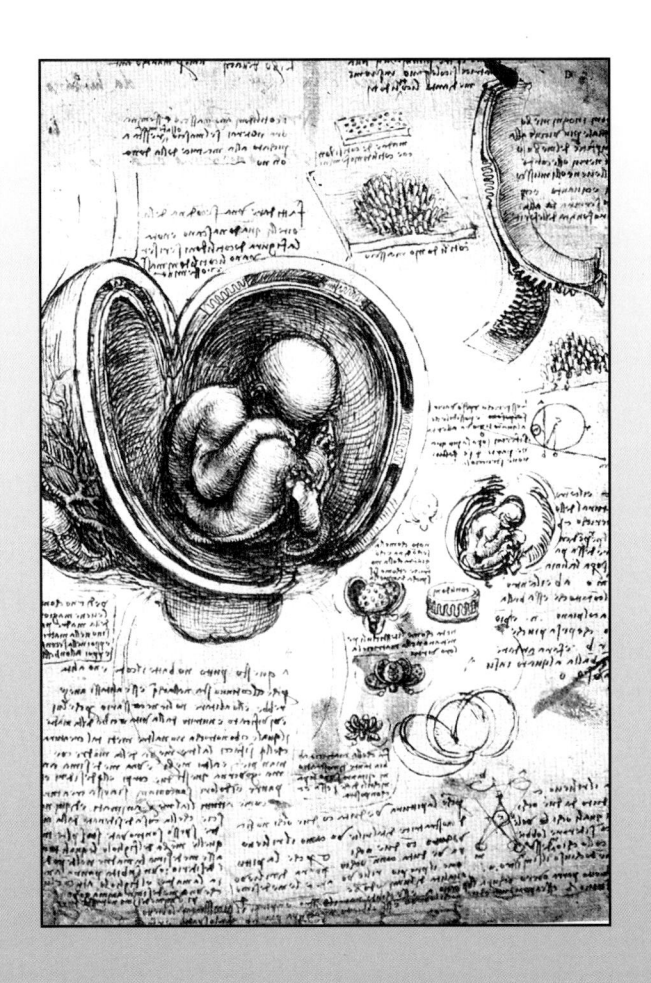

Chapter 57
Fertility

Eric Simons and Kamal Ahuja

Introduction

Since many more patients are now surviving long term after treatment for haematological malignancies and bone-marrow failure syndromes, and since these patients are often young when they undergo therapy, the problem of their probable subsequent infertility is often of great significance. Most patients of childbearing age, or the parents of children who need intensive chemo radiotherapy, require information prior to the procedure concerning chances of a future pregnancy. If they do not request such information spontaneously, the issue should be addressed prior to treatment to enable a male patient to make a decision concerning sperm cryopreservation. For female patients, the problem is more complex since it is currently not possible technically to offer an ovum cryopreserving programme, and most female bone-marrow transplant patients will require ovum donation if they subsequently wish to become pregnant. This aspect is described later.

Fertility after bone-marrow transplantation: gender issues

There are many anecdotal case reports in the literature concerning pregnancies occurring subsequent to high-dose chemotherapy sometimes associated with total lymph-node irradiation or total body irradiation (TBI) in patients transplanted for aplastic anaemia or leukaemia [1–6], but pregnancy is much less likely to occur following TBI. However, Samuelsson et al. [7] reported the case of a 28-year-old woman treated for acute lymphoblastic leukaemia who received total body irradiation and high-dose chemotherapy as conditioning. She had a healthy girl four years later. Also, Lipton et al. [8] report on four pregnancies occurring in three women in their twenties after total body irradiation, although one of these women suffered two miscarriages. Up until 1993, however, there were only six live births reported in the literature which had occurred after total body irradiation, and all of these patients were under 25 years of age when transplanted.

In 1988, Sanders et al. [1] evaluated ovarian function in 187 women between 13 and 49 years of age from 1 to 15 years (median, 4 years) after marrow transplant for aplastic anaemia or leukaemia. Among 43 women transplanted for aplastic anaemia following 200 mg/kg cyclophosphamide, all 27 under 26 years of age, but only 5 of 16 greater than 26 years of age recovered normal ovarian function. Nine of the 43 have had 12 pregnancies, resulting in 8 live births, and 2 elective and 2 spontaneous abortions. All 8 children are normal. Nine of 144 women transplanted for leukaemia following 120 mg/kg cyclophosphamide and 9.20–15.75 Gy TBI recovered ovarian function. Two of these 9 have had 3 pregnancies, resulting in 2 spontaneous and 1 elective abortion. The probability of having ovarian failure was 0.35 by seven years for patients receiving cyclophosphamide alone and 1.00 at one year for patients receiving cyclophosphamide plus TBI ($P < 0.0001$). By seven years after transplant the probabilities of having normal ovarian function were 0.92 after cyclophosphamide alone and 0.24 after cyclophosphamide plus TBI ($P < 0.0001$). Multivariate analysis showed that TBI was the only factor significantly influencing ovarian failure and that both TBI and greater patient age at transplant were significantly associated with a decreased probability of recovering normal ovarian function.

More recently, Maruta et al. [9] reported a woman of 23 years who received fractionated total body irradiation 2.5 Gy × five doses as part of her conditioning therapy prior to an allogeneic bone-marrow transplant for acute lymphoblastic leukaemia. Her menses recurred spontaneously four years later and a healthy child was born six years later.

An excellent analysis of various aspects of pregnancy after bone-marrow transplantation has been carried out by the Seattle group [10] on a large number of men and women who had undergone a transplant procedure with or without TBI as part of the conditioning regimen. Here, 1522 disease-free survivors after bone-marrow transplantation for either aplastic anaemia or haematological malignancies treated between August 1971 and January 1992, were examined. Of 708 women who were post-pubertal at the time of transplant, 110 recovered normal ovarian function and 21 became pregnant. Also, 9 girls prepubertal at the time of transplant who had normal gonadal function became pregnant. Table 57.1 summarizes the situation with pregnancy after bone-marrow transplantation and Table 57.2 summarizes some of the problems which may be encountered during pregnancy.

Table 57.1 Problems after bone-marrow transplantation

- Spontaneous abortion rate increased after total body irradiation, after abdominal irradiation or after high-dose alkylating agents
- Increased incidence of preterm labour
- Increased incidence of low birthweight babies
- No increase in congenital malformations
- To date, no increase in later medical problems

Table 57.2 Factors contributing to pregnancy problems*

- 'Hostile' vaginal environment
- Reduced tubal patency
- Reduced elasticity of uterine musculature
- Poor tissue perfusion (foetus and uterus)
- Altered elasticity/competence/patency of cervix
- Infection
- Distorted uterine cavity

*These may occur in association with previous irradiation, alkylating agent therapy, or chronic graft-versus-host disease.

Pregnancies of women who had received a marrow transplant, particularly if TBI was included in the conditioning regimen, were accompanied by an increased risk of spontaneous abortion, of preterm labour and of low birthweight babies. These infants, however, did not appear to be at increased risk of congenital abnormalities.

In a report published in 1994 [11], Spinelli *et al.* carried out a prospective follow-up of ovarian recovery in 79 females who had undergone BMT with TBI used as part of the conditioning. They underwent regular gynaecological examinations, including plasma levels of luteinizing hormone (LH), follicle-stimulating hormone (FSH), 17 β-oestradiol and pelvic ultrasonography. The authors attempted to ascertain: (1) early and late effects of TBI on ovarian function; (2) compliance and results of hormonal replacement therapy (HRT); and (3) predictive events for ovarian recovery. During the first year after BMT, there was a decrease in 17β-oestradiol levels and an increase in FSH–LH (4% of the women complained of deterioration in their sexual function). Forty-nine adult females were selected to receive systemic HRT on the basis of age (<45 years), absence of medical contraindications or refusal. Compliance and tolerability were good overall: 65% never stopped HRT; this was discontinued in 14 patients for medical reasons and in 3 because they no longer wished to take it. Forty-three females completed six months of HRT; vasomotor symptoms disappeared in 91% of 58 women who previously experienced these symptoms. Improvement of genitourinary symptoms was seen both with local and systemic hormonal therapy. However, sexual symptoms were reduced in 21 of 26 women (81%) given HRT compared with 8 of 19 (42%) women given local treatment ($P = 0.02$). The actuarial chance of having a menstrual period 10 years after BMT was 43%. It was 100% in patients who had been prepubertal at the time of BMT and 36% in post-menarchial females. In the latter group, it was 100% if under 18 years of age at the time of BMT and 15% in those over 18 years. It was therefore concluded that:

- adult women undergoing TBI before BMT experience loss of ovarian function immediately after treatment associated with vasomotor and gastrointestinal symptoms and loss of libido;
- 13.5% of all post-menarchial females experience ovarian failure;
- this recovery is related to age and menarchial status at the time of BMT;
- HRT should be started as soon as possible after BMT to reduce menopausal symptoms and to minimize the long-term effects of oestrogen deficiency;
- HRT should be stopped at regular intervals to ascertain whether there has been recovery of ovarian function;
- contraceptive counselling may be relevant where recovery of ovarian function has occurred.

As far as males are concerned, there are fewer reported cases where recovery after total body irradiation or high-dose chemotherapy has occurred and the patient has fathered children [12–14.] Of post-pubertal male patients, 157 of 618 recovered testicular function and the partners of 33 became pregnant. Pakkala *et al.* [12] report the case of an azoospermic patient who fathered a child four years after receiving fractionated TBI and his paternity was proven with DNA methodology. Sanders *et al.* [13] report 2 male patients who regained fertility after BMT following conditioning with cyclophosphamide and TBI. Both patients received single-fraction TBI. Recovery of fertility led to a pregnancy in both cases.

In 1991, Sanders [15] reported only 2 men who recovered sperm production after TBI and cyclophosphamide at what was at the time seven to eight years from BMT. In 1992, Shiobara *et al.* [16] reported the complete recovery of sperm production in a man who had undergone BMT, although radiation was not included in his preparative regimen.

Barker *et al.* [17] have recently reviewed 25 males who had undergone a bone-marrow transplant procedure, with or without TBI as part of the conditioning therapy. They found that, of these 25 patients, 3 recovered normal sperm counts. Of these three, one had had an allo-BMT for aplastic anaemia with cyclophosphamide and TBI conditioning and two had undergone allo-BMT for acute myeloid leukaemia. One had received cyclophosphamide and TBI and one had had cyclophosphamide, Adriamycin, carmustine, 6-thioguanine and cytosine, but no radiotherapy. This group had previously reported the two men discussed above who recovered their fertility, [14], making a total of 5 of 46 patients.

Hinterberger-Fischer *et al.* [18] undertook hormonal assessment of a number of BMT patients one to six years after allogeneic, syngeneic and autologous bone-marrow transplantation. Among 6 male patients transplanted for haematological malignancies, 4 had elevated FSH but normal LH and thyroxine levels, while two had normal LH, FSH and thyroxine levels or elevated LH and FSH levels but decreased thyroxine levels, respectively. One male transplanted for severe aplastic anaemia who did not therefore receive TBI, parented a healthy child. These investigators however, found a relatively high incidence of offspring complications, including (i) persistence of foetal circulation syndrome, (ii) erythroblastosis foetalis and (iii) prolonged newborn icterus, unlike Sanders *et al.* in 1996 who found no increase in foetal abnormalities on a much larger study population [10].

Conclusion

In summary, therefore, it seems from the published data that females have a much better chance than males of regaining their fertility after BMT, particularly if TBI has not been included in the conditioning programme. However, their chances of recovering fertility are strongly age-related. Men, however, are much less likely to recover fertility after a BMT programme even if TBI has been excluded from the conditioning programme, although single fraction radiotherapy is more likely to be associated with recovery of gonadal function [19]. Age of the male patient at BMT does not appear to be related to recovery of gonadal function, although the time that has elapsed post-transplant is likely to be relevant, in terms of allowing a sufficiently long period for recovery of spermatogenesis. The development of assisted reproduction technology, particularly the micromanipulation of gametes, has opened an exciting new avenue for the treatment of male infertility (see below).

Assessment of recovery of gonadal function

Females

After treatment, the best index of recovery of gonadal function in women is a day 3 profile of FSH–LH–17β-oestradiol in a natural cycle (Table 57.3). When the 17β-oestradiol is > 90 pmol/litre and FSH is < 8 IU/litre with LH ≤ 8 IU/litre, the chance of a future pregnancy is average. However, it should not be overlooked that there is no absolute link between hormone profiles and eggs, which may well be of poor quality even in the presence of adequate hormone levels. Fertility is a complex issue and depends in equal measure upon the quality of both eggs and sperm, and upon a number of other issues.

Bone-marrow transplantation should have little effect upon tubal patency but other unrelated causes of

Table 57.3 Criteria for normal gonadal function in women

- Return of spontaneous menses
- Normal FSH, LH and oestradiol levels

tubal blockage should be excluded in a female who appears to have a hormone profile compatible with ovulation but who fails to conceive.

When counselling patients before or after bone-marrow transplantation about fertility issues, it is as well to be prudent when making prognostications without being unnecessarily pessimistic; there are many issues in operation after bone-marrow transplantation which may make the chances of a patient becoming pregnant extremely remote.

It seems that in patients who are under 17 years of age, spontaneous menstruation may well recur and patients may be fertile. For the remainder, and particularly for older patients, fertility is permanently lost and these patients require ovum donation.

Ovum donation

Indications for ovum donation are as follows. Premature menopause: amenorrhoea for at least one year, FSH >20 IU before the age of 40 years and desire for pregnancy in selected older women. In practice, most units offering a service will do so up to the age of 45 years and many up to the age of 50 years. See Table 57.4.

All types of donation are controlled by the Human Fertilization and Embryology Authority in the UK (HFEA). Tables 57.5 to 57.9 summarize the possible types of ovum donation.

Ovum donors may be known or unknown to the recipient [20]. If unknown, donors may be fertile, or infertile and participating in a shared-egg scheme [21]. Finally, donors may be a mixture of the above. Each of these sorts of donation offers advantages and disadvantages. With known donors, the principal advantage is that the offspring will derive from a known source of genes. Disadvantages include the

Table 57.4 Indications for ovum donation

- Premature menopause
    - Amenorrhoea one year
    - FSH > 20 IU before age 40
- Desire for pregnancy
- Selected older menopausal patients

Table 57.5 Types of ovum donation*

- Known
- Unknown
    - Fertile
    - Infertile (shared-egg scheme)
- Mixture of known/unknown

*Controlled by Human Fertilization and Embryology Authority in the UK (HFEA).

Table 57.6 'Known' ovum donation

Advantages

- Known source of genes

Disadvantages

- Child may grow up with confused ideas about its origin
- Contrary to desire of the HFEA
- Recipient might be under pressure to donate
- Drugs administered to donor may have unanticipated risks

Table 57.7 'Unknown fertile' ovum donation

Advantages

- Altruistic non-patients who donate to a unit
- Conform to HFEA ideal

Disadvantages

- Need for drugs and egg collection operation with known risks
- Family dislocation with no prospect of compensation
- Drugs might be proven to carry a cancer risk
- Few donors of this type

Table 57.8 'Unknown infertile'* ovum donation

Disadvantage
- Moral risk of donor enticement

Advantages
- Two infertile groups are helped
- Large number of worthy donors
- Recipient does not need to recruit her own donor

*Infertile, i.e. shared egg donation: recipient pays the cost of donor's egg collection operation in return for half the eggs.

Table 57.9 Mixed 'known/unknown' ovum donation

Advantages
- Well-established method of donation
- Anonymity between donor and recipient

Disadvantages
- Drugs might have unforeseen risks e.g. hyperstimulation syndrome
- Whilst donor and recipient do not know each other, others know when the recipient is pregnant after donation
- Risk of manipulation of child
- Recipient must recruit donor for anonymous third party: loss of dignity

As far as unknown fertile donors are concerned, the advantages include the fact that they are sufficiently altruistic to donate to a unit and that they conform to the HFEA ideal. There are few patients of this type. Disadvantages include the need for drugs and egg-collection operations with their known associated risks. Also, family dislocation could occur with no prospect of compensation. The stimulatory drugs might also prove to confer a cancer risk.

In the unknown, infertile situation, shared-egg donation is carried out. The recipient pays the cost of the donor's egg collection operation in return for half of the eggs. Advantages are that two infertile parties are helped and that there is a large pool of worthy donors. Also, the recipient does not need to recruit her own donor, and hence anonymity is preserved. A potential disadvantage is the perceived moral risk of donor enticement.

As far as the mixed known and unknown situation for ovum donation is concerned, advantages are that this is a well-established method of donation which maintains anonymity between donor and recipient. Disadvantages include the fact that the drugs may also have unforeseen risks in addition to the known risks such as hyperstimulation syndrome. Also, although the donor and recipient do not know each other, there are other people who perceive that the recipient is pregnant after donation, and subsequent manipulation of the child could occur. Finally the recipient has to recruit a donor for an anonymous third party, possibly resulting in loss of dignity.

Ideally, eggs could be harvested and cryopreserved before treatment with irradiation or anticancer drugs commences. However, cryopreservation of eggs for clinical purposes is not feasible at present and it is not licensed by the HFEA. Also, the necessary delay to mature follicles and harvest eggs might jeopardize the efficacy of primary therapy for the malignant process. However, current research directed at ovarian biopsy with late individual follicle maturation may become available in the future.

There are thus several methods of egg donation available to those who lose their reproductive capability. All methods must be carried out in a HFEA-controlled centre selected to meet the personal needs of the recipient. A publication from the Authority is available covering legal and technical aspects.

perceived risk for the child as it grows up with possibly a conflicting understanding of its origin. Such donations are also currently contrary to the wishes of the HFEA, one reason for this being that the recipient might be under pressure to donate. Also, drugs administered to the donor might have unforeseen risks, although this pertains to all donors of ova who require stimulation to hyperovulate.

Males

The criteria for normal gonadal function in men are normal FSH, LH and testosterone levels, and the presence or absence of a normal sperm count (Table 57.10).

> **Table 57.10 Criteria for normal gonadal function in men**
>
> - Normal FSH, LH and testosterone levels
> - Presence of a normal sperm count

Late effects of bone-marrow transplantation in females

Although loss of reproductive capability is foremost in the minds of patients and attendants alike, it is a loss of follicular activity and oestrogen production which is of greater importance in terms of later health problems. The loss of ovarian function impinges upon reproduction (loss of eggs may be temporary or permanent) and oestrogen production. The latter may result in loss of follicles and/or follicular activity may be temporary or permanent. If permanent or protracted, the effects of oestrogen loss will be experienced (vasomotor problems, osteoporosis, possible early cardiovascular disease, etc).

Age-dependent functional groups

Age-dependent functional groups include:
- premenarchial patients;
- patients who have experienced the menarche and who are of reproductive age;
- postmenopausal patients.

Premenarchial (up to age 13 years)

Loss of ovarian tissue may lead to stunting of growth. Monitoring should be carried out by the haematologist, paediatrician and gynaecologist. *Beware of oestrogen deficiency which is needed for growth.* Commencement of menses is a good prognostic sign. Await follicular activity. If this occurs, no treatment is needed. Reproductive potential can be regarded as unimpaired.

From menarche (age 13 years) into reproductive age

All patients should be on a low-dose combined oral contraceptive pill. If contraindicated, cyclical progesterone should be prescribed. Hormone replacement therapy should be given if there is no ovarian activity. Cyclo-Progynova or Dimagest, for example, are commonly used commercial products and will conserve normal growth.

Selection of patients for hormone replacement therapy (HRT).
If FSH rises without a 17β-oestradiol response:
- a scan will show no ovarian activity;
- quarterly FSH, LH and 17β-oestradiol levels should be carried out;
- when FSH is above 20 IU with little ovarian response, i.e. low 17β-oestradiol and no follicles on scan, start routine HRT.

There is a wide choice of regimes, and the regime must contain both 17β-oestradiol and progesterone to prevent abnormal bleeding and the risk of endometrial atypia. Ovarian scan should be repeated every three months.

Monitoring of HRT is as follows:
- twice-yearly review of FSH and 17β-oestradiol levels;
- stop treatment for three months, then recheck FSH and 17β-oestradiol levels;
- restart HRT if menses do not restart or FSH rises without response;
- if patient is sexually active, contraception is needed.

Table 57.11 summarizes the current options for hormone replacement therapy.

Sexually active patients desiring pregnancy

There is no simple test to confirm egg production or quality of eggs. A low 17β-oestradiol level must not be allowed to continue for more than six months as bone matrix loss will occur.

Amenorrhoeic patients

The procedure is:
- monitor 17β-oestradiol every two to three months;
- scan with 17β-oestradiol < 100 pmol/litre;
- HRT for six months, then stop.

Table 57.11 Current options for hormone replacement therapy

- Contraceptive pill
- Oral administration of conjugated oestrogens with progestogens
- Transdermal oestrogen with oral progestogens (good compliance, less gastrointestinal hepatic side effects, delivers physiological hormone 17β-oestradiol).

Regular menstruation
Monitor as follows:
- day 3: FSH and 17β-oestradiol;
- day 21: plasma progesterone.

If the patient has been trying for 12 months or more to become pregnant, offer routine infertility investigations. These include:
- Hormones:
    day 3: FSH, LH and 17β-oestradiol levels
    day 21: progesterone level;
- Tubes:
    hycosy: least invasive way to establish tubal patency;
    hysterosalpingogram;
    laparoscopy only if other pelvic pathology suspected;
- Semen analysis:
    including sperm count, morphological examination and bacterial and viral culture;
    post-coital test.

Post-menopausal
The diagnosis includes amenorrhoea for six months, elevated FSH and a 17β-oestradiol level <60 pmol/litre. Treatment is with HRT, tibolone and biphosphonates.

Reproduction after bone-marrow transplantation

When oestrogen replacement therapy is being administered with monitoring of menstruation, the following situations can occur.

Patient on HRT
If under 35 years old, ovarian recovery is possible. When reproductive needs become dominant:
- stop hormone replacement therapy;
- wait for three months for recovery of menses;
- then, on day 3, perform a profile of FSH: 17β-oestradiol levels.

If FSH:
- is < 9 IU/litre, oocytes are likely to be satisfactory;
- is > 9 but < 12 IU/litre and 17β-oestradiol is 60–90 fertility is impaired: repeat tests to establish trend;
- is > 12 IU/litre and 17β-oestradiol is < 60 pmol/litre consider donor eggs, especially if repeat tests give similar results.

Menses not recurring
Random profile FSH–LH–17β-oestradiol (probability is that FSH > 20 IU/litre and 17β-oestradiol < 60 pmol/litre). If repeat test is similar or worse, donor eggs are required.

Patient menstruating regularly
Perform a day 3 profile FSH: 17β-oestradiol levels.

Irregular menstruation
Polycystic ovaries (PCO) or perimenopause are possible. Diagnosis is by:
- day 3: profile FSH–LH–17β-oestradiol. Results will differentiate between these two conditions;
- ultrasound scan: PCO has diagnostic characteristics;
- treat as routine for PCO patients or as above if perimenopausal.

Diagnosis of polycystic ovaries
- raised 17β-oestradiol level;
- LH:FSH is reversed, > 2:1;
- ultrasound scan.

Diagnosis of perimenopause
- 17β-oestradiol depressed or low normal (< 60 pmol/litre);
- FSH elevated >10 IU/litre;
- LH might also be >10 IU/litre.

Ovarian tissue freezing

Research is currently taking place into the storage possibilities and cryopreservation of ovarian tissue. This has been successful in sheep and could offer an excellent solution for patients requiring BMT. Tissue could be re-implanted or individual follicles cultured to provide single eggs for *in vitro* fertilization followed by embryo transfer.

Testicular function and microassisted fertilization (MAF) in cancer patients

Declining semen quality

During the last two decades, a significant decline in the reproductive capacity has been reported in a number of studies. The incidence of cancer of the testes has also increased. This may be unilateral, and is often associated with other abnormalities of the testis including undescended testes, hypospadias and spermatogenic arrest. Falling sperm quality and increased incidence of cancer may be influenced by similar genetic and environmental factors causing a dramatic overall increase in male infertility [22,23].

When a male infertility factor becomes apparent, special sperm preparation techniques are employed to improve sperm performance such as Percoll gradient separation, microdrop culture and pentoxyfylline addition, and these are then used during assisted conception procedures. In those who fail to fertilize eggs *in vitro*, however, the emotional blow may be severe. For many decades, donor sperm was the only way to treat severe problems such as oligoasthenoteratozoospermia but this was not universally acceptable. The recent arrival of microassisted fertilization (MAF) has dramatically changed that situation for many patients.

MAF techniques

The term 'micromanipulation' covers a range of techniques that involve the handling of individual sperm and egg cells (Table 57.1). Micromanipulation techniques work by bringing the genetic material of sperm and eggs into very close contact, thus aiding fertilization. Couples, including many cancer patients who have had poor fertilization during previous *in vitro* fertilization (IVF) attempts, or who have been discouraged from trying IVF because of a severe male problem, may have a much greater chance of conception through MAF techniques.

- ICSI (intracytoplasmic sperm injection)
  This is the most successful of these techniques. Eggs are taken from the ovary as in a normal IVF operation. A single sperm is then 'caught' and injected into the centre of each egg using a very fine glass needle.
- SUZI (subzonal sperm injection)
  Where one to ten sperm are placed just inside the egg zona pellucida or 'shell'. This method is not as successful as ICSI and so is now less commonly used.
- PZD (partial zone dissection)
  This is where a small slit is made in the zona pellucida to either facilitate sperm entry, or to later help the embryo to 'hatch'.

Spermatozoa retrieved from sites which were previously considered 'unphysiological' for fertilization have been shown to produce significant success with ICSI, sometimes even better than routine IVF using ejaculated spermatozoa. (Table 57.12). Testicular spermatozoa, immotile spermatozoa and even undifferentiated spermatids have been successful in generating viable embryos and pregnancies. [24] Children born following MAF treatment have been shown to produce no disconcerting neonatal evidence of genetic abnormalities to date [25].

MAF and patients treated for malignant diseases

Cancer and its treatment both contribute to male factor infertility by lowering sperm quality, as judged

Table 57.12 ICSI and IVF in assisted conception

Type of spermatozoa	Percentage success per embryo transfer
Epididymal (ICSI)	25.5%
Testicular (ICSI)	23.3%
Ejaculated (IVF)*	14.8%

*Data from the Human Fertilization and Embryology Authority (1995)

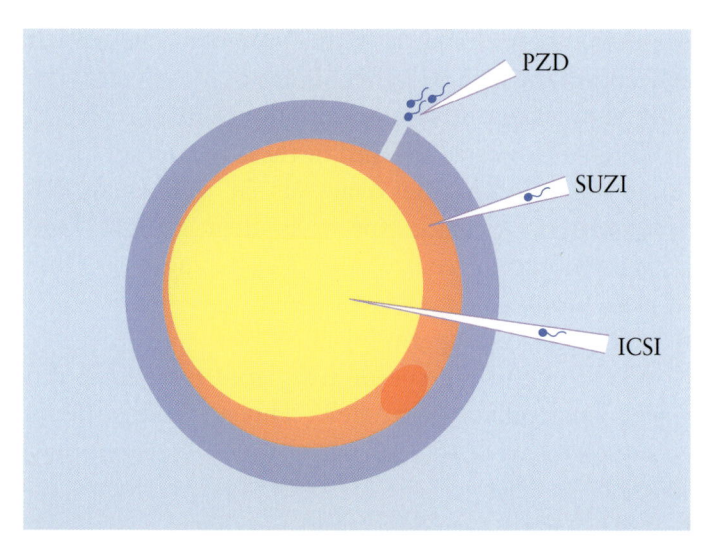

Figure 57.1 Microassisted fertilization (MAF) techniques. PZD = partial zone dissection drilling of zona pellucida; SUZI = subzonal sperm injection; ICSI = intracytoplasmic sperm injection.

by a number of morphological (i.e. count, abnormal appearance, motility, progression) and physiological (i.e. antibodies) criteria. MAF techniques are therefore increasingly applied to overcome infertility amongst post-therapy cancer patients, particularly cases of testicular cancer [26]. It is not unreasonable to speculate that in the future these techniques may be applied to BMT patients with an equal degree of success.

The posthumous use of sperm cryostored prior to the initiation of radiotherapy or chemotherapy, has been available for some time but the chances of success were low [27]. The MAF techniques are also likely to have a significant impact in this area because of the poor quality of sperm in cancer patients. In the UK, the HFEA Act 1990 allows women to use their deceased husband's sperm, provided appropriate consents are available [28]. Bone-marrow transplantation patients, unlike those who may suffer sudden illness leading to death, are unlikely to have any problems with providing consent for the posthumous use of their spermatozoa to initiate a pregnancy in a named partner. Ethical complications which are envisaged in cases of acute illnesses leading to death are therefore unlikely to arise in BMT patients.

References

1. Sanders JE, Buckner CD, Amos D et al. Ovarian function following marrow transplantation for aplastic anemia or leukemia. *J Clin Oncol* 1988; **6**(5): 813–818.
2. Hirabayashi N, Goto S, Isogai C, Tomita A and Ohno T. Successful pregnancy after allogeneic bone marrow transplantation: two case reports. *Rinsho Ketsueki (Jap J Clin Hematol)* 1996; **35**(7): 710–712,
3. Eliyahu S and Shalev E. A successful pregnancy after bone marrow transplantation for severe aplastic anaemia with pre-transplant conditioning of total lymph-node irradiation and cyclophosphamide. *Br J Haematol* 1994; **86**(3): 649–650.
4. Kang BJ, Tzeng CH, Chen LY et al. Normal full-term pregnancy after allogeneic bone marrow transplantation for severe aplastic anemia: a case report. *Chung Hua i Hsueh Tsa Chih (Chinese Med J)* 1991; **48**: 404–407.
5. Hinterberger-Fischer M. Pregnancy and fetal complications after bone marrow transplantation. *Wiener Med Wochenschr* 1991; **141**: 228–231.
6. Milliken S, Powles R, Parikh P, Whitehead M, Mayes I and Prentice A. Successful pregnancy following bone marrow transplantation for leukaemia. *Bone Marrow Transplant* 1990; **5**: 135–137.
7. Samuelsson A, Fuchs T, Simonsson B and Björkholm M. Successful pregnancy in a 28-year-old patient autografted for acute lymphoblastic leukemia following myeloablative treatment including total body irradiation. *Bone Marrow Transplant* 1993; **12**: 659–560.
8. Lipton JH, Derzko C, Fyles G, Meharchand J and Messner HA. Pregnancy after BMT: three case reports. *Bone Marrow Transplant* 1993; **11**: 415–418.
9. Maruta A, Matsuzaki M, Miyashita H et al. Successful pregnancy after allogeneic bone marrow transplantation following conditioning with total body irradiation. *Bone Marrow Transplant* 1995; **15**: 637–638.
10. Sanders JE, Hawley J, Levy W et al. Pregnancies following high-dose cyclophosphamide with or without high-dose busulfan or total body irradiation and bone marrow transplantation. *Blood* 1996; **87**: 3045–3052.
11. Spinelli S, Chiodi S, Bacigalupo A et al. Ovarian recovery after total body irradiation and allogeneic bone marrow transplantation: long-term follow up of 79 females. *Bone Marrow Transplant* 1994; **14**: 373–380.
12. Pakkala S, Lukka M, Helminen P, Koskimies S and Ruutu T. Paternity after bone marrow transplantation following conditioning with total body irradiation. *Bone Marrow Transplant* 1994; **13**: 489–490.
13. Sanders JE, Buckner DC, Leonard JM et al. Late effects on gonadal function of cyclophosphamide, total body irradiation and marrow transplantation. *Transplantation* 1983; **36**: 252–255.
14. Jacob A, Goodman A, Holmes J. Fertility after bone marrow transplantation following conditioning with cyclophosphamide and total body irradiation. *Bone Marrow Transplant* 1995; **15**: 483–484.

15. Sanders JE. The impact of marrow transplant preparative regimens on subsequent growth and development. *Semin Hematol* 1991; **28**: 244–249.
16. Shiobara S, Nakao S, Yamaguchi M *et al*. Complete recovery of sperm production following bone marrow transplantation for leukemia. [Letter.] *Bone Marrow Transplant* 1992; **10**: 313.
17. Barker H, Jacob A, Newton J, Goodman A and Holmes J. Recovery of fertility in males following bone marrow transplantation. *Bone Marrow Transplant* 1997. In press.
18. Hinterberger-Fischer M, Kier P, Kalhs P *et al*. Fertility, pregnancies and offspring complications after bone marrow transplantation. *Bone Marrow Transplant* 1991; **7**: 5–9.
19. Heimpel H, Arnold R, Hetzel WD *et al*. Gonadal function after bone marrow transplantation in adult male and female patients. *Bone Marrow Transplant* 1991; **8**(Suppl): 21–24.
20. Ahuja KK and Simons EG. Anonymous egg donation and dignity. *Human Reproduction* 1996; **11**: 1151–1154.
21. Ahuja KK, Simons EG, Figmanya W, Dalton M, Armar NA, Kirkpatrick P and Sharp S. Egg sharing in assisted conception: ethical and practical considerations *Human Reproduction* 1996; **11**: 1126–1131.
22. Skakkeback NE and Keiding N. Changes in semen and the testes. *Br Med J* 1994; **309**: 1316–1317.
23. Adami H-Q, Bergsstrom R, Mohner M, Zatonski W, Storm H and Ekbom A. Testicular cancer in nine Northern European countries. *Int J Cancer* 1994; **59**: 33–38.
24. Fishel S, Islam I and Tesarik J. Spermatid conception: a stage too early, or a time too soon? *Hum Reproduction* 1996; **11**: 1371–1375.
25. Bonduelle M, Legein J, Brysse A *et al*. Prospective follow-up study of 423 children born after ICSI. *Hum Reproduction* 1996; **11**: 1558–1564.
26. Challis E, Ochinger S, Acosta AA, Morshedi M, Veeck L, Bryzyski RG and Mansher SJ. Successful fertilisation and pregnancy outcome in *in vitro* fertilisation using cryopreserved/thawed spermatozoa for patients with malignant diseases. *Hum Reproduction* 1992; **7**: 105–108.
27. Bahadur G. Posthumous assisted reproduction (PAR): cancer patients, potential cases, counselling and consent. *Hum Reproduction* 1996; **12**: 2573–2575.
28. Ahuja KK, Mamiso J, Emerson G, Bowen-Simpkins P, Seaton A and Simons EG. Pregnancy following ICSI treatment with dead husband's spermatozoa: ethical and policy consideration. *Hum Reproduction* 1997; **12**: 6, 1360–1363.

Part 4

Other considerations

Setting up the transplant unit

Nursing management in the BMT unit

Outpatient management

Multicentre observational databases in bone-marrow transplantation

Ethnic considerations

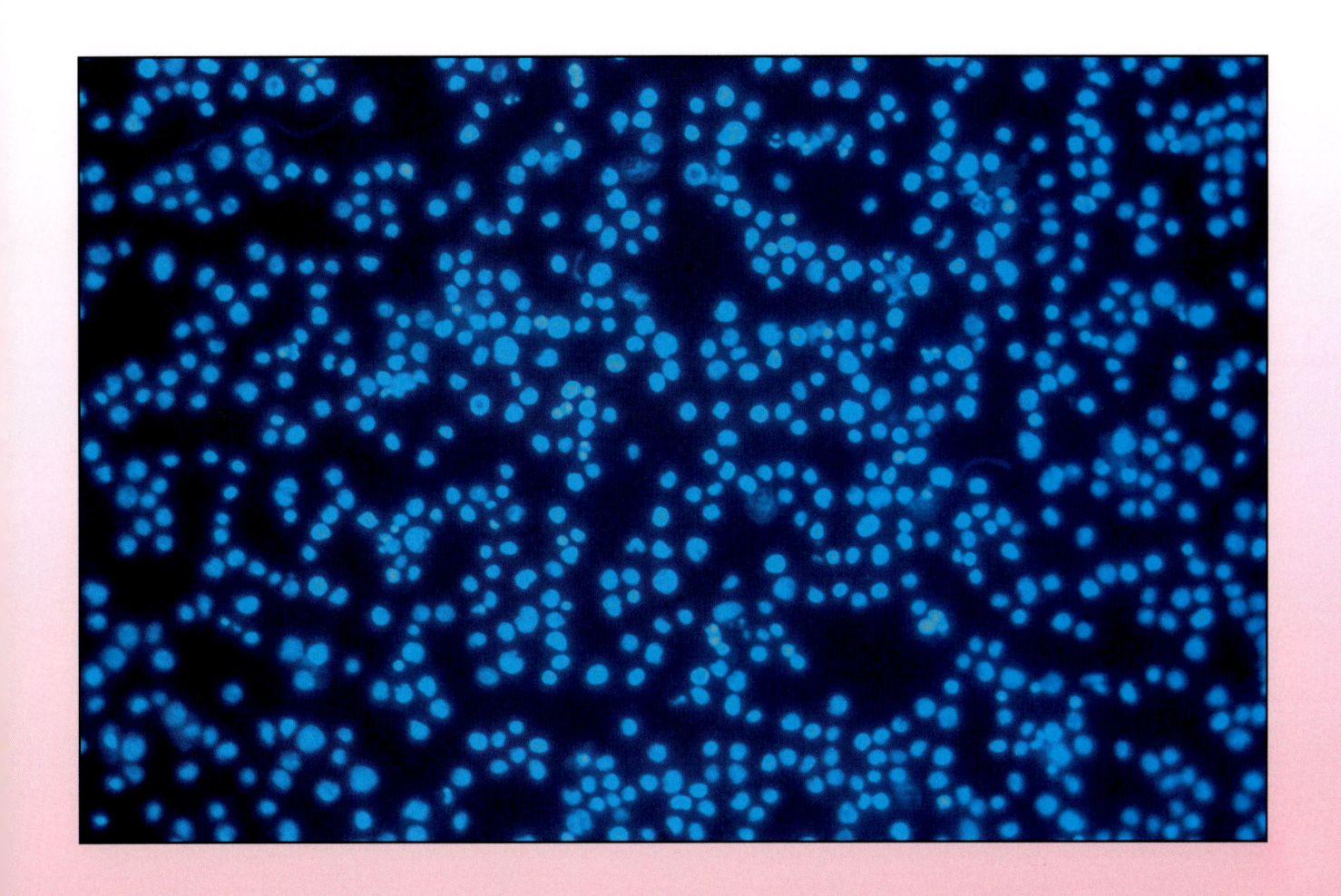

Chapter 58

Setting up the transplant unit

Sarah Hart

Introduction

Infection remains the most significant complication of cancer therapy [1] and is related to the physical and immune status of the patient, the underlying disease of the patient and the proposed treatment plan [2]. Diseases associated with immunological disorders such as aplasia and leukaemia, coupled with treatment programmes which cause profound and protracted granulocytopenia, such as bone-marrow transplantation (BMT), are associated with an increased risk of acquiring an infection [3]. Hiemenz and Green [4] suggest that the immune system may take as long as one to two years to recover after BMT, with factors such as graft-versus-host disease (GvHD) influencing this recovery. Such information suggests that when planning a BMT unit suitable accommodation for re-admission and outpatient facilities should be included in the plans, with infection-control principles and good practices featuring high on the list of priorities for the planned unit.

Protective isolation

When Young and Rubin [5] listed areas of controversy in the management of infection in the immuno-compromised host, they included in their list: 'Elements of protected environment, antibiotic prophylaxis and selective microbial decontamination most useful in preventing infections in compromised hosts.' Today, these issues continue unresolved, which makes planning a BMT unit an arduous task.

In 1994, Poe and colleagues [6] undertook a survey of BMT units in the USA to identify and describe specific BMT infection prevention measures: the sample included 91 BMT units. It was found that all units used some type of protected environment. These researchers concluded that little standardization of practices existed and efforts should be made to test the cost-effectiveness and benefits of the various measures used prior to national standards being compiled. The variation in infection prevention facilities may be related to the Centers for Disease Control and Prevention (USA) recommendations regarding protective isolation [7] that suggested:

> Certain patients are highly susceptible to infection and require special protective care regimes, intended to reduce the risk of infection. However, protective isolation does not appear to reduce this risk, any more than strong emphasis on appropriate hand-washing during patient care. [However, the recommendations go on to say] Compromised patients should be put in private rooms whenever possible.

As protective isolation units have been commissioned since this time, it suggests that planners are not confident that compliance with hand-washing policies can be achieved. Studies of hand-washing in other care settings support these concerns [8,9].

Many researchers have undertaken trials attempting to evaluate protective isolation, mainly in the 1970s and early 1980s. Yates and Holland in 1973 [10] undertook a prospective randomized controlled clinical trial where patients with acute myeloid leukaemia were randomized into four groups, which included standard ward care versus three different types of barrier nursing. The results indicated that there was no difference in the incidence of infection within the first 21 days but after that time patients in the protected environment developed fewer infections. This suggested that for patients whose length of immunosuppression was expected to be long, a protective environment may be beneficial.

Around the same time, Levine et al. [11] studied 88 patients with acute leukaemia who were divided into three groups. These included protective isolation with topical and oral non-absorbable antibiotics and a low microbial diet, or oral non-absorbable antibiotic only, or standard ward care without prophylactic oral or topical antibiotics. The results demonstrated a marked reduction of infection in the group in protective isolation receiving topical and oral non-absorbable antibiotics and a low microbial diet. These findings are supported by the studies from Dietrich et al. [12] and Ribas-Mundo and colleagues [13].

While protective isolation has been seen to reduce the incidence of bacterial infections and therefore to reduce the costs of treating infections, long-term survival has not been improved by the use of protective isolation except in the cases of patients with aplastic anaemia who received their BMT in protective isolation and were seen to develop less GvHD [14].

Outpatient transplants

There has been a move towards non-continuous confinement of patients in hospital who have received allogeneic bone-marrow transplants, (see also Chapter

6). Russell et al. [15] evaluated 20 patients who lived locally and spent time at home. These patients continued with their dietary restrictions, antibiotic prophylaxis and avoidance of crowds whilst at home. The mortality data for this study compared favourably with that from other institutions. This suggests that there are some educated and competent patients and relatives who are pleased to take advantage of such an arrangement, but there are many more who prefer to remain within the safe environment of the hospital, continuously supported by highly skilled staff, in addition to those who either live too far away, have unsuitable living accommodation, or are too ill to take advantage of such arrangements. The authors of this study support this view suggesting that there is no point in relaxing isolation policies if patients are unable to go home.

Psychosocial aspects of protective isolation

The implications of the psychosocial impact of protective isolation have been much debated, and need to be considered when planning a BMT unit. Winters and colleagues [16] reviewed the literature related to depression and social isolation of BMT and undertook a study to reveal the psychosocial needs of patients and relatives. This study provided a list of five psychosocial concepts associated with BMT, concerning the nursing approach to patient needs (Table 58.1).

Ahles and Shedd [17] support the view that prolonged hospitalization and isolation are major stress factors confronting BMT patients, but suggest that these problems are relatively transient and often resolve as the patient begins to improve medically. They conclude by stating that effective psychosocial intervention practices for BMT programmes have yet to be established. Wilkins et al. [18] suggest that anxiety is related to illness rather than to the imposed isolation unless patients have a past psychiatric history. The more recent study of Knowles in 1993 [19] points out that if patients in protective isolation have been involved in the decision making and are able to be prepared for the experience over a period of time, they may cope better during their admission in hospital. Interestingly, Wade and Schimpff [20] consider that patients can believe protective isolation represents a special attempt to treat them as individuals, and compliance with prophylactic antibiotics, for example, can be improved by the constant reminder of the precautions being used.

Antibiotic resistance

A further factor to be considered is the major increase in antibiotic-resistant organisms [21], for example methicillin-resistant *Staphylococcus aureus* (MRSA) [22] and vancomycin-resistant *Enterococcus* (VRE) [23]. These trends suggests that infection control practices within a haematology–oncology unit should be maintained, and may need to be increased since nosocomial infections due to antibiotic-resistant organisms are potentially life-threatening and problems associated with halting an outbreak of infection caused by antibiotic-resistant organisms is immense [24]. The recent increases in infections caused by antibiotic-resistant organisms dispels the hope of Hathorn [3] that new therapeutic agents might render the value of protective measures obsolete.

It can generally beaccepted that protective isolation does not significantly reduce the number of endogenous nosocomial acquired infections, while exogenous nosocomial acquired infections are reduced by relatively simple infection control precautions. Hathorn [3] suggests using a comprehensive approach, taking into account both exogenous and endogenous sources of pathogens. Wade and Schimpff [20] point out that if protective isolation facilities are available it is logical to use them.

Table 58.1 The five core concepts contributing to provisional practice (after Winters et al., 1994 [16])

- Discovering the lived reality: the BMT experience seen through the eyes of patient and family
- Emerging awareness: awareness by nurse of interfamily and interstaff relationships
- Behind closed doors: nurse–patient interactions not fully documented in hospital notes
- Managing the flow: actions taken by patient or nurse to structure interpersonal relations
- Keeping watch: nurse ascertains whether patient's family will help or hinder patient's well-being

Logistics

When planning a BMT facility, the benefits of protective isolation should be correlated with the disadvantages already discussed, in addition to the major cost implications of building, equipping and staffing such a unit and the difficulty in recruiting and maintaining specially trained staff within the nursing [25,26], housekeeping, engineering, dietary and catering departments [4].

A rational approach for the planning team to take is to make the many major decisions before embarking upon any structural work. This includes predicting the future numbers and types of patients who will require care, and budgeting for treatment programmes, available space and other back-up facilities such as catering. When these issues have been addressed, the many existing studies relating to infection control can be used as a basis for determining the features of the planned BMT unit.

The care for single rooms

After the number of beds has been determined a decision as to whether this accommodation will be for single or for shared use must be made. Wade and Schimpff [20] are clear with their advice, stating that if the proposal is for profoundly neutropenic patients to be in single rooms after their white counts have dropped, these patients should enter single rooms on admission to prevent the acquisition of potentially pathogenic hospital organisms which could cause infections after they have become neutropenic. A study of wound infection rates supports this view. Cruse and Foord [27] found that patients who were admitted to hospital some time before their operation were more likely to develop wound infections. Wilson [28] suggested that a single room acts as a reminder that special precautions are required. However, Ayliffe et al. [29] point out that single rooms require a higher nurse/patient ratio than do general wards, and that this set-up will require forward planning.

Other considerations include issues relating to the level of dependency of BMT patients, as sick patients generally find that the peace and quiet of a single room is beneficial. Also, relatives and friends will wish to visit and may even need to stay in the room during the night for compassionate reasons, which can be disturbing for other patients in shared rooms. This information suggests single-room accommodation is preferable to shared rooms.

Room requirements

Patient rooms must be well-lit and large enough to allow space for clinical procedures to be carried out. They require a lavatory, hand-wash-basin and shower, since facilities such as these, if shared, can easily become contaminated with microorganisms such as *Clostridium difficile* which can cause significant outbreaks of cross-infection [30]. Showers are marginally preferable to baths [31] and take up less space. They are easier to clean [29] and for those patients with hair, hair is easier to wash under a shower. The floors and other surfaces of hospital wards can easily become contaminated with bacteria [32] and need to be of an impervious, non-slip, hard-wearing, easy-to-clean and maintain substance. There has been a move away from the use of carpets [33], mainly because they are harder to keep stain-free and clean, and because they take some time to dry following steam cleaning. Table 58.2 summarizes the basic patient requirements to be taken into account when setting up a new BMT unit.

A hand-wash basin should be situated outside each patient room where staff and visitors can wash their hands on the way in and out of the rooms. To prevent incorrect use, taps which can be turned on by knee, foot or automatic means are preferable to wrist-operated taps which are likely to become contaminated if used incorrectly. The flow of water should be

Table 58.2 Considerations for patients when setting up a new BMT unit

- Single rooms preferable, with HEPA air flow
- Access to oxygen and suction equipment
- En suite shower and lavatory
- Supply of nutritious, palatable food
- Entertainment facilities: video, television
- Exercise facilities: exercise bicycle
- Communication facilities: intercom, telephone

controlled to provide a steady stream of hand-hot water which will not splash the user or the environment. An adequate supply of good quality paper towels must always be available. These are preferable to hot-air electric driers where the drying time can be inadequate, resulting in persons drying their hands on their clothes or not washing their hands at all [34]. Liquid bactericidal hand soap should be provided for routine use. However, in an emergency, staff may not have the necessary time to wash and dry their hands by the conventional means, and therefore an alcoholic hand rub must also be available at the entrance and inside each room for quick and convenient cleaning of hands.

Plastic aprons should be placed by the hand-basin to be worn by all persons entering the room. Plastic aprons provide a barrier impervious to bacteria and fluid between the patient and the uniform of the staff member. This should prevent contamination of the uniform and its subsequent dissemination to other patients during further contacts [35].

Each patient room requires suction, oxygen equipment and patient-monitoring equipment; larger equipment should be conveniently situated near to the BMT unit.

Patient rooms should contain some means whereby the patient can exercise, such as an exercise bicycle. The patient will also require entertainment and communication facilities, including a telephone, intercom, television, video recorder and radio. These will relieve boredom, and music can be very effective in counteracting feelings of isolation and discouragement [36].

Water supply

Consideration should be given to the water supply, as hot-water systems in hotels and hospitals have been the most common source of legionellosis in the UK [37]. Legionnaires' disease is caused by inhalation of fine aerosols which are contaminated with the Gram-negative bacillus, *Legionella pneumophilia*, and are therefore a potential hazard for persons in their vicinity. Outbreaks have been associated with air-conditioning systems, in particular those with cooling towers, and hot-water systems [38,39]. Prevention relies upon the hospital engineers following a regular monitoring programme. Cooling towers should be chlorinated, water tanks should be emptied and cleaned, and a pipe system installed which is free of dead legs. Water pipes should be lagged to keep the temperature of the cold water below 20°C and the hot water supply at 50°C at the taps after they have run for one minute [40]. Table 58.3 outlines the precautions which should be taken to prevent *Legionella* infection.

Air

Air supplied to a BMT unit should be free from dust, spores and bacteria. Air-conditioning systems allow air to be filtered, humidified and warmed, which provides not only clean air but a comfortable environment for patients and staff. Invasive *Aspergillus* is a potential problem for severely immuno-compromised patients [41], and this risk is increased during building work when *Aspergillus* spores are liberated into the air. Rhame [42] recommends that all BMT units are provided with filtered air, involving the use of high-efficiency particulate air (HEPA) filters. These remove 99.97% of particles as small as 0.3 μm in diameter and so prevent airborne bacteria and spores entering the BMT unit. Ideally, the system should be capable of providing a supply of both negative and positive pressure air. This allows the flexibility to care for immunocompromised patients in the positive pressure air-conditioning, since air from the general area will not enter these rooms.

Patients infected with airborne diseases such as varicella-zoster can be cared for within the negative pressure rooms, since air from these rooms is prevented from passing out into the general areas and

Table 58.3 Preventing Legionella infection

- Water-cooling towers should be chlorinated
- Water tanks should be emptied and cleaned regularly
- Pipe systems should be free of dead legs
- Water pipes should be lagged, and temperature of cold water maintained below 20°C
- Hot water should be 50°C at taps after they have run for one minute [4]

other patients' rooms. For such a system to function correctly, doors and windows must be kept shut [43]. Such a system is very expensive to install and requires regular maintenance.

Catering

When planning catering facilities for a BMT unit the side-effects of treatment must be considered. For example, the initial nausea and vomiting associated with the radiotherapy and chemotherapy and the oral pain which commonly develops later. Gaston-Johansson *et al.* [44] studied pain and psychological distress in patients undergoing BMT and found that all patients complained of oral pain. Such problems necessitate small, soft, nutritious meals and drinks at times which coincide with their doses of analgesics. Flexibility within the food service is therefore essential; as Van der Meer [45] indicates, a poor diet has a major impact on host defence against infection.

Bone-marrow transplantation units require a ward kitchen for drinks and snack production, and if the main hospital kitchen catering facilities are not near enough or suitable for the provision of a clean diet, the ward kitchen should be sufficiently large and well equipped to provide patients' meals.

Food is a potential source of infection. Hathorn [3] suggests the most effective means of infection prevention in immunocompromised patients is the maintenance of a cooked food diet during the period of granulocytopenia. Pattison [46] undertook a survey of clean diets in BMT centres in the UK and found restrictions varied, but there was a trend away from sterile diets to a modified diet. Such a diet involves excluding foods known to be potentially problematic, such as raw fruit and vegetables, undercooked eggs and delicatessen-type foods which have been extensively handled during manufacture. Barrie [47] suggested ways of avoiding contamination of food which include good hygiene, proper cooking, handling and storage of food, all of which can be achieved by appropriate training and supervision. Training in food safety for food-handlers is essential, with all cooking, temperature control, serving and storage of food complying with the Food Safety Act 1990 [48]. The Food Safety (General Food Hygiene) Regulations 1995 [49] and the Food Safety (Temperature Control) Regulations 1995 [50].

Drinking water is generally safe to drink. However, outbreaks of infection associated with contaminated water have occurred and some units provide boiled water for patients, which is more reliable than bottled water which may contain organisms [51]

Other requirements

Other areas to be included are a clinical room with lockable cupboards for drugs and disinfectant, a designated drug refrigerator and adequate storage space where medical and surgical supplies can be stored safely and cleanly. A hand-wash-basin must be conveniently sited to ensure compliance with hand-washing prior to handling sterile stock and drugs.

It is essential that all body fluids and used equipment can be processed quickly and conveniently. The sluice area should be placed away from the kitchen and clinical room, near enough to the patients to facilitate disposal of bed-pans. The sluice will need storage space for used items such as non-disposable equipment and linen, but clean equipment must not be stored in the sluice as airborne contamination of clean stock can occur. A disinfecting bed-pan washer, clinical sink and hand-wash-basin will also be required.

Adequate storage space and a top-up supplies system will be needed so that stock items can be replenished daily. This is preferable to using valuable ward space for storage of vast amounts of linen and other stock.

Equipment for the unit should be chosen with care, taking into consideration all relevant health and safety recommendations. For example, ice machines have been the source of cross-infection and must be chosen with care, efficiently installed and regularly serviced, and correctly used [52].

Costs

When equipping a BMT unit, the capital costs and running costs of the supplies have to be taken into consideration. For example, the decision between a washer disinfecting bed-pan machine with reusable bed-pans and a macerator and disposable bed-pans makes little difference in terms of revenue cost, but issues such as existing drainage systems, water supply and storage space collectively often makes the preference for a certain item of equipment clear [53].

In general, manufacturers and suppliers of equipment as diverse as beds and intravenous pumps should supply details of their product. Results from clinical trials may allow comparison between different products so that informed decisions can be made regarding the most appropriate items of equipment.

Accomodation for relatives

Provision should be made to accommodate relatives and close friends of BMT patients since many relatives wish to stay in the hospital if their patient is particularly ill or distressed; occasionally, a relative may wish to sleep in an armchair in the patient's room, although such arrangements are not ideal for protracted periods of time due to a lack of toilet facilities and facilities for preparing food and washing clothes. Relatives' accommodation is therefore best situated near to the BMT unit so that they can obtain sufficient rest and therefore be more likely to cope with the demands of visiting and supporting their sick relative. It is also essential that visitors are able to maintain scrupulous personal hygiene to minimize the chances of patients acquiring exogenous infections. Within the BMT unit, a room should be available where staff can have the opportunity to provide help and support to relatives and friends away from the patient's room, since family and close friends of patients undergoing BMT may well experience great stress and feelings of helplessness [17].

Staff

Staff accommodation should include lavatories and washing facilities, as well as areas to store personal property needed during the working shift, office space for preparing reports and carrying out other paper work, and holding meetings. A quiet room should be provided where staff can receive counselling and support, as stress and burn-out among oncology nurses is common [54–56] and is increasing due to the shortage of nurses (see Chapter 59). Table 58.4 summarizes the major considerations when setting up a new BMT unit.

Many issues relating to the provision of inpatient accommodation for BMT patients remain unsolved. However, an association between protective isolation and the reduction in bacterial infections was seen in studies undertaken in the 1970s and early 1980s and these have resulted in most hospitals providing BMT accommodation which adheres to the infection-control principles which will reduce the risk of acquiring an infection during the BMT procedure.

Table 58.4 Considerations for staff when setting up a new BMT unit

- Layout of rooms
- Water supply
- Kitchen
- Sluice facilities
- Storage space
- Facilities for relatives
- Staff accommodation

Anecdotal evidence and common sense suggest that single rooms with *en suite* lavatories and showers, clean air, clean food, adequate supplies and scrupulous cleaning and maintenance of BMT units are essential for those hospitals in the fortunate position of being able to plan and build a new BMT unit. Such provisions should ensure that BMT patients proceed as smoothly as possible through their treatment, and allow carers a more comfortable working day and with increased job satisfaction.

References

1. Chanock S. Evolving risk factors for infectious complications of cancer therapy. In: *Haematology/Oncology Clinics of North America. Infectious Complications in the Immunocompromised Host. 1.* PA Pizza (ed.), 1993; 7: 771–794 (Philidelphia: WB Saunders).
2. Bowell B. Protecting patients at risk. *Nursing Times* 1992; 88: 32–35.
3. Hathorn JW. Critical appraisal for antimicrobials for prevention of infection in immunocompromised hosts. In: *Hematology/Oncology Clinics of North America. Infectious Complications in the Immunocompromised Host. 2.* PA Pizza (ed.). 1994; 7: 1051–1099 (Philidelphia: WB Saunders).
4. Hiemenz JW and Green JN. Special consideration for the patient undergoing allogenic or autologous BMT. In: *Hematology/Oncology Clinics of North America. Infectious Complications in the Immunocompromised Host. 2.* PA Pizza (ed.), 1993; 7: 961–1002 (Philidelphia: WB Saunders).
5. Young LS and Rubin RH. Introduction. In: *Clinical Approach to Infection in the Compromised Host*, 2nd edn. RH Rubin and LS Young (eds), 1987; 1: 1–5 (New York: Plenum Medical).

6. Poe SS, Larson E, McGuire D and Krumm S. A national survey of infection prevention practices on bone marrow transplant units. *Oncology Nursing Forum* 1994; **21**: 1687–1693.
7. Centres of Disease Control Guidelines for Isolation Precautions in Hospital. *Infect Control* 1983 (special supplement); **4**: 325.
8. Taylor L. An evaluation of handwashing techniques. *Nursing Times* 1978; **74**: 54–55.
9. Sedgewick J. Handwashing in hospital wards. *Nursing Times* 1984; **80**: 64–67.
10. Yates JW and Holland JF. A controlled study of isolation and endogenous microbial suppression in acute myeloid leukaemia patients. *Cancer* 1973; **32**: 1490–1498.
11. Levine AS, Siegel SE, Schrieber AD *et al*. Protected environment and prophylactic antibiotics. A perspective controlled study of their utility in the therapy of acute leukaemia. *New Engl J Med* 1973; **288**: 477–483.
12. Dietrich M, Rosche H, Rommel K and Hochapfel G. Antimicrobial therapy as part of the decontamination procedure for patients with acute leukaemia. *Eur J Cancer* 1973; **9**: 443–447.
13. Ribas-Mundom, Granena A and Rozman C. Evaluation of a protective environment in the management of granulocytopenic patients. A comparative study. *Cancer* 1981; **48**: 419–424.
14. Buckner CD, Clift RA, Sanders JE *et al*. Protective environment for marrow transplant recipients. *Ann Intern Med* 1978; **89**: 893–901.
15. Russell JA, Poon MC, Jones AR, Woodman RC and Ruether BA. Allogenic bone marrow transplantation without protective isolation in adults with malignant disease. *Lancet* 1992; **339**: 38–40.
16. Winters G, Miller C, Maracich L, Compton K and Haberman MR. Provisional practice: the nature of psychosocial bone marrow transplant training. *Oncol Nursing Forum* 1994; **21**: 1147–1154.
17. Ahles TA and Shedd P. Psychosocial impact of bone marrow transplantation in adult patients: prehospitalization and hospitalization phases. In: *Bone Marrow Transplantation. Principles, Practices and Nursing Insights*. MB Wheldon (ed.), 1991: 280–292 (Boston: Jones and Bartlett).
18. Wilkins EGL, Ellis ME, Dunbar EM and Gibbs A. Does isolation of patients with infections induce mental illness? *J Infect* 1988; **17**: 43–47.
19. Knowles H. The experience of infectious patients in isolation. *Nursing Mirror* 1993; **89**: 53–56.
20. Wade JC and Schimpff SC. Epidemiology and prevention of infection in the compromised host. In: *Clinical Approach to Infection in the Compromised Host*, 2nd edn. RH Rubin and LS Young (eds), 1987; **2**: 5–40 (New York: Plenum Medical).
21. Kelly J and Chivers G. Built-in resistance. *Nursing Times Supplement J Infect Control Nursing* 1996; **92**: 23: 1–5.
22. Cox RA, Conquest C, Mallaghan C and Marples RR. A major outbreak of methicillin resistant Staphylococcus aureus caused by a new phage-type (EMRSA-16). *J Hosp Infect* 1995; **29**: 87–106.
23. Hospital Infection Control Practices Advisory Committee. Recommendations for preventing the spread of vancomycin resistance. *Infect Control Hosp Epidemiol* 1995; **16**: 105–113.
24. Duckworth G. Revised Guidelines for the Control of Epidemic Methicillin-Resistant *Staphylococcus aureus*. *J Hosp Infect* 1990; **16**: 351–377.
25. Gulatte MM and Levine N. Recruitment and retention of oncology nurses. *Oncol Nursing Forum* 1990; **17**: 419–427.
26. Department of Health. *NHS Workforce in England*. 1989 (London: HMSO).
27. Cruse PJE and Foord R. The epidemiology of wound infection in a 10-year prospective study of 62 939 wounds. *Surg Clin North Am* 1980; **60**: 27–40.
28. Wilson J. The immune system and the immunocompromised patients. In: *Infection Control in Clinical Practice* 1995; **4**: 77–105 (London: Baillière Tindall).
29. Ayliffe GAJ, Lowberry EJL, Gedded AM and Williams JD. Prevention of infection inwards. 11. Isolation of patients, management of contacts and infection precautions for ambulances. In: *Control of Hospital Infections. A Practical Handbook*, 1992, 3rd edn **8**: 142–169 (London: Chapman & Hall Medical).
30. Worsley M. A major outbreak of antibiotic-associated diarrhoea. *Public Health Lab Service Microbiol Digest* 1993; **10**: 97–99.
31. Mitchell NJ. Whole body disinfection with chlorhexidine. Is shower bathing more effective than bathing? *J Hosp Infect* 1984; **5**: 96–99.
32. Ayliffe GAJ, Collins BJ and Lowbury EJL. Ward floors and other surfaces as reservoirs of hospital infection. *J Hygiene (Cambridge)* 1967; **65**: 515–536.
33. Anderson RL, Mackel DC, Stoler BS and Mallison GF. Carpeting in hospitals: an epidemiological evaluation. *J Clin Microbiol* 1982; **15**: 408–415.
34. Matthews JA and Newson WB. Hot air electric hand driers compared with paper towels for potential spread of airborne bacteria. *J Hosp Infect* 1987; **9**: 85–88.
35. Hambraeus A. Transfer of *Staphylococcus aureus* via nurses uniforms. *J Hygiene (Cambridge)* 1973; **71**: 799–814.
36. Cook JD. Music as an intervention in the oncology setting. *Cancer Nursing* 1986; **9**: 23–29.
37. Bartlett CLR, Macrae AD and Macfarlane JT. *Legionella Infections*. 1986 (London: Edward Arnold).
38. Health and Safety Executive. *The Control of Legionellosis Including Legionnaires' Disease*, 1991 (HMSO Publication Centre: Department of Health).
39. Health and Safety Executive Working Group on Legionellosis, 1992 (HMSO Publication Centre: Department of Health).
40. Fallon RJ. How to prevent an outbreak of legionnaires' disease. *J Hosp Infect* 1994; **27**: 247–256.
41. Khardoni N. Host–parasite interaction in fungal infection. *Eur J Clin Microbiol Infect Dis* 1989; **8**: 331–352.
42. Rhame FS. Prevention of nosocomial aspergillosis. *J Hosp Infect* 1991; **18**(Suppl A): 466–472.
43. Anaissie E. Opportunistic mycoses in the immunocompromised host: experience at a cancer centre and review. *Clin Infect Dis* 1992; **14**(Suppl 1): S43–53.
44. Gaston-Johansson F, Franco T and Zimmerman L. Pain and psychological distress in patients undergoing autologous bone marrow transplantation. *Oncol Nurses Forum* 1992; **19**: 41–47.
45. Van de Meer JWD. Defects in host defense mechanisms. In: Clinical Approach to Infection in the Compromised Host 3rd

edn. RH Rubin and IS Young (eds.) New York Plenum Medical 1994; **3**: 33–44.
46. Pattison AJ. Review of current practice in clean diet in the UK. *J Human Dietetics* 1993; **6**: 3–11.
47. Barrie D. The provision of food and catering service in hospital. *J Hospital Infect* 1996; **33**: 13–33.
48. Food Safety Act 1990 (London: HMSO).
49. Food Safety (General Food Hygiene) Regulations 1995 (London: HMSO).
50. Food Hygiene (General) Regulations 1995 (London: HMSO).
51. Communicable Disease Report: Surveillance of Waterborne Disease and Water Quality. *Public Health Laboratory Service* 1996; **6**: 73–74.
52. Burnett IA, Weeks GR and Harris DM. A hospital study of ice making machines: their bacteriology, design, usage and upkeep. *J Hosp Infect* 1994; **28**: 305–313.
53. Johnson A. Bedpans: disposables or reusables? *Nursing Times* 1989; **85**: 72–74.
54. Sadler C. Bone marrow patients can place extra stress on nurses. *Nursing Mirror* 1985; **160**: 6.
55. Wolf GA. Nursing turnover – some causes and solutions. *Nursing Outlook* 1981; **29**: 233–236.
56. Cronin-Stubbs D. Professional impairment strategies for managing the troubled nurse. *Nursing Admin* 1985; **9**: 44–45.

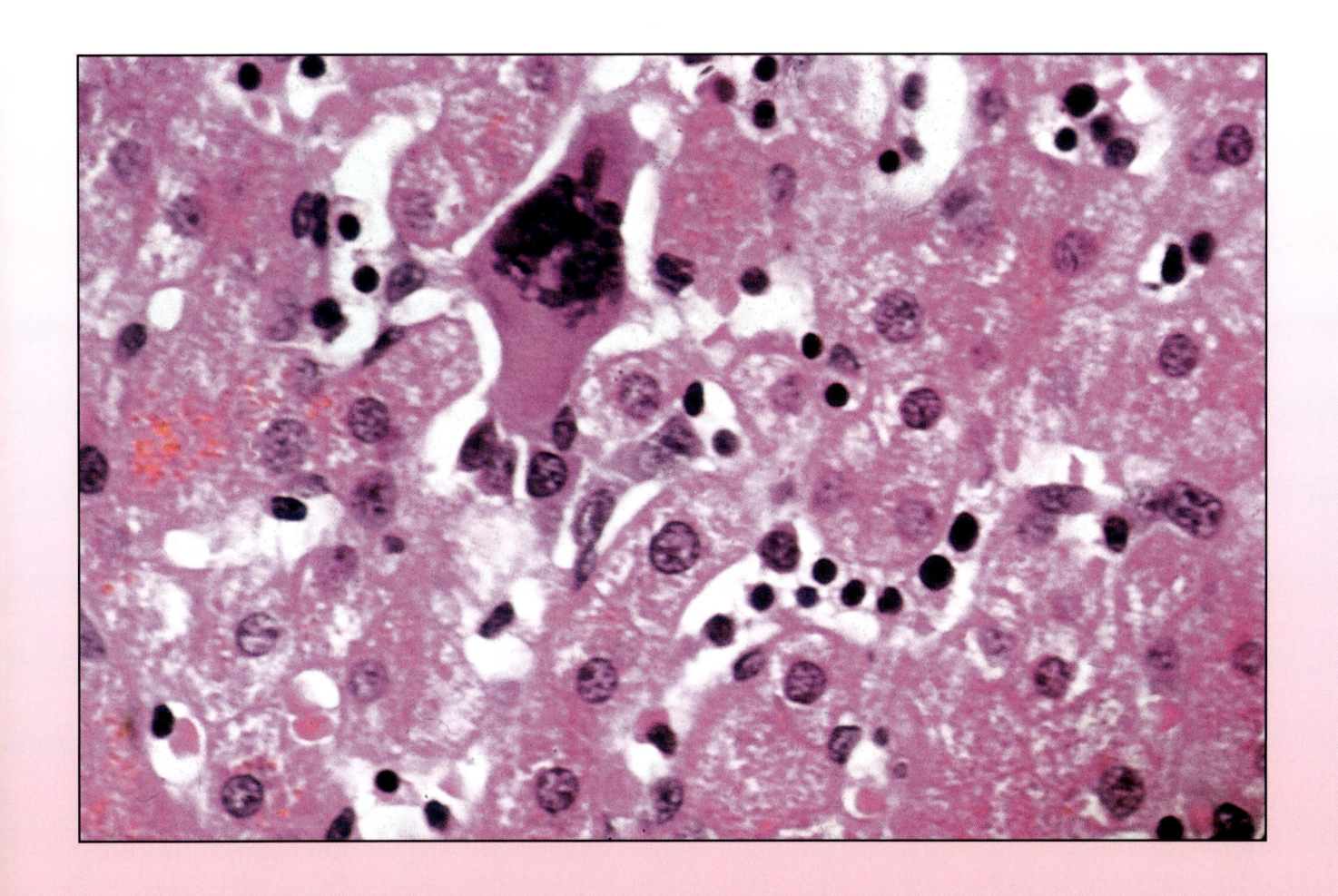

Chapter 59

Nursing management in the BMT unit

Helen Porter

Introduction

The last three decades have seen the development of blood and bone-marrow transplantation (BMT) from an experimental treatment to an established therapeutic modality for a large number of malignant and non-malignant disorders. Medical advances in tissue typing, blood product support, antibiotic therapy and growth factors have facilitated this growth. In line with these developments, nursing has faced new challenges and has seen the rapid advancement of BMT nursing as a speciality in its own right. Nursing management of these patients requires a high level of specialized knowledge and skills to optimize patient care. Bone-marrow transplantation nursing is, however, not just one speciality. It encompasses acute medicine, intensive care, palliative care, infection care, wound management, paediatrics and, with the widening age boundaries, care of the elderly. Nursing management in the bone-marrow transplant unit is both a complex and creative challenge.

Nursing administration

Strategic planning

Bone-marrow transplantation is a complex treatment. It requires the provision of expert medical and nursing personnel, specialized environment and equipment and the utilization of resources. Change and development in this field is constantly occurring and strategic planning involving the whole team is crucial to ensure safe and effective delivery of treatment and care within the available resources of the institution. The nurse manager plays an important part in this team, reflecting the vital role of the nurse in the care of the BMT patient.

Collaboration between medical, nursing and other related disciplines (Table 59.1), recognizes the role each has in the service provision. All disciplines should be involved in developing the goals and philosophy of the unit.

Human resource management

Bone-marrow transplant nursing is a speciality which primarily combines the elements of oncology with critical care. The BMT nurse needs to develop expert knowledge and skills and to be able to function as part of a team. This nursing team includes the nurse manager, clinical nurse specialist, registered nurses and support workers. There is little guidance on the nursing establishment of the BMT unit. The British Committee for Standards in Haematology Task Force (BCSHCHT) [1] provide guidelines on the provision of facilities for the care of adult patients with haematological malignancies. They define four levels of care and advise on the extent of knowledge, training and expertise that is required in nursing but do not specify establishment numbers. Similarly, the standards set by the European Blood and Marrow Transplantation group (EBMT) [2] specify that staff numbers should reflect the amount of activity in the transplant unit and that these should be comparable to those of an intensive care unit. Campbell and Foody [3] recommend a high ratio of registered nurses to unregistered nurses, with a registered nurse:patient ratio of 1:2. In determining the level and skills required for the BMT unit, the manager may find it useful to visit other similar units. Provision of the nursing establishment needs to take into consideration:

- type of transplants performed;
- number of transplants performed per week;
- patient age range;
- whether intensive care is performed on the unit;
- number of beds;
- isolation procedures;
- extended role of the nurse;
- support services available.

Nurse recruitment for BMT units commonly involves nurses with a background in oncology. In planning the workforce, the nurse manager may also

Table 59.1 Related disciplines

- Chaplaincy
- Community liaison
- Dietetics
- Occupational therapist
- Oral hygiene
- Physiotherapy
- Psychological medicine
- Social work

look at the skills provided by other specialities and recruit from paediatrics and intensive care, for example, to ensure a diverse, multiskilled team. The role and function of the BMT nurse will vary according to the individual unit. However, the role is one that is constantly expanding its boundaries to improve patient care. In some units, this extended role incorporates placement and removal of venous access devices, administration of intravenous drugs, apheresis procedures, bone-marrow harvesting, nurse prescribing and venepuncture. The BCSHCHT also identifies the need for the provision of expert nursing in the form of nurse specialists. The remit of a BMT clinical nurse specialist includes clinical support, education, advice and clinical leadership. The clinical nurse specialist assists with developing standards of care, policies and procedures, orientation and staff development programmes and research [3]. Other clinical nurse specialists such as those dealing with pain control, critical care and infection control provide valuable support for the unit staff.

Orientation, education and staff development

Orientation, education and training should be provided in a structured programme for both new and existing staff. Bone-marrow transplant nurses are working in a rapidly changing environment and need to keep abreast of these developments to ensure optimum patient care [4–5]. The programme should provide the opportunity for didactic, experiential and self-directed learning. Learning resources include videos, critical pathways, policies and procedures, programmed texts, textbooks and unit-generated written information, together with input from medical, pharmacy and nursing personnel (Table 59.2). Core learning objectives defined by the unit with specialized input from the clinical nurse specialist and nurse manager form the basis for the orientation and education programme. Table 59.2 summarizes the issues to be considered.

The BMT unit is an acute care environment which new members of the team often find stressful and frightening. Provision of systems of support such as 'buddy' systems, preceptorship and mentoring go a long way in guiding the new nurse through the first few weeks of work. As well as providing support, this facilitates experiential learning 'at the bedside' under the direction and supervision of an experienced practitioner. An on going continuing education programme aimed at the experienced members of the team will continually update and recognize the learning needs of the team.

Table 59.2 Orientation programme

Experiential	Case review*	Didactic
Admission of patient	Detection of infection	Overview of malignancies
Attend transplant talk	Management of sepsis	Haemopoiesis
Observe apheresis	Fluid and electrolyte imbalance	Indications for BMT
Observe bone-marrow harvest	Mucositis	Types of BMT
Attend total body irradiation	Graft-versus-host disease	Conditioning regimens
Administer conditioning regimen	Nausea and vomiting	Laboratory values
Administer transplant	Multisystem organ failure	Infection control
Care for patient in protective isolation	Multiple drug therapy	Psychological issues
Discharge planning		Emergency procedures

*With preceptor/clinical nurse specialist.

Together with unit-based education strategies, there are a number of recognized haematology, BMT, oncology and critical care courses that are available. Education, research and practice can also be shared through the medium of conferences and study days such as those run by the EBMT Nurses Group and the Royal College of Nursing Leukaemia and Bone Marrow Transplant Forum.

Staff stress

It is well recognized that nurses working within a bone-marrow transplant unit are subjected to many stressors [3,6,7]. The patients are often young and of a similar age group to the nursing staff. The treatment is aggressive and the nurse has to support and care for the patient and his family through a major life crisis. The treatment carries significant morbidity and mortality and the patient requires a high level of acute care, which is often similar to that of an intensive care environment. The nurse will develop close relationships with the patient and the family over the prolonged treatment period. If the patient is dying, the nurse will need to support the patient through the change from being orientated to cure and life to being death-orientated, and there is often a feeling among the staff that they have failed. All these issues can lead to a high emotional cost paid by the nurse, causing 'burn-out'. When stress is prolonged, this can lead to significant staff problems such as repeated errors, poor judgement, decreased productivity, increased illness and absenteeism [8].

There are many approaches to minimizing or treating staff stress. Emphasis should be placed by the nurse manager on team-building strategies. It should be recognized that all members of the team are subject to the stressors. The team should have a common goal and philosophy of care, as group cohesion and unity provide a supportive network for the individual nurse. Within this framework, 'buddy' or mentor systems are valuable in providing support from peers. Regular support group meetings allow the nurse to express the issues causing stress and to be able to discuss them freely. These groups can be led internally, for example by the nurse manager or externally, perhaps by a member of the psychological support team. Other strategies for decreasing stress include reflective practice, staff-friendly shift patterns and orientation and continuing education programmes.

Resource issues

Bone-marrow transplant patients require frequent complex monitoring. Adequate numbers of non-invasive blood pressure and pulse monitoring devices, pulse oximetry and electronic thermometers are required. Provision should be available for cardiac monitoring and electrocardiography (ECG) recording. Other equipment such as intravenous therapy devices are essential. The numbers of these are determined by the type of transplant performed and patient numbers. Systems should be in place for evaluation of devices in use, as should maintenance programmes.

Planning and organization of care

Nursing care of the BMT patient is diverse. Ford and Ballard [9] identified concepts that are essential in understanding the nursing care of BMT patients:

- The chemoradiation therapy the patients receive would be fatal if they were not 'rescued' with an infusion of stem cells.
- Major complications in patients after transplant are usually iatrogenic.
- Complications often occur simultaneously.
- Clinical manifestations of some complications, although often of sudden onset, may be subtle.
- The clinical manifestations of different complications can be the same.
- One complication can cause or exacerbate another.
- The treatment of one complication can cause or exacerbate another.
- Prophylaxis or treatment for one complication may have to be modified or terminated because of the development of another complication.

The function of the BMT nurse must encompass patient education, and prevention, early detection and treatment of patient problems. The nurse must develop diagnostic skills to ensure prompt treatment, as many clinical situations are acute in onset and potentially life-threatening. The nurse must work in collaboration with the medical team in both diagnosis and treatment. The patient traverses a number of stages during the transplant and exhibits different needs and problems at these various stages.

Table 59.3 highlights the main patient problems during the acute phase after transplantation.

Table 59.3 Problems in the acute phase post-BMT

Gastrointestinal	Renal	Pulmonary	Skin	Haematological	Gonadal	Neurological	Cardiac	Liver
Mucositis	Acute failure	Fibrosis	GvHD	Infection fungal viral bacterial protozoal	Dysfunction	Leukoencephalopathy	Atrial fibrillation (A.F)	GvHD
Diarrhoea	Fluid and electrolyte imbalance	Pneumonia	Radiation changes	Thrombocytopenia	Infertility	Cognitive changes	Cardiomyopathy	Veno-occlusive disease
Nausea and vomiting	Radiation nephritis	Interstitial pneumonitis	Drug allergies	Anaemia			Endocarditis	Drug-induced liver damage
GvHD	Acute haemolytic reaction	Pulmonary oedema	Alopecia	Disseminated intravascular coagulopathy				
Salivary gland damage	Haemorrhagic cystitis	Pulmonary haemorrhage		Graft failure				
Taste changes		Acute respiratory failure						
Malnutrition								

Policies and procedures

Policies and procedures should be developed to provide direction for care that should reflect current research, and the individual needs of the unit. Policies and procedures ensure safe, standardized practice and may provide a forum for quality assurance and audit. Development of policies and procedures should be carried out within a multidisciplinary framework. Policies and procedures for a BMT unit include the issues summarized in Table 59.4.

Patient education

The bone-marrow transplant is a complex and intensive treatment which can carry a significant morbidity and mortality rate. To ensure fully informed consent to the procedure from the patient and his family, the nurse will need to spend time giving education and support. Culture, socioeconomic background and locus of control [10] are three critical factors that impinge upon patient and family education concerning the BMT procedure.

Owing to the complexity of the information needs of the patient, it is important that the nurse sees the patient on a number of occasions. Pretransplant information is given by the transplant coordinator (medical) and this requires support by the nurse. The clinical nurse specialist is well placed to see the patient and family prior to admission to the unit. Information should encompass the various phases of the transplant: donor selection, admission to the unit, preparative regimen, transplant infusion, aplasia, treatment complications and engraftment, discharge planning and ambulatory follow-up [10]. This amount of

Table 59.4 Policies and procedures for a BMT unit

Control of infection	Clinical practice access services	Clinical treatment	Nursing practice
Preparation of room and equipment	Cell separator services	Intravenous therapy	Nursing documentation
Protective isolation	Sperm banking and ovum storage	Administration of therapeutic substances	Admission procedure
Low microbial diet	Blood product support	Oral care	Discharge procedure
Microbiology and surveillance cultures	Rehabilitation services	Skin care	Orientation and new staff education
Hand-washing	Community liaison	Venepuncture	Nursing establishment and skill mix
Decontamination		Administration of bone marrow	Philosophy of nursing
Patient and family education		Cardiopulmonary resuscitation	
		Anti-emetics	
		Pain control	
		Management of sepsis	
		Nurse-assisted medical procedures	

information may be frightening and overwhelming for the patient and family. Education in these matters should be individualized, with various strategies such as one-to-one teaching, family/group teaching as well as the use of learning aids such as written information and video recordings. Some units allow the patient to tape-record the transplant talk so that the information can be repeated. The nurse should use this time to assess the patient for any specific physical or psychological problems which may affect the transplant process. These may include previous problems with nausea and vomiting, and needle phobias. The patient should be assessed for the amount of information that he requires and should be given the opportunity to discuss specific queries and concerns. As well as providing information on the phases of the transplant, the patient may require teaching about procedures that he may be asked to undertake. These include care of the skin-tunnelled catheter and administration of subcutaneous growth factors. With the advent of ambulatory/home care, the patient may also undertake self-administration of chemotherapy via ambulatory infusion devices, and antibiotic therapy.

Documentation of care

Many different methods of documenting planned and administered nursing care have been used in BMT units. Pre-written standing orders, protocols, care plans, computer programmes and critical pathways [11] do much to streamline and direct nursing care. Patient assessment is simplified by the use of assessment tools such as the Oral Assessment Guide [12]. Whichever form of documentation is chosen, it should be sufficiently flexible to meet the diversity of patient problems together with the individual patient needs.

An example of a proforma of pretransplantation critical issues is shown in Table 59.5.

The future

Ambulatory care

Recent developments have seen the dramatic shift from caring for BMT patients in a specialized BMT unit to ambulatory home care. An increasing number of patients are receiving all or part of their transplant as an outpatient. Due to the nature and severity of potential side-effects, such care has been undertaken with great caution. The BMT nurse plays a crucial role in ensuring safe delivery of care through the strategic planning of the ambulatory care service.

The development of an ambulatory care service involves environmental concerns, patient education initiatives, patient selection criteria, selection of appropriate venous access and infusion devices, community support services, resource implications and available backup from the inpatient BMT service.

Research

The last three decades have seen many advances in the field of bone-marrow transplantation. This, together with the development of refinements in patient care such as improved antibiotic regimens and improved blood product support, has necessitated that the nurse continually advance the boundaries of her knowledge of patient care issues. We have already seen development of the extended role for the nurse in the advent of the BMT clinical nurse specialist role. BMT nurses must ensure that these changes in patient care are effected through research and they must continually investigate how nursing can help the patient cope with the considerable physical and psychological morbidity associated with this procedure. Nurses must also ensure that taking on an increasing amount of the traditional medical role is not at the detriment of nursing care guidelines as outlined in the UKCC *Scope of Practice* [13].

Table 59.5 Example of pretransplant critical pathway

Patient name .... Consultant ....

Hospital number .... Regime ....

Date of birth ....

Blood group .... CMV status ....

Date	Patient activity	Comments/signature
	Referral to transplant team Initial assessment	
	Pretreatment authorization obtained	
	Pretransplant appointment with clinical nurse specialist	
	PRETREATMENT DISEASE EVALUATION: CT scan Bone marrow aspirate and trephine Tumour markers Other	
	PRETREATMENT PHYSICAL EXAMINATION: History and physical examination Renal function Pulmonary function Cardiac function Blood tests (full blood count; urea and electrolytes (U&E); coagulation; viral screen, etc.) Infection screening Allergy and drug reaction history	
	TRANSPLANT TALK WITH MEDICAL AND NURSING STAFF: Consent	
	REFERRAL TO MULTIDISCIPLINARY TEAM: Dietician Dental hygienist Physiotherapist Other	
	APPOINTMENT WITH CLINICAL NURSE SPECIALIST TO EXPLAIN: Apheresis procedure Teach growth factor self-administration (or arrange community support) Evaluate venous access Apheresis procedure for two consecutive days Evaluate harvest count; if necessary repeat harvest Assess patient for suitability for ambulatory/home care	

Table 59.5 Continued

Date	Patient activity	Comments/signature
	High-dose chemotherapy Referral to day care unit Arrange admission date Insertion of venous catheter Teach patient to care for catheter Visit BMT unit and meet named nurse	
	CHEMOTHERAPY SCHEDULE:	
	Day of peripheral blood stem-cell transplant	
	RECORD OF WRITTEN INFORMATION GIVEN TO PATIENT: Stem-cell harvesting Care of skin-tunnelled catheter Chemotherapy High-dose chemotherapy and autologous transplantation Mouth care Hospital admission booklet Isolation procedures Going home after transplant	

References

1. British Committee for Standards in Haematology Clinical Haematology Task Force. Guidelines on the Provision of Facilities for the Care of Adult Patients with Haematological Malignancies (including Leukaemia and Lymphoma and Severe Bone Marrow Failure). *Clin Lab Haematol* 1995; **17**: 3–10.
2. Link H, Schmitz N, Gratwohl A and Goldman J for the Accreditation Sub-Committee of the European Group for Blood and Marrow Transplantation (EBMT). Standards for specialist units undertaking blood and marrow stem cell transplants – recommendations from the EBMT. *Bone Marrow Transplant* 1995; **16**: 733–736.
3. Campbell LR and Foody MC. Administrative issues of an inpatient BMT unit. In: *Bone Marrow Transplantation, Administrative and Clinical Strategies*. PC Buchsel and MB Whedon (eds), 1995: 39–68 (Boston: Jones and Bartlett).
4. Kelleher J and Jennings M. Nursing management of a marrow transplant unit: a framework for practice. *Semin Oncol Nursing Bone Marrow Transplant* 1988; **4**: 60–68.
5. Porter H. Educational developments for nurses working in bone marrow transplantation. In: *Proceedings of the Bone Marrow Transplantation Symposium, 7th International Conference on Cancer Nursing, Vienna August 1992*, 51–52 (SCUTART PROJECTS Ltd, Harrow, Middx).
6. Thomas S. The bone marrow transplant unit and nursing management. In: *Bone Marrow Transplantation in Practice*. J Treleaven and J Barrett (eds), 1992: 353–359 (Edinburgh: Churchill Livingstone).
7. Ford R. Reducing nursing-staff stress through scheduling, orientation and continuing education. *Nursing Clin North Am* 1983; **18**: (3) 597–602.
8. Sarantos S. Innovations in psychological staff support: a model program for the marrow transplant nurse. *Semin Oncol Nursing Bone Marrow Transplant* 1988; **4**: 69–73.
9. Ford R and Ballard B. Acute complications after bone marrow transplantation. *Semin Oncol Nursing Bone Marrow Transplant* 1988; **4**: 15–24.
10. Jassak PF and Porter NL. Strategies for education of the BMT patient. In: *Bone Marrow Transplantation, Administrative and Clinical Strategies*. PC Buchsel and MB Whedon (eds), 1995: 351–364 (Boston: Jones and Bartlett).
11. Burns JM, Tierney K, Long GD, Lambert SC and Carr BE. Critical pathway for administering high-dose chemotherapy followed by peripheral blood stem cell rescue in the outpatient setting. *Oncol Nursing Forum* 1995; **22**: 1219–1224.
12. Eilers J, Berger AM and Peterson MC. Development and testing of the Oral Assessment Guide. *Oncol Nursing Forum* 1988; **15**: 325–330.
13. United Kingdom Central Council for Nursing, Midwifery and Health Visiting. *The Scope of Practice*, 1992 (London UKCCNMHV).

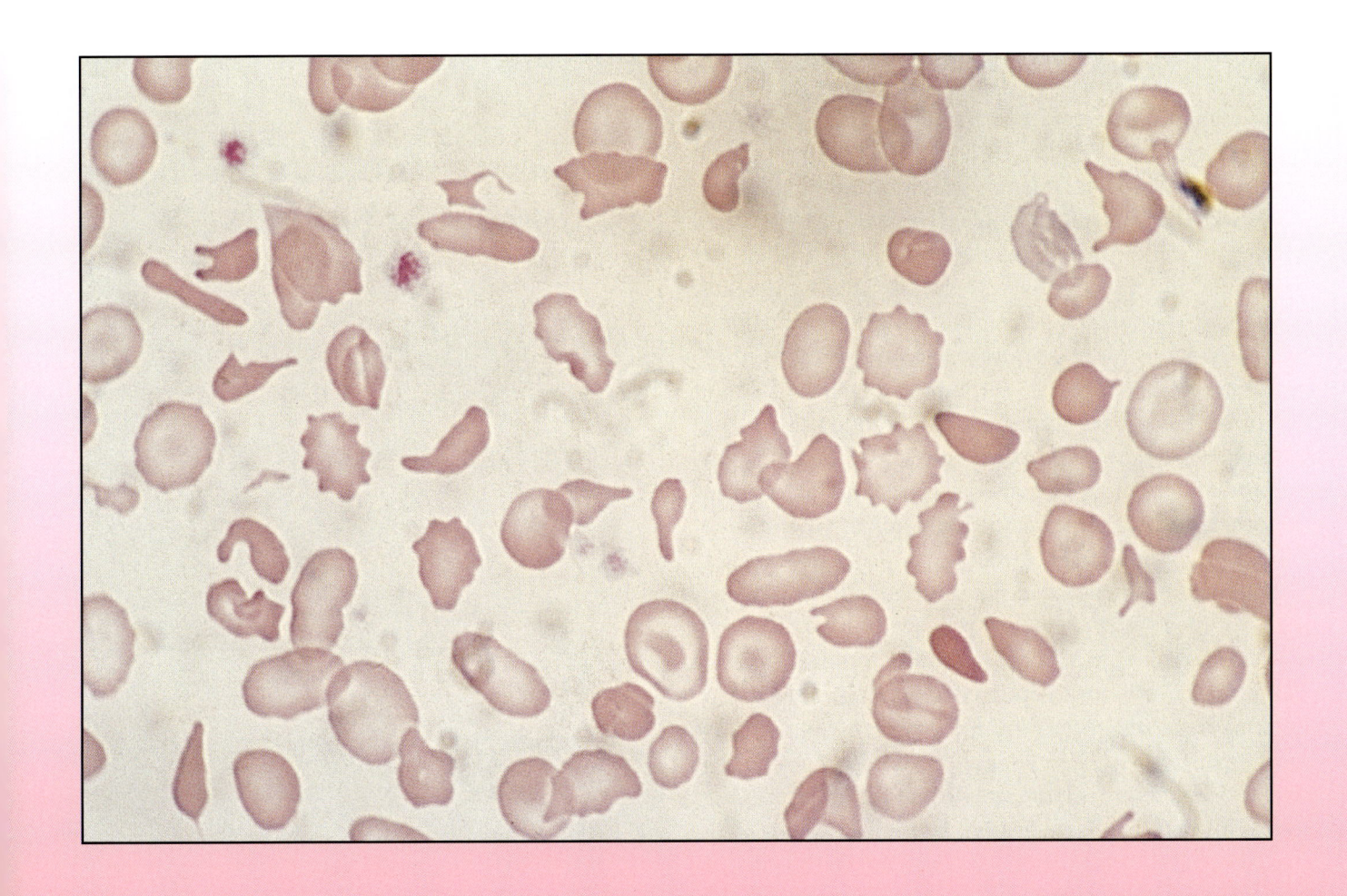

Chapter 60

Outpatient management

James A. Russell

Introduction

Bone-marrow transplants and blood cell (PBPC) transplants are complex and expensive procedures placing the highest demands on healthcare delivery systems. Recent technological developments are helping to make these procedures easier and safer. At the same time, economic pressures are increasing. While it is particularly expensive to occupy a hospital bed during the more critical stages, the incentives to care for these patients as outpatients depend to some extent on the system under which one operates. If the patient or a third party is paying the bill then outpatient care, if feasible, becomes very attractive. On the other hand, if a bed is already available in a public system, the immediate incentive is less, although a restructuring of the system may still be indicated. Until then, it may be just as convenient to care for the patient on the inpatient unit and allow frequent passes. The preparatory work before conditioning is given can be done from the outpatient clinic for most patients in most institutions. Thereafter the needs of autologous and allogeneic transplant patients are different enough to merit separate consideration.

There are substantial advantages in having a dedicated team take over patient care from the time of planning until follow-up ends. The way in which outpatient care is organized will depend on a variety of factors including, for example, the overall size of the programme, whether both autologous and allogeneic transplants are done and whether both children and adults are treated. Although all members of the nursing team need to be familiar with all aspects of the procedure, once a certain 'critical mass' is reached there may be some advantages to some specialization of responsibilities (Table 60.1).

As in so many other areas, good communication is essential to a smoothly functioning programme. There are advantages to frequent personnel interaction. In our programme, for example, regular team meetings will include representatives from several disciplines including psychosocial services, tissue typing, radiotherapy and the apheresis programme.

Autologous transplants

Pretransplant period

Preparation and counselling of patients before transplant is addressed in Chapter 23. Suffice it to say

Table 60.1 The bone-marrow transplant/blood cell transplant outpatient nursing team – examples of division of responsibilities

- Unrelated donor registry
- Related donor recruitment
- Donor processing or booking, granulocyte colony-stimulating factor, apheresis
- Autologous transplants
- Allogeneic transplants
- Subspeciality clinics
- Regular follow-up clinics
- Intravenous therapy

Table 60.2 Pre-transplant arrangements for autologous transplant patients

- Assessment of disease status – radiology blood tests, clinical, etc.
- Bone-marrow examination
- Organ function, e.g. heart, lung, liver, renal
- Venous access (apheresis and support)
- Mobilizing chemotherapy
- Growth factors
- Leukapheresis

that the pretransplant planning is largely an exercise in coordinating a number of activities at different times and in different places with the least inconvenience and delay (Table 60.2).

Peritransplant period

Historically, autologous bone-marrow transplant patients required admission to hospital from the start of conditioning to the point at which neutrophils were recovering and the patient was no longer dependent on intravenous therapy. The use of peripheral blood progenitor cells (PBPC) instead of bone marrow has resulted in decreased morbidity, expense and duration of hospitalization [1]. The consequent shift of care to outpatient delivery has offered further cost savings without sacrificing the safety and efficacy of these procedures. In some centres, outpatient care of such patients is now routine [1–3]. The majority of admissions can usually be limited to a few days and many patients can be treated entirely as outpatients (Table 60.3).

Autologous transplant patients, the majority of whom are now receiving PBPC, have a relatively short period of pancytopenia with median recovery times of 10–14 days for granulocytes and platelets. Other complications depend in part upon the conditioning regimen used. Stomatitis may be severe and necessitate intravenous analgesia but parental nutrition is not usually needed. Transfusions and antibiotics can be given on an outpatient basis.

There are some advantages to integrating early outpatient care with the inpatient unit. In particular, continuity of care and communication among staff will be better during this particularly critical time when immediate attention should always be available. Whatever the administrative structure there are some fundamental requirements. These are outlined in Table 60.4.

Long-term follow-up

After the acute toxicities are over, routine management of the autologous transplant patient can be returned to the referring physician as the care is essentially that of any intensive chemotherapy patient.

Table 60.3 Factors encouraging outpatient autologous transplantation

Social	Technical
Economic pressures	Mobilized PBPC accelerate engraftment
Patient preference	Improved anti-emetics
	Antibiotics every 24h

Table 60.4 Requirements for an outpatient autologous transplant unit

- Proximity of accommodation, inpatient and outpatient areas
- Emergency medical cover
- Guaranteed inpatient beds available
- Rapid laboratory results
- Prompt access to blood bank

Allogeneic transplants

Before transplant

The same principles apply as for autologous transplants but the list is somewhat more extensive (Table 60.5).

Peritransplant period

Each conditioning regimen presents its own challenges when delivered to outpatients. None of these, however,

Table 60.5 Pretransplant arrangements for allogeneic transplant patients

Recipient	Donor
Assessment of disease status (radiology, blood tests, clinical)	Screening tests
Screening tests (serology etc.)	Venous access*
Material for engraftment studies	Growth factor mobilization*
Organ function (heart, lung, liver, renal)	Leukapheresis*
Subspecialty consultations	Operating room
Venous access	
Protocol, admission	
*Blood cell transplants	

should be insuperable. Repeated doses of cyclophosphamide may need intensive hydration and/or mesna which may be difficult to administer on a 24-hour basis. Convulsions associated with busulphan, sometimes occurring despite anticonvulsants, may make care givers uneasy about outpatient care, and patients should always be accompanied. On the other hand, agents such as VP16 and total body irradiation can easily be delivered to outpatients [4]. Bone marrow and blood cells can be infused in the clinic although some precautions are necessary if large volumes of dimethylsulphoxide are given with cryopreserved products.

Because the maximal effects of conditioning take a few days to develop, many patients remain relatively well the first few days after transplant and can be managed with a daily outpatient visit. They need instruction to return to the clinic or inpatient unit quickly if problems arise.

Our experience is that patients often need to be in hospital when stomatitis occurs and frequent intravenous administration of analgesics and other medications is needed. After the patient is able to eat, discharge is feasible unless other complications occur. Thus, much of the time spent out of hospital before discharge is during neutropenia, the period when isolation would be used in many institutions. Outpatient care in the early post-transplant period is therefore only feasible for institutions who have decided that isolation is unnecessary. The limited data available suggest that this may be the case in some centres [5]. On the other hand, a recent study from the International Bone Marrow Transplant Registry (IBMTR) indicates a significant survival benefit from the use of high energy particulate air (HEPA) filtration and/or laminar air flow (LAF) units [6]. While there may be a number of explanations for this observation it will clearly make many centres reluctant to abandon isolation if they have not already done so. It is also possible that newer developments such as the use of growth factors will shorten the neutropaenic period sufficiently to render any benefits of isolation undetectable.

We have attempted to address the question of how much treatment can be delivered to allogeneic transplant recipients as outpatients in the immediate post-transplant period. A group of BMT and blood cell transplant patients were studied who were treated without isolation after 1988 [7]. Passes were taken as desired, but it must be remembered that some patients could not take advantage of this because they lived too far away. The data illustrate our belief that the need for admission is essentially independent of engraftment *per se* (Table 60.6).

If isolation is not used, our data suggest that, while feasible to some extent, it will be harder to administer most of the early post-transplant care to allogeneic transplant patients as outpatients than has been the case for autologous PBPC transplants. Thus, although 83% of patients took passes at some time, this represented only a median of 25% of their inpatient days. On the other hand, we have treated the occasional patient without any overnight stay in hospital. If early indications that the use of PBPC or blood cell transplant in the allogeneic setting are borne out, a move to outpatient care in the early post-transplant phase may be facilitated [8–12]. There are indications that earlier discharge, fewer transfusions and accelerated engraftment can be achieved [12] although it is unlikely that the proportional savings will be as impressive as with autologous transplants. Nevertheless, if conditioning can be given on an outpatient basis (instead of admitting the patient on day −5), and if 5 of 20 (our current median stay for family donor blood cell transplant [12]) outpatient days can be achieved post-transplant then we could still shorten hospital stay for the average patient by 40%.

As with autologous transplants there may be some advantages in having outpatient care of allogeneic transplant patients carried out on or close to the inpatient unit by the inpatient team. This allows

Table 60.6 Hospitalization is not directly dependent on neutrophil count

- Passes were taken for a median of 25% of inpatient days
- In patients who took passes, a median of 78% were before engraftment
- In 27%, all passes were before engraftment
- 23% of patients were discharged before engraftment

continuity of care and facilitates communication during a particularly critical period.

Long-term follow-up

Immediately after discharge, it is important to have clear communication between outpatient and inpatient teams. Close monitoring may still be necessary and patients need to stay in the vicinity of the transplant centre until they are stable and the team is comfortable that they can be followed from a greater distance.

Allogeneic BMT patients are best supervised by a dedicated team specializing in the care of these patients. Graft-versus-host disease and other longer term toxicities demand close monitoring so that they can be detected and treated early. The requirements for the unit are similar to those for autologous transplant patients where facilities for intravenous therapy, diagnostic testing and minor surgery should be readily available.

Printed information is useful for patients after discharge so that they can be advised about which problems to report and whom to contact. We prefer patients to report any issues directly to the BMT team and to be persistent. They are advised against going to emergency departments or seeking help from elsewhere before contacting the team.

There are advantages to maintaining a group of subspecialists with a special interest in BMT. This allows them to develop expertise which is not available in the wider community. Our own programme has developed clinics in hepatology and pulmonology medicine attended by BMT physicians as well as the relevant subspecialists. This provides the most efficient method of sharing and concentrating expertise. Such clinics become valuable if a significant number of patients need frequent subspecialty consultations. For example, in our programme, about one-third of all patients are seen in the pulmonary clinic (Table 60.7).

When a rapid response from other departments is required, this may sometimes be best achieved by admitting the patient to hospital, but this should be discouraged if there are no other pressing medical reasons to do so. It is important to establish a system whereby consultations can take place promptly. Waiting several days for an appointment is invariably unacceptable for transplant patients.

Some issues are so universal that regular screening of all patients by a dedicated subspecialist before and after transplant is advisable (Table 60.8). Data gathering presents a formidable challenge in the long-term care of these patients. Whether for routine clinical management or research studies, well-defined protocols are essential. A system of ensuring that routine tests are performed, results obtained and appropriate action taken is fundamental. Follow-up protocols and records should be as straightforward as possible to assist data managers.

The duration of follow-up of allogeneic BMT patients depends to some extent upon whether the programme is regional or whether patients come from far afield. Whether all patients need indefinite follow-up by the transplant team is debatable, but some kind of basic information, such as that collected by the IBMTR, may be useful for delineating the true long-term morbidity of these procedures.

Table 60.7 Subspecialists in follow-up of allogeneic bone-marrow and blood cell transplant patients

On demand (rapid response):
- Dermatology
- Hepatology
- Gastroenterology
- Pulmonology
- ENT
- Renal

Table 60.8 Subspecialists in management of allogeneic bone-marrow and blood cell transplant patients. Routine pre- and post-transplant assessment

- Endocrine (paediatrics)
- Ophthalmology
- Gynaecology
- Psychosocial
- Dental

References

1. Peters WP, Ross M, Vredenburgh JJ et al. The use of intensive clinic support to permit outpatient autologous bone marrow transplantation for breast cancer. *Semin Oncol* 1994; **21**(Suppl 7): 25–31.
2. Gluck S and Des Rochers C. High-dose chemotherapy followed by blood cell transplantation: a safe and effective outpatient approach. *Bone Marrow Transplant* 1997: **20**; 431–434.
3. Burns JM, Tierney DK, Long GD, Lambert SC and Carr BE. Critical pathway for administering high-dose chemotherapy followed by peripheral blood stem cell rescue in the outpatient setting. *Oncol Nursing Forum* 1995; **22**: 1219–1224.
4. Algara M, Valls A, Vivancos P and Granena A. Outpatient total body irradiation for bone marrow transplantation. *Bone Marrow Transplant* 1995; **14**: 381–382.
5. Russell JA, Poon M-C, Jones AR, Woodman RC and Reuther BA. Allogeneic bone marrow transplantation for adults with malignancy without protective isolation. *Lancet* 1992; **339**: 38–40.
6. Passweg J, Rowlings PA, Atkinson KA et al. Influence of protective isolation on outcome of allogeneic bone marrow transplantation for leukemia. *Bone Marrow Transplantation*. In Press.
7. Stotts M and Bouchard M. Allogeneic bone marrow and blood cell transplantation without protective isolation: a seven-year retrospective review. *Bone Marrow Transplant* 1996; **17**(Suppl 1): S152.
8. Körbling M, Przepiorka D, Huh YO et al. Allogeneic blood stem cell transplantation for refractory leukemia and lymphoma: potential advantage of blood over marrow allografts. *Blood* 1995; **85**: 1659–1665.
9. Schmitz N, Dreger P, Suttorp M et al. Primary transplantation of allogeneic peripheral blood progenitor cells mobilized by filgrastim (granulocyte colony-stimulating factor). *Blood* 1995; **85**: 1666–1672.
10. Bensinger WI, Weaver CH, Appelbaum FR et al. Transplantation of allogeneic peripheral blood stem cells mobilized by recombinant human granulocyte colony-stimulating factor. *Blood* 1995; **85**: 1655–1658.
11. Azevedo WM, Aranha FJP, Gouvea JV et al. Allogeneic transplantation with blood stem cells mobilized by rh-G-CSF for hematological malignancies. *Bone Marrow Transplant* 1995; **16**: 647–653.
12. Russell JA, Brown C, Bowen T et al. Allogeneic blood cell transplants for haematological malignancy: preliminary comparison of outcomes with bone marrow transplantation. *Bone Marrow Transplant* 1996; **17**: 703–708.

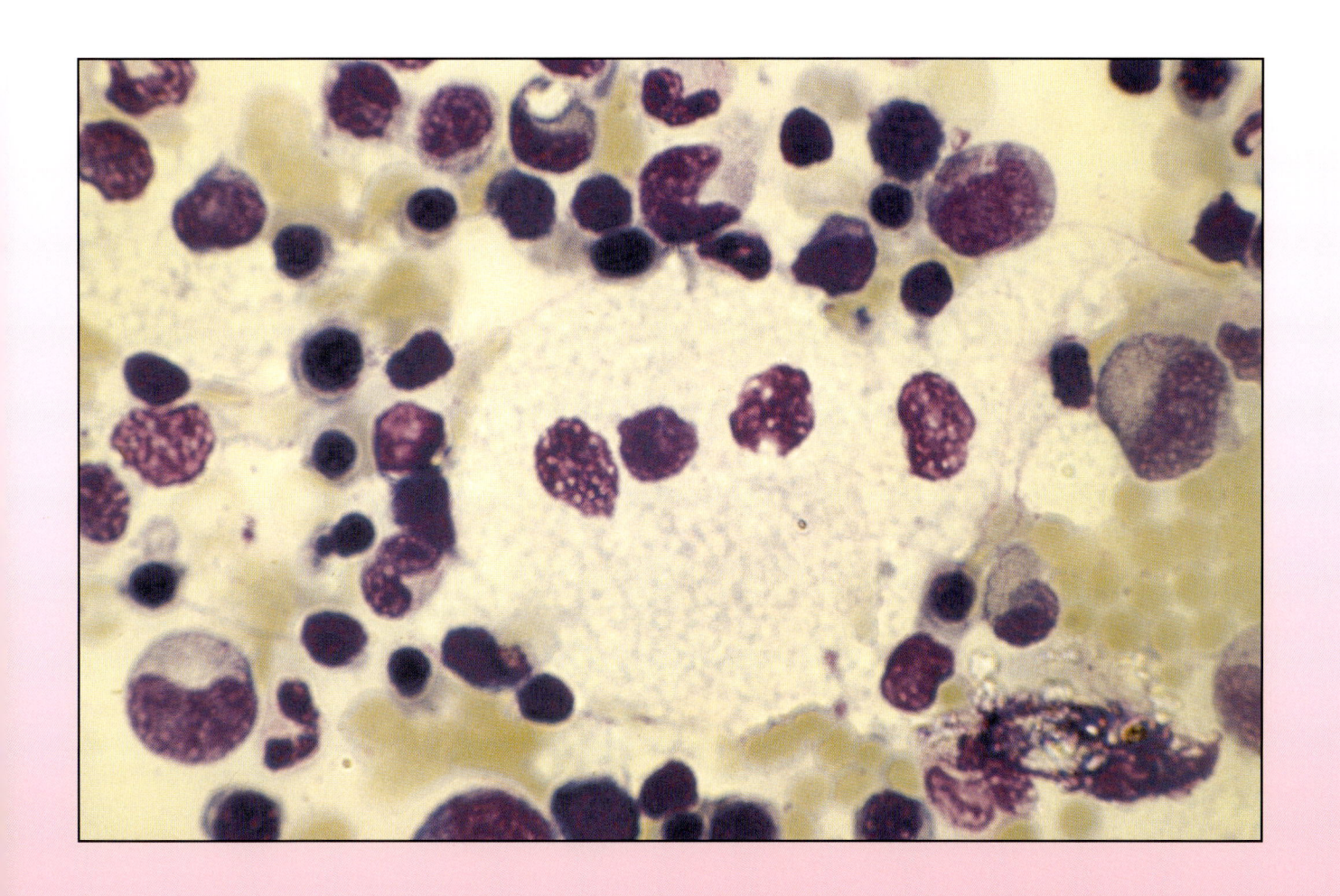

Chapter 61

Multicentre observational databases in bone-marrow transplantation

Philip A. Rowlings, Kathleen A. Sobocinski, Mei-Jie Zhang,
John P. Klein and Mary M. Horowitz

Introduction

The first successful allogeneic bone-marrow transplants in humans were performed in 1968. Since then, use of allogeneic or autologous hematopoietic stem-cell transplantation has increased dramatically, with an estimated 40 000 blood and bone-marrow transplants worldwide in 1996. Concomitant with development and diffusion of this technology has been a coordinated, international effort to collect and analyze data on transplant outcome through the International Bone Marrow Transplant Registry (IBMTR) and the Autologous Blood and Marrow Transplant Registry – North America (ABMTR). The IBMTR, established in 1972, and the ABMTR, established in 1990, are voluntary organizations involving more than 400 transplant centres in 47 countries (Appendices 1 and 2). Participating centres submit data on their consecutive allogeneic and/or autologous haematopoietic stem-cell transplants to the IBMTR/ABMTR Statistical Center, a division of the Health Policy Institute of the Medical College of Wisconsin. These registries now have data on over 65 000 transplants performed worldwide. The largely voluntary efforts of the participating centres have resulted in the establishment of a unique resource of data and statistical expertise for studying haematopoietic stem-cell transplantation.

Another large consortium of blood and marrow transplant teams exists in Europe, the European Group for Blood and Marrow Transplantation (EBMT). The EBMT was formed in 1973 and now has a membership of over 350 teams. Unlike the IBMTR/ABMTR with a single centralized statistical centre focusing mainly on analyses of observational data, the EBMT performs multiple functions, including providing a forum for interaction among individuals, institutions and groups involved in clinical transplantation, conducting prospective randomized clinical trials and establishing standards for transplant centres practising in Europe [1]. However, the EBMT also maintains several disease-specific observational databases used to analyze transplant outcomes.

---

*For the Advisory Committees of the International Bone Marrow Transplant Registry and Autologous Blood and Marrow Transplant Registry – North America Medical College of Wisconsin

The need for multicentre observational databases in bone-marrow transplantation

Assessing transplant outcome is complex. Outcomes are influenced by many patient- and disease-related factors such as age, disease stage and prior treatment, as well as transplant-related factors such as stem-cell source, conditioning regimen and graft-versus-host disease (GvHD) prophylaxis. Ideally, most transplant issues would be addressed by large randomized clinical trials. However, many factors limit the application of randomized trials in haematopoietic stem-cell transplantation. Many diseases treated with transplants are uncommon; single centres may treat only a few patients with a given disorder. This makes randomized trials difficult and also limits the ability to perform non-randomized (phase II) trials with sufficient power to detect meaningful effects. Small trials, even when randomized, may give misleading results [2]. New transplant technologies are being introduced rapidly, so results of prospective clinical trials may be obsolete before they are published. Autologous transplants, increasingly used to treat more common cancers such as breast cancer, have rapidly diffused into the non-academic setting since the early 1990s, where randomized trials are rarely done and results of therapy infrequently published. Some important transplant issues are not amenable to randomization, such as differences in outcome associated with differences in donor type.

In a systematic review of 255 transplant-related studies published between 1990 and 1992, only 16 (6%) were randomized trials; most had fewer than 100 patients [3]. Even when randomized trials are performed, enrolled patients may represent only a small proportion of the target population and may not be representative of the larger group [4–6]. Results of treatments administered in these trials may differ from those obtained when the technology is more widely applied.

The most common type of bone-marrow transplant study published is a single-centre series of consecutively treated patients [3]. These studies generally focus on a particular conditioning regimen or other treatment in a cohort of patients where other factors may or may not be uniform. Many lack sufficient numbers to adjust for heterogeneity in prognostic factors and treatment regimen. Most clinical trials focus on short- and intermediate-term outcomes (one to five years). However, there is a need for long-term follow-up of transplant recipients, since high-dose therapy may be associated with important effects, such as therapy-related cancers, that may not occur until many years after transplant.

Observational databases may facilitate analysis of transplant outcomes in many ways by focussing on questions difficult to address in randomized trials. These include descriptions of transplant results in various disease states and patient groups, analysis of prognostic factors, comparison of transplant regimens, comparison of transplant with non-transplant therapy, intercentre variability in diagnosis, practice and outcome, analytical approaches to evaluating transplant outcome and evaluation of costs of different types of transplants. Collaboration of groups maintaining separate databases may further facilitate such studies. The IBMTR and EBMT have collaborated on several studies. A recent example was an analysis of patients receiving human leukocyte antigen (HLA)-identical sibling transplants for chronic lymphocytic leukaemia [7]. Each group had small numbers of patients (<30), limiting the power of conclusions. By collaborating, results in 54 patients were published. Further cooperative analyses are ongoing.

Descriptive studies

Databases which include a very large proportion of centres involved in allogeneic and autologous transplantation are uniquely suited to descriptive studies. This is particularly important for rare diseases, or for more common conditions where transplants are infrequent. Single centres often have only one or a few cases, precluding meaningful assessment of outcome. Registries, by combining data from many centres, provide a more precise estimate of results and may identify efficacy or call attention to problems with transplants. Examples of descriptive studies using IBMTR/ABMTR data are analyses of transplants for Philadelphia-positive chromosome (Ph+) acute lymphoblastic leukaemia [8], for Diamond–Blackfan anaemia [9] and for Hodgkin's disease [10].

Identification of prognostic factors

Large numbers, and heterogeneity of patients, allow use of multivariate regression techniques to evaluate associations of patient- and disease-related variables with outcome. This is an important use of large observational databases, since many prognostic factor studies are limited by small numbers, non-representative populations, and/or insufficient detail on patient and disease characteristics [11–14]. Examples of such studies include assessment of risk factors for acute and chronic GvHD [15,16], interstitial pneumonia [17,18] and veno-occlusive disease of the liver [19], prognostic factors for relapse and leukaemia-free survival after transplants for acute myelogenous leukaemia (AML), acute lymphoblastic leukaemia (ALL) and chronic myelogenous leukaemia (CML) [20–23], risk factors for graft failure after transplants for severe aplastic anemia [24] and factors associated with outcome of T-cell-depleted transplants for leukaemia [25].

Comparison of transplant regimens

Ideally, new conditioning regimens, GvHD prophylaxis regimens and other transplant manoeuvres would be tested in large randomized trials. However, as discussed above, these trials are often difficult to perform [26,27]. It is possible to compare results of various strategies among concurrently treated patients using observational data, if there is sufficient clinical information for each patient to allow adjustment for potentially confounding effects of important prognostic variables. The IBMTR used this approach to compare transplant regimens for aplastic anaemia [28], to compare GvHD prophylaxis regimens in leukaemia [29], to compare results of HLA-identical sibling, HLA-mismatched related and unrelated donor transplants for leukaemia [30,31], and to compare purged and unpurged autotransplants for acute myelogenous leukaemia [32]. It can also be used to study the effect of specific patient or disease characteristics as in the IBMTR analysis of the impact of age over 40 years on transplant outcome [33,34].

Comparing transplant with alternative treatments

In some instances, transplants treat diseases where there is no other effective therapy, e.g. Fanconi anaemia. In other diseases, e.g. acute leukaemia, there are other potentially curative treatments. The question then arises whether transplants are better than alternative treatments. Rarity of the diseases treated, variable treatment philosophies, and limited availability of donors, technologies and resources make evaluating these questions in randomized trials difficult. It is also difficult to compare published results of transplant and non-transplant treatments directly because of differences in patient selection and inherent delay in performing transplants, leading to truncation of early failures from most transplant series (time-to-treatment bias) [35–38]. Comparisons of transplant versus alternative therapies can be done by combining observational transplant data with primary data compiled by groups studying chemotherapy regimens [35–43]. The IBMTR has conducted several studies comparing transplant with non-transplant therapy in adults with acute myelogenous leukaemia in first remission [44], adults with acute myelogenous leukaemia in second remission [45], adults with acute lymphoblastic leukaemia in first remission [46], children with acute lymphoblastic leukaemia in second remission [47] and adults with chronic myelogenous leukaemia in first chronic phase [48]. Chemotherapy data for these studies were contributed by several cooperative oncology groups including the Eastern Cooperative Oncology Group [44], the Pediatric Oncology Group [47], the German Multicenter Acute Leukemia Therapy Trials Groups [43], the German Acute Lymphoblastic Leukemia Therapy Group [45,46], the British Medical Research Council [44], and the Italian CML Study Group [48].

Determining late consequences of transplant

The large, longitudinal databases are uniquely suited to study late and infrequent effects of transplantation. The IBMTR/ABMTR has information on >10 000 persons surviving three or more years after transplantation. The IBMTR/ABMTR, in collaboration with the National Cancer Institute and the Fred Hutchinson Cancer Center and members of the EBMT recently completed a study of solid tumours developing after allogeneic bone-marrow transplants [49]. Late (two or more years after transplant) causes of death in allograft recipients are currently being examined and preliminary data from this study were recently presented [50].

Developing statistical methodology for transplant outcomes

Large databases are a rich resource for developing mathematical models of post-transplant outcomes. Examples include addressing the problems of adjusting for centre effects following a proportional hazards regression analysis [51], comparing transplant and non-transplant therapies [35] and comparing therapies with diverging outcomes over time (for example, comparing autologous and allogeneic transplants where autologous transplants tend to have fewer early deaths but higher late failure from relapse) [52].

It is important to emphasize that studies of observational data from multiple centres do not replace the need for carefully conducted single centre phase I and II studies or single or multicentre randomized studies. Rather, they offer a complementary approach for addressing issues in BMT. The remainder of this chapter summarizes current use and outcomes of haematopoietic stem-cell transplantation using data from the IBMTR/ABMTR.

Current use and outcomes of bone-marrow transplantation

Figure 61.1 shows how use of blood and marrow transplants continues to increase. We estimate 12 000 allogeneic and 18 000 autologous transplants were done in 1995, worldwide. Most autotransplants use haematopoietic progenitor cells collected from blood (Figure 61.2). Fewer than 20% are done with bone marrow alone. In contrast, over 90% of allografts use bone marrow. Despite recent interest in collecting allogeneic cells from peripheral blood or umbilical cord blood, few such transplants have yet been done.

Most allogeneic transplants are from HLA-identical sibling donors (Figure 61.3). However, only about 30% of transplant candidates have such a donor. Increasing availability of HLA-typed volunteers through large national and international registries has enabled increasing use of unrelated donors for bone-marrow transplants. Transplants from unrelated donors now account for about 25% of allogeneic transplants.

The most common indications for allogeneic and autologous transplants differ (Figure 61.4). Among cases reported to the IBMTR/ABMTR, 74% of

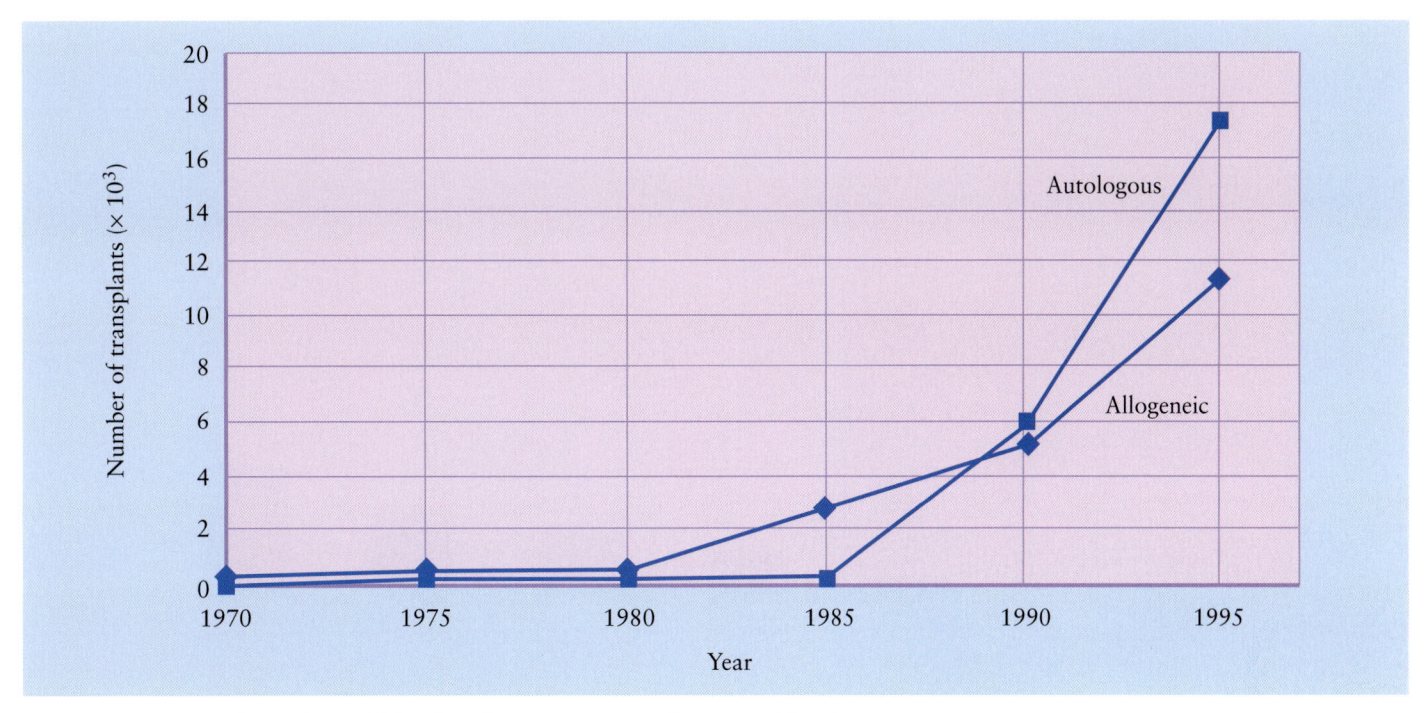

Figure 61.1 Annual number of blood and marrow transplants worldwide (1970–1995).

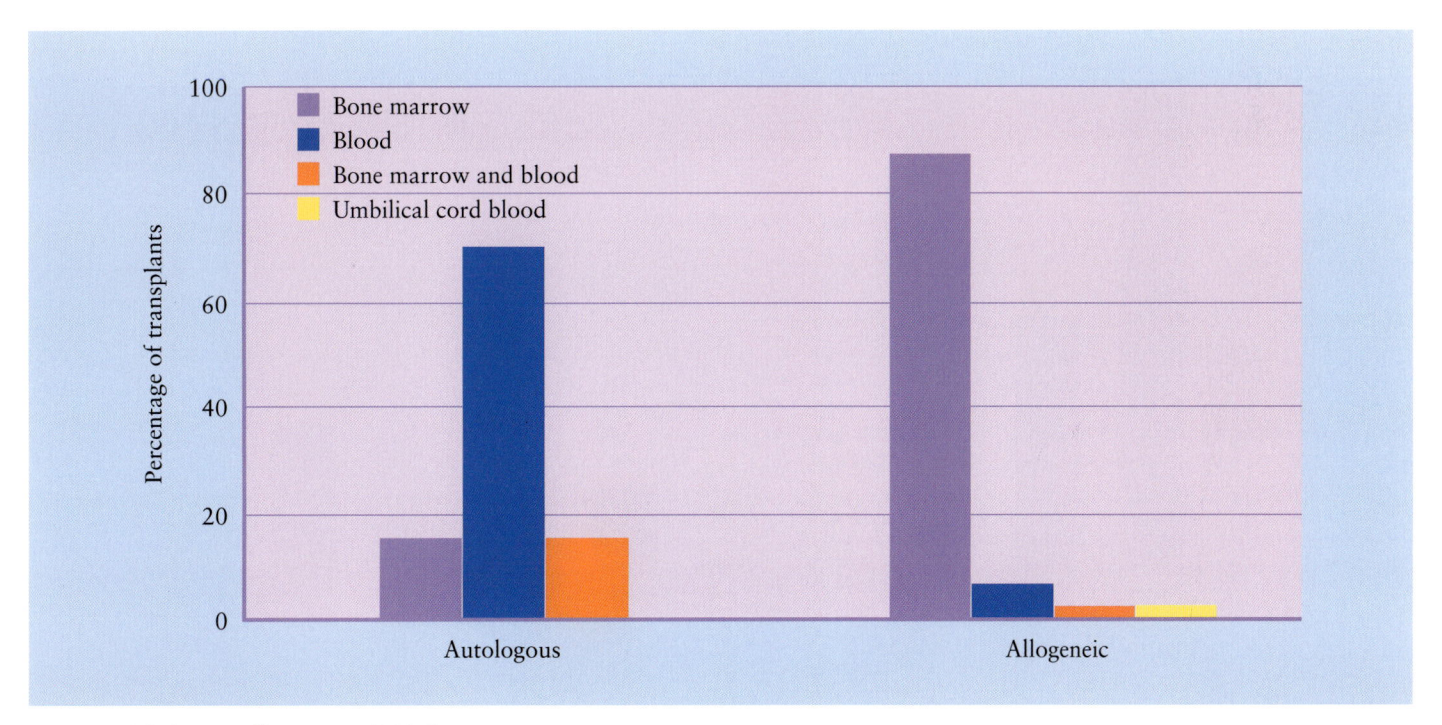

Figure 61.2 Stem-cell sources (1995).

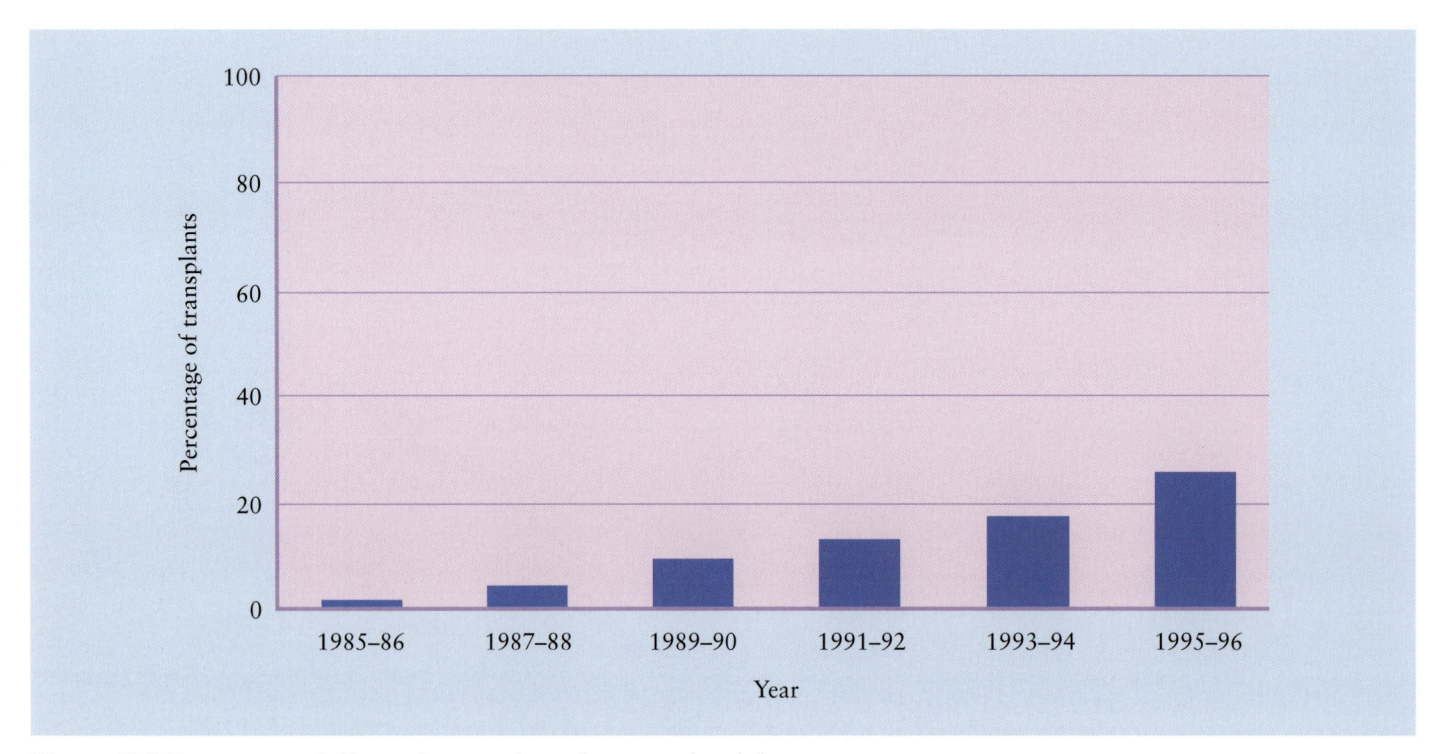

Figure 61.3 Percentage of allogeneic transplants from unrelated donors.

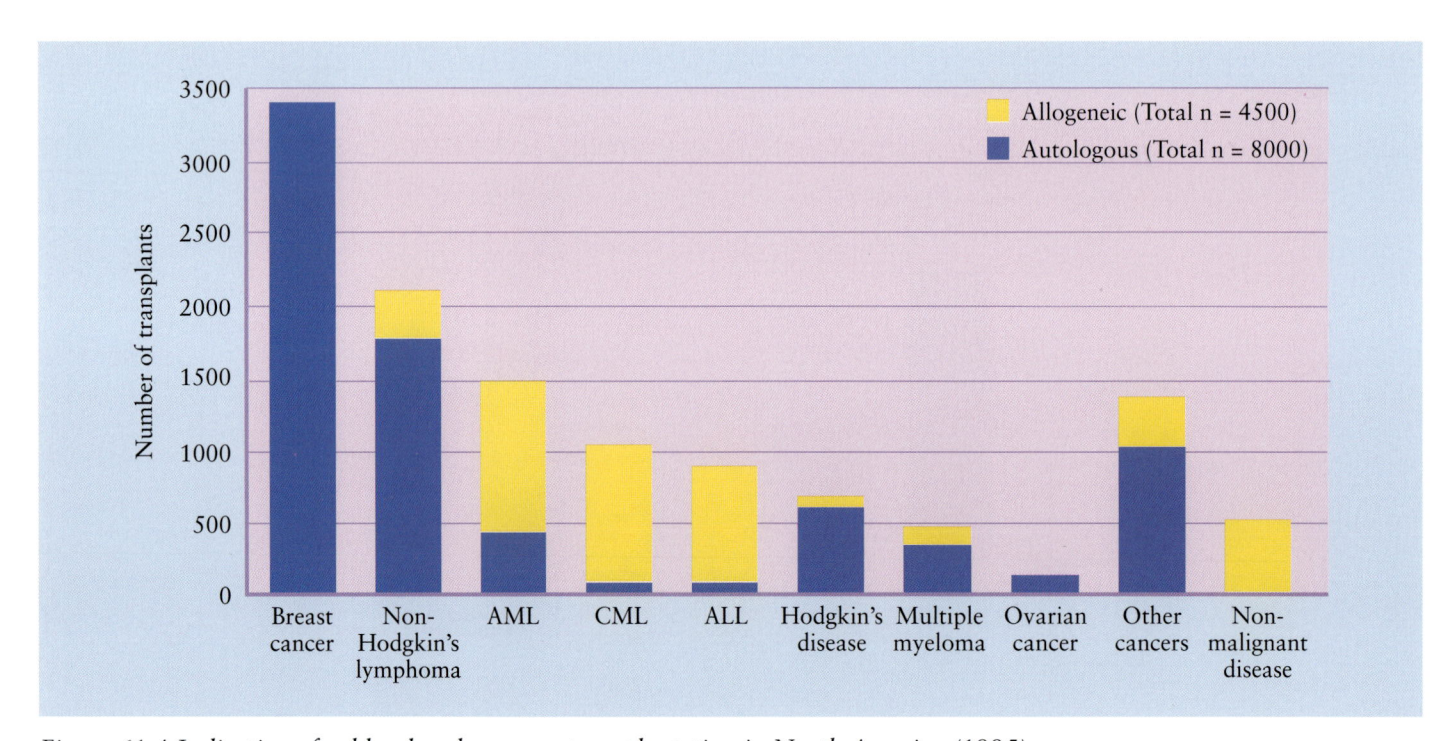

Figure 61.4 Indications for blood and marrow transplantation in North America (1995).

allogeneic transplants are for leukaemia or preleukaemia: 22% for CML, 23% for AML, 19% for ALL, 7% for myelodysplastic syndromes and 3% for other leukaemias. Ten per cent are for other cancers including non-Hodgkin's lymphoma (6%), multiple myeloma (3%), and Hodgkin's disease (<1%). The remainder are for aplastic anaemia (7%), immune deficiencies (2%), inherited disorders of metabolism (1%) and other non-malignant disorders (6%). Until recently, autotransplants were used solely to treat cancer. The most common indications for autotransplants in North America in 1995 were breast cancer (42%), non-Hodgkin's lymphoma (23%), Hodgkin's disease (9%), multiple myeloma (8%), AML (6%), ovarian cancer (2%), ALL (1%), CML (1%), with 8% for a variety of other cancers. The most striking recent change in autotransplant use in North America is the dramatic increase in autotransplants for breast cancer. In 1989, about 15% of autotransplants in North America were for breast cancer while in 1995, the figure was over 40%. One hundred-day mortality is often used as a gauge of procedure-related toxicity (Figure 61.5). Allogeneic transplants are associated with high risks of GvHD, infections and liver toxicity, resulting in relatively high early mortality. Among HLA-identical transplants done in 1995 and reported to the IBMTR, 100-day mortality rates range from about 10% for persons with acute leukaemia in first remission to almost 40% for those with advanced leukaemia. Progressive leukaemia contributes to the early mortality rates among patients transplanted with advanced disease. Early mortality is generally lower after auto- than allotransplants (Figure 61.6). Among autotransplants done in 1995 and reported to the ABMTR, 100-day mortality ranges from <5% in women with stage II–III breast cancer to about 15% in persons with advanced lymphoma.

Chronic myelogenous leukaemia is the most frequent indication for allogeneic bone-marrow transplantation. Among 3409 recipients of HLA-identical sibling transplants done between 1989 and 1995, reported to the IBMTR, three-year probabilities of relapse (95% confidence interval) were 16 ± 2% for 2753 transplants done in first chronic phase, 36 ± 6% for 490 in accelerated phase, and 61 ± 11% for 166 in blast phase. Three-year probabilities of leukaemia-free survival (LFS) were 59 ± 2%, 37 ± 5% and 17 ± 7%, respectively (Figure 61.7). Of interest, persons

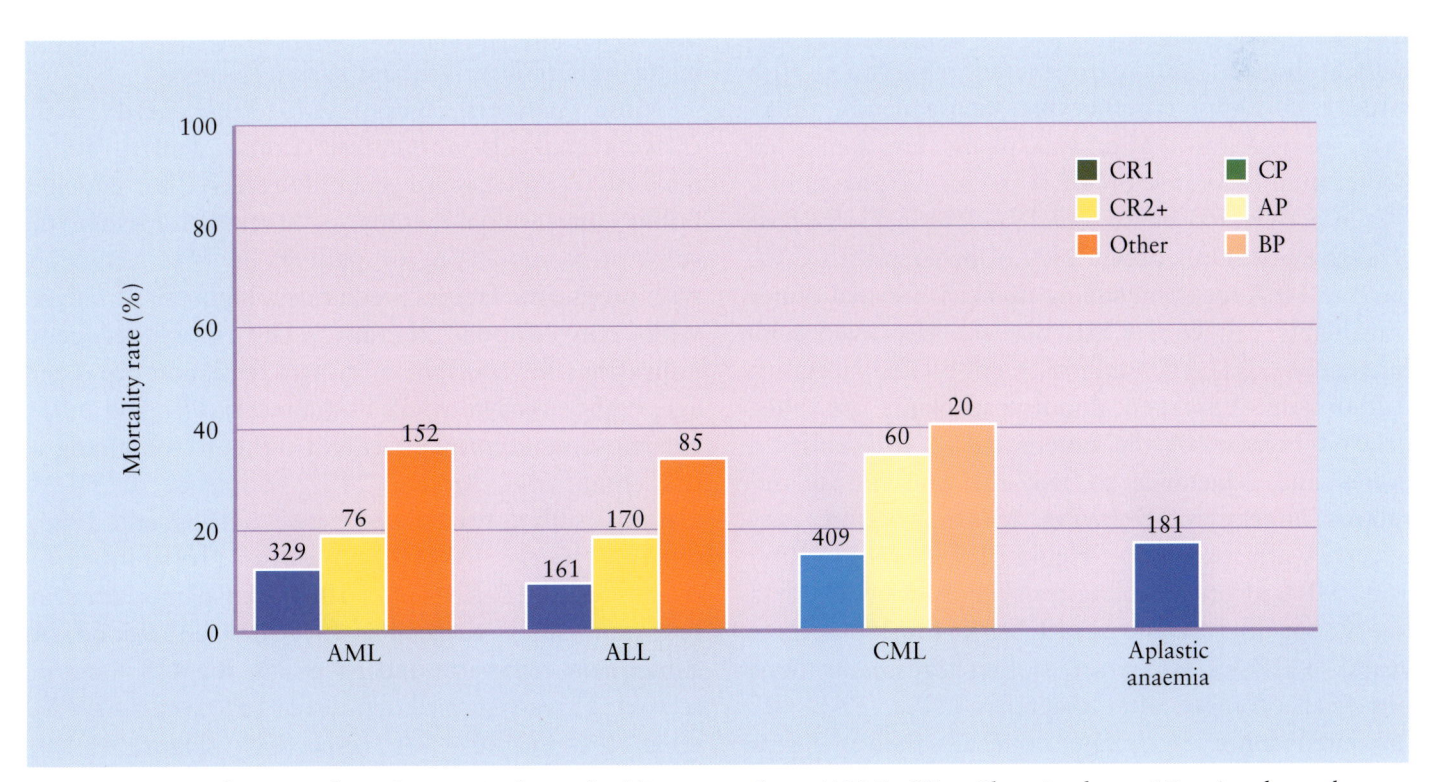

Figure 61.5 100-day mortality after HLA-identical sibling transplants (1995). CP = Chronic phase; AP = Accelerated phase; BP = Blast phase. Numbers on bars = numbers of patients evaluable.

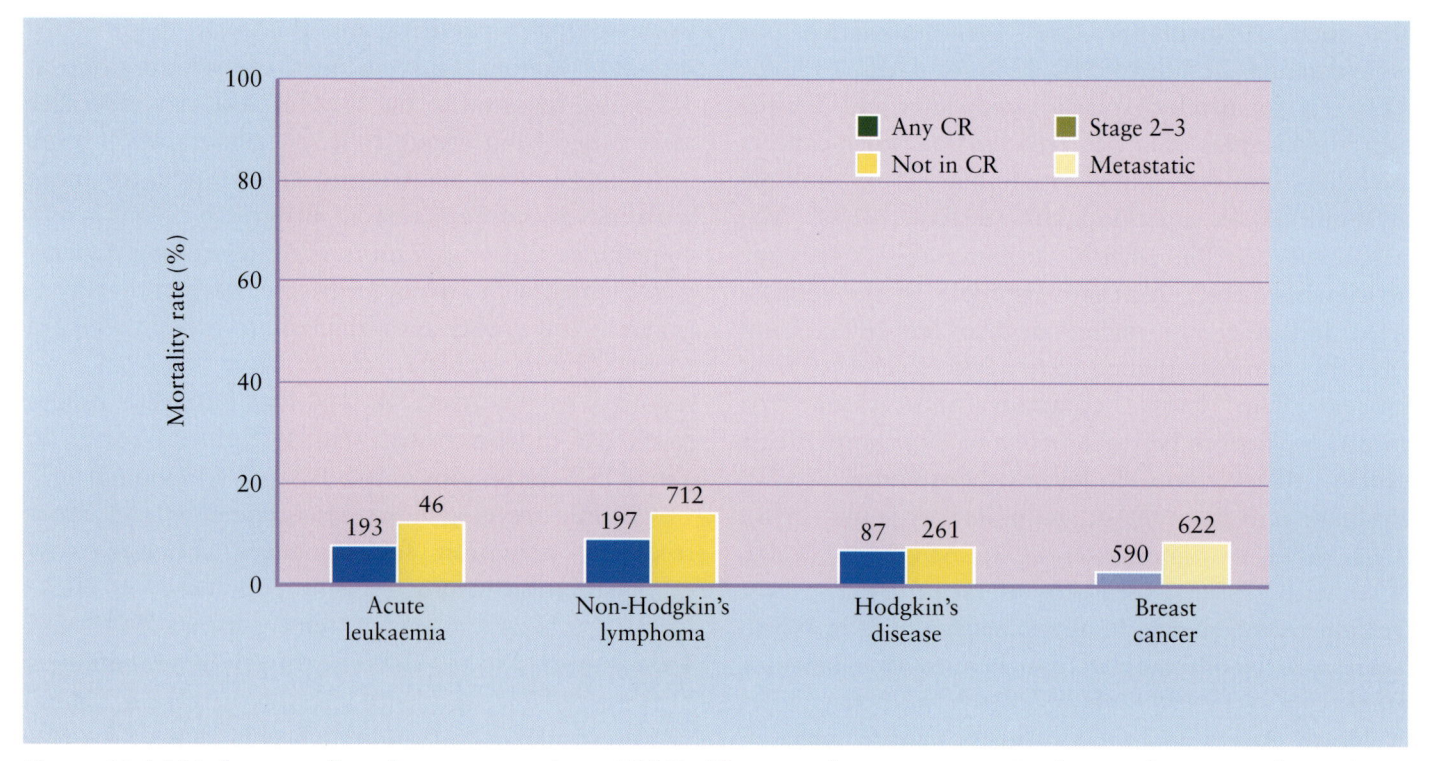

Figure 61.6 100-day mortality after autotransplants (1995). CR = complete remission. Numbers on bars = numbers of patients evaluated.

relapsing after an HLA-identical sibling transplant for CML often survive for long intervals with conventional treatment. Many achieve durable haematological and cytogenetic remissions with infusion of donor lymphocytes. Consequently, three-year survival rates after transplants are somewhat higher than LFS rates: 66 ± 2% in chronic phase, 44 ± 5% in accelerated phase and 19 ± 7% in blast phase (Figure 61.8). Only about 30% of persons with CML have an HLA-identical sibling donor. Unrelated donor transplants can cure CML but are associated with higher risks of GvHD and transplant-related mortality. Additionally, unrelated donor transplants are often delayed because of the time required to identify a donor and reluctance to risk the high transplant-related mortality. Delaying transplantation may adversely affect outcome. Figure 61.9 shows LFS after 1623 HLA-identical sibling transplants done less than one 1 year after diagnosis of CML (64 ± 3% at three years), 1127 HLA-identical sibling transplants done one year or more after diagnosis (51 ± 3%), 122 unrelated donor transplants done less than one year after diagnosis (47 ± 13%), and 497 unrelated donor transplants done one year or more after diagnosis (35 ± 5%). Outcome of unrelated donor transplantation may be affected by factors other than interval between diagnosis and transplant such as donor–recipient histocompatibility, recipient age and others.

Most patients with ALL are cured with conventional chemotherapy. Consequently, bone-marrow transplants are generally reserved for patients failing conventional therapy, i.e. in relapse or second or subsequent remission, or patients in first remission with prognostic factors predicting a high risk of failure with conventional therapy. The most frequent indications for transplants in first remission are older age, high leukocyte count at diagnosis, Ph+ and other chromosome abnormalities and difficulty obtaining a first remission. Among 2497 recipients of HLA-identical sibling transplants between 1989 and 1995, reported to the IBMTR, three-year probabilities of relapse were 25 ± 4% for 1005 transplants done in first remission, 46 ± 4% for 1074 in second or subsequent remission and 68 ± 7% for 418 done in relapse. Three-year probabilities of LFS were 54 ± 4%, 40 ± 13% and 20 ± 5%, respectively (Figure 61.10). Among 357 recipients of autotransplants for ALL done between 1989 and 1995, reported to the ABMTR,

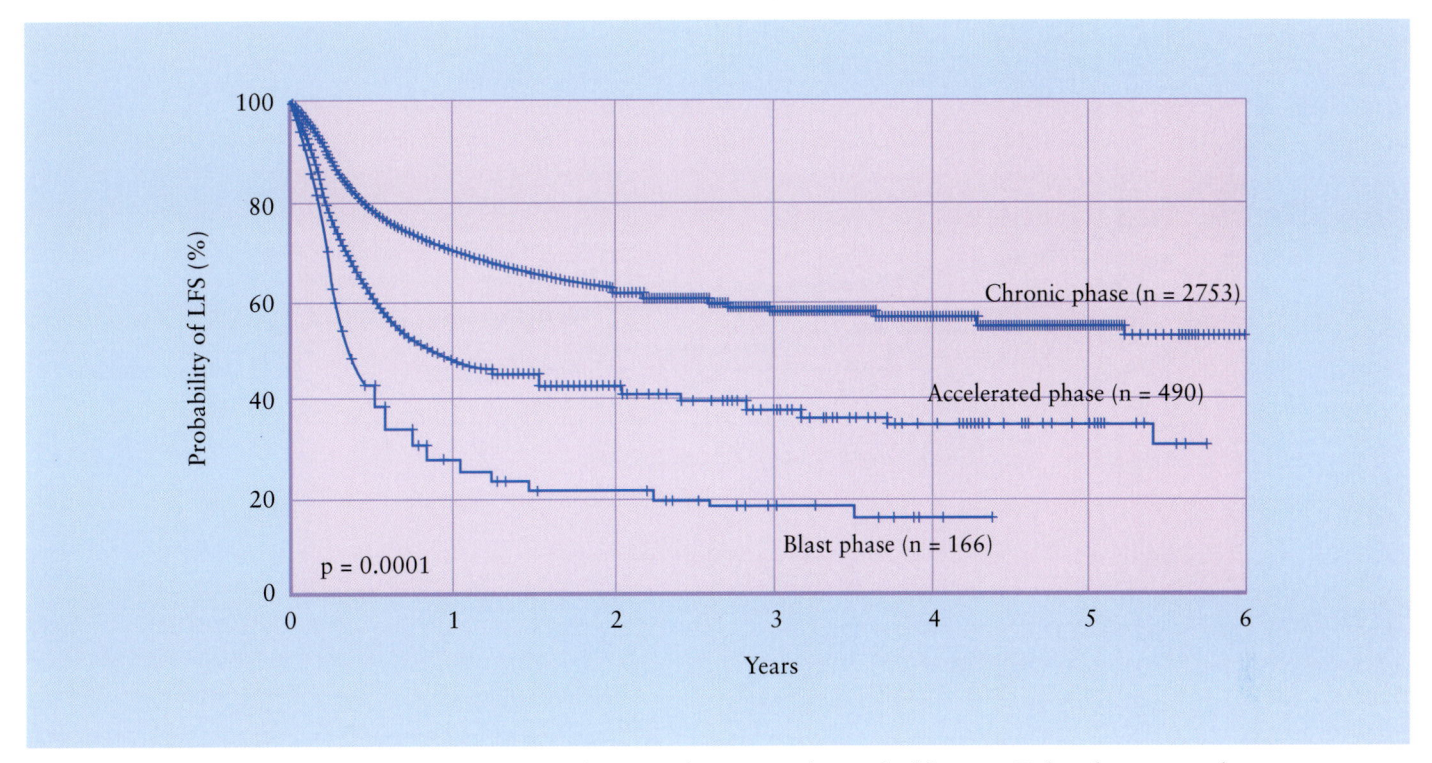

Figure 61.7 Probability of leukaemia-free survival (LFS) after HLA-identical sibling BMT for chronic myelogenous leukaemia (1989–1995).

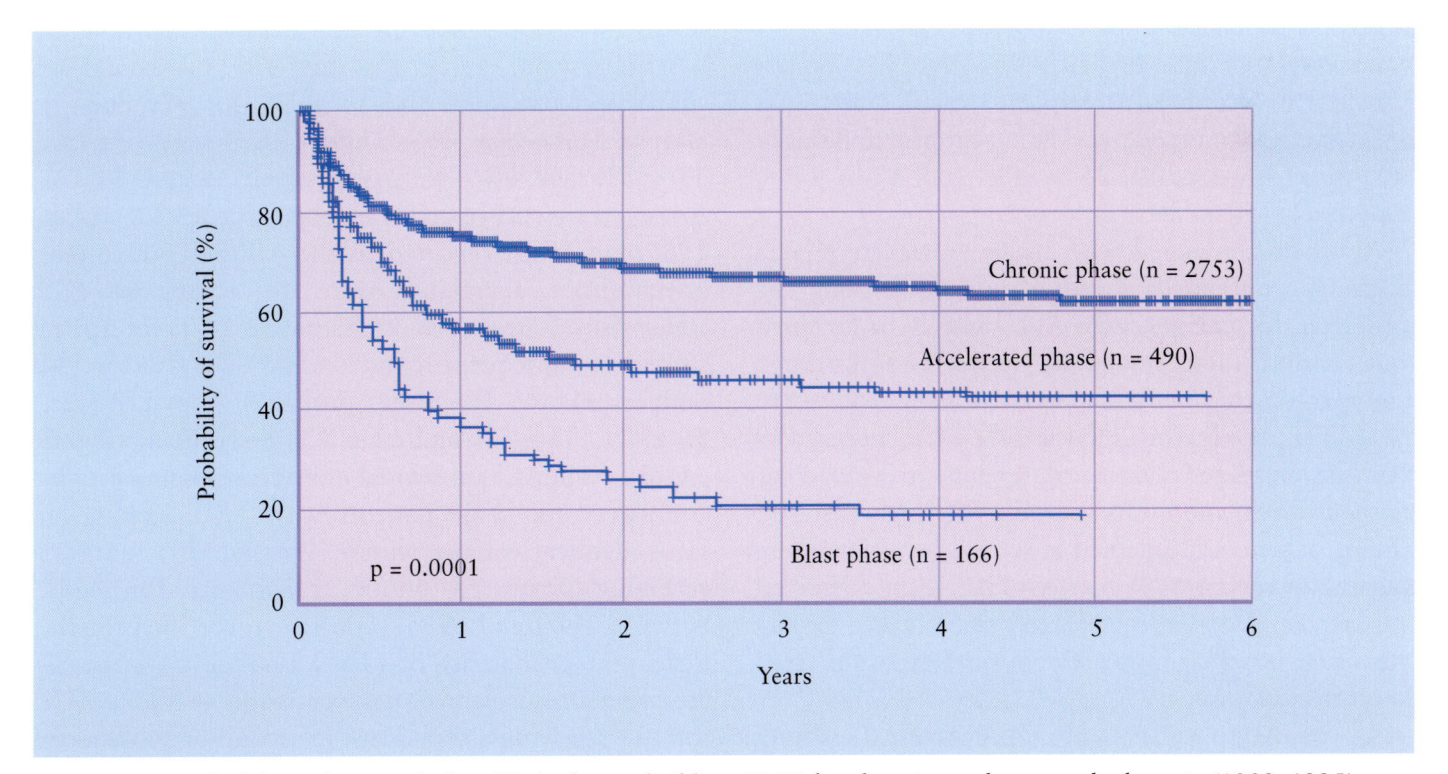

Figure 61.8 Probability of survival after HLA-identical sibling BMT for chronic myelogenous leukaemia (1989–1995).

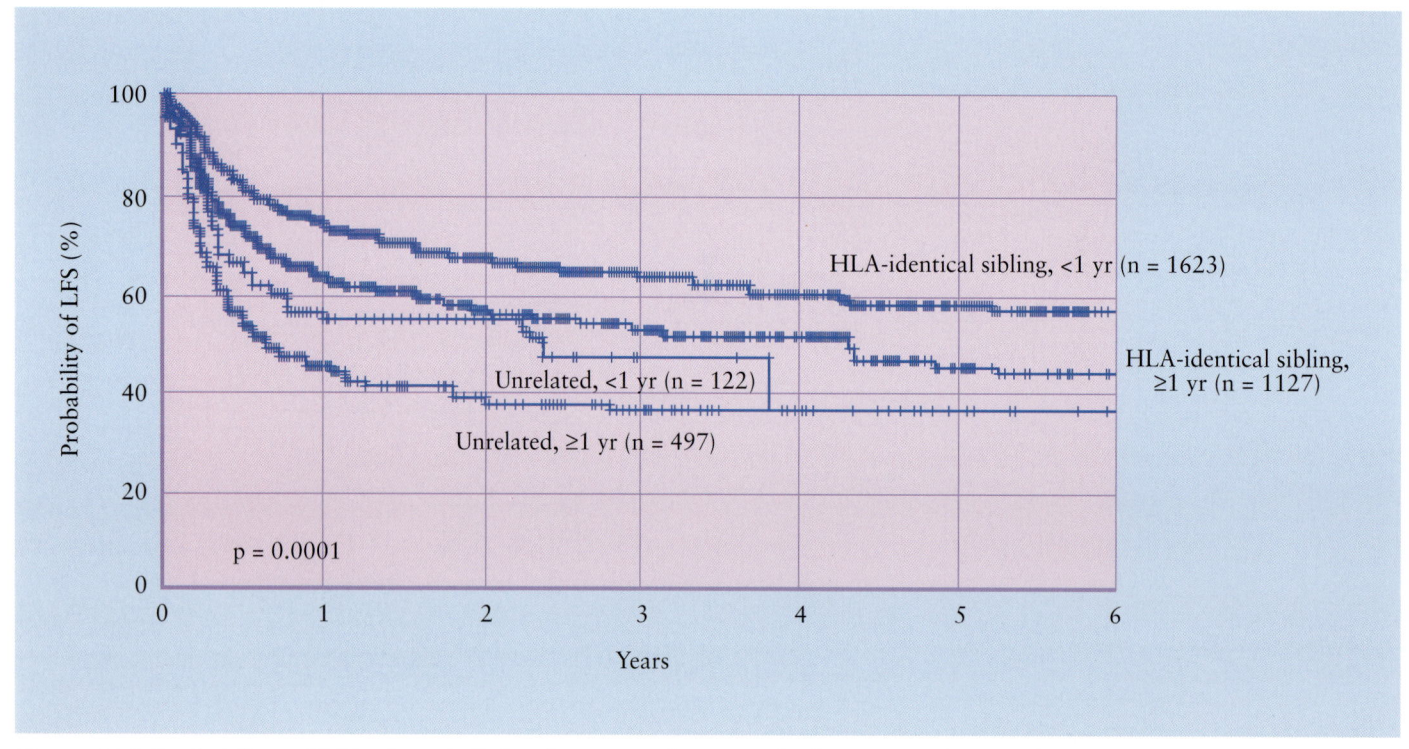

Figure 61.9 Probability of LFS after BMT for chronic myelogenous leukaemia in chronic phase. Interval from diagnosis to transplant.

three-year probabilities of relapse were 49 ± 14% for 102 transplants done in first remission, 70 ± 7% for 228 done in second or subsequent remission and 76 ± 24% for 27 done in relapse. Three-year probabilities of LFS were 43 ± 12%, 25 ± 6% and 17 ± 17%, respectively (Figure 61.11).

Although associated with higher transplant-related mortality, unrelated donor transplants may be considered for patients with ALL unlikely to be cured with chemotherapy. Among 102 recipients of unrelated donor transplants for ALL in first remission reported to the IBMTR, three-year LFS was 37 ± 14%; among 300 receiving unrelated donor transplants in second or subsequent remission, LFS was 36 ± 6% (Figure 61.10). Among patients transplanted in second remission, there was no difference in LFS between HLA-identical sibling and unrelated donor transplants, since higher GvHD rates were offset by lower relapse rates after unrelated donor transplants.

As in ALL, results of HLA-identical sibling transplants for AML correlate with remission state. Among 3503 recipients of HLA-identical sibling transplants done between 1989 and 1995, and reported to the IBMTR, three-year probabilities of relapse were 24 ± 2% for 2247 transplants done in first remission, 45 ± 8% for 459 in second or subsequent remission and 57 ± 5% for 979 done in relapse. Three-year probabilities of LFS were 59 ± 2%, 35 ± 5% and 26 ± 4%, respectively (Figure 61.12). Among recipients of autotransplants for AML between 1989 and 1995, reported to the ABMTR, three-year probabilities of relapse were 44 ± 4% for 858 transplants done in first remission, 56 ± 6% for 401 in second or subsequent remission and 83 ± 8% for 144 done in relapse. Three-year probabilities of LFS were 50 ± 4%, 38 ± 5% and 12 ± 7%, respectively (Figure 61.13). As in ALL, unrelated donor transplants may be considered for some patients with AML lacking an HLA-identical sibling donor. Among 208 patients receiving unrelated donor transplants for AML between 1989 and 1995, reported to the IBMTR, the three-year probability of LFS was 57 ± 13% for 87 receiving a transplant in first remission and 25 ± 12% for 121 receiving a transplant in second or subsequent remission (Figure 61.12).

Allotransplants are the treatment of choice for young patients with aplastic anaemia who have an HLA-identical sibling. Three-year probabilities of

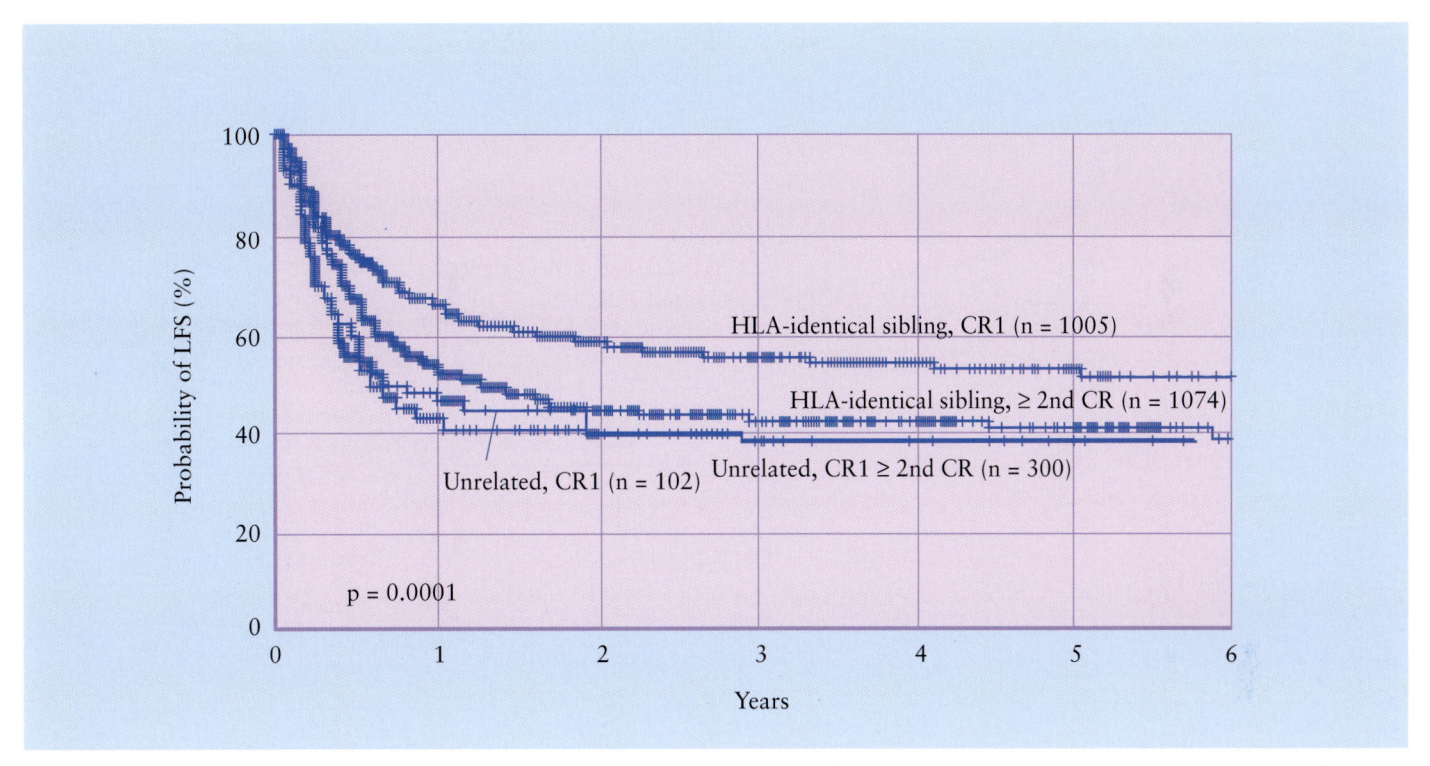

Figure 61.10 Probability of LFS after allogeneic BMT for acute lymphoblastic leukaemia (1989–1995). CR = complete remission.

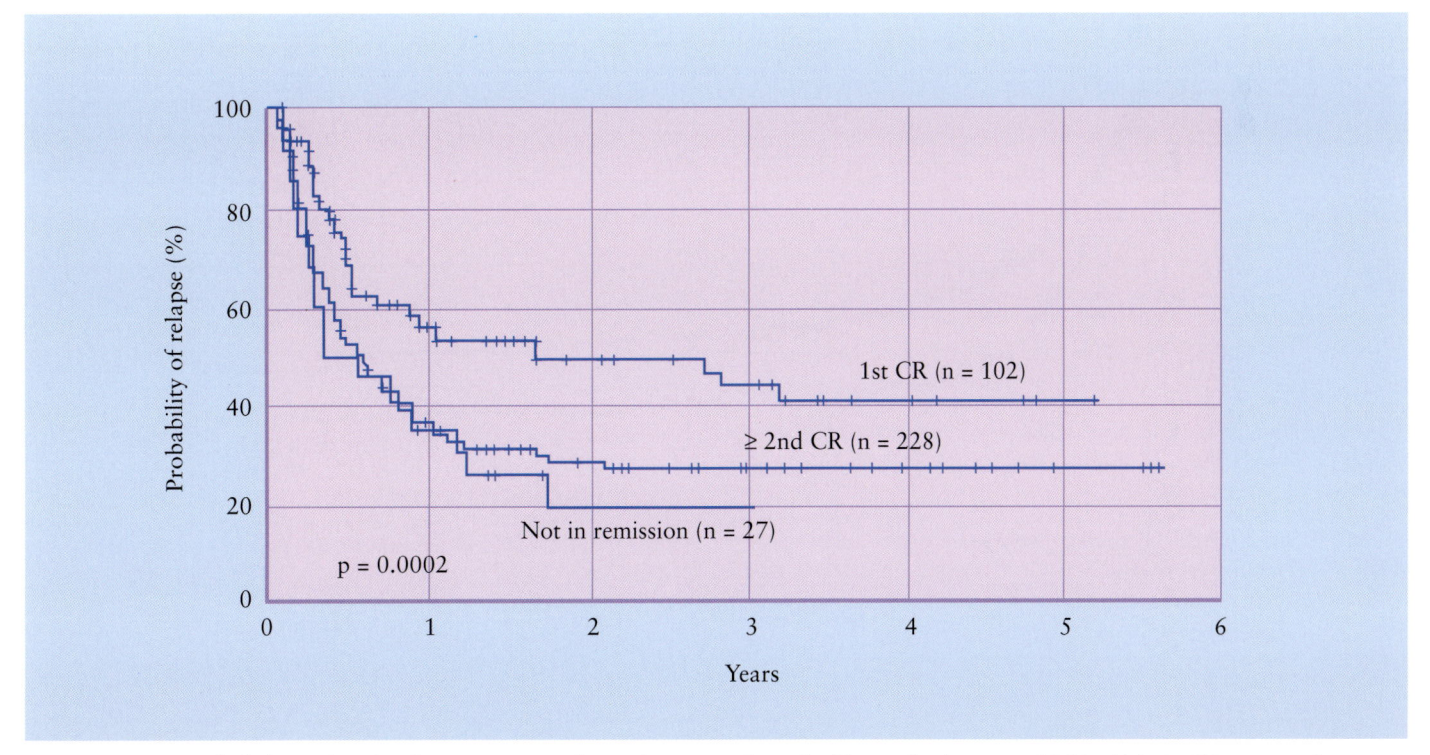

Figure 61.11 Probability of LFS after autotransplants for acute lymphoblastic leukaemia (1989–1995). CR = complete remission.

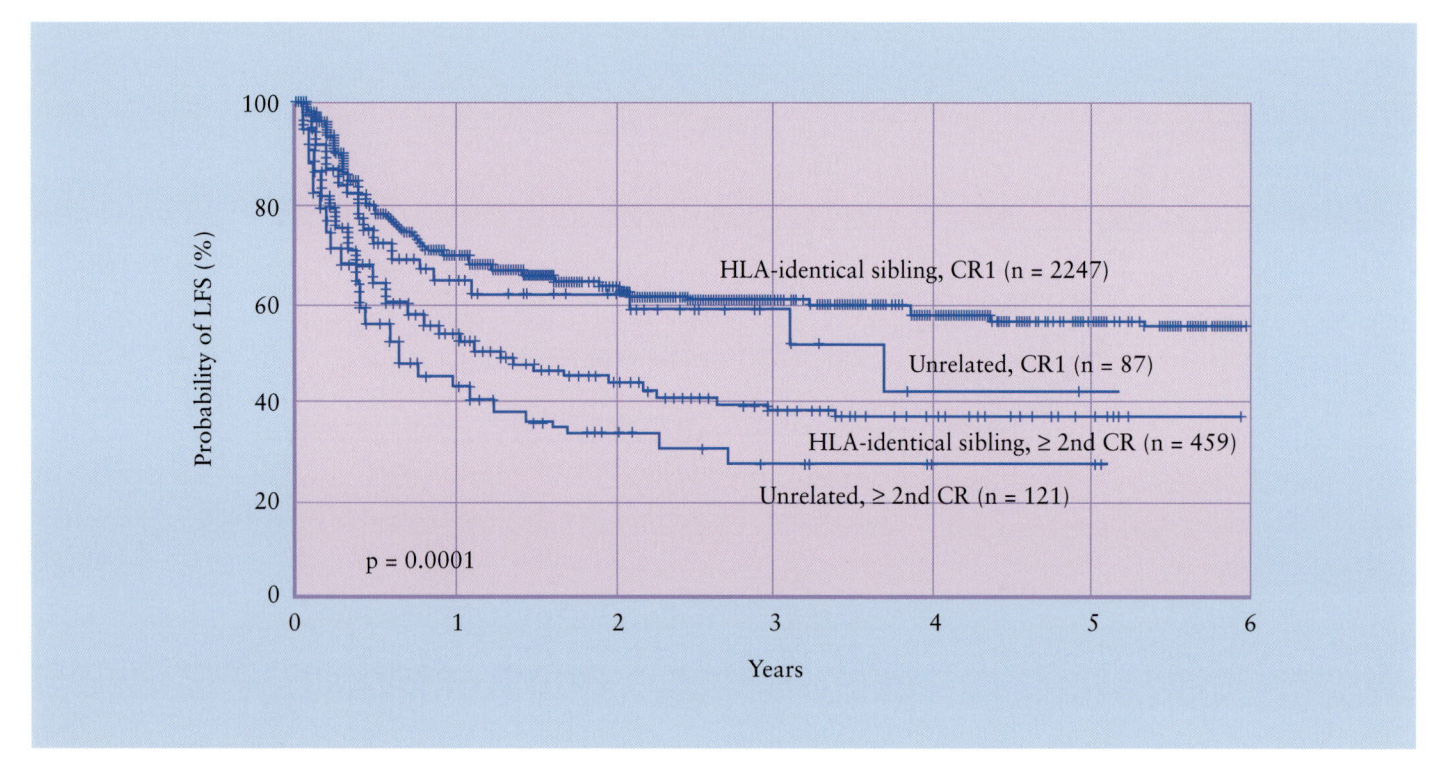

Figure 61.12 Probability of LFS after allogeneic BMT for acute myelogenous leukaemia (1989–1995). CR = complete remission.

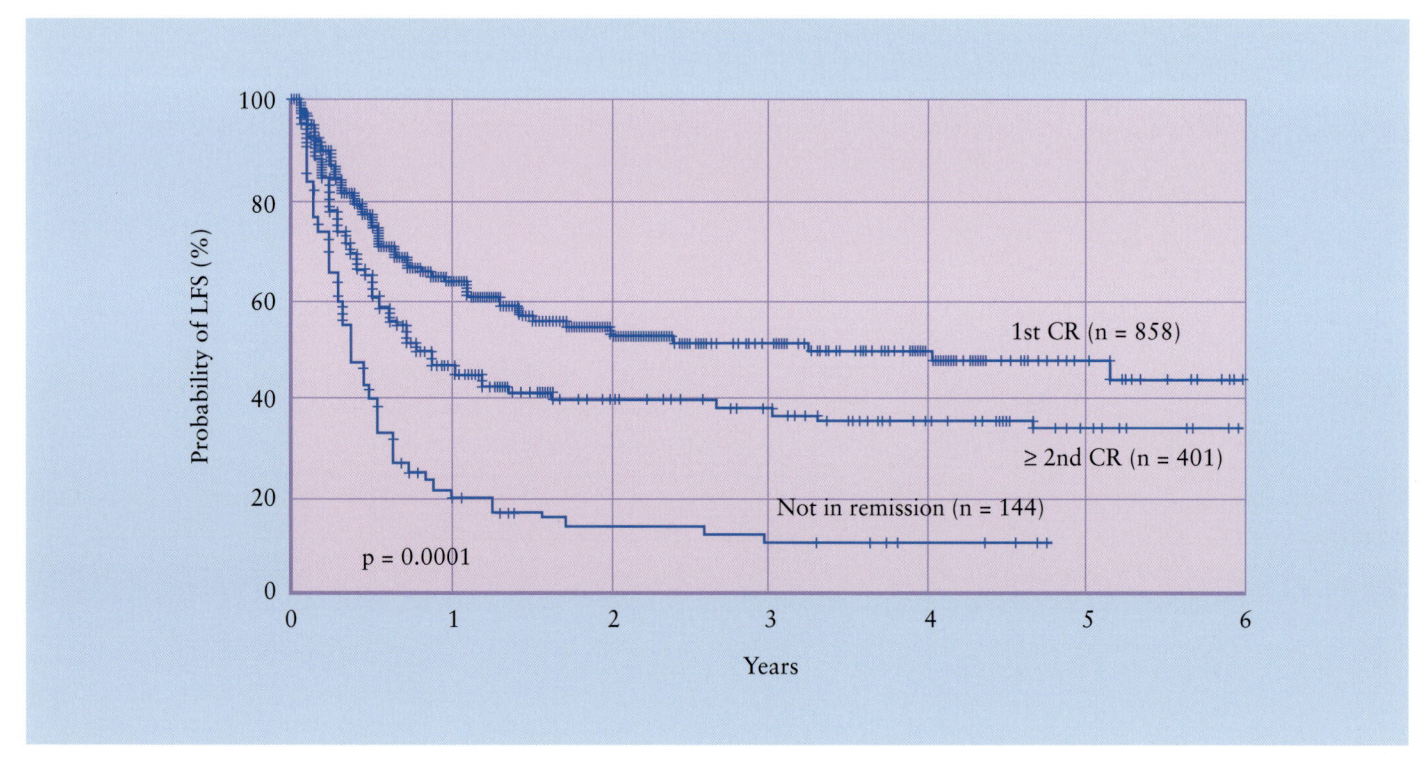

Figure 61.13 Probability of LFS after autotransplants for acute myelogenous leukaemia (1989–1995). CR = complete remission.

survival after 1477 HLA-identical sibling transplants between 1989 and 1995, reported to the IBMTR, were 73 ± 4% for patients <20 years of age and 61 ± 5% for those older (Figure 61.14). Results were not as good in 200 recipients of unrelated donor transplants: 41 ± 10% in 136 patients <20 years and 40 ± 13% in 64 older patients.

Most patients with Hodgkin's disease are cured with conventional chemotherapy. However, for the 20–30% failing conventional therapy, autotransplants are effective salvage therapy. Among 993 autotransplants between 1989 and 1995 reported to the ABMTR, three-year probabilities of survival were 86 ± 12% for 49 patients transplanted in first remission, 60 ± 6% for 463 transplanted in first relapse and 76 ± 8% for 224 transplanted in second or subsequent remission and 49 ± 9% for 257 patients never in remission (Figure 61.15).

Autotransplants are also commonly used for non-Hodgkin's lymphoma. Among 407 patients receiving autotransplants for low-grade lymphoma, three-year probabilities of survival were 83 ± 14% for 64 patients transplanted in first remission, 67 ± 11% for 159 in first relapse, 65 ± 16% for 64 in second remission and 52 ± 16% for 120 never achieving remission with standard chemotherapy (Figure 61.16). Among 1413 patients receiving autotransplants for intermediate grade or immunoblastic lymphoma, three-year probabilities of survival were 68 ± 10% for 143 patients in first remission, 45 ± 5% for 594 in first relapse, 60 ± 8% for 250 in second remission and 40 ± 7% for 426 never achieving remission with conventional chemotherapy (Figure 61.17). Most failures after autotransplants for non-Hodgkin's lymphoma are owing to relapse.

Breast cancer is the most frequent indication for autotransplants in North America. Among 5705 women receiving autotransplants for breast cancer between 1989 and 1995 and reported to the ABMTR, three-year probabilities of survival were 74 ± 6% in 888 women with stage II disease, 70 ± 7% in 749 women with stage III disease, 51 ± 11% in 314 women with inflammatory breast cancer and 31 ± 2% in 3754 women with metastatic breast cancer (Figure 61.18). Outcome in metastatic breast cancer is significantly better for women achieving a complete response with conventional therapy prior to transplant. Among the 3220 women transplanted for metastatic disease in

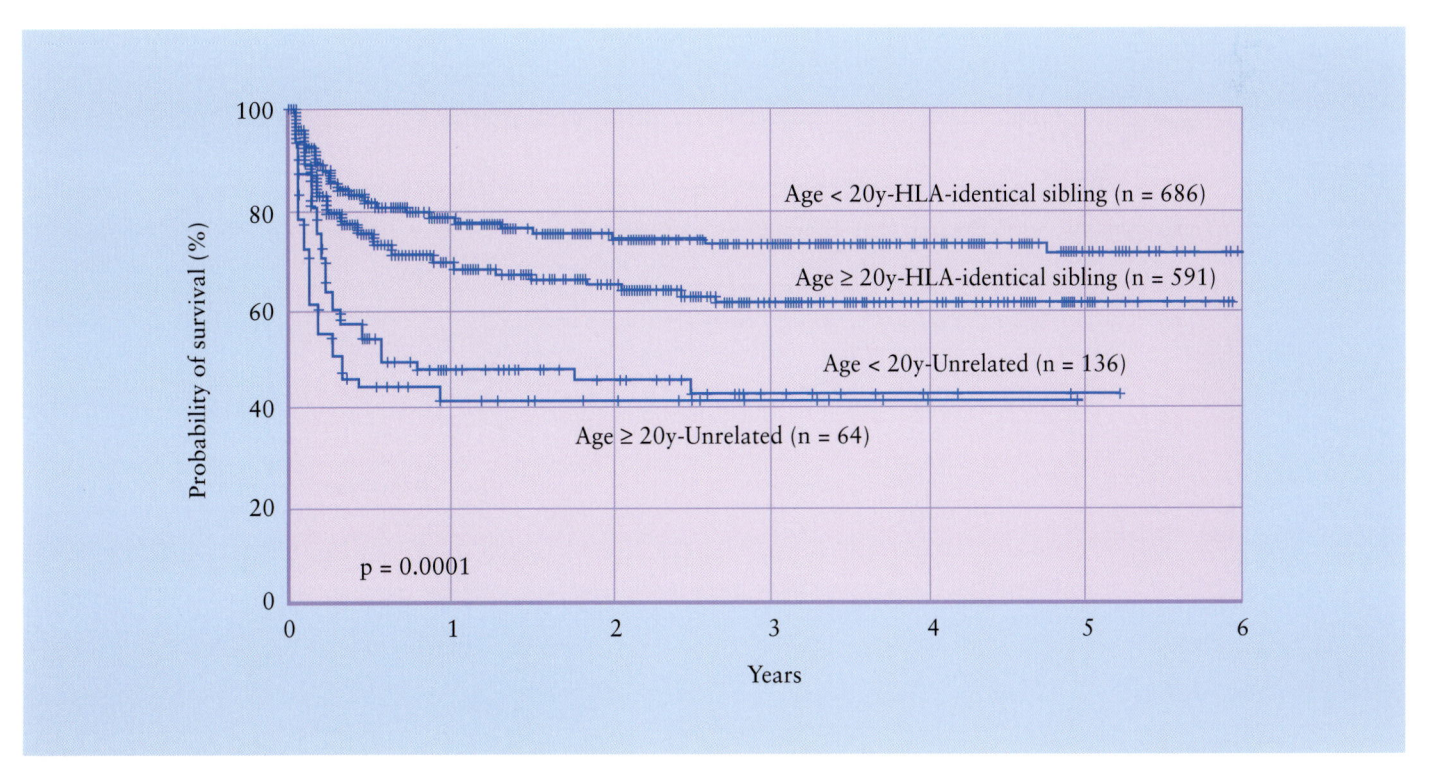

Figure 61.14 Probability of survival after HLA-identical sibling and unrelated BMT for severe aplastic anaemia (1989–1995).

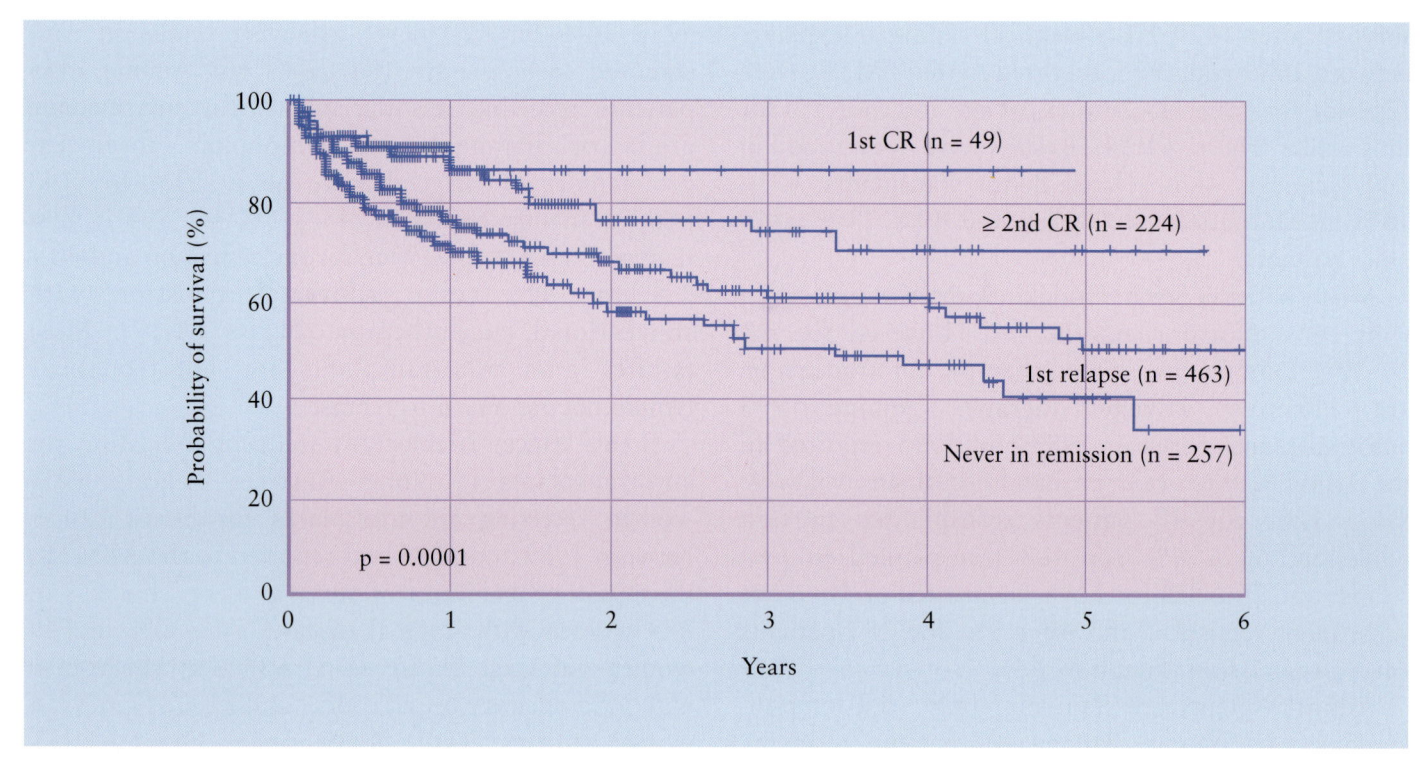

Figure 61.15 Probability of survival after autotransplants for Hodgkin's disease (1989–1995). CR = complete remission.

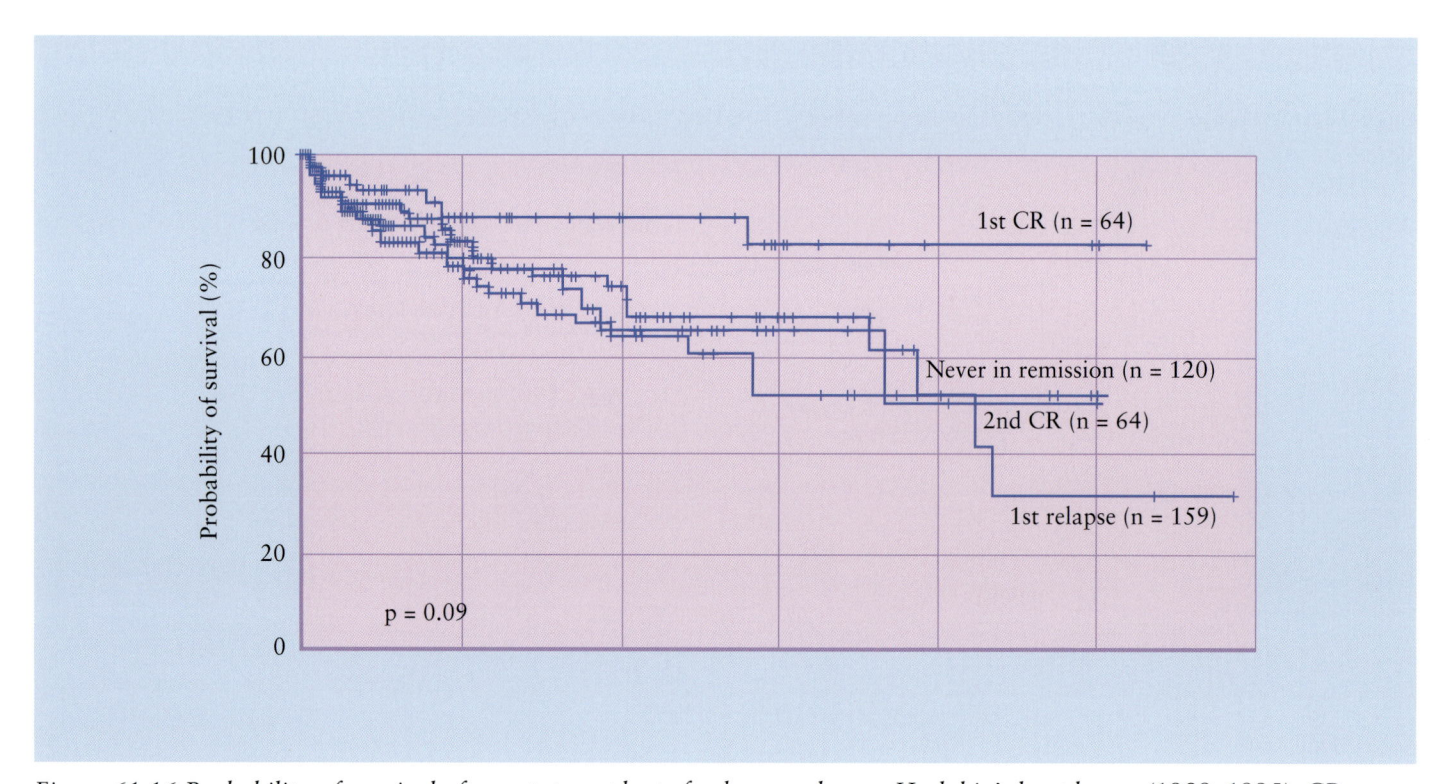

Figure 61.16 Probability of survival after autotransplants for low-grade non-Hodgkin's lymphoma (1989–1995). CR = complete remission.

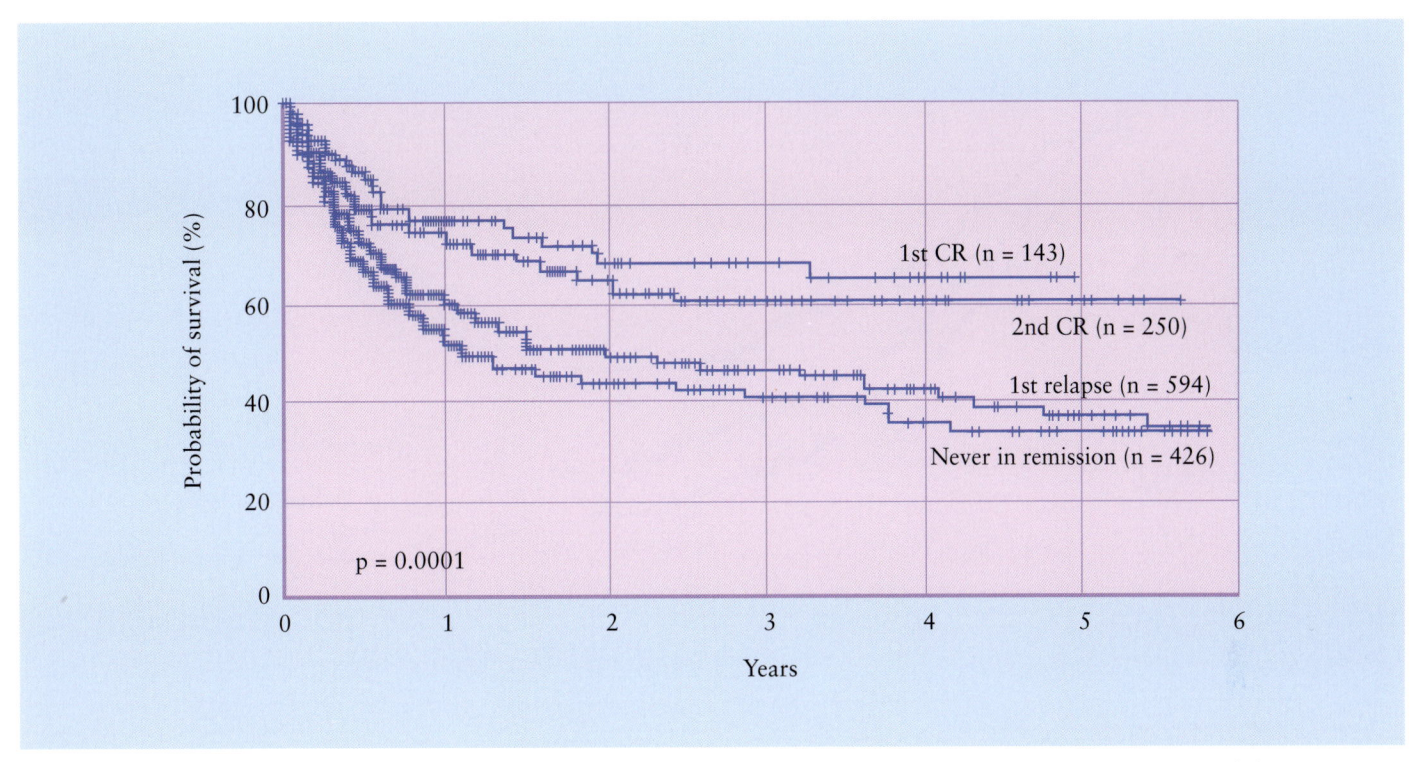

Figure 61.17 Probability of survival after autotransplants for intermediate grade or immunoblastic non-Hodgkin's lymphoma (1989–1995). CR = complete remission.

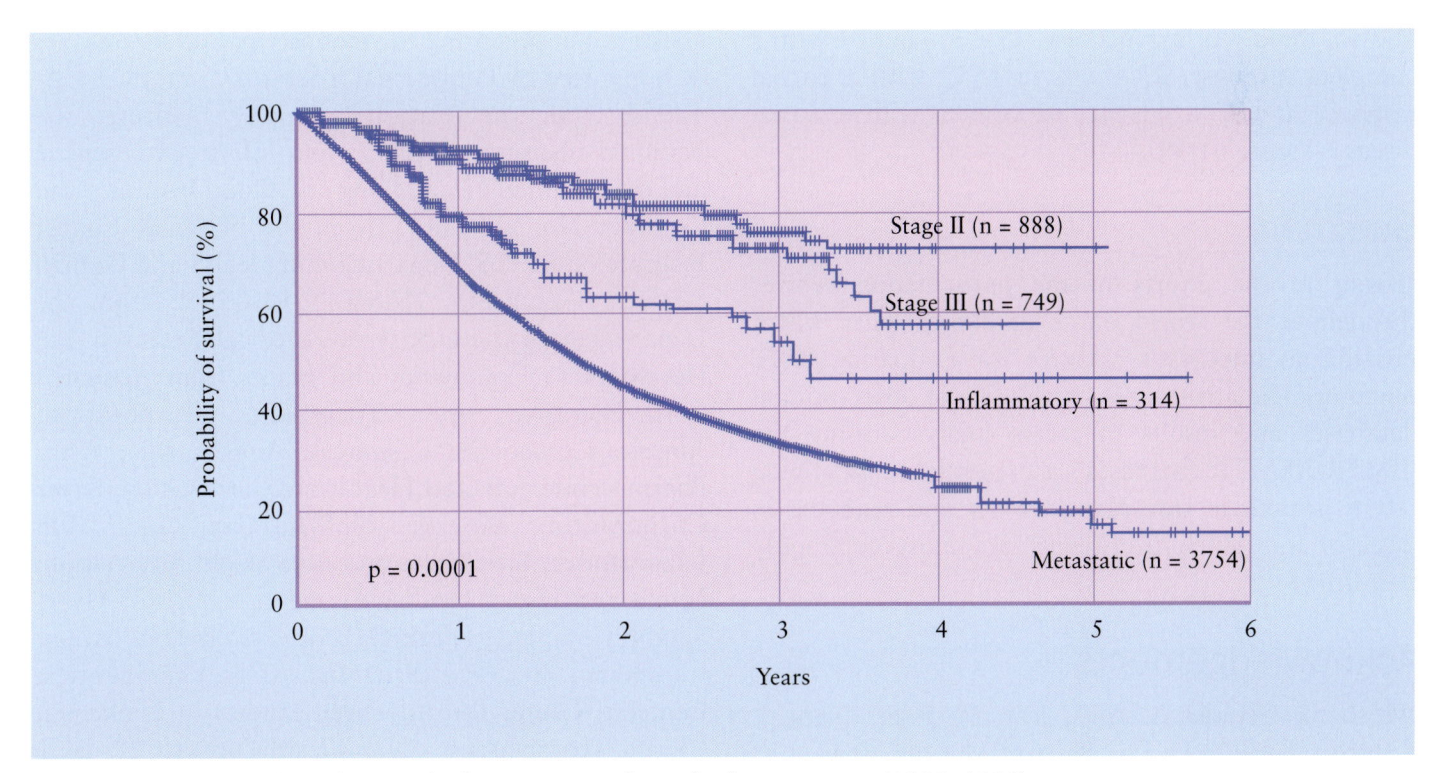

Figure 61.18 Probability of survival after autotransplants for breast cancer (1989–1995).

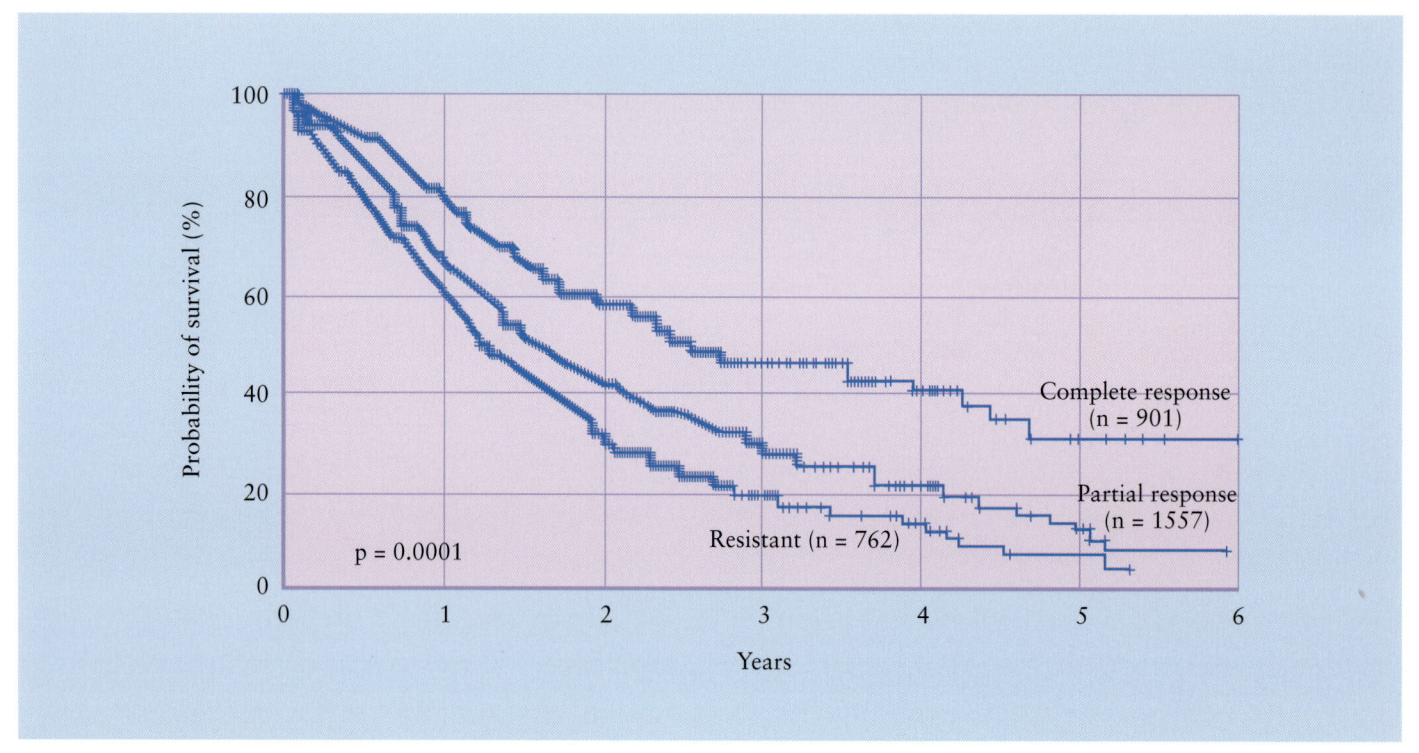

Figure 61.19 Probability of survival after autotransplants for metastatic breast cancer. Pretransplant chemosensitivity (1989–1995).

whom pretransplant response to chemotherapy was known, three-year survival was 45 ± 5% in 901 with a complete response, 27 ± 4% in 1557 with a partial response and 17 ± 4% in 762 women with resistant disease (Figure 61.19).

Summary

Owing to the efforts of the participating centres throughout the world, large databases exist which provide an important resource for evaluating BMT outcome. The advantages of using large observational databases and results of recent analyses using the IBMTR/ABMTR databases are presented summarizing recent growth in transplant activity and outcome in diseases for which transplants are most commonly performed.

Acknowledgements

We thank Claudia A. Abel, Jean M. Eder, Diane J. Knutson, Barbara H. Liu, Barbara McGary, Sharon K. Nell, Melodee L. Nugent, Jane E. Rebro, Janelle M. Stano, Hongyu Tian and Patty A. Vespalac for help with data management and analysis. We thank Kim R. Hyler, Lisa J. Lehrmann and Linda Schneider for assistance in preparing the manuscript and figures.

Supported by Public Health Service Grant PO1-CA-40053 from the National Cancer Institute, the National Institute of Allergy and Infectious Diseases, and the National Heart, Lung and Blood Institute, and Contract No. CP-21161 from the National Cancer Institute of the U.S. Department of Health and Human Services; Grant No. DAMD17-95-I-5002 from the Department of the U.S. Army Medical Research and Development Command; and grants from Activated Cell Therapy; Alpha Therapeutic Corporation; American Oncology Resources; Amgen, Inc.; Astra Pharmaceutical; Baxter Healthcare Corporation; Bayer Corporation; Biogen; BioWhittaker, Inc.; BIS Laboratories; Blue Cross and Blue Shield Association; Lynde and Harry Bradley Foundation; Bristol-Myers Squibb Company; Frank G. Brotz Family Foundation; Caremark, Inc.; CellPro, Inc; Cell Therapeutics; Centeon; Center for Advanced Studies in Leukemia; Chiron Therapeutics; Cigna HealthCare; COBE BCT Inc.; Coulter Corporation; Coram Healthcare; Charles E. Culpeper Foundation; Eleanor Naylor Dana Charitable Trust; Deborah J. Dearholt Memorial Fund;

Eppley Foundation for Research; Fujisawa USA, Inc.; Genentech, Inc.; Glaxo Wellcome Company; Hewlett-Packard Company; Hoechst Marion Roussel, Inc.; Immunex Corporation; Janssen Pharmaceutica; Kettering Family Foundation; Kirin Brewery Company; Robert J. Kleberg, Jr. and Helen C. Kleberg Foundation; Herbert H. Kohl Charities; Lederle Laboratories; Life Technologies, Inc.; Eli Lilly Company Foundation; The Liposome Company; Nada and Herbert P. Mahler Charities; Medical SafeTEC; MGI Pharma, Inc.; Milstein Family Foundation; Milwaukee Foundation/Elsa Schoeneich Research Fund; NCSG and Associates, Inc.; NeXstar Pharmaceuticals, Inc; Samuel Roberts Noble Foundation; Ortho Biotech Corporation; John Oster Family Foundation; Elsa U. Pardee Foundation; Jane and Lloyd Pettit Foundation; Alirio Pfiffer Bone Marrow Transplant Support Association; Pfizer, Inc.; Pharmacia and Upjohn; QLT PhotoTherapeutics; Quantum Health Resources; RGK Foundation; Roche Laboratories; RPR GenCell; Sandoz Oncology; SangStat Medical Corporation; Schering-Plough International; Walter Schroeder Foundation; Searle; SEQUUS Pharmaceuticals Inc.; Stackner Family Foundation; Starr Foundation; StemCell Technologies; Joan and Jack Stein Charities; SyStemix; Therakos; TS Scientific and Planer Products; Wyeth-Ayerst Laboratories; and Xoma Corporation.

Appendix 1 Institutions participating in the International Bone Marrow Transplant Registry (in alphabetical order according to country)

British Hospital of Buenos Aires	Buenos Aires	Argentina
Hospital de Pediatria, S.A.M.I.C.	Buenos Aires	Argentina
Institutos Médicos Antartida	Buenos Aires	Argentina
Navy Hospital Pedro Mallo	Buenos Aires	Argentina
Alexander Fleming Institute	Buenos Aires	Argentina
Hospital Privado de Cordoba	Cordoba	Argentina
Fundacion Dr. Jose Maria Mainetti	Gonnet	Argentina
Hanson Center for Cancer Research	Adelaide	Australia
Royal Brisbane Hospital	Brisbane	Australia
Royal Children's Hospital Brisbane	Brisbane	Australia
Royal Prince Alfred Hospital	Camperdown	Australia
Royal Children's Hospital	Parkville	Australia
Royal Melbourne Hospital	Parkville	Australia
Princess Margaret Hospital for Children	Perth	Australia
Royal Perth Hospital	Perth	Australia
Alfred Hospital	Prahran	Australia
Sydney Children's Hospital	Randwick	Australia
Royal North Shore Hospital	St. Leonards	Australia
St. Vincent's Hospital	Sydney	Australia
The New Children's Hospital	Westmead	Australia
Westmead Hospital	Westmead	Australia
Queen Elizabeth Hospital	Woodville	Australia
St. Anna Children's Hospital	Vienna	Austria
Universität Klinik für Innere Medizin I	Vienna	Austria
AZ Sint-Jan	Brugge	Belgium
Children's University Hospital	Bruxelles	Belgium
Cliniques Universitaires Saint-Luc	Bruxelles	Belgium
University Hospital Antwerp	Edegem	Belgium
University Ziekenhuis Gasthuisberg	Leuven	Belgium
Universitaire De Liege/Centre Hospitalier	Liege	Belgium
Hospital de Clinicas	Curitiba	Brazil
Universidade de São Paulo	Ribeirao Preto	Brazil
Instituto Nacional de Cancer	Rio de Janeiro	Brazil
Instituto do Coracao – INCOR	São Paulo	Brazil
Santa Casa Medical School	São Paulo	Brazil
Alberta Children's Hospital	Calgary	Canada
Tom Baker Cancer Centre	Calgary	Canada
Victoria General Hospital/Dalhousie University	Halifax	Canada
Chedoke-McMaster Hospitals	Hamilton	Canada
University Hospital	London	Canada
Hôpital Sainte-Justine	Montreal	Canada
Montreal Children's Hospital	Montreal	Canada
Royal Victoria Hospital	Montreal	Canada
Hôpital du Saint-Sacrement	Quebec City	Canada
Hospital for Sick Children	Toronto	Canada
Princess Margaret Hospital	Toronto	Canada
British Columbia's Children's Hospital	Vancouver	Canada
Vancouver Hospital & Health Science Centre	Vancouver	Canada
Health Science Centre	Winnipeg	Canada
Hospital Militar	Santiago	Chile
Universidad Católica de Chile	Santiago	Chile
Beijing Medical University	Beijing	China
Bei Tai Ping Lu Hospital	Beijing	China
Lanzhou General Hospital	Lanzhou	China
Institute of Hematology, CAMS	Tianjin	China
Hospital Mexico	San Jose	Costa Rica
Klinika za Unutrasnje bolesti KBC-Rebro	Zagreb	Croatia
Hermanos Arneijeiras Hospital	Havana	Cuba
Instituto de Hematologia e Immunologia	Havana	Cuba
Charles University Hospital	Pilsen	Czech Republic
Institute of Hematology & Blood Transfusion	Prague	Czech Republic
University Hospital Motol	Prague	Czech Republic
Rigshospitalet	Copenhagen	Denmark
NCI Cairo University	Cairo	Egypt
Helsinki University Central Hospital	Helsinki	Finland
Türkü University	Türkü	Finland
Universitaire d'Angers	Angers	France
Centre Hospitalier Universitaire Besançon	Besançon	France
Universitaire de Caen	Caen	France
Hospital A. Michallon	Grenoble	France
Centre Hospitalier Regional de Lille	Lille	France
Hôpital Debrousse	Lyon	France
Hôpital Edouard Herriot	Lyon	France
Institut J. Paoli I. Calmettes	Marseille	France
De l'Hôpital Cochin	Paris	France
Hôpital des Enfants Malades	Paris	France
Hôpital Robert Debre	Paris	France
Hôpital Saint-Antoine	Paris	France
Hôpital Saint-Louis	Paris	France
Hôtel Dieu de Paris	Paris	France
Groupe Hospitalier du Hau Leveque	Pessac	France
Hôpital Jean Bernard	Poitiers	France
Centre Henri Becquerel	Rouen	France
Hôpital Nord	St. Etienne	France
Hôpital de Purpan	Toulouse	France
Hospital Regional de Toulouse	Toulouse	France
Universitatsklinikum Rudolf Virchow	Berlin	Germany
Universität Hospital Charite	Berlin	Germany
Heinrich-Heine Universität/Children's Hop Med Ctr	Düsseldorf	Germany
University of Hamburg	Hamburg	Germany
Medizinische Hochschule Hannover (Adults)	Hannover	Germany
Medizinische Hochschule Hannover (Paediatrics)	Hannover	Germany
Christian-Albrechts-Universität	Kiel	Germany
University of Leipzig	Leipzig	Germany
Universitäts Kinderklinik	München	Germany
Universität München/Klinikum Grosshadern	München	Germany

Medizinische Universitätsklinik	Tübingen	Germany	Dr. Daniel Den Hoed Cancer Center	Rotterdam	Netherlands
Children's Hospital	Tübingen	Germany	University Hospital Utrecht	Utrecht	Netherlands
Universität Ulm	Ulm/Donau	Germany	Auckland Hospital	Auckland	New Zealand
Deutsche Klinik für Diagnostik	Wiesboden	Germany			
Evangelismos Hospital	Athens	Greece	Auckland Medical School	Auckland	New Zealand
Prince of Wales Hospital/Chinese University-HK	Hong Kong	Hong Kong	Starship Children's Health Center	Auckland	New Zealand
Queen Mary Hospital	Hong Kong	Hong Kong	Christchurch Hospital	Christchurch	New Zealand
National Institute of Haematology	Budapest	Hungary			
Tata Memorial Hospital	Bombay	India	Wellington School of Medicine	Wellington	New Zealand
All India Institute of Medical Science/Institute Rotary Ca Hosp	New Delhi	India	Silesian Medical Academy	Katowice	Poland
Med Science Univ of Tehran/ Dr. Shariati Hospital	Tehran	Iran	Academy of Medicine	Poznan	Poland
			I Klinika Chorob Dzieci	Poznan	Poland
St. James's Hospital	Dublin	Ireland	Postgraduate Medical Center	Warsaw	Poland
Hadassah University Hospital	Jerusalem	Israel	Instituto Portugues de Oncologia	Lisbon	Portugal
S. Orsola University Hospital	Bologna	Italy	Instituto Portugues de Oncologia-Centro de Porto	Porto	Portugal
Universita di Bologna	Bologna	Italy			
Spedali Civili – Brescia	Brescia	Italy	Clinical Hospital Number 6	Moscow	Russia
Ospedale San Martino	Genoa	Italy	National Research Center for Hematology	Moscow	Russia
Ospedale Cervello	Palermo	Italy			
Ospedale di Pesaro	Pesaro	Italy	Petrov Research Institute of Oncology	St. Petersburg	Russia
Ospedale Civile	Pesaro	Italy	Russian Institute of Hematology & Blood Transfusion	St. Petersburg	Russia
Ospedale S. Camillo	Rome	Italy			
Università degli Studi, La Sapienza	Rome	Italy	King Faisal Specialist Hospital & Research Centre	Riyadh	Saudi Arabia
Università Delgi Studi Di Roma	Rome	Italy			
Di Midollo Osseo Ospedale Molinette	Torino	Italy	Riyadh Armed Forces Hospital	Riyadh	Saudi Arabia
University of Torino	Torino	Italy			
Udine University Hospital	Udine	Italy	University Hospital	Bratislava	Slovak Republic
Chiba University School of Medicine	Chiba	Japan			
Hyogo College of Medicine – Blood Transfusion	Hyogo	Japan	University of Cape Town Medical School	Cape Town	South Africa
Hyogo College of Medicine – Internal Medicine	Hyogo	Japan	Wynberg Hosp/Capetown Haematology Clinic & BMT	Cape Town	South Africa
Tokai University School of Medicine	Kanagawa	Japan	University of Witwatersrand Medical School	Johannesburg	South Africa
Kanazawa University School of Medicine	Kanazawa-shi	Japan			
Nagoya Daini Red Cross Hospital	Nagoya	Japan	Hospital General Vall d'Hebron	Barcelona	Spain
Niigata University Medical Hospital	Niigata	Japan	Hospital Infantil Vall d'Hebron	Barcelona	Spain
Center For Adult Diseases	Osaka	Japan	Hospital de la Santa Creui Sant Pau	Barcelona	Spain
Jichi Medical School	Tochigi-ken	Japan	University of Barcelona	Barcelona	Spain
National Cancer Center Hospital	Tokyo	Japan	Hospital Reina Sofia	Cordoba	Spain
Keio University	Tokyo	Japan	Hospital Ntra Sra Del Pino	Islas Canarias	Spain
Nihon University	Tokyo	Japan	Hospital Puerta de Hierro	Madrid	Spain
University of Tokyo/Institute of Medical Science	Tokyo	Japan	Hospital de la Princesa	Madrid	Spain
			Hospital Ramon y Cajal	Madrid	Spain
Kanagawa Cancer Center	Yokohama	Japan	Hospital Regional 'Carlos Haya'	Malaga	Spain
Jordan University Hospital	Amman	Jordan	Son Dureta Hospital	Palma de Mallorca	Spain
Asan Medical Center	Seoul	Korea			
Samsung Medical Center	Seoul	Korea	Hospital Marques De Valdecilla	Santander	Spain
The Catholic University of Korea	Seoul	Korea	Hospital La Fe	Valencia	Spain
Hospital Kuala Lumpur Institute of Paediatrics	Kuala Lumpur	Malaysia	University of Göteborg	Goteborg	Sweden
			Huddinge Hospital	Huddinge	Sweden
University of Malaya	Kuala Lumpur	Malaysia	University of Lund	Lund	Sweden
Hospital Especialidades Centro Medico	Mexico D.F.	Mexico	University Hospital Uppsala	Uppsala	Sweden
Centro de Hematologia y Medicina Interna	Puebla	Mexico	Kantonsspital	Basel	Switzerland
			Kantonsspital Zurich	Zurich	Switzerland
Leiden University Hospital (Paediatrics)	Leiden	Netherlands	Kinderspital Zurich	Zurich	Switzerland
Academic Hospital Maastricht	Maastricht	Netherlands	National Taiwan University Hospital	Taipei	Taiwan
University of Nijmegen	Nijmegen	Netherlands	National Yang-Ming Medical College	Taipei	Taiwan

Tri-Service General Hospital NDMC	Taipei	Taiwan	Richland Memorial Hospital	Columbus	USA
Ankara University Medical School	Ankara	Turkey	Children's Hospital	Columbus	USA
Gulhane Military Medical Academy	Ankara	Turkey	The Ohio State University Medical Center	Columbus	USA
SSK Tepecik Teaching Hospital	Izmir	Turkey			
Birmingham Heartlands Hospital	Birmingham	UK	Baylor University Medical Center	Dallas	USA
Queen Elizabeth Medical Centre	Birmingham	UK	Children's Medical Center of Dallas	Dallas	USA
University Hospital of Wales	Cardiff	UK	Medical City Dallas Hospital	Dallas	USA
Royal Infirmary of Edinburgh	Edinburgh	UK	Presbyterian/St. Luke's Medical Center	Denver	USA
Glasgow Royal Infirmary	Glasgow	UK	University of Colorado Health Sciences Center	Denver	USA
HCI International Medical Centre	Glasgow	UK			
Royal Hospital for Sick Children	Glasgow	UK	Wayne State University	Detroit	USA
St. James's University Hospital	Leeds	UK	City of Hope National Medical Center	Duarte	USA
Charing Cross Hospital/Westminster Medical School	London	UK	Duke University Medical Center	Durham	USA
			Cook-Fort Worth Children's Medical Center (Pediatrics)	Fort Worth	USA
Great Ormond Street Hospital for Children	London	UK	Harris Methodist Fort Worth (Adults)	Fort Worth	USA
London Clinic	London	UK	Harris Methodist Fort Worth	Fort Worth	USA
Royal Free Hospital	London	UK	University of Florida (Adult) – JHMHC	Gainesville	USA
Royal London Hospital Whitechapel	London	UK	University of Florida (Paediatrics) – JHMHC	Gainesville	USA
Royal Postgraduate Medical School	London	UK			
St. George's Hospital Medical School	London	UK	St. Francis Medical Center	Honolulu	USA
Royal Victoria Infirmary	Newcastle	UK	Baylor College of Medicine	Houston	USA
City Hospital	Nottingham	UK	M.D. Anderson Cancer Center	Houston	USA
John Radcliffe Hospital – University of Oxford	Oxford	UK	St. Joseph's Hospital Medical Center	Houston	USA
			Texas Children's Hospital	Houston	USA
Royal Marsden Hospital	Sutton	UK	Indiana University Hospitals	Indianapolis	USA
British Hospital & Faculty of Medicine	Montevideo	Uruguay	Methodist Hospital of Indiana Cancer Center	Indianapolis	USA
IMPASA, Centro de Trans. de Medula Osea	Montevideo	Uruguay	Mayo Clinic Jacksonville	Jacksonville	USA
			University of Kansas	Kansas City	USA
Albany Medical Center	Albany	USA	Children's Mercy Hospital #128	Kansas City	USA
Don & Sybil Harrington Cancer Center	Amarillo	USA	University of Tennessee Medical Center	Knoxville	USA
University of Michigan Women's Hospital	Ann Arbor	USA	Wilford Hall USAF Medical Center	Lackland AFB	USA
Emory University	Atlanta	USA	University of California-San Diego	La Jolla	USA
The Johns Hopkins Oncology Center	Baltimore	USA	University of Arkansas for Medical Sciences	Little Rock	USA
University of Maryland Cancer Center	Berkeley	USA			
Alta Bates Medical Center	Berkeley	USA	Children's Hospital of Los Angeles	Los Angeles	USA
National Institutes of Health	Bethesda	USA	Southern California Permanente Medical Group	Los Angeles	USA
University of Alabama at Birmingham	Birmingham	USA			
Massachusetts General Hospital	Boston	USA	UCLA – Centre for Health Sciences	Los Angeles	USA
Roswell Park Cancer Institute	Buffalo	USA	University Louisville/James Graham Brown Cancer Centre	Louisville	USA
Medical University of South Carolina	Charleston	USA			
Children's Memorial Hospital	Chicago	USA	University of Wisconsin	Madison	USA
Michael Reese Hospital and Medical Center	Chicago	USA	Marshfield Clinic	Marshfield	USA
			Loyola University Medical Center	Maywood	USA
Northwestern Memorial Hospital/ N.W. University	Chicago	USA	St. Jude Children's Research Hospital	Memphis	USA
			Miami Children's Hospital	Miami	USA
Rush-Presbyterian-St. Luke's Medical Center	Chicago	USA	Froedtert Hospital/Medical College of Wisconsin	Milwaukee	USA
Wyler Children's Hospital	Chicago	USA	University of Minnesota	Minneapolis	USA
Children's Hospital Medical Center	Cincinnati	USA	West Virginia University Hospitals	Morgantown	USA
Jewish Hospital of Cincinnati	Cincinnati	USA	Children's Hospital – Louisiana State University	New Orleans	USA
University of Cincinnati Medical Center	Cincinnati	USA	Louisana State Medical Center	New Orleans	USA
Rainbow Babies and Children's Hospital	Cleveland	USA	Memorial Medical Center	New Orleans	USA
			Tulane University Medical Center	New Orleans	USA
Case Western Reserve University Hospital	Cleveland	USA	Memorial Sloan-Kettering Cancer Center	New York City	USA
Cleveland Clinic	Cleveland	USA	Mt. Sinai Hospital	New York City	USA

Medical Center of Delaware	Newark	USA	University of Utah Medical Center	Salt Lake City	USA
University of Oklahoma Health Sciences Center	Oklahoma City	USA	South Texas Cancer Institute	San Antonio	USA
			University of Texas Health Science Center	San Antonio	USA
Bishop Clarkson Memorial Hospital	Omaha	USA			
University of Nebraska Medical Center	Omaha	USA	University of California Moffitt Hospital	San Francisco	USA
Children's Hospital of Orange County	Orange	USA			
St. Joseph Hospital	Orange	USA	Mayo Clinic Scottsdale	Scottsdale	USA
St. Joseph's Hospital and Medical Center	Paterson	USA	Louisiana State University Medical Center	Shreveport	USA
Children's Hospital of Philadelphia	Philadelphia	USA	Cardinal Glennon Children's Hospital	St. Louis	USA
Hahnemann University Hospital	Philadelphia	USA	St. Louis Children's Hospital	St. Louis	USA
Temple University Comprehensive Cancer Center	Philadelphia	USA	St. Louis University Health Sciences Center	St. Louis	USA
Thomas Jefferson University Hospital	Philadelphia	USA	All Children's Hospital	St. Petersburg	USA
Children's Hospital of Pittsburgh	Pittsburgh	USA	Stanford University Medical Center	Stanford	USA
Montefiore University Hospital	Pittsburgh	USA	H. Lee Moffitt Cancer Center	Tampa	USA
Western Pennsylvania Cancer Institute	Pittsburgh	USA	University of Arizona Cancer Center	Tucson	USA
Oregon Health Sciences University (Adults)	Portland	USA	Children's National Medical Center	Washington	USA
			George Washington University Medical Center	Washington	USA
Oregon Health Sciences University (Paediatrics)	Portland	USA			
			Georgetown University Medical Center	Washington	USA
Roger Williams Medical Center	Providence	USA	The Westlake Comprehensive Cancer Center	Westlake Village	USA
Washoe Medical Center	Reno	USA			
Medical College of Virginia	Richmond	USA	Cancer Center of Kansas	Wichita	USA
Mayo Clinic	Rochester	USA	Wake Forest University	Winston-Salem	USA
Strong Memorial Hospital	Rochester	USA	University of Massachusetts Medical Center	Worcester	USA
Sutter Memorial Hospital	Sacramento	USA			
LDS Hospital	Salt Lake City	USA	Hospital Central de Valencia	Valencia	Venezuela

Appendix 2 Institutions participating in the Autologous Blood and Marrow Transplant Registry (in alphabetical order according to city)

Albany Medical Center	Albany	USA	Centro de Internacion e Investigation	Buenos Aires	Argentina
Alberta Children's Hospital	Alberta	Canada	Hospital Privado De Oncologia	Buenos Aires	Argentina
Presbyterian Health Care Services	Albuquerque	USA	ITMO Fundacion Mainetti	Buenos Aires	Argentina
Don & Sybil Harrington Cancer Center	Amarillo	USA	Navy Hospital 'Pedro Mallo'	Buenos Aires	Argentina
C.S. Mott Children's Hospital	Ann Arbor	USA	Roswell Park Cancer Institute	Buffalo	USA
University of Michigan Medical Center	Ann Arbor	USA	Lahey Hitchcock Clinic	Burlington	USA
Gulhane Military Medical Academy	Ankara	Turkey	University of Calgary	Calgary	Canada
Arlington Cancer Center	Arlington	USA	Royal Prince Alfred Hospital	Camperdown	Australia
Emory Clinic	Atlanta	USA	The Wynberg Hospital	Cape Town	South Africa
Emory University	Atlanta	USA	University of North Carolina Chapel Hill	Chapel Hill	USA
Northside Hospital	Atlanta	USA			
Southwest Regional Cancer Center	Austin	USA	Hollings Cancer Center	Charleston	USA
Johns Hopkins Hospital	Baltimore	USA	University of Virginia Medical Center	Charlottesville	USA
University of Maryland Cancer Center	Baltimore	USA			
Hosp. General Vall d'Hebron	Barcelona	Spain	Children's Memorial Hospital	Chicago	USA
Mary Bird Perkins Cancer Center	Baton Rouge	USA	Rush Presbyterian/St. Luke's Medical Center	Chicago	USA
Alta Bates Hospital	Berkeley	USA			
University of Alabama at Birmingham	Birmingham	USA	University of Chicago Medical Center	Chicago	USA
Dana-Farber Cancer Institute	Boston	USA	Children's Hospital Medical Center	Cincinnati	USA
Montefiore Medical Center	Bronx	USA	Jewish Hospital of Cincinnati	Cincinnati	USA
Alexander Fleming Institute	Buenos Aires	Argentina	University Hospital Cincinnati	Cincinnati	USA

Case Western Reserve University Hospital	Cleveland	USA
Cleveland Clinic Foundation	Cleveland	USA
Rainbow Babies and Children's Hospital	Cleveland	USA
Rocky Mountain Cancer Center	Colorado Springs	USA
University of South Carolina	Columbia	USA
Columbus Children's Hospital	Columbus	USA
Ohio State University Hospital	Columbus	USA
Hospital Privado de Cordoba	Cordoba	Argentina
Hospital de Clinicas	Curitiba	Brazil
Hospital Nossa Senhora Das Gracas	Curitiba	Brazil
Baylor University Medical Center	Dallas	USA
Children's Medical Center Dallas	Dallas	USA
Medical City Dallas Hospital	Dallas	USA
Miami Valley Hospital	Dayton	USA
Halifax Medical Center	Daytona Beach	USA
Presbyterian St. Luke's Hospital	Denver	USA
Henry Ford Hospital	Detroit	USA
Wayne State University	Detroit	USA
City of Hope National Medical Center	Duarte	USA
Duke University Medical Center	Durham	USA
Northwest Oncology & Hematology Associates	Elk Grove Village	USA
University of Connecticut Health Center	Farmington	USA
Bone Marrow & Stem Cell Institute of Florida	Fort Lauderdale	USA
Cook-Fort Worth Children's Medical Center	Fort Worth	USA
Harris Methodist Oncology Program	Fort Worth	USA
University of Florida, Shands Hospital	Gainesville	USA
Cancer & Hematology Centres of Western Michigan	Grand Rapids	USA
East Carolina University School of Medicine	Greenville	USA
Cancer Centers of the Carolinas	Greenville	USA
Hackensack Medical Center	Hackensack	USA
Victoria General Hospital	Halifax	Canada
James River Transplant Center	Hampton	USA
Hermanos Ameijeiras Hospital	Havana	Cuba
Instituto de Hematologia e Immunologia	Havana	Cuba
Hinsdale Hematology-Oncology Associates	Hinsdale	USA
Queen's Medical Center	Honolulu	USA
St. Francis Medical Center	Honolulu	USA
Baylor College of Medicine	Houston	USA
M.D. Anderson Cancer Center	Houston	USA
Indiana University Hospital & Outpatient Center	Indianapolis	USA
Methodist Hospital of Indiana	Indianapolis	USA
St. Vincent Hospital & Health Care Center	Indianapolis	USA
Baptist Regional Cancer Center	Jacksonville	USA
Mayo Clinic Jacksonville	Jacksonville	USA
Children's Mercy Hospital	Kansas City	USA
University of Kansas Medical Center	Kansas City	USA
University of Tennessee Medical Center	Knoxville	USA
Scripps Clinic & Research Foundation	La Jolla	USA
Dartmouth-Hitchcock Medical Center	Lebanon	USA
University of Kentucky Medical Center	Lexington	USA
Arkansas Cancer Research Center	Little Rock	USA
London Health Sciences Centre	London	Canada
Kaiser Permanente of Southern California	Los Angeles	USA
UCLA Center for Health Sciences	Los Angeles	USA
USC/Norris Cancer Hospital	Los Angeles	USA
James Graham Brown Cancer Center	Louisville	USA
University of Wisconsin	Madison	USA
North Shore University Hospital	Manhasset	USA
Marshfield Clinic	Marshfield	USA
Loyola University Medical Center	Maywood	USA
Methodist Hospital Central	Memphis	USA
Response Technologies	Memphis	USA
St. Jude Children's Research Hospital	Memphis	USA
Baptist Hospital of Miami	Miami	USA
Miami Children's Hospital	Miami	USA
Froedtert East Hospital	Milwaukee	USA
St. Luke's Medical Center	Milwaukee	USA
Abbott Northwestern Hospital	Minneapolis	USA
University of Minnesota	Minneapolis	USA
British Hospital & Faculty of Medicine	Montevideo	Uruguay
Hosp. Naciel Ministere of Public Health	Montevideo	Uruguay
IMPASA, Centro de Trans. de Medula Osea	Montevideo	Uruguay
Hôpital Sainte-Justine	Montreal	Canada
Jewish General Hospital	Montreal	Canada
Montreal Children's Hospital	Montreal	Canada
Royal Victoria Hospital	Montreal	Canada
Sacre Coeur Hospital	Montreal	Canada
West Virginia University	Morgantown	USA
Vanderbilt University Medical Center	Nashville	USA
All India Institute of Medical Sciences	New Delhi	India
Louisiana State University Medical Center	New Orleans	USA
Memorial Medical Center	New Orleans	USA
Tulane University Medical Center	New Orleans	USA
Columbia University	New York	USA
Memorial Sloan-Kettering Cancer Center	New York	USA
Mt. Sinai Medical Center	New York	USA
New York Hospital Cornell Medical Center	New York	USA
Medical Center of Delaware	Newark	USA
Hoag Cancer Center	Newport Beach	USA
University of Oklahoma Health Sciences	Oklahoma	USA
Immanuel Cancer Center	Omaha	USA
University of Nebraska Medical Center	Omaha	USA
Children's Hospital of Orange County	Orange	USA
Saint Joseph Hospital	Orange	USA
UCI Medical Center	Orange	USA
Ottawa General Hospital	Ottawa	Canada
The Desert Hospital Comprehensive Cancer Center	Palm Springs	USA
Clínica Universidad de Navarra	Pamplona	Spain
Lutheran General Hospital	Park Ridge	USA
Hematology Associates	Peoria	USA

Children's Hospital of Philadelphia	Philadelphia	USA	Hospital Especialidades Centro Medico	San Mateo	Mexico
Hahnemann University Hospital	Philadelphia	USA	Mayo Clinic Scottsdale	Scottsdale	USA
Temple University Comprehensive Cancer Center	Philadelphia	USA	LSU Medical Center-Shreveport	Shreveport	USA
			Dakota Midwest Cancer Institute	Sioux Falls	USA
Thomas Jefferson University Hospital	Philadelphia	USA	Baystate Medical Center	Springfield	USA
University of Pennsylvania Hospital	Philadelphia	USA	Memorial Medical Center	Springfield	USA
Children's Hospital of Pittsburgh	Pittsburgh	USA	Cardinal Glennon Children's Hospital	St. Louis	USA
Shadyside Hospital	Pittsburgh	USA	St. Louis Children's Hospital	St. Louis	USA
University of Pittsburgh	Pittsburgh	USA	St. Louis University Medical Center	St. Louis	USA
The Cancer Center of Boston	Plymouth	USA	Methodist Hospital/Nicollet Cancer Center	St. Louis Park	USA
St. Charles & John T. Mather Hospital	East Setauket	USA	All Children's Hospital	St. Petersburg	USA
Legacy Good Samaritan Hospital	Portland	USA	Petrov Research Institute of Oncology	St. Petersburg	Russia
Oregon Health Sciences University	Portland	USA	Bennett Cancer Center	Stamford	USA
Providence Portland Medical Center	Portland	USA	Stanford University Hospital	Stanford	USA
Instituto Portugues de Oncologia-Centro do Porto	Porto	Portugal	Northeastern Ontario Regional Cancer Centre	Sudbury	Canada
Alfred Hospital	Prahran	Australia	SUNY-Health Science Center	Syracuse	USA
Roger Williams Medical Center	Providence	USA	H. Lee Moffitt Cancer Center	Tampa	USA
Centro de Hematologia Y Medicina Interna	Puebla	Mexico	Scott & White Clinic	Temple	USA
			Hospital for Sick Children	Toronto	Canada
Hopital du Saint-Sacrement	Quebec City	Canada	Toronto General Hospital	Toronto	Canada
Cancer & Blood Institute of the Desert	Rancho Mirage	USA	Arizona Cancer Center	Tucson	USA
Riverview Medical Center	Red Bank	USA	St. Francis Hospital	Tulsa	USA
Washow Regional Cancer Center	Reno	USA	New York Medical College	Valhalla	USA
Medical College of Virginia	Richmond	USA	British Columbia's Children's Hospital	Vancouver	Canada
Universidade Federal de Rio de Janeiro	Rio de Janeiro	Brazil	Vancouver General Hospital	Vancouver	Canada
Mayo Clinic Rochester	Rochester	USA	Donauspital	Vienna	Austria
University of Rochester	Rochester	USA	Georgetown University Medical Center	Washington DC	USA
Sutter Memorial Hospital	Sacramento	USA			
University of California Davis Cancer Center	Sacramento	USA	George Washington University Medical Center	Washington DC	USA
LDS Hospital	Salt Lake City	USA	Walter Reed Army Medical Center	Washington DC	USA
University of Utah School of Medicine	Salt Lake City	USA			
South Texas Cancer Institute	San Antonio	USA	Westlake Comprehensive Cancer Center	Westlake Village	USA
University of Texas Health Sciences Center	San Antonio	USA			
Children's Hospital San Diego	San Diego	USA	St. Francis Hospital	Wichita	USA
University of California, San Diego	San Diego	USA	Manitoba Cancer Treatment Center	Winnipeg	Canada
Instituto Nacional de Cancerologia	San Fernando	Mexico	Wake Forest University	Winston-Salem	USA
University of California, San Francisco Medical Center	San Francisco	USA	University of Massachusetts Medical Center	Worcester	USA
University of California, San Francisco Pediatrics	San Francisco	USA			

References

1. Gratwohl A, Gorin C, Apperley J et al. The European Group for Blood and Marrow Transplantation (EBMT): A report from the President and the Chairmen of the Working Parties. *Bone Marrow Transplant* 1996; **18**: 677–691.
2. Fayers PM and Machin D. Sample size: how many patients are necessary? *Br J Cancer* 1995; **72**: 1–9.
3. Niland, JC, Gebhardt JA, Lee J and Forman SJ. Study design, statistical analyses, and results reporting in the bone marrow transplantation literature. *Biol Blood Marrow Transplant* 1995; **1**: 47–53.
4. Begg CB. Selection of patients for clinical trials. *Semin Oncol* 1988; **15**: 434–50.
5. Schmucker DL and Vesell ES. Underrepresentation of women in clinical drug trials. *Clin Pharm Therap* 1993; **54**: 11–15.
6. Gorkin L, Schron EB, Handshaw K et al. Clinical trial enrollers vs. nonenrollers: the Cardiac Arrhythmia Suppression Trial (CAST) Recruitment and Enrollment Assessment in Clinical Trials (REACT) project. *Controlled Clinical Trials* 1996; **17**: 46–59.
7. Michallet M, Archimbaud E, Bandini G et al. for the European Group for Blood and Marrow Transplantation and the International Bone Marrow Transplant Registry. HLA-identical sibling bone marrow transplantation in younger patients with chronic lymphocytic leukemia. *Ann Intern Med* 1996; **124**: 311–315.

8. Barrett AJ, Horowitz MM, Ash RC *et al*. Bone marrow transplantation for Philadelphia chromosome-positive acute lymphoblastic leukemia. *Blood* 1992; **79**: 3067–3070.
9. Mugishima H, Gale RP, Rowlings PA *et al*. Bone marrow transplantation for Diamond–Blackfan anemia. *Bone Marrow Transplant* 1995; **15**: 55–58.
10. Gajewski JL, Phillips GL, Sobocinski KA *et al*. Bone marrow transplants from HLA-identical siblings in advanced Hodgkin's disease. *J Clin Oncol* 1996; **14**: 572–578.
11. Harrell FE, Lee KL, Matchar DB and Reichert TA. Regression models for prognostic prediction: advantages, problems, and suggested solutions. *Cancer Treat Rep* 1985; **69**: 1071–1077.
12. Simon R and Altman DG. Statistical aspects of prognostic factor studies in oncology. *Br J Cancer* 1994; **69**: 979–998.
13. Greenland S. Power, sample size and smallest detectable effect determination for multivariate studies. *Stat Med* 1985; **4**: 117–127.
14. Starmer CF and Lee KL. A data-based approach to assessing clinical interventions in the setting of chronic disease. *Cancer Treat Rep* 1982; **66**: 1077–1082.
15. Gale RP, Bortin MM, van Bekkum DW *et al*. Risk factors for acute graft-vs-host disease. *Br J Haematol* 1988; **67**: 397–406.
16. Atkinson K, Horowitz MM, Gale RP *et al*. Risk factors for chronic graft-vs-host disease after HLA-identical sibling bone marrow transplantation. *Blood* 1990; **75**: 2459–2464.
17. Weiner RS, Bortin MM, Gale RP *et al*. Interstitial pneumonitis after bone marrow transplantation: assessment of risk factors. *Ann Intern Med* 1986; **104**: 168–175.
18. Weiner RS, Horowitz MM, Gale RP *et al*. Risk factors for interstitial pneumonia following bone marrow transplantation for severe aplastic anemia. *Br J Haematol* 1989; **71**: 535–543.
19. Rozman C, Carreras E, Qian C *et al*. Risk factors for hepatic veno-occlusive disease following HLA-identical sibling bone marrow transplants for leukemia. *Bone Marrow Transplant* 1996; **17**: 75–80.
20. Gale RP, Horowitz M and Bortin M. IBMTR analysis of bone marrow transplants in acute leukemia. *Bone Marrow Transplant* 1990; **4**: 83–85.
21. Gale RP, Horowitz MM, Weiner RS *et al*. Impact of cytogenetic abnormalities on outcome of bone marrow transplants in acute myelogenous leukemia in first remission. *Bone Marrow Transplant* 1995; **16**: 203–208.
22. Barrett AJ, Horowitz MM, Gale RP *et al*. Marrow transplantation for acute lymphoblastic leukemia: factors affecting relapse and survival. *Blood* 1989; **74**: 862–871.
23. Goldman JM, Gale RP, Horowitz MM *et al*. Bone marrow transplantation for chronic myelogenous leukemia in chronic phase: increased risk of relapse associated with T-cell depletion. *Ann Intern Med* 1988; **108**: 806–814.
24. Champlin RE, Horowitz MM, van Bekkum DW *et al*. Graft failure following bone marrow transplantation for severe aplastic anemia: risk factors and treatment results. *Blood* 1989; **73**: 606–613.
25. Marmont AM, Horowitz MM, Gale RP *et al*. T-cell depletion of HLA-identical transplants in leukemia. *Blood* 1991; **78**: 2120–2130.
26. Feinstein AR. An additional basic science for clinical medicine. II. The limitations of randomized trials. *Ann Intern Med* 1983; **99**: 544–550.
27. Graham-Pole J. Treating acute lymphoblastic leukemia after relapse: bone marrow transplantation or not? *Lancet* 1989; i: 1517–1518.
28. Gluckman E, Horowitz MM, Champlin RE *et al*. Bone marrow transplantation for severe aplastic anemia: influence of conditioning and graft-versus-host disease prophylaxis regimens on outcome. *Blood* 1992; **79**: 269–275.
29. Ringden O, Horowitz MM, Sondel P *et al*. Methotrexate, cyclosporine, or both to prevent graft-versus-host disease after HLA-identical sibling bone marrow transplants for early leukemia? *Blood* 1993; **81**: 1094–1101.
30. Ash RC, Horowitz MM, Gale RP *et al*. Bone marrow transplantation from related donors other than HLA-identical siblings: effect of T-cell depletion. *Bone Marrow Transplant* 1991; **7**: 443–452.
31. Szydlo R, Goldman JM, Klein JP *et al*. Results of allogeneic bone marrow transplants for leukemia using donors other than HLA-identical siblings. *J Clin Oncol* 1997; **15**: 1767–1777.
32. Miller CB, Rowlings PA, Jones RJ, Keating A, Zhang MJ and Horowitz MM. Autotransplants for acute myelogenous leukemia (AML): effect of purging with 4-hydroperoxycyclophosphamide (4HC). *Proc Am Soc Clin Oncol* 1996; **15**: 338a.
33. Ringden O, Horowitz MM, Gale RP *et al*. Outcome after allogeneic bone marrow transplant for leukemia in older adults. *J Am Med Ass* 1993; **270**: 57–60.
34. Lazarus HM, Horowitz MM, Nugent ML. Outcome of autotransplants in older adults. *Proc Am Soc Clin Oncol* 1996; **15**: 338a [abstr. 977].
35. Klein JP and Zhang MJ. Statistical challenges in comparing chemotherapy and bone marrow transplantation as a treatment for leukemia. In: *Lifetime Data: Models in Reliability and Survival Analysis*. NP Jewel, AC Kimber, M-LT Lee and GA Whitmore (eds), 1996: 175–186 (Norwell, MA: Kluwer Academic Press).
36. Begg CB, McGlave PB, Bennett JM, Cassileth PA and Olan MM. A critical comparison of allogeneic bone marrow transplantation and conventional chemotherapy as treatment for acute myelogenous leukemia. *J Clin Oncol* 1984; **2**: 369–378.
37. Hermans J, Suciu S, Stijnen T *et al*. Treatment of acute myelogenous leukaemia: An EBMT–EORTC retrospective analysis of chemotherapy versus allogeneic or autologous bone marrow transplantation. *Br J Cancer Clin Oncol* 1989; **25**: 545–550.
38. Messerer D, Neiss A, Horowitz MM, Hoelzer D and Gale RP. Comparison of chemotherapy and bone marrow transplants using two independent clinical databases. *J Clin Epidemiol* 1994; **47**: 1119–1126.
39. Moon TE, Jones SE, Bonadonna G, Powles TJ, Rivkin S, Buzdar A and Montague E. Using a database of protocol studies to evaluate therapy: a breast cancer example. *Stat Med* 1984; **3**: 333–339.
40. Davis K. The comprehensive cohort study: the use of registry data to confirm and extend a randomized trial. *Recent results. Cancer Res* 1988; **111**: 138–148.
41. Mantel N and Byar D. Evaluation of response-time data involving transient status: an illustration using heart-transplant data. *J Am Stat Ass* 1974; **69**: 81–86.

42. Turnbull BW, Brown BW and Hu M. Survivorship analysis of heart transplant data. *J Am Stat Ass* 1974; **69**: 74–80.
43. Gale RP, Büchner T, Zhang MJ *et al*. HLA-identical sibling bone marrow transplants versus chemotherapy for acute myelogenous leukemia in first remission. *Leukaemia* 1996; **10**: 1687–1691.
44. Gale RP, Horowitz MM, Rees JKH *et al*. Chemotherapy versus transplants for acute myelogenous leukemia in second remission. *Leukaemia* 1996; **10**: 13–19.
45. Horowitz MM, Messerer D, Hoelzer D *et al*. Chemotherapy compared with bone marrow transplantation for adults with acute lymphoblastic leukemia in first remission. *Ann Intern Med* 1991; **115**: 13–18.
46. Zhang MJ, Hoelzer D, Horowitz MM *et al*. for the Acute Lymphoblastic Leukemia Working Committee. Long-term follow-up of adults with acute lymphoblastic leukemia in first remission treated with chemotherapy or bone marrow transplantation. *Ann Intern Med* 1995; **123**: 428–431.
47. Barrett AJ, Horowitz MM, Pollock BH *et al*. Bone marrow transplants from HLA-identical siblings as compared with chemotherapy for children with acute lymphoblastic leukemia in a second remission. *New Engl J Med* 1994; **331**: 1253–1258.
48. Zhang MJ, Baccarani M, Gale RP *et al*. Survival of patients with chronic myelogenous leukemia relapsing after bone marrow transplantation: comparison with patients receiving conventional chemotherapy. *Br J Haematol* 1997; **99**: 23–29.
49. Curtis RE, Rowlings PA, Deeg HJ *et al*. Solid cancers after bone marrow transplantation. *New Engl J Med* 1997; **336**: 897–904.
50. Socié G, Sobocinski KA, Veum-Stone J and Horowitz MM. Long-term survival and analysis of late causes of death after allogeneic bone marrow transplantation (BMT). *Blood* 1996; **88**: 643a [abstr. 2561].
51. Commenges D and Andersen PK. Score test of homogeneity for survival data. *Lifetime Data Analysis* 1995; **1**: 145–160.
52. Klein JP and Zhang M. Technical Report #12: Confidence regions for the equality of two survival curves. July 1996.

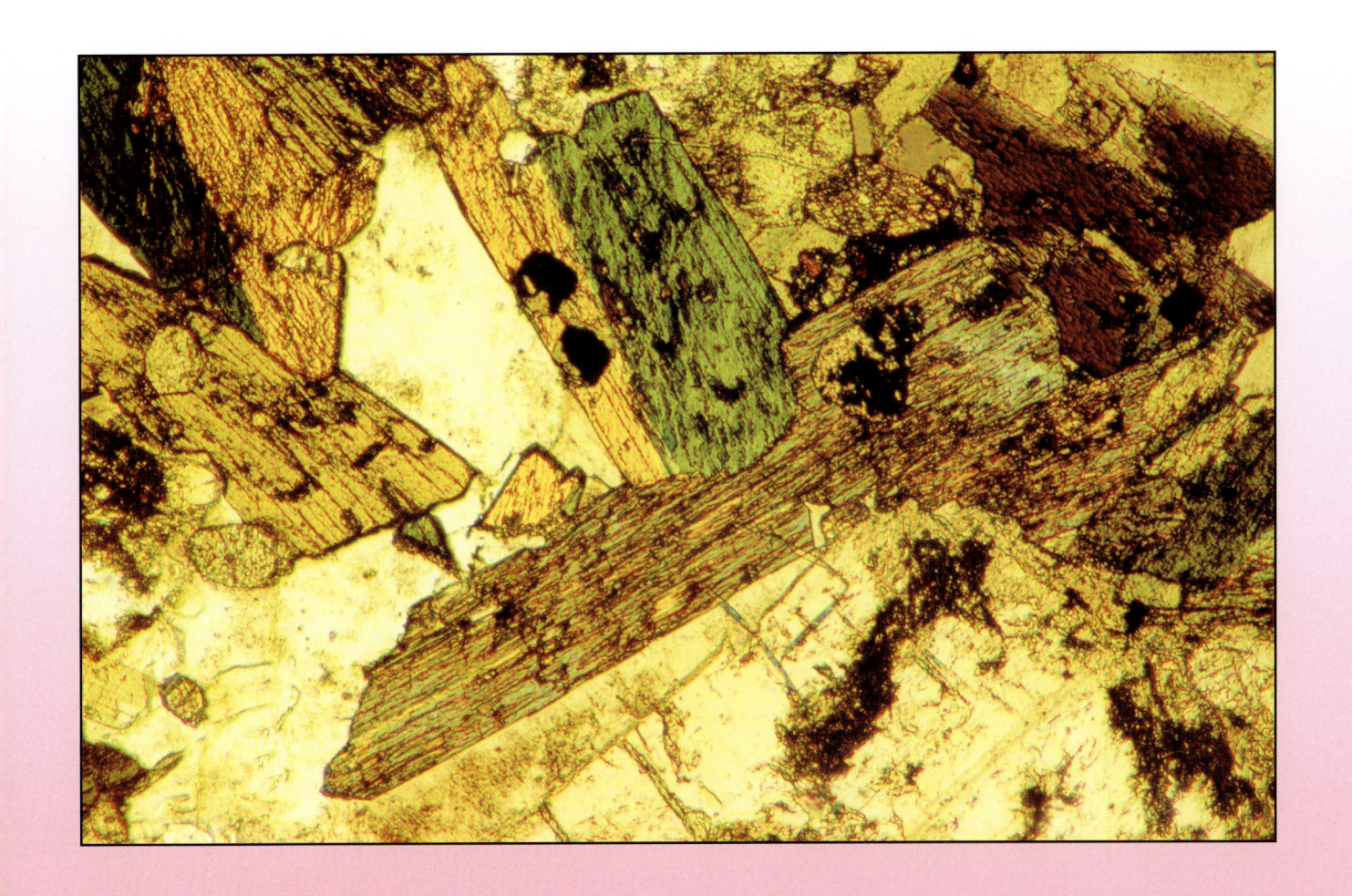

Chapter 62

Ethnic considerations

James Smith

Introduction

We live in an increasingly multicultural and multireligious society, and those who are involved in the care of patients who are candidates for bone-marrow transplantation need to become more aware of the cultural, social and religious issues which are of major importance to those for whom they care. Ease of travel, the ageing and increasing number of people born in the USA and Europe within established immigrant communities, refugees from a wide range of countries where persecution and conflict of one sort or another have caused them to seek asylum, all contribute to the increasing richness of community life. These factors also place a burden of responsibility upon those who work within the healthcare sector. Approach to patient care has to cease being ethnocentric and become more open and embracing of different ideas, cultures and lifestyles.

E.B. Taylor [1] in his seminal work on anthropology defines culture thus: 'Culture is that complex whole which includes knowledge, beliefs, art, morals, law, custom and any other capabilities and habits acquired as a member of society.' If we examine Taylor's definition, it can be seen that it encapsulates most of the facets of the cultural make up of the individual. Cultural behaviour is a set of evolved guidelines which an individual member of a group inherits as a member of a particular group within society. It is through such guidelines that an individual's view of the world is moulded and influenced, and is the baseline whereby life experience is interpreted. Cultural or ethnic background often provides the template for an individual persons' behaviour patterns.

Unless it has been displaced by AIDS, cancer is probably today's most feared disease [2]. Many people fear the word 'cancer' and will try to avoid using it. Within many ethnic groups, not only the word, but the disclosure of the diagnosis, contravenes strict social taboos. Because cancer as a disease is frequently invisible, a culture of myth and fear has sprung up around such a diagnosis, and a language of metaphor such as 'killer disease' or 'the big C' is commonplace. Conversely, within the medical and associated professions a language of euphemism may accompany the diagnosis of cancer; words such as 'tumour' or 'lump' are still used to disguise the reality of the disease from the patient.

There are, however, some cultures where the diagnosis of cancer causes loss of hope, not only for the patient, but also the patient's family. In his study of the needs of ethnic Chinese patients, Ho [3] suggests that 'cancer is a punishment for some "sin" or evil act committed by the patient, and a cancer diagnosis could bring shame or ridicule on the family'. Within many Asian and Chinese communities there is also a fear of contagion. This fear may well stem from a confusion between lung cancer and tuberculosis which in some circumstances can exhibit similar symptoms. The effect on a family from such ethnic backgrounds may be socially devastating. Poliakoff [2] makes the point that 'in many cases sexual relationships are ended between husband and wife for fear of contagion, or a patient is no longer welcome at social activities. It is not the cancer *per se* that is feared, but that the sick person will spread bad luck to the rest of the family'. There is no doubt that cancer in any of its many forms is feared by most people across the spectrum of races and cultures, however, with an increasing awareness of the efficacy of education, and the growing availability of literature in a diversity of languages, barriers are slowly being broken down. Although progress in education is evident, there remains a need for healthcare professionals to acquire knowledge pertinent to the needs of patients from ethnic minority communities.

This chapter is an attempt to draw attention to the major issues and concerns which may affect the care of the patient from an ethnic minority and to offer some explanation for various problems and misunderstandings which may arise from such a relationship.

Communication

Within the world of illness, communication between patient and professional needs to be established quickly and efficiently. Various writers have made studies of the ability or inability of healthcare workers to establish well understood dialogue with patients. Quereshi [4] states that: 'English health care professionals tend to regard everyone as English, and to assume that patients have similar needs.' He continues: 'Even Americans do not speak the same language as the English, so how can an overseas patient express himself in a way that sounds English to English ears?' Verbal communication is an essential part of everyday existence, but it is true to say that within the world of medicine there is language which is both unique to the medical world and everyday language which is used in medical context which is not easily understood, even by patients for whom English is a first language. Szasz [5] suggests that a patient's understanding of the nature of his or her disease is interpreted and understood through the information conveyed to him by healthcare workers, and the individual's interpretation of this information has enormous implications for the way in which the patient responds to his or her disease and to those who care for them.

Our ability to communicate freely and on equal terms with those around us plays a major part in our ability to be self-determining. It follows, then, that when our ability to communicate is restricted by new and technical language, in what is, for many, a socially hostile environment, patients lose confidence in their ability to be self-determining with a degree of environmental and social control. Volosinov [6] maintains that the 'process which defines a person as an individual can be explained in terms of the individual's normal social environment'. The hospital ward or outpatients department is rarely such an environment for a patient and is such only in part for staff [7]: 'Health care workers should be aware of the fact that medicine is a cultural entity in itself, with a language of its own, and understanding of this reality may well be the first step in effectively communicating with a patient.'

Although the majority of ethnic minority groups resident within the UK originate from both the new and old Commonwealth, there are still a considerable number of people for whom English is at best a second language. Often, it is the women within such communities who have less understanding of English, as many spend their lives within a very tightly knit community where the normal language of conversation is that of their old home. Men usually have a greater grasp of English, simply because they are required to be the bread-winners, and as such are more exposed to the need to learn English. Naturally, the younger members of most communities speak English as a first language as many are born in the UK, and they are frequently also able to speak the mother tongue of the parents. This offers some assistance when an interpreter is required for a parent or a grandparent.

However, it is unfair to burden a young person with translation of issues of an intimate nature, especially if the patient is of the opposite sex. For this reason it is important for hospital departments to have interpreters available who have a ready knowledge of medical language and who will translate questions accurately. It is not sufficient, nor is it ethical, to have members of staff translating on an ad hoc basis, especially when there is a risk of breaching confidentiality.

For patients whose command of English is minimal or even non-existent, it is always important to have an interpreter who is able to provide accurate translation in both directions. It is also more acceptable to have an interpreter of the same sex as the patient.

The availability of explanatory leaflets in a variety of the more usual minority languages is a great step forward in patient care, and it is important to have a selection of such leaflets or booklets available for patients so that some of their questions can be answered and fears allayed before more complicated procedures are undertaken. It is equally important to be aware that some professionals within the healthcare sector use English as a second language, and that this may lead to increased anxiety for patients from other linguistic backgrounds as it is possible to misunderstand subtle changes in nuance within conversation.

Although verbal communication is the norm for most patients of Caucasian origin, and patients from this group are usually happy to respond to direct questions with direct answers, this may not always be the case with patients from ethnic minority groups. Often it is seen as impolite to respond directly to questions posed by a person viewed as having authority, and therefore answers may need to be negotiated. This may be the cause of some impatience on the part of the professional, but gradual disclosure of information by the patient is very much part of the patient's need to build a relationship of trust and confidence with the person who will be responsible for his care. In the same way, gestures which may be perceived as normal in a white Western society may be viewed otherwise by certain groups. Eye contact, for example, is perceived as a normal part of conversational behaviour in white societies, whereas it is seen as disrespectful by many Middle Eastern, Indian and Chinese communities. Similarly, patients from these groups may feel ill at ease if greeted in a traditionally English way by a handshake. Physical contact, especially with members of the opposite sex, is viewed as improper especially at a first meeting; a simple greeting, followed by an invitation to sit down is much preferred.

Dress, modesty and the medical examination

For many patients, the doctor–patient consultation is an experience which promotes high levels of anxiety, particularly when the consultation is to take place in the unfamiliar surroundings of a hospital, rather than the more familiar surroundings of their general practice. The hospital is an environment which promotes an array of competing emotions within the patients who are attending: anxiety, fear, uncertainty, threat, hope and the possibility of cure. Singer [8] writes: 'The hospital calls up some of our deepest anxieties – about pain, decay and death – in the promissory rhetoric of the remedial.' When patients enter a hospital, they enter a mostly unfamiliar world, where a new set of rules apply, their most intimate bodily functions are discussed openly and their bodies become objects of intimate scrutiny and examination. For most patients from any cultural background, this disruption to their normal ability to be self-determining results in a feeling of diminished status, as the boundaries of public and private space and behaviour is dissolved.

For many ethnic minority communities, the prospect of a medical examination is viewed with apprehension and, for some, horror. In many cultures, to convey and reveal intimate details about oneself without some form of negotiation is seen as impolite and immodest. It is important to establish a relationship of trust and respect before details of physical disease are disclosed. Within the Western mind there is an expectation of examination by the doctor; this will either be preceded or followed by a series of incisive and often intimate questions. There is frequently disappointment in the Western patient when they are not 'examined' and the more thorough the examination, the more elevated the status of the examiner becomes in the minds of many patients.

Such openness about examination and bodily functions is not the case for the majority of non-white Western Europeans. Negotiated, delicate questioning is quite alien to many doctors within the Western tradition, and patients who do not respond to direct questions with equally direct answers may be perceived as difficult.

The importance of a negotiated style of examination cannot be overemphasized, nor can the fact that many patients from ethnic minority communities will wish to be accompanied by family members or friends at all times. This is most true in the case of the female patient especially as Western medicine is still dominated by male doctors. Examination by a male may well be perceived by the female patient as a threat to her modesty and status. Female patients being examined by a male should be chaperoned as a matter of course.

In addition to expecting a negotiated interview, the patient from an ethnic minority group may have minimal understanding of the language of questioning, and in such cases the patient may withdraw into a state of non-verbal communication where gestures, facial expression and vague hand movements become the language of the interaction. Such non-verbal communication may be well understood by a family member who is present and it is important that their contribution to the dialogue be given credence.

The desire for modesty among many groups may be considered as obsessive and obstructive by some in the health service, but the preservation of a patient's modesty is a vital part in the building of a relationship of trust between patient and potential carers. Although the strictest rules concerning exposure and examination apply to the women of many ethnic groups, there are many groups of men for whom modesty is equally important. It is not unknown for a man from a Middle Eastern and Islamic tradition to ask for a male doctor or male nurse, or where exclusively female carers are available, a male chaperone. Although this may appear strange to the Western mind, it is an important part of maintaining integrity, modesty and autonomy for the patient and such a desire should be accorded respect.

Those who work in large centres in major cities are used to the sight of women dressed in the chador with faces veiled, or in one of the many varieties of dress from the African and Indian traditions. Such forms of dress frequently display not only a cultural and religious significance, but also community and family status. To demand their removal without due consideration for the patient's modesty may be perceived as an assault on all these factors. It is also important to be aware that in many cultures the status of the women is very different from that of the woman in Western society. The status of the woman may not be as highly valued, and they may be seen by their male partner as property, rather than as an equal within a relationship. This subordinate relationship may well be carried over into the medical interview.

Certain aspects of the woman's life, such as menstruation, may be areas where there is a major cultural or religious taboo. The menstruating woman is viewed as unclean by many societies, and to touch or examine a woman who is menstruating may be viewed as polluting the examiner. Further, questions about such an intimate function addressed to a woman in front of her husband or a male relative or interpreter will remain unanswered and cause major distress to all concerned.

As many women from the Middle East are aware of the critical view held in the West concerning female circumcision, there is often profound reluctance by women to undergo intimate examination where any degree of genital mutilation has taken place.

Use of language must be precise. Those who speak English as a second language or communicate through an interpreter will not understand much medical language, nor use of everday language which has been adapted by the medical profession to mean a specific condition. For example, 'incontinent' in its medical use means an inability to control voiding of urine or faeces. However the *Pocket Oxford Dictionary* defines the word as a 'lack of self restraint especially in relation to sexual appetite'.

For patients who seek treatment in this country, yet come from an area where modesty is highly esteemed, the idea of a bodily examination of any sort may be one which has not been previously encountered. Allowances must be made for reluctance to comply with the Western medical model and the distress which will occur as a result of such a shock to the patient's cultural norms.

It is important, then, for the person involved in conducting the medical interview to be aware of sensitivities which exist, and whenever possible to take the opportunity to understand why modesty is so valued within so many cultures.

Altered body image and function

Since the beginning of time, people of diverse cultures have sought and found ways of altering their body image by many means and for various purposes. Of the many such rites, some were easy to initiate and transient in their effect. For example, the cutting of a lock of hair from a male child on the eighth day of life in early Semitic cultures. Other methods such as tattooing, body piercing or puberty initiation rites took much longer, were more painful, and had permanent results.

The circumcision of a male child, usually soon after birth, but in some cultural groups at puberty, was – and still is – probably the most commonly practised of all such rites, and is still a cause of great celebration among many cultures, especially those of the Jewish and Islamic communities. While such a practice is considered acceptable within most societies, many societies, especially in the West condemn its female counterpart, although according to the *World Health Organization Chronicle* [9], over 84 000 000 women worldwide are estimated to have undergone some form of genital mutilation. Whatever one feels about such birth or puberty initiation rites, their tradition and history are deeply rooted within a cultural ideal and are seen as desirable for many reasons.

Change of body image which is related to medical intervention and treatment is frequently treated with grave suspicion, and may well have a permanent effect on the way an individual is treated and accepted within his community. To try and understand why such suspicions occur, it is important to acquire some background knowledge about how the disease process is understood within different communities. What, for instance, determines an individual's status within a cultural hierarchy? According to Comeroff [10], 'illness of any kind constitutes a threat to the body of a patient and their understanding of themselves. If the illness is severe in nature, the change of status for the patient may be threefold: that of a movement of understanding from well person to patient to one who is less well and able than before'. Further, irrespective of cultural tradition or background, dysfunction of the body may disturb the harmony existing between physical, social and moral aspects of being. Change of body image or function may well become a constant reminder to the subject of the altered or dysfunctional state.

Some change of body image or function is inevitably involved when a patient undergoes bone-marrow transplantation. Hair loss from chemotherapy, infertility from total body irradiation and loss of weight during treatment are examples. Some of these may well be temporary, but changes such as infertility may be permanent and may cause individuals to alter their notions of themselves as useful beings, and to address changes in social roles and activities. This may well have a profound effect on the psychological outlook of the patient. However, for some patients, such changes also affect their social standing within both their family and community. Capacity for employment may be affected as may the ability to be financially independent or insurable. Also marriageability in communities where arranged marriage is practised can be influenced.

The needs of patients whose body image has been changed by such measures as amputation or stoma formation are well understood and supported, but for those whose body changes are hidden, perhaps by changes in fertility status, needs are often misunderstood and neglected.

In his book *Culture, Health and Illness*, Helman [11] suggests that cultural concepts surrounding the issue of body image may be perceived in the categories shown in Table 62.1.

Each of these three factors can influence, either singularly or plurally, the way in which both the patient and their family perceive the patient's altered status within a community. This altered status may be either permanent or temporary depending on the nature of the illness causing the change.

Within the realms of bone-marrow transplantation, one of the more obvious and often immediate changes which can affect a patient's self-image is that of hair loss. Visually, hair loss in women patients is often perceived by the carer as being more serious than for men, as many men tend to lose hair within the ageing process. This may not always be the case, however, and hair loss in men from the Sikh community, the Orthodox Jewish community or the Rastafarian community, may cause profound distress which is misunderstood and possibly underemphasized by carers. The loss of hair for many patients from ethnic minority groups mave have lasting effects on their psychological and spiritual conditions, as such a loss may be symbolic of a future which is bleak. It can also be a visible manifestation of a progressive and unrelenting disease process within.

The reassurance that hair usually regrows after chemotherapy may often not be as helpful as we imagine. Although temporary, this dramatic change may have permanent effects on the way that patients understand themselves. Many cultures ascribe great significance to hair. Watson [12] writes of the beliefs about hair function within traditional Cantonese society. It is commonly held that hair has both the ability to absorb life forces and also that it is a vehicle for the excretion of toxins arising from disease. For the patient and the family of a patient from such a community, there may well be concerns about the ability of the patient to recover from his disease when such an important medium for recovery is lost.

As previously stated, hair loss for members of the Sikh community may cause a profound sadness for patient and family. For members of the Sikh community, the integrity of the body is of great religious significance. According to Guru Gobind Singh [13]: 'Sikhs shall be in their natural form, that is, without loss of hair, and in the case of men, without loss of foreskin, in opposition to the ordinances of the Hindus and the Mohammedans.' Of the many significances of hair within the Sikh tradition, the most important is that it is a visible sign of the great gift of life which they are given. Uberoi [14] suggests that for Sikhs to lose hair is to be diminished as an individual, and for some, to experience diiminished status within the community. For a Sikh woman, her hair is a visible sign and barometer of her health and status. Furthermore, it is a visible statement of her beliefs and community identity. Loss of her hair, then, is a visible sign of her illness and, in terms of her role within a community or family, of her ability to bear children. After bone-marrow transplantation, this may well be the case.

Table 62.1 Cultural concepts concerning body image (after Helman 1992 [11]

- Beliefs about the optimal shape and size of the body, including clothing and surface decoration
- Beliefs about the inner structure of the body
- Beliefs about how the body functions

Beliefs about hair and its significance are not confined to Indian and Chinese communities. Leach [15], Strathern [16] and Soyinka [17] write independently about the variety of significances which hair conveys within the wide spectrum of African cultures. Hair loss is perceived in many African cultures as a sign of poor health or infertility. It is also seen as an indicator of hidden and sinister disease which may be the result of a curse or the breaching of a taboo. In such cases the patient's status within a community will almost certainly be diminished, occasionally to the point of ostracism. In such a traditionally centred community folk myths continue to play a part in the maintenance of cultural identity. Within certain sub-Saharan groups, one of the underlying fears attendant upon hair loss is that hair provides a barrier of protection from the harmful spirits of the air, and the loss of hair removes that protective barrier.

The care of hair for most black communities within the UK is a matter of great importance, and induced hair loss is a matter of concern. There is, however, one group for whom hair loss is of major religious significance. Although Rastafarianism is, in religious terms, a recent development [18], it has as its heart a very African orientation. Inspired by Marcus Garvey in Jamaica during the 1930s, the Rastafarian movement advocated pride in black consciousness, and growth of the movement was an inevitable consequence of unjust white domination of black society. Garvey exhorted his followers to look to Africa for the crowning of a black king as a sign for the redemption of the black community. The hope was realized when King Haile Selassie, the first King of Ethiopia was crowned. He was Ras Tafari. Thereafter, the movement grew rapidly through the Caribbean, white dominated countries of the Commonwealth in Africa, and within the UK and USA. The 'dreadlocks' became the outward sign of commitment to the movement, to Ras Tafari, the Lion of Judah. The dreadlocks became a symbol of the lion's mane, black dignity, and the right of the black person to become self-determining. The induced loss of hair is for some members of the Rastafarian community a surrender of their black freedom and dignity.

As previously mentioned, religion is one of the major determinants of cultural identity. This does not simply refer to the issue of whether a person practises a religion or not, but involves the often long intermingling of religion and culture in the establishment of group identiy. According to Spector [19], it is frequently difficult to distinguish between those aspects of a person's belief system arising from a religious background and those that stem from their ethnic and cultural heritage. This is certainly the case in terms of assessing the trauma of hair loss within sections of the Jewish, Christian and Muslim communities. The importance of hair, especially to women of 'peoples of the book' is attributed by some to the Old Testament reference to the fact that hair is the crowning glory of the woman. Although the custom within Orthodox Judaism is to have either very short or shorn hair, frequently covered by a wig, Jewish women from other traditions value their hair very highly.

Within the Christian tradition there is an enormous breadth of tradition and observance, but within the more austere traditions who interpret biblical teaching literally, there is enormous distress at the induced loss of hair, as it may be viewed by an individual as a sign of disfavour or punishment. Such groups include members of the Exclusive Brethren and Taylorite sects, who maintain a very insular community network.

Helman [11] writes that 'in every society, the human body has a social as well as a physical reality. That is, size, shape and adornment of the body are a way of communicating information about the owners status within society.' This statement supports the research of Freedman [20] who, in her study of hair loss in white women in American society, states 'hairstyle reflects a personal message about self concept and self identity . . . the loss of hair is an extremely traumatic experience precisely because it is the precursor to loss of self'.

Although the problems of hair loss are usually connected with the status and personhood of adult patients, when looking at such problems in relation to bone-marrow transplantation, one also needs to look at the effects on paediatric patients in terms of cultural status and identity. White, Western European society is by and large a self-determining or 'I' -centred culture. This is especially true when it comes to selecting partners for a permanent or married relationship. In many African, Arabic, Asian and Chinese communities this is not the case. The arranged marriage frequently remains the normal procedure, and complex interfamily negotiations take place to secure marriage for eligible offspring.

Of the many factors which are taken into account within the negotiations for arranged marriage, the main considerations are frequently the potential of the couple to continue a family line by producing children and the intactness of the bodies of potential partners. Dowry payment, which is the property or money which the bride brings with her into the marriage, is the subject of intense negotiation, and is still common practice within Middle Eastern, Indian and some South Asian communities. Part of dowry negotiation is dependent on scrutiny of family lines, especially the potential to produce male children. Bridewealth, which is a more common practice in sub-Saharan Africa, is that payment which the potential groom takes into the bride's family upon betrothal, but the potential liaison is subject to similar scrutiny.

Scott [21] writes: 'in many races it is customary for betrothal to take place during infancy, and indeed there are some instances where this occurs at the moment of birth. In such instances, of course, the arrangements are made either directly by parents or through a professional matchmaker'. These early arrangements will enable families to begin the process of either paying dowry or bridewealth, or at least setting aside wealth to finance the arranged marriage when it happens.

In the case of the child who has been rendered sterile by bone-marrow transplant-related issues, a declaration of infertility may incur financial penalty for the parents, or at least loss of status within their cultural community. A similar situation may apply in the case of arranged bridewealth.

Although hair loss is the most obvious of the alterations to body image in the process of bone-marrow transplantation, other factors should be considered. Skin changes as a result of graft-versus-host disease may be of a permanent or semi-permanent nature, and scarring from Hickman line insertion or similar access devices may cause permanent, albeit minimal, scarring. Such scarring, especially in young girls, is of concern to parents, especially when scars are is in the area of a potentially developing breast. In many cultures, notably the Cantonese and Vietnamese, breast integrity is vitally important. Watson [12] writes of the importance of breast milk in traditional Chinese society as an essential part of preparation of an infant for growth in the world of disease. The integrity of the breast is important in that it is a sign to both the woman and her partner that all is well within: it is barometer of good health. Scarring or deformation of the breast is conversely a sign that all is not well, and that the bearer of such marks may not be the ideal mother. Beliefs in the regenerative power of breast milk are not confined to Chinese or Vietnamese cultures; similar beliefs about breast integrity are held within some African cultures, as are those of the magical powers of breast milk.

Strathern [16] writes of the parallel symbolism of the power of semen which is the creative element in the production of children. This power continues to be passed to the neonate through the breast milk of the mother. The life force is perceived as cyclical, from father to mother, mother to boy child.

The possibility for infertility, then, is also a major issue for the parents of a male child, especially if he is either the oldest or an only son. If parents are involved in bridewealth negotiations, the financial burden of withdrawing from a marriage contract may be ruinous. Although such issues apply in the main to cultures where arranged marriage is the norm, iatrogenic infertility of a son continues to have major repercussions on family status in groups where no such arrangements apply.

Profound grief reactions have been observed in families from Mediterranean countries, when it has been learned that the oldest or only son will be infertile as a result of treatment. The mother of such a male child will frequently blame herself for his condition, and see his infertile state as a reflection of her defectiveness. It has also been observed that both young men and women from some Mediterranean communities, who prior to treatment have been engaged to be married, have terminated their relationship. This was not because of a desire to seek a new partner, but rather to allow the fit partner to proceed with a relationship where the birth of a family would be more likely.

When a male patient is likely to be rendered sterile and he is post-pubertal, the issue of sperm banking is important as the hope of a future family may be an important factor in his psychologial well-being . There are problems with this procedure, however, and these will be dealt with briefly below in the discussion on religious considerations.

Cultural influence on the behaviour of pain and distress

'Pain,' writes Morrell [22], 'is in one form or another, an inseparable part of everyday life. It is also probably the commonest symptom encountered in clinical practice.' Pain in some form or another has been experienced by almost everyone, yet its presentation is uniquely individual. It is well understood that pain is not simply a neurophysiological process, but an experience which occurs at the amalgamation of a variety of factors. It may be that pain which results from a minor injury is localized, and that the neurophysiological response is most dominant, but where a disease process is more life threatening, a greater variety of factors play increasingly important parts in the way that a patient and the patients family display pain behaviour.

Much has been written about the variety of factors which intermingle to produce what we define as pain. Physical, psychological, spiritual, social and financial aspects all play their part. However, the cultural and historical facets of the patient's background should also be taken into account. Helman writes 'not all social and cultural groups respond to pain in the same way; how people respond to and perceive pain, both in themselves and in others can be largely influenced by their cultural background. How and whether people communicate their pain to health care professionals and to others may also be influenced by cultural factors' [11]. These words must be taken seriously. If they are not, then the accusation of an ethnocentric and exclusive approach to healthcare is justified. Further, in the interpretation of pain behaviour, and the patient's needs in terms of assistance, the fact that health carers also come from a variety of different cultural and ethnic backgrounds may well make precise needs difficult to deal with.

In their study of attitudes to pain in patients with similar illness, Davitz and Samesima [23] invited 554 nurses from six ethnic groups to answer a complex questionnaire about pain in their patient subjects. Among the many interesting propositions and conclusions drawn from the study, the following is most pertinent to this section. Japanese and Chinese nurses believed that their patients suffered from a greater degree of physical pain than their Caucasian and Hispanic counterparts. This caused surprise in the Caucasian group who hitherto had thought that a feature of the oriental demeanour was to suffer physical pain with stoicism and lack of emotion. Caucasian and Hispanic nurses thought that oriental patients were less prone to pain, whereas oriental nurses indicated that oriental patients were more prone to pain.

The above illustrates well the frequent misunderstandings which we hold about the behaviour of people from other cultures, and also how 'public' pain display is interpreted. Within oriental society, great value is placed upon control of expressive behaviour, and children may well be taught from early childhood to control expression of feelings. This does not mean that pain is absent, and with sympathetic and gentle negotiation, it is possible to enable the patient to admit to pain without any loss of personal discipline.

Interestingly, the converse of the above study of physical pain was true, when psychological issues surrounding pain were assessed by the same group of nurses. Thus, although all shared a common goal, that of high-quality care with pain in all its manifestations well controlled and understood, the interpretation of how these aims were to be achieved was markedly different.

According to Fabrega and Tyma [24]: 'Pain behaviour includes changes in facial expresssion, grimaces and changes in demeanor or activity, as well as certain sounds made by the victim, or words used to describe the condition or appeal for help.' This may be the case generally, but when one examines cultural understandings of pain, it can be observed that in some cultures pain behaviour may be displayed in the absence of physical pain, or conversely, persons do not exhibit what we would consider normal reactions to painful events. To clarify this apparent conflict, it is useful to look at two types of pain behaviour, or reactions to pain, those of private and public pain displays.

Engel [25] stresses that pain is often 'private data', in other words, for carers to be aware of a patient's pain or distress they are dependent on the type and level of signalling which the patient conveys either verbally or non-verbally. When this happens, the private perception and experience of pain become a social or public event; private pain becomes public pain. In some circumstances, the pain that a patient is suffering may remain a private event, totally interiorized by the sufferer. This form of reaction is present in those societies which place high value on stoicism and fortitude, including the Oriental cultures as mentioned above, and some sections of the white community where the 'stiff upper lip' reaction in the presence of pain, distress and grief is highly valued. Similarly, those who are unable to communicate with ease in the language of the carer may sometimes be assumed not to be in any pain or distress. The absence of pain behaviour as we understand it within our society does not mean the absence of private pain in those societies for whom we care.

It is with the interpretation of public pain expression that carers play a major role. The degree of comfort which the patient may experience may depend upon the carer's reaction to and help with such pain. By his or her understanding of the social and cultural expectations of patients' in relation to their disease, carers will be able to offer either poor- or high-quality care.

Undoubtedly, pain behaviour, particularly in its voluntary aspects, is highly influenced by psychological, social and cultural factors. These determine whether private pain becomes manifest as public pain. Further, the form such behaviour takes is dependent upon the social setting of the patient, and the degree of confidence the patient has in his or her new environment. An additional and important factor which deserves consideration is the patient's ability to translate private into public pain, the significance that the patient attaches to the pain and whether the pain is considered to be 'normal' or 'abnormal'. Zbrowski [26] writes: 'a culture's expectations and acceptance of pain as a normal part of life will determine whether it is seen as a clinical problem requiring a clinical solution'.

If it is accepted that cultural backgound exercises an influence on the nature, understanding and expression of pain, it can be appreciated that those caring for patients in the field of bone-marrow transplantation should be open and mindful to differing pain displays and attitudes to suffering. This is essential to provide an optimal level of care. Each culture or ethnic group possesses its own language of distress. Members of such groups have their own ways of signalling both in verbal and non-verbal ways to show that pain and or distress are present. Both the form of pain behaviour and/our response to it have a cultural component. Landy [27] writes: 'pain behaviour depends on whether the individual's culture values or disvalues the display of emotional expression as a response to pain'.

Those who are involved in the care of patients should be aware of both the differences and the similarities in pain behaviour within diverse ethnic groups and, with such awarenes and acute observation, sensitivity to patients of a cultural group different to our own can be enhanced and care become more effective. As Brink [28] states: 'healing does not take place in a clinical vacuum'.

Stereotyping of pain behaviour within particular ethnic groups should be avoided. Healthcare professionals should recognize the needs of others in what is basically a white-orientated health service. Mares [29] describes the effective healthcare professional as 'one who is equipped with knowledge and appreciation of diversity of values and beliefs'. Only when one is equipped in such a way will effective understanding and control of pain in patients from ethnic groups different to our own exist at an optimal level.

Cultural and spiritual aspects of pain and pain display are interwoven at a very deep level in the person's understanding of his personhood. Although the individual may not exercise, practise or ritualize his or her faith, customs, family and community expectations are very important. Within the various religious traditions that exist, there may be patients from the Buddhist tradition who refuse pain control simply on religious grounds. This refusal is part of the patient's desire to remain wholly in control of his being, an important feature of the concept of living the life of Buddhist awareness. Swerdlow and Stjernsward [30] make a similar point about the desire of some Hindu patients to refuse pain control and 'quietly accept pain' so that the balance of karma is not disturbed. Other patients may refuse analgesia for a variety of personal reasons.

Relatives may express the pain for some patients from ethnic minority groups, either by requesting pain control or by displaying overt pain behaviour. The white Western concept of 'self' is usually expressed in terms of independence from a community, whereas the concept of 'self' in Chinese, Indian, African, Arabic, Caribbean and Mediterranean communities is frequently expressed in terms of interdependence on an extended family or community. Decision-making is often shared by the patient with other members of the family and social group. The patient may wish to be surrounded by as many members of the family as possible at times of consultation, treatment and pain, so that the experience can be shared throughout the family.

Constant visitors, often asking questions or seeking attention, must be accepted by those who care for patients from ethnic minority groups as normal pain behaviour. It is rarely a desire to be disruptive, but is born out of true compassion for a sick relative or friend. Also, to be accepted by carers is that behaviour of pain or distress may be displayed by relatives, especially if the patient is isolated, and his or her physical demeanour is markedly changed. It is rare for hospitals to have a place where disorientated and emotionally vulnerable families can be offered support, or even a degree of privacy from others who may be in a similar situation. Laussaniere and Auzanneau [31] write that developing palliative care within a haematology department 'calls for a number of preliminary factors, among them ensuring the patient's participation in decisions which concern them, giving information and support to the family, and assessing the psychological effects of informing patients of their diagnosis'. In an ideal world, these factors should come into play at the beginning of a treatment programme, and not at the palliative stage.

Ouaknin [32] writes: 'the ethics of caring are the ethics of a caress; the caressing hand remains open, never tightening its grip, never "getting hold of"; it touches without pressing, it moves obeying the shape of the caressed body'. This statement certainly offers a model for the understanding and control of pain within the haematological setting.

Table 62.2 shows the principal areas which may cause concern for different ethnic groups.

Religious considerations

As previously stated, cultural and religious issues relating to understanding of the disease process and its treatment are interwoven at a very deep level. Although the individual patient may not exercize, practise or ritualize his or her faith, customs and community expectations are nevertheless very

Table 62.2 Issues of concern for patients from different ethnic backgrounds when undergoing bone-marrow transplantation

- Diet
- Blood product transfusion
- Hair loss
- Sterility
- Body scars
- Body image changes
- Necessity for removing sacred garments
- Modesty issues
- Origin of medications

significant. Neuberger [33] writes: 'labels are important. It is not uncommon to find people who describe themselves as agnostic Jews, Muslims, or Hindus, but cultural roots are very important, regardless of beliefs or current religious practice'.

Within this section, it is intended to give a brief introduction to the major religious faiths, and also to annotate areas where blood or blood products may be problematic for patients or relatives. The religions are presented in alphabetical order.

Baha'i

The Baha'i religion was founded in Iran in 1863 when Baha'u'llah declared himself to be the new prophet proclaimed by the 'Bab'. Bab (literally 'Gate to the Truth') had been one of the leaders of the millenarian 'Babi' movement in Iran. Although the roots of Baha'i are steeped firmly in the Shi'a Islamic tradition, the millenarian movement was hounded and persecuted in Iran because of the radically modernizing ideas that it embraced. Bab was executed in 1850 in an attempt to suppress what was seen as a heretical Islamic sect. Contrary to expectations, the Baha'i movement continued to flourish, and after the 1863 declaration by Baha'u'llah, the Baha'i faith began to grow outside Iran. It is now estimated that there are more than five million followers of the Baha'i faith worldwide.

Although Baha'is accept that Jesus and Mohammed were prophets, they hold that the identity of God must be retaught through prophecy in each generation. One of the main ideals of Baha'i is the belief in a spiritual pilgrimage which will unite the world as a global community, and share a common language.

There is no formal ministry within the Baha'i faith, and the teachings stress the right of equality for women. Monogamous family life is a social ideal, although the community is very supportive towards those who divorce. For the practising Baha'i, daily prayers are an important part of their observance, and frequently patients wish family or friends to be with them at this time of prayer. The most important date within the Baha'i religious calendar is 21 March, the Baha'i New Year (Nawruz). Some Baha'is wish to fast prior to the New Year celebrations. The period of fasting begins on 2 March and food is not consumed between dawn and dusk.

Diet is a matter of personal choice although alcohol is not taken. There are no ethical problems for Baha'i patients with regard to blood products. Blood donation and organ donation is actively encouraged by Baha'i assemblies. Sperm banking is a matter of personal choice, but it is not prohibited. Patients of the Baha'i faith derive from a large number of ethnic groups so it is likely that some patients may follow certain cultural behaviour patterns in addition to the requirements of religious practice.

Buddhism

Buddhism is a philosophy and an ethical system which has its origins in the Hindu world of India about 600 years CE. There are many sects within Buddhism, but the two main groups are the Mahayana school which is prevalent in China and Japan and the Theravada school prevalent in South-East Asia. Like many other religions, Buddhist practice is influenced by the cultures within which it exists. Specific religious practices are prayer, chanting and meditation. Some Buddhists may fast on the first and fifteenth days of the month (full and new moon), but for some the fast may simply mean abstaining from meat.

There are a considerable number of Buddhists who adopt either a vegetarian or vegan diet, but this is much a matter of choice. Although there has always been a fascination with the Buddhist way in the West, it was not until the latter part of this century that significant numbers of Caucasians converted to Buddhism.

Some Buddhists will refuse pain control of any kind as it 'clouds the mind' and will possibly prevent the achievement of nirvana, the higher state of understanding which exists when the eternal cycle of life and death is broken. Although there are no specifically religious problems associated with blood or blood products, Dinh and Ganesan [34] suggest that Vietnamese patients may fear blood tests that require even small samples of blood, mainly because they believe that the body contains a finite and irreplaceable amount of blood.

Lai and Yue [35] make similar observations about Kampuchean, Laotian and Chinese patients because of the belief that loss of blood will weaken their bodies, and may even be life-threatening: 'In the Chinese culture, loss of blood may be connected with the loss of "Chi" which is thought of as a finite substance within the body and is contained in the blood.' Ho [3] suggests that the offering of a red drink such as cranberry juice may alleviate some of the patient's anxieties. He also makes the point that 'these particular groups have high levels of fear about contagion'.

Sperm banking is a matter of personal choice; there are no specific regulations which condemn the practice.

Many Buddhists are wary of donating blood or bone marrow, which is partly a philosophical ideal of keeping the body inviolate and also a cultural issue for many as explained above.

Christianity

Just as many Christians view other faiths as homogeneous, united faiths, so many non-Christians have this view of Christianity. This not the case. The diversity of Christian belief and practice varies greatly. The three main strands of observance may be said to be the Orthodox tradition, the Roman Catholic tradition and the Reformed tradition, but this is a simplistic division. Within the Orthodox tradition, each patriarchate has a degree of autonomy which means a variety of liturgical practice and tradition. The Roman Catholic tradition, although having the most Christian churches, and being essentially united in practice and belief through the authority of the Pope, has major variations in liturgical practice throughout the world. It often embraces the richness of indigenous culture within its ceremony. In the Reformed tradition, which includes the Church of England and the 'Free' churches, there probably exists the widest variance in belief and practice, from the essentially liberal 'Middle Church of England' to the biblical fundamentalist and literalist schools of the Pentecostal and Charismatic movements. It would be impossible in a section such as this to define each of the denominational practices and the variations within their beliefs. It is important for the persons reponsible for patient care to investigate with sensitivity any particular problems which the patient may have or forsee. The following is a summary of issues which may arise from patients within the 'Christian' umbrella.

Sperm banking for male patients may be a problem for some; the more traditional interpretations of both the Orthodox and Catholic churches teach that masturbation is an unnatural act, and that conception should only be accomplished through penetrative intercourse. For many men, however, the possibility of becoming a father after treatment means that they will follow their own conscience. Similar restrictions on sperm banking may also apply to males from charismatic and literalist traditions including some Pentecostal and Brethren groups especially the Exclusive Brethren, who hold to the Old Testament concept that 'spilling one's seed' is an abomination in the sight of God.

Chemotherapy-induced hair loss has posed problems for female members of the Brethren groups. The hair of the women in such groups usually remains uncut (or long), is partially covered by a headsquare, and is perceived to be her 'crowning glory'. Loss of hair may be interpreted as a sign of God's disfavour or punishment. This will be compounded if , as a result of treatment, the woman is also rendered infertile.

Some of the Charismatic and Fundamentalist Christian congregations are very concerned about methods used in the development of drugs, and may ask if any of the drugs which they are to receive have been developed either through animal experiments or by using human tissue. Usually members of such groups are very well-informed and may use such questions to test the honesty of those who will be responsible for their care.

Problems associated with blood products are usually culturally based, although some patients may seek reassurance that blood from unrelated sources has tested negative for HIV.

Many Christians will be willing donors of blood or bone marrow, but the more futuristic Christian groups such as the Exclusive Brethren and similar small groups are usually unwilling unless the blood is for a member of their own group, and only then after much serious thought and prayer.

Christian Science

If the Christian Science patient is in hospital voluntarily, it is likely that he or she will accept minimal conventional treatment, and will request that any medical treatment be kept to a minimum. Usually the patient will be in contact with a Christian Science practitioner who will offer support and advice.

It is unlikely that a Christian Scientist would consent to any treatment which altered the body image, as members of this group wish to keep the body inviolate. Members of the Christian Science movement are also unlikely to accept blood products or to donate them.

Children of Christian Scientists fall under the provision of the Children's Act 1989. Therefore, parents would be unable to stop treatment on their child that was deemed essential by medical practitioners.

Hinduism

Hinduism is the probably the most difficult of the major religions to define. Unlike other faiths, it did not have a single founder. As Sen states [36]: 'It grew gradually over a period of five thousand years, absorbing and assimilating all the religious and cultural movements in India.' Hinduism possesses many authorative scriptures, but none is exclusive. Hinduism [36] is 'more like a tree that has grown gradually, than like a building which has been erected by some great architect at a particular point in time'.

In Hinduism, all particular religious truths are manifestations of the One Truth. Krishna declares in The *Bhagavad Gita* [37]: 'however men approach me, even so do I accept them; for on all sides, whatever path they may choose is mine'. The knowledge and acceptance of this vital truth is the ultimate inner mystical experience which Hindus express in their regular prayers, 'from delusion lead me to truth, from darkness lead me to light, from death lead me to immortality' [38].

As a way of life, the path of Hinduism is both eclectic and syncretic. It has no problems selecting and absorbing elements from other religious traditions and adapting them. Hinduism is essentially a faith of India rooted in India's cultural, literal and philosophical history and tradition.

Hindu practices and customs vary a great deal depending on the area of origin, the significance of caste and local deities within a specific area. Nicholls [39] suggests that Hinduism is a social system as well as a set of beliefs. Many Hindus are vegetarians, some are vegan, usually women. Fasting on a regular basis, especially Holy Days, is performed mostly by women. Fasting may vary from a strict fast to the consumption of 'pure' foods such as fruit and yoghurt.

Qureshi [4] makes the point that hospital staff should be aware that chapatis which are a staple of many people from the Indian subcontinent, are made from flour which contains phytic acid and binds with serum calcium to form calcium phytate. This substance is excreted, and consequently serum calcium levels may fall and calcium absorption is inhibited.

Although the majority of Hindus are vegetarians, some eat meat, but not beef which is from a sacred animal, or pork which is considered unclean and from a scavenging animal. Strict Hindus may enquire about the origin of drugs used in their treatment and be especially concerned about accepting those which have been developed using either porcine or bovine products.

Jewellery worn by Hindus often has both religious and ornamental significance. Gold worn next to the skin is believed to ward off disease. Both men and women wear jewellery, and those of Brahmin caste, a sacred thread (janeu) over the right shoulder and around the body. Patients wearing such articles may be reluctant to remove them and, if these are removed, they will require assurance that they will be treated with reverence, respect and care. This is particularly important when preparing a patient for total body irradiation and its effects.

Blood transfusions and bone-marrow transplants are usually acceptable, although some Hindus, especially women, have anxieties about donating either blood or bone marrow. This is normally a cultural issue concerned with weakness caused by loss of blood. Some Hindu women also have great anxiety about induced alopecia, as it may be seen as a sign of punishment or disfavour.

Some older Hindu women are very self-conscious about medical examination as they possess religious tattoos, sometimes around the neck, or upper chest, but more frequently on the forearms. These tattoos are most common in Hindus from Gujarat [4] and most often centre around what at first appear to be swastikas. These symbols are, in fact, sacred symbols representing the name of God in Hindi script, and are the reverse of the infamous swastika.

Traditional Hindu medicine such as Ayurvedic practice may be used by patients alongside Western medicine.

Humanism

In an increasingly secular society, more people are calling themselves Humanists. The *Oxford Dictionary of Peoples and Cultures* suggests that 'humanism is an outlook of a kind which in some sense places people at the centre of the universe'. This implies and means, in fact, that humanism is by definition open to individual interpretation of great variety.

No specific theory of humanism exists, but a world view which claims that the only source of value in creation is humanity may be called humanist. In some ways humanism opposes religious belief by virtue of the fact that humanism accepts that humans can be perfected. In this way humanism also has connexions with individualism as a philosophy of life. The first articulate writings concerning humanist thought were written by the Dutch humanist Erasmus in the fifteenth century. Some commentators would suggest that Marx could be more accurately described as a humanist. Existentialism, which has emerged both within both secular and religious societies in the twentieth century is also a form of humanist thought.

In relation to medical treatment there is no constant line of thought running through the humanist view. Although humanism by some definitions would possess a very utilitarian ethic in terms of medical care, many individuals who have adopted the humanist label are very sensitive about such issues as animal experimentation in pharmacological research and are well informed about such issues. As individualism is a major feature in humanist observance, careful and sensitive enquiry concerning the individual's needs are required of medical staff.

Islam

Nicholls [39] states that the religion of Islam 'is one of the outstanding phenomena of history. Within a century of the death of its founder, the muslim empire stretched from Southern France, through Spain, North Africa, the Levant and Central Asia to the margins of China'. Although Islam is not a major religion in white Western Europe, it has continued to advance through Africa, India and South-East Asia.

Many of the migrant communities within Western Europe espouse the Muslim faith. There are now estimated to be some 800 000 000 followers of Islam throughout the world.

In common with other major faiths, Islam is not a homogeneous faith in that there are various groups within it. It is influenced by the culture within which it is set. The two main Islamic groups are those of the Shi'a and Sunni schools which consititute by far the majority of Muslims worldwide. Parallel to both schools is the smaller, but important Sufi or mystical tradition of Islam. All these groups fully accept the Koran as their teaching, although interpretation may be different in certain areas. Several splinter groups emerged from the Shi'a school over the centuries, the influential Isma'lis who are not accepted as true Muslims by the mainstream of Islam being the most numerous. Over the centuries various groups also emerged from the Sunni school. The most numerous, though tiny in comparison to the major schools of Islam, is the Ahmadiyya movement centred in Kashmir which again is not accepted as true Islam.

As with all other religions, there are varying degrees of adherence to the tenets of Islam, so some of the special considerations which are listed below will not necessarily apply to all patients of the faith. Adult Muslims are required to pray five times a day. These prayers are preceded by ritual ablutions which require running water. There is an obligation to fast between dawn and dusk during the holy month of Ramadan, the ninth month of the Muslim calendar. Although people who are ill are exempted from this obligation, many devout Muslims wish to observe the fast. Some pious Muslims will refuse injections or eye drops during periods of fast though there is no religious ruling on the matter. It is helpful to Muslim patients if a compass is available to determine the direction of the Holy City of Mecca from the hospital where they are a patient.

Muslims are forbidden to eat the flesh of the pig in any form. Other meat can be eaten provided it is *halal*, or ritually slaughtered in the way prescribed by Islamic law. Alcohol is forbidden.

Depending on the tradition and adherence to the Islamic faith, sexual segregation is exercised and many Muslims would prefer to be examined and cared for by members of the same sex. Both men and women are required to dress modestly, and sometimes, particularly where Muslim women are concerned, this is perceived by Westerners to be taken to extremes. This may be a source of contention, when many people involved in healthcare would be perceived by modestly attired Muslims as being immodestly clad and therefore lacking authority or being deserving of respect. Some Muslim women will be reluctant to remove jewellery as this holds both cultural and economic significance.

Hair loss for some is seen as loss of status and a source of shame. Women who are menstruating may be seen as unclean by their male partners so will not be visited during this time. Female circumcision is practised in some Muslim countries. This is not a religious practice, but culturally based. However, women who have experienced genital mutilation are often reluctant to undergo intimate examination, particularly if they are aware of the attitude to this practice in the West.

In many Muslim countries where arranged marriages are the normal practice, there will be much concern about changed body image in children who are being treated by bone-marrow transplantation. Main concerns will be about scarring and changes in fertility status.

There are no specific rulings prohibiting blood transfusions or use of blood products although some reluctance may occur when male-to-female sibling donation is suggested.

Some Muslims may enquire about methods used in development of drugs used, the main concerns being about either use of porcine products or human tissue. Abortion is forbidden in Islamic law, as is sperm banking. The latter may well cause great distress to unmarried males and their families, particularly if they are either an oldest or an only son. The continuation of a family line is very important within many Islamic social groups.

Jainism

There are some three million adherents to the Jainist religion and philosophy found mainly within the Indian states of Gujarat and Maharashtra, and there are a substantial number of Jainists within the UK, mainly in London. The Jainist philosophy of non-violence emerged from the teaching of the twenty-four conquerors or *jinas*, the last and greatest being Mahavira who lived about 550 years BC. Central to Jainist thought is the concept of 'Ahimsa', or respect for all life. This concept demands strict vegetarianism and prohibits any action which causes suffering to any living creature or plant. This means that diet in the strictest of Jains is limited to vegetable products and the plant must not be killed or damaged by its removal.

Although relatively small in size, the Jainist faith has exercised a major influence in India's history, particularly in the case of Gandhi's non-violent movements. Although many Jainists are involved in the healthcare professions, the strictest adherents of the faith would probably not wish to receive major interventions into their illness.

Bone-marrow transplantation may well be refused on the grounds that it would cause pain to the donor and even shorten the donor's life. Diet would equally be problematic, unless relatives provided all the patient's food. Concerns about origins of drugs used may also cause ethical dilemmas for the more devout. Jainism is tolerant towards other religions, is not in any way evangelical, and seeks peaceful coexistence between all peoples.

The devout Jain patient who is seriously or terminally ill may with the permission of family and spiritual elders take a vow of 'Sallekhana' which is a ritual fast preparing them for and leading them to death. The taking of such a vow is of great importance to the patient and the patient's family and is of great spiritual merit.

Jehovah's Witnesses

Of all blood product taboos, those of the Jehovah's Witnesses are most widely known by staff involved in healthcare. According to the precepts of the Watch Tower Bible and Tract Society, any treatment which includes the use of blood products is according to Singelenberg [40] 'a transgression of divine precepts. Additionally, in the judgement of believers, secular proof [of this transgression] is abundant these days, AIDS is a powerful justification to abstain from blood'. Singelenberg's article gives both history and detail surrounding such pronouncements, and is a comprehensive document.

It is therefore unlikely that a memeber of the Jehovah's Witnesses would present themselves for a bone-marrow transplant. However, pressure may be exerted upon non-Witness members of a family where such a treatment has been accepted, and in the case of children of Jehovah's Witness families, the provisions of the Children's Act 1989 would require enforcing. It has been noted on occasion that where this has been enforced, children who have received treatment have been rejected by their families.

Judaism

The Jewish faith is the oldest of the three 'religions of the book', the other two being Christianity and Islam. In addition to being members of a particular faith, many Jews also consider themselves as part of a distinct ethnic group. Most Jews in the UK originated from Eastern and Central Europe and migrated to this country during the nineteenth and twentieth centuries. However, there are small Jewish communities from several countries who have migrated or sought refugee status within the last fifty years. These include Jews from Turkey, Cyprus, Yemen and Ethiopia.

As with other religions, there are varying degrees of adherence and practice by individuals and there are also cultural accretions which are not necessarily Jewish in nature. Some members of the Jewish community have abandoned all ritual practices.

The vast majority of the Jewish community in the UK (over 95%) speak English, although Yiddish is spoken by older members of the community and members of the Orthodox religious (Hasidic) group. Depending on country of origin, other languages such as Polish or Hungarian may be spoken.

The three main traditions within the Jewish community are the Orthodox, Liberal and Reform traditions. While members of the Orthodox group obey the laws of the Torah and the Rabbinic tradition strictly, the Liberal and Reform traditions make concessions to a modern lifestyle.

The Sabbath, the Jewish Holy Day, begins at sunset on Friday and ends on Saturday evening. The Sabbath is both an important religious and family occasion, and for non-practising Jews the Sabbath is often kept as a special family time. For Orthodox Jews, no work of any kind is done on the Sabbath.

For some very devout Jewish patients, the fast prior to Yom Kippur (the Day of Atonement) is kept so strictly that alternatives to oral medication may be necessary.

Modesty is important for many members of the Jewish community and for Orthodox Jews it is essential to preserve modesty. It is immodest for men to touch women other than their wives, so it is preferred by Orthodox women to have female carers. Orthodox men likewise prefer to be attended by males. Women may wish to keep their hair covered at all times and men may also either wear a *yarmulke* or skullcap, or in some cases a shawl. All practising Jews observe a Jewish dietary regulations to some degree. Pork and its derivatives, shellfish and fish without fins and scales are prohibited. Other meat is permitted provided it is kosher, i.e. slaughtered and prepared according to Jewish law. Orthodox Jews will wish to eat a kosher diet, which is prepared in a special kitchen containing separate utensils for the preparation of meat dishes and those which contain dairy products. Meat and dairy products must not be served simultaneously, nor within several hours of each other.

As Judaism is a very life-affirming faith, most patients will accept medication without question. However, some patients may wish to consult their rabbi in consultation with their doctor when a treatment is either a trial, or if the medication concerned has a porcine derivation. The patient's right to self-determination has long been a subject for debate among Hebrew scholars and it continues to be so. Sinclair [41] writes: 'it is noteworthy that Rabbi Yisraeli is one of the few *halakhic* commentators who recognises a person's right to their own body. The majority of authorities are of the opinion that people hold their bodies in trust from God, and hence patient autonomy is not a legitimate value in Jewish tradition'. (Rabbi Yisraeli's position is cited in *Biomedical Legal Decisions* 194 [Heb], Israel Medical Association, Tel Aviv, 1989.)

Blood transfusions and blood products are permitted for Jewish patients, but Jews of the Orthodox tradition are unlikely to donate such products unless they are for members of their own families – definitely not for gentiles.

As the Jewish faith is family-centred, infertility caused by preparation for bone-marrow transplantation is a great sadness for the family, particularly when it involves an oldest or only son. Sperm banking is not permitted by Jewish law, and will not be undertaken by members of the Orthodox community. Some members of the other traditions may well donate sperm for banking, but such a decision is likely to be made in consultation with family and rabbi.

In the case of children undergoing treatment, Jewish families will invariably give support to all attempts by medical staff to halt or cure the disease.

Rastafarianism

Brief mention has already been made about members of the Rastafarian faith and its origins. The following points, however, are pertinent to the care of Rastafarian patients. Rastafarians will not eat any product of the pig and many are vegetarians. Usually, only natural food is eaten and tinned or preserved food is eschewed. Blood or blood products are normally refused, although some Rastafarians may consider receiving such products from members of their own families. Many Rastafarians are reluctant to take western medicines, especially if they feel that these will contaminate or damage their bodies. Hair loss in chemotherapy is an example of such a fear.

Maintainance of modesty is very important especially for women. Women prefer to be examined by carers of the same sex. Children of strictly devout Rastafarian families may come under the provisions of the Children's Act 1989.

Sikhism

The word 'Sikh', from the sanskrit *shishya* meaning 'pupil', describes a monotheistic faith which has its origins in both the Hindu and Islamic traditions of India. Sikhism teaches an equality of people and rejects the caste system. Uberoi [42] states 'the custom of wearing long and unshorn hair [*kes*] is among the most cherished and distinctive signs of an individual's membership of the Sikh path, and it always seems to have been so. This distinctive anti-depilatory injunction was established early as one of the four taboos that are impressed upon the neophyte at the ceremony of initiation into Sikhism'. Unshorn hair is one of the five symbols of Sikh identity. The other four are the comb, the bracelet, special undergarments and the sword (usually miniature). All these symbols possess great significance and there may be a marked reluctance by members of the Sikh faith to remove them. Sensitive negotiation, with assurance that good care will be taken of the objects, will usually reassure the patient, as removal is vital when scans or total body irradiation are undertaken.

Maintaining modesty is important for Sikh patients, and women especially prefer to be examined and cared for by the same sex. Removal of the *kaccha* or special underwear worn by many may be done with reluctance and a desire to replace the garment as quickly as possible. As with other faiths there are degrees of adherence to the precepts of Sikhism, and this applies especially to diet. While many devout Sikhs eat a vegetarian diet, many Sikhs eat most foods without demur, as long as none of the foods consumed are offensive to others with whom they are eating.

Hair loss induced by medical treatment may be the cause of profound sadness to members of the Sikh faith, but such a loss does not usually prevent the patient from undergoing treatment. It is a matter of personal choice, as is the issue of sperm banking. There is no objection to the use of blood products within the Sikh tradition.

Zoroastrianism (Parsi)

Of Zorastrianism, Zaehner [43] writes: 'the religion of Zoroaster has today almost vanished from the face of the earth, and is now professed by less than 120 000 souls'. Although this may be the case, it was the national religion of the Persian Empire from the third to the seventh century CE, and it is still practised by an influential minority in India, particularly around Bombay, and in London. The Parsi community in London migrated to the UK mainly from former colonies in East Africa, where they were very influential in commerce and trade, notably the spice trade in Zanzibar.

Children are initiated into the faith between the ages of seven and fifteeen, and it is at this time that the sacred shirt (*sadra*) and girdle (*kusti*) are worn for the first time. These garments, which are worn at all times, are treated with great respect. Sensitivity is required when these articles are removed for medical examination.

Parsis maintain a very high standard of personal hygiene and running water is always preferred. A high standard of modesty is also preserved. Although there are no particular dietary restrictions, some Parsis elect to be vegetarians, and some will eat only vegetables whilst in hospital. Blood transfusion and bone-marrow transplantation are not permitted by the Parsi faith as they are considered pollutant and therefore against the will of God. Less orthodox members, however, may permit such procedures. Children of orthodox families may fall under the provisions of the Children's Act 1989.

As preservation of genetic purity is important to members of the Parsi faith, and marriage outside the faith is not permitted, any treatment which may render a patient sterile, especially one who is unmarried, may well be refused.

Conclusion

This chapter is intended only as an introductory guide to the complexeties of cultural and religious issues which may be relevant for patients undergoing bone-marrow transplanation. It is not intended to be an exhaustive study, nor does it contain many of the more esoteric beliefs about blood which abound in many of the worlds cultures. However, it is hoped that it may both introduce and explain some of the more commonly held beliefs, and also give some explanation for the more common taboos.

References

1. Taylor EB. *Primitive Culture; Research into the Development of Mythology, Philosophy, Art and Customs*, 1871 (London: John Murray).
2. Poliakoff M. Cancer and cultural attitudes. In: *Health and Cultures*, Vol 1. R Masi, L Mensah and K Macleod (eds), 1995 (Ontario: Mosaic Press).
3. Ho AKH. *Report on the Study Assessing the Needs of Ethnic Chinese Patients*, 1990. (Vancouver: Canadian Cancer Society).
4. Quereshi B. *Transcultural Medicine*, 1994 (Dordrecht: Kluwer Academic).
5. Szasz T. *The Myth of Mental Illness*, 1961. (London: Harper and Row).
6. Volosinov VN. Freudianism. *A Marxist Critique*, 1976. (London: Academic Press).
7. Smith JW. Non-medical culture and the language of medical culture. In: *Clinician in Management*, 1995; 4: 3 (London: Churchill Livingstone).
8. Singer L. *Erotic Warfare, Sexual Politics and Theory in the Age of the Epidemic*, 1993. (New York: Routledge).
9. *World Health Organization Chronicle*, 1986 (Geneva: WHO).
10. Comaroff J. Medicine, symbol and ideology. In: *The Problem of Medical Knowledge*. P Wright and A Treacher (eds), 1982 (Edinburgh: Edinburgh University Press).

11. Helman C. *Culture, Health and Illness*, 1992 (London: Wright).
12. Watson J. Pollution in Cantonese society. In: *Death and the Regeneration of Life*. M Bloch and J Parry (eds), 1994 (Cambridge: Cambridge University Press).
13. Singh R. *The Sikh Way of Life*, 1968 (New Delhi: India Publishers).
14. Uberoi J. Symbols of Sikh identity. In: *Religion in India and New Delhi*. T Madan (ed.), 1992 (New Delhi: Oxford University Press).
15. Leach E. Magical hair. *J Roy Anthropol Inst* 1968; **77**: 164–167.
16. Strathern A. Witchcraft, greed, cannibalism and death. In: *Death and the Regeneration of Life*. M Bloch and J Parry (eds), 1982 (Cambridge: Cambridge University Press).
17. Soyinka W. *Myth, Literature and the African World*, 1992 (Cambridge: Cambridge University Press).
18. Smart N. *The World's Religions*, 1994 (Oxford: Oxford University Press).
19. Spector R. *Cultural Diversity in Health and Illness*, 1991 (New York: Appleton and Lange).
20. Freedman T. Social and cultural dimensions of hair loss in women. *Cancer Nursing* 1994; **17**: 334–341.
21. Scott GR. *Curious Customs of Sex and Marriage*, 1995 (London: Senate House, University of London).
22. Morrell DC. Symptom interpretation in general practice. *J Royal Coll Gen Pract* 1977; **22**: 297–309.
23. Davitz L and Samesima Y. Suffering as viewed in six different cultures. *Am J Nursing* 1976; **76**: 1296–1297.
24. Fabrega H and Tyma S. Language and cultural influences in the description of pain. *Br J Med Psychol* 1976; **47**: 349–371.
25. Engel GL. Psychogenic pain and the pain-prone patient. *Am J Med* 1980; **26**: 899–909.
26. Zbrowski M. Cultural components in response to pain. *J Social Issues* 1952; **8**: 16–30.
27. Landy D. *Culture, Disease and Healing*, 1977 (New York: Macmillan).
28. Brink PJ. *Transcultural Nursing*, 1976 (London: Prentice Hall).
29. Mares P. *Health Care in Multiracial Britain*, 1985 (Cambridge: National Extension College).
30. Swerdlow M and Stjernsward J. Cancer pain relief – an urgent problem. *World Health Forum* 1982; **3**: 325–330.
31. Laussaniere JM and Auzanneau G. The quality of terminal care in haematology. *Eur J Palliative Care* 1995; **2**: 169–172.
32. Ouaknin MA. *Méditations Erotiques*, 1992 (Paris: Ballard).
33. Neuberger J. *Caring for Dying People of Different Faiths*, 1987 (London: Austen Cornish).
34. Dinh DK and Ganesan S. The Vietnamese. In: *Cross Cultural Caring*. N Waxler Morrison et al (eds), 1990 (Vancouver: University of British Columbia).
35. Lai MC and Yue KMK. The Chinese. In: *Cross Cultural Caring*. N Waxler Morrison et al (eds), 1990 (Vancouver: University of British Columbia).
36. Sen KM. *Hinduism*, 1967 (London: Pelican).
37. Mascaro J [translator]. *The Bhagavad Gita*, 1962 (London: Penguin).
38. Mascaro J [translator]. *The Upanishads*, 1963 (London: Penguin).
39. Nicholls BJ. Hinduism. In: *The World's Religions*. N Anderson (ed), 1975 (London: Intervarsity Press).
40. Singelenberg R. The blood transfusion taboo of Jehovah's Witnesses: origin, development and function of a controversial doctrine. *J Soc Sci Med* 1990; **31**: 515–523.
41. Sinclair DB. *Non-Consensual Medical Treatment of Competent Individuals in Jewish Law within Tel Aviv University. Studies in Law*, 1992, Vol 2 (Tel Aviv: The Cegla Institute for Comparative International Law, University of Tel Aviv).
42. Uberoi JPS. *Five Symbols of Sikh Identity*, 1992 (New Delhi: Oxford University Press).
43. Zaehner RC. Zoroastrianism. In: *The Concise Encyclopaedia of Living Faiths*, 1979 (London: Open University/Hutchinson).

Index

A

100-day mortality after autotransplants (table) 902
100-day mortality after HLA-identical sibling transplants (figure) 901
2-chlorodeoxyadenosine 298
4-hydroperoxycyclophosphamide 198
4-hydroperoxycyclophosphamide 514
AA *see* Acquired aplastic anaemia
ABO compatibility in blood transfusions 796–98
   HLA compatibility and 796
     major 796–97
     minor 797
   major incompatibility 797, 799
   major and minor incompatibility 799
   minor incompatibility 798, 799–800
   red-cell aplasia 797–98
ABVD 131, 140
Aciclovir 702, 703, 704, 714, 775
Ackland *et al* (1988) 24
Acquired aplastic anaemia 238–55
   aetiology 241
   alloimmunization 242
     prevention of 243–44
   blood product support 243
     CMV screening 244
     irradiation of 244
   BMT for 13, 239
     age and 247
     alternative donor 247
     assessment prior to 242–43
     children in 372
     conditioning regimen 250–51, 252–53
     fertility and pregnancy following 254
     graft rejection 249–50
     graft-versus-host disease and 248, 253–54
     indications for 246–49
     non-sibling 247
     patient selection 245–46
     second malignancies after 254
     second transplants for graft rejection 251
     stem-cell dose 251
     syngeneic twins and 248–49
     T-cell depletion of donor bone marrow 251
   criteria 246
   cytogenetics 239–40, 242
   definition 246–47
   diagnosis
     cytogenetics 239–40
     inherited 241
     marrow-cell culture studies 240
     morphology 239
     PNH clone 240
     X-chromosome inactivation studies 240
   Fanconi's anaemia 241, 242, 248, 254, 260–65, 372
   febrile neutropenia 244
   graft failure 651
   graft-versus-host disease and 248, 253–54
   granulocyte transfusions 244–45
   haemopoietic growth factors 245
   HLA antigen screening 242
   infection prophylaxis 244
   inherited 241
   marrow-cell culture studies 240, 242
   PNH clone 240, 242
   treatment results 245
   virological screening 242
   see also Severe aplastic anaemia
Acute GvHD prophylaxis after HLA-identical sibling BMT: combined immunosuppression (table) 606
Acute GvHD grading Thomas *et al* (table) 603
Acute GvHD, incidence in unrelated transplant and impact of HLA-matching (table) 600
Acute hepatic GvHD showing bile duct damage (figure) 641
Acute renal failure 774–75
   aetiology 774
   conditioning therapy and incidence of 775
   definition 774
   drugs and 775
   graft-versus-host disease and 775
   incidence 774
   intravascular volume depletion 774
   TBI and 775
Acute subdural haematoma (figure) 789
Acute tumour lysis syndrome 776
Adaptive tasks in chronic illness (table) 828
Adenosine deaminase deficiency *see* Severe combined immunodeficiency
Adenosine deaminase negative SCID 233
Adenoviruses 716–17
Adhesion molecules in GvHD (table) 637
Adjunctive therapy 734–35
Adrenal gland problems 851
Adriamycin 131, 153, 200, 858
Advani *et al* (1992) 461
Advantages of using a family donor (allogeneic stem-cell transplantation (table) 409
Adverse prognostic factors (cGvHD) 628
AEIOP trial 43
Ahles and Shedd (1991) 871
AHPCS, breast cancer and high-dose chemotherapy 192–97
Air filtration 760, 873
   high-efficiency particulate air filtration 760
ALG 374
Alkylating agents used for autografting (table) 582
Alkylating agents 18
   autografting 582
   neurological problems and 788
Alkyl-lysophospholipids, purging graft 514–16
ALL
   adult and childhood compared 64–65
   adult subtypes 65
   allogeneic BMT 67–79
     adults in 377–80
     children in 88–91, 367, 369
     non-HLA-identical sibling donors 70, 378–80
     PH-chromosome and 69
     primary induction failure in 69–70
     resistant relapse and 70
     results 72
     risk factors in remission 68–69
   autologous BMT and 70–71
     Dana Farber study 91
     children in 91–92
     Tiley *et al* (1993) 92
   B-ALL 64
   chemotherapy in adults 64, 66
   childhood 64–65, 88–91
     first remission 366
     outcome 366
     second remission and beyond 367–70
     unrelated donor transplantation in 366–70
   CNS involvement in adults 64, 65–66, 71
   Copelan and McGuire (1995) 65
   cytosine arabinoside and 65
   donor lymphocyte transfusions 73
   extramedullary relapse 72
   Gorin (1995) 71
   graft-versus-host disease and 72–73
   GvL effect 32
   HLA-identical siblings and 74–77
   Hoelzer (1994) 65
   Linker *et al* (1991) 65
   MRD detection using immunophenotyping 661–63
   PH-chromosome and 49, 64
     BMT for 69
   preparative regimens 72
     Chao *et al* (1989) 72
   pretransplant intensification and 71
   prognostic features 65
     BMT and 65
   purging the graft 508, 512
   relapse after BMT 73–74, 76–77
   remission in 66
     BMT 67–69
   TBI 71, 72
   transplant related mortality 73
   treatment in adults 65–67
     BFM Cooperative Group 65
     comparisons 75
     decisions about 73–79
     strategy 77–79
Allogeneic bone-marrow transplants 6–7
   acquired aplastic anaemia and 239, 372
   ALL and 67–79, 367–70
   AML and 32
     children 34–36, 84–87, 371
     timing 36–37
   autoimmune disorders and 307–10
   CLL and 298–301
   CNL and 49
   CML and 51, 375–77
     atypical 49
     children in 93, 364–75
     cytoreductive regimens 52
     relapse 53–55
     survival rates 51, 56
     T-cell depletion 54
     timing 51–52
     unrelated donor 375–77
   compared with autologous transplants 6, 143
   complications of 15
   composition 7
   drawbacks 286–87
   enzyme distribution following 287–88
   follicular lymphoma and 158
   Gaucher's disease and 288
   high grade non-Hodgkin's lymphoma 167–68
   Hodgkin's lymphoma in 143
   immune deficiency and 15
   immunodeficiencies of the lymphoid system and 224
   immunodeficiencies of the phagocytic system and 224
   immunological rejection 15
   jCML and 373
   lymphoblastic lymphoma and 168
   mechanisms by which effective 286

MDS and 102–105
mucopolysaccharidoses and 288
multiple myeloma and 110–15
outpatient care 891–93
preparative regimen 12, 15, 550–61
risk stratification 37
   Ferrant *et al* (1995) study 37
   IBMTR study 37
   UK MRC AML-10 trial 37
sAML and 102, 103–104
small lymphocytic lymphoma and 159
Allogeneic stem-cell transplantation
  composition of harvests from normal donors 465
  conditioning therapy 397–98
  disease-free survival 407–408
  donors 392
    access to alternative 394–96
    clinical transplantation using alternative 397–408
    compatibility with host 394
    composition of harvests from normal 465
    considerations when choosing 396–97
    cord blood units 396
    definition of matching with host 393–94
    genetics of histocompatibility 392–93
    haplo-identical 408
  engraftment 397–99, 407–408
    kinetics 467
  graft
    failure 398–99
    manipulation 398
    T-cell depletion of 474–504
  graft-versus-host disease 399–401, 407–408, 468–69, 474–76
    late complication 404–406
    T-cell depletion 399–400, 474–76
  history 463
  immune reconstitution 467–68
    delay 405
  infection and 401–404
    evaluation of 403
    late 405
    prohylactic treatment 403–404
  lymphoproliferative disorder 404
  mobilization and collection of cells 463–65
    side effects 465–67
  quality of survivorship 407
  recurrent leukaemia 405–406
  T-cell depletion 492–96
Allogenic reaction (figure) 613
Alloresponse 10
  antigen stimulating 10
  GvHD and 9, 11
  interaction of donor and patient 8
Allo-SCT *see* Allogeneic stem-cell transplantation 392
Alternative systemic treatment of chronic GvHD (table) 631
Alternative treatment comparison 897–99
Alyea *et al* (1996) 114
Alymphocytosis *see* Severe combined immunodeficiency
Ambulatory care *see* Outpatient care
American National Cancer Institute protocols 208
AML
  allogeneic BMT and 32, 378
    BFM Study Group 85
    children in 84–87
    relapse risks 33
    timing of 36–37
  autologous BMT and 87–88
    AIEOP 87–88

EBMT report 88
POG 87
relapse and 87–88
Barnes and Loutit (1956) 32
busulfan and 32
children in 34–36, 84–88, 371
  chemotherapy compared with BMT 84–87
  cord blood 88
  preparative regimen 84
  remission 85
DFS 104
donor lymphocyte infusions and 32
Down's syndrome and 87
graft-versus-leukaemia and 32–34
GvHD and 32
MDS and 100
MRD detection using immunophenotyping 663
purging the graft 508–509
prognostic features 38
relapse and 33, 87–88
sAML 102, 103–104
syngeneic transplants
Amphotericin B 730, 731–34, 735, 775
  lipid preparations of 732–34, 736
    efficacy 734
  prophylactic treatment in neutropenia 758
Anaemia
  bone marrow in treatment of 2–4, 15
  iron administration and 2
  pernicious 2
Anasetti *et al* (1990, 1992, 1994) 608
Anatomic barrier disruption 690
Anderson *et al* (1989) 198
Anderson *et al* (1993) 113, 117
Andre *et al* (1996) 139
Andrykowski *et al* (1992) 407
Annual number of blood and marrow transplants worldwide (figure) 899
Anorexia 812
Anthony Nolan Bone Marrow Trust (ANBMT) 352
  maintenance of register 358
  number of transplants using donors from (table) 356
  success rates using donors from 355–57
  world distribution of transplants performed using donors from (table) 356
Anthony Nolan Research Centre 4, 364
Anthracycline 66, 298
Anti TNFα 608
Anti-αβ 486–87
Antibiotic-resistant organisms 871
Antibody targeted purging 517–19
  antibody and complement 517–18
  immunotoxins 518–19
    pokeweed antiviral protein (PAP) 519
    ricin 519
Anti-CD2 485, 608
Anti-CD20 153
Anti-CD25 608
Anti-CD3 484, 608
Anti-CD5 608
Anti-CD6 485–86
Antigen
  alloresponse and 10
  human histocompatibility (HLA) 3–4, 10, 14
  major histocompatibility complex (MHC) 10
  minor histocompatibility 10
  presentation 9
  T-cell receptor interaction with peptide 9
Anti-IL-2R 608
Antila *et al* (1992) 819
Antin *et al* (1994) 608

Antisense oligonucleotides 516
  combined with mafosamide 516
Antithymocyte globulin 270
Anti-tumour treatment *see* Malignancies
Antiviral agents
  CMV and 701, 702
Antilymphocyte globulin 570
Aplastic anaemia *see* Acquired aplastic anaemia, Severe aplastic anaemia
Appelbaum (1978) 164
Applicability of MRD techniques in acute leukaemias (table) 672
Archimbaud *et al* (1994) 35
Area infiltrated by local anaesthetic, showing the entry and exit sites of the catheter (figure) 424
Arteriovenous fistulae and grafts 421
Asparaginase 66
Aspergillus 724, 725, 728–29, 762
  diagnosis 726
Associazone Italiana Ematologia et Oncologia Pediatrica, 87, 90
  AML and allogeneic BMT trials 34
ATG 607, 608
Atkinson *et al* (1991) 703
Atovaquone 736
Attal *et al* (1992) 116, 124
Autografting
  CML and 57–58
    Hammersmith results 57
  in vitro manipulation 57, 58
    antisense oligodeoxynucleotides 58
    tyrosine kinase inhibitors 58
    Vancouver group 58
  in vivo approach 57
    Uppsala and Genoa groups 57
Autoimmune diseases (AID) 306–10
  allogeneic BMT and 307–308, 310
  autoimmune haemolytic amaemia 307
  autologous BMT and 308–10
    relapse after 309
    T-cells and 309–10
  conditioning regimens 308–309
  immunoblative therapy and 307–08
  ITP 307
  microscopic polyangiitis 307
  mobilization of blood progenitor cells 308
  prevalence 306
  rheumatoid arthritis 306
    current treatment 306
  systemic lupus erythematosus 306, 307
  systemic necrotizing vasculitis 307
  systemic sclerosis 306, 307
  TBI and 309
  Wegener's granulomatosis 307
Autoimmune haemolytic anaemia 306
Autoimmune haemolytic amaemia 307
Autologous Blood and Marrow Transplant Registry
  institutions participating in 915–17
Autologous bone-marrow cells
  IL-2 for and for purging graft 513
Autologous bone-marrow transplants 38–43
  AEIOP trial 43, 87
  ALL and 70–71
    children in 87–88
  AML and
    purging the graft 40
    trials 42–43
  appropriate use of 17
  autoimmune disorders and 308
  background rationale 38–39
  BGMT trial 43
  bone-marrow failure and 15

Index

CCG trial 43
chemotherapy and 39
CLL and 298–99, 300
compared with allogeneic transplants 6, 143
complications of 15, 39
composition 7
epithelial ovarian cancer and 208
EORTC trial 42, 43
first remission, in 39
germ-cell tumours and 215, 219
GOELAM trial 43
graft failure and 652
Hodgkin's lymphoma and 138–41, 143
HOVON trial 42, 43
immune deficiency and 15
malignant melanoma and 209
MDS and 102
MRC trial 42, 43
multiple myeloma in 115–21
  purged 116–17
myeloablative therapy and 153–54
neuroblastoma and 176
outpatient care and 890–91
POG trial 42, 43, 87
purging the graft 40–41
relapse 39
  primary treatment of 40
rhabdomyosarcoma 181
sarcoma 208
second remission, in 39–40
  busulfan-cyclophosphamide and 39
selection biases 42
small-cell lung cancer 209
solid tumours
  in adults 206
  in children 174–90
timing of 41–42
Autologous PBSC transplant 454–63
CD 34+ cells 462–63
characteristics of blood stem cells 454
engraftment following 456–62
  factors affecting 459
  kinetics and quality of graft 457–59
European Group for Blood and Marrow Transplantation data 454
growth factors
  following transplant 459–60
  mobilization of cells and 455–56
high dose regimens for 572–77
mobilization of cells
  chemotherapy with 455
  factors affecting 459
  growth factors with 454–56
  kinetics of 456
Avanzini et al (1995) 751
Axathioprine 241
Ayash et al (1994) 193
Ayliffe et al (1981) 872
Azathioprine 629
Azevedo et al (1995) 463, 468
Azoles 730–31

B

Bach et al (1968) 224
Bacteraemia (complication of catheters) 427–28
Bacterial infections 690–94
  anatomic barrier disruption 690
  antibiotic therapy 692–94, 759
  diagnosis 692
  empirical antimicrobial chemotherapy 692–94
  infecting organisms 690–94
  neutropenia 690, 758–59
  prophylactic treatment 758–63
  surveillance cultures 692
Baha'i faith 931–32
  diet and 932
  sperm banking 932
Balduzzi et al (1995) 600
Baltimore Group, CML cytoreductive regimens 52
Barker et al (1996) 858
Barlogie et al (1984) 115, 116
Barnes and Loutit 3
Bastion et al 155
BAVC 576
Baxter Isolex 300i large-scale separator for immunomagnetic enrichment of CD34+ cells (figure) 525
Baxter MaxSep™ large-scale separator for negative immunomagnetic separation (figure) 523
B-cell lymphomas *see* non-Hodgkin's lymphoma
BCNU *see* Carmustine
BCNU 141, 209
BCNU 185, 578
BCR gene
  PH-chromosome and 48
BCR/ABL gene 48–49
  CML and 49
  CNL and 49
BEAM 135, 136, 138, 141, 144, 157, 166, 167, 300, 309, 577, 578–81
BEAM regimen results (table) 580
Bearman et al (1990) 772
Benedetti-Pancini et al (1995) 206
Bensinger et al (1995) 464
Bensinger et al (1996) 463, 468
BEP 220
BFM Cooperative Group 65, 85
BGMT trial 43
Bhagavad Gita, The 933
Bibbington et al (1993) 816, 817
Bierman et al (1993) 140
Billingham (1966) 596
Billings (1894) 2
Bioelectrical impedance 818
Bitran et al (1996) 193
Blaise et al (1992) 545
Bleomycin 131, 214, 215, 218, 219, 300, 788
Blood Transfusion Service Register 352
Blood transfusion 796–807
  ABO compatibility 796–98
  antibody testing 798–99
  blood grouping 798–99
  ethnic considerations 932, 936, 938
  febrile neutropenic post-transplant patient and 805–806
  graft-versus-host disease and 804
  Jehovah's witnesses 936
  passive immune therapy and 804
  platelet transfusion 801–804
  red-cell transfusions 796
  Rh blood groups 798
  risks 796
  selection of blood groups 799–801
  Zoroastrianism 938
Body image 925–26
Body weight
  nutritional status and 817–18
Bolger et al (1986) 654
Bone Marrow Donors Worldwide 353
Bone-marrow transplantation (pregnancy) (table) 857
Bone-marrow harvest problem (table) 477
Bone-marrow transplant/blood cell transplant outpatient nursing team (table) 890
Bone-marrow transplants (Europe) as registered to the EBMT group (table) 364
Bone-marrow
anaemia and 2
animal
  extraction of 2
CD34+ cells 5, 7
collection 434–38
contamination during harvest 477
donor panels 4
engraftment 12–13
failure syndrome
  nuclear weapons and 2
  primary 2–3
  secondary 2–3
  spleen cells and 2
graft rejection 9, 11, 14–15, 249–52
  treatment where high risk 14
graft-versus-host disease (GvHD) 3–4, 4–6, 11, 13, 14
  acute 596–612
  alloresponse and 9, 13
  ALL and 70
  AML and 32–34
  CML and 52, 55, 59, 376
  cyclosporin treatment 4, 33
  immune recovery and 11–12
  mHag and 334–35
  prophylactic treatment 14, 604–606
  unrelated donors and 55
graft-versus-marrow effect 13
haematopoietic stem-cell transplantation 3, 8
harvesting problems 477
parasitic infections and 2
purging 508–531
  AML and 40, 508–509
  breast cancer and 196–200
  childhood solid tumours 185–86
  Hodgkin's lymphoma and 143
  multiple myeloma and 116–17
radiation 2
sources 435
T-cells and 5, 8–9, 11, 14, 229, 251, 476–508, 611
transplants (BMT)
  acquired aplastic anaemia for 13, 239, 372
  adaptation to 830
  allogeneic 6, 13, 32, 34–38, 49, 110–15, 224, 373–74, 375–86
  ALL and 65, 67–69, 367–370
  AML and 32, 371
  aplastic anaemia and 13, 239, 372
  application of 4
  appropriate type 316
  autoimmune disorders and 307–11
  autologous 6–7, 13–14, 15, 38–43, 70–71, 87–88, 102, 174, 208, 209, 215, 219, 298–99, 300
  blood transfusion support for 796–807
  cartilage-hair hypoplasia for 229
  children in 84–95
  clinical management of 13
  CLL and 298–302
  CML and 49, 51–57
  colony-forming units 3
  complications 15, 94–95, 768–80
  composition 7
  current use and outcomes of 898–910
  database information 14
  disease-free survival (DFS) 14
  disease relapse 14
  donors 14
  drawbacks 286–87
  early attempts 2

enzyme distribution following 287–88
Epstein-Barr virus-associated
  lymphoproliferative disorders 94
ethnic considerations 922–38
European Bone Marrow Transplant Group
  4, 14, 41, 67, 88, 102, 103, 104, 110,
  114, 130, 142, 143, 144, 154, 155, 176,
  179, 181, 208, 306, 310, 367, 376, 455,
  577, 596, 651, 880
Fanconi's anaemia and 260–64, 372–73
fitness for 318–20
follicular lymphoma and 158
follow-up 15
Gaucher's disease and 288
graft failure see Graft failure
graft-versus-host disease 3–4, 3–5, 11–13,
  14, 32, 52, 55–56, 59, 70, 72–73, 111,
  225, 248, 376, 596–612, 620–34
graft-versus-leukaemia (GvL) effect see
  Graft-versus leukaemia
high grade non-Hodgkin's lymphoma and
  167–68
Hodgkin's lymphoma in 143
human histocompatibility antigen (HLA)
  and 3–4, 10
immune deficiency following 15
immunodeficiency diseases 227–37
immunological considerations 8–12
International Bone Marrow Transplant
  Registry (BMTR) 4, 17, 33, 36, 51, 67,
  90, 113, 114, 596
jCML and 93, 373
leukaemia and 3, 6
lymphoblastic lymphoma and 168
lysosomal enzyme defects and 13
lysosomal storage diseases and 286–90
malignancies and 3–4, 13
MDS and 93–94
mechanisms by which effective 286
mucopolysaccharidoses and 288
multiple myeloma and 110–19
  mechanism 3
metabolic disorders and 13
MHC class II deficiency for 229
neuroblastoma 176
non-malignant disorders and 13
nutritional support 812–23
Omenn's syndrome for 229
pancytopenia following 646–55
patient selection 13–14, 245–46, 316
phagocytic cell disorders for 229–31
preparative regimen 12, 15, 550–61
pretransplant consultation 317–18
pretransplant investigations 318–20
procedure 287–90
purine nucleoside phosphorylase deficiency
  for 229
radiation-induced failure syndrome and 2–3
relapse following 15, 52–54
religious considerations 931–38
risk factors 14
sAML and 102, 103–104
second malignancies 94–95, 845
sensitization against donor antigens 336
sickle-cell disease and 14, 15, 278–83
small lymphocytic lymphoma and 159
solid tumours in children and 174–86
source of cells 320
stem cells and 3, 7, 320
supportive care 14–15
T-cell immunodeficiencies for 229, 231
thalassaemia major and 15, 268–74
time off work 318
transplant-related mortality 15

transplant talk 308–18
twins and 3
venous access 420–429
Wiskott-Aldrich syndrome for 228–29
X-linked hyper IgM syndrome 229
X-linked proliferative syndrome 229
transplantation history 2
see also Marrow
Boulad et al (1995) 851
Brain infections post stem-cell transplant
  (figure) 719
Brain tumours see Malignant brain tumours in
  childhood
Breast cancer 192–201
  AHPCS 192–97
  graft purging 196–200
    negative 198
    positive selection 298–200
    rationale 196–197
  high-dose chemotherapy
    Adriamycin 200
    AFM 192
    autologous haematopoietic progenitor cell
      support 192–95
    busulfan 200
    CAF 192
    carboplantin 194, 200
    cisplatin 193
    CPA/cDDP/BCNU 192, 193, 194, 201
    cyclophosphamide 193, 194, 200, 201
    etoposide 193, 200
    ifosfamide 200
    LOMAC 192
    melphalan 193
    multi-cycle 192–95
    new regimens 200–201
    rationale 192
    results with primary breast cancer 194
    single-cycle and metastatic breast cancer
      192–93
    thiotepa 193, 194
  metastatic 192–93
  PBPCs 196
Breast carcinoma
  high dose chemotherapy and 19, 20
Brenner et al 91, 197
Brink (1976) 930
British Bone Marrow and Platelet Donor Panel
  352
British Bone Marrow Registry 364
British Committee for Standards in
  Haematology Task Force 880, 881
British Medical Research Council 898
British National Lymphoma Investigation
  (BNLI) registry 130, 131, 133, 144
Broad irregular hyphae with wide angle
  branching in brain tissue in mucormycosis
  (figure) 730
Broviac et al (1973) 423
Brown Sequard and D'Arsenoval 2
Buckner et al (1994) 466
Buddhists 930, 932
  diet 932
  pain control 932
Buffy coat preparations 436–37, 802
Busulfan 18, 22, 552, 567, 576, 582
  acquired aplastic anaemia and 241
  administration 23–24
  children and 23
  ALL and 72
  AML and 32
  bioavailability of 20
  breast cancer and 200
  CLL and 300

CML and 50, 52, 375
  children in 92
Ewing's sarcoma 182
graft failure and 652
growth and endocrine disturbances and 94
haemorrhagic cystitis and 776
Hodgkin's lymphoma and 135
immunodeficiency diseases and 226, 228
multiple myeloma and 111, 113, 117, 119,
  121
myelodysplastic syndromes in childhood and
  374
neurological problems and 788
PBSC transplantation and 463
phagocytic cell disorder and 230
relapse and 678
TBI and 544–45
thalassaemia 270
veno-occlusive disease and 22, 771
Byers et al (1990) 608

C

CAF 192
Campath 1G 374, 569–70, 652
CAMPATH antibodies 481, 482–84
  series of rat monoclonal antibodies (table) 482
  (table) 483
Canal et al (1993) 25
Cancer in South East England 1992 (Thames
  Cancer Registry) 130
Candida 724, 725, 726–28, 762
  diagnosis 726
  treatment 730–36
Canellos et al (1992) 131
Capillary leak syndromes
  complication of BMT 15
Capsular yeasts in a skin biopsy in cutaneous
  cryptococcosis (figure) 729
Carbopec 219
Carboplatin 18, 22, 180, 194, 200, 215–16,
  218, 219, 788
  administration 25
Cardiovascular complications
  children of 843
  conditioning-related toxicity 777
  endocarditis 778
  hypertension 778
  pericarditis 778
Care see Patient
Carella et al (1991) 143
Carmustine 18, 22, 117, 209, 568, 582, 788,
  858
  administration 24
  pharmacology 583
  Jones et al (1993) 24
Cartilage-hair hypoplasia 229
Casper et al (1995) 375, 600
Cataract formation after total body irradiation
  (figure) 844
Cataracts 544
  children and 844
Catering facilities 874
Catheter-related complications (table) 427
Catheters 420
  Broviac 423
  central venous 421–22
  non-tunnelled 422
  complications of long-term 426–29
    bacteraemia 427–28
    infection 427
    insertion complications 426–27
    migration 428–29
    occlusion 428

septicaemia 427–28
thrombosis 428
endogenous flora and 758
Hickman 422, 423–25
implantable devices 422
indwelling vascular 320–21
long-term tunnelled lines 423–25
lumen 421–22
maintenance 425
occlusion 428
Raaf 423
removal 426
thrombosis 428
Causes of post-BMT acute renal failure (table) 774
Causes of pulmonary complications post-BMT (table) 773
Causes of skin and mucosa disruption (table) 690
CBL1 608
CBV 134, 578–81
CCG trial 43
CD34 198, 457–59, 462, 519, 520
CD34+ cells 6, 9, 455, 457–59, 462, 469
  graft-versus-host disease and 610–611
  isolation and transplantation of 462–63
CD40 ligand deficiency see X-linked hyper IgM syndrome
CECC 186, 187
Cell kill 539
Cell Pro CEPRATE™ SC clinical-scale device (figure) 521
CellPro column 200
Cellular assays 340
Central nervous system see Neurological complications
Central venous catheter 421–22
Centrifugal elutration 480, 511–12
Centrocytic lymphoma see Mantle cell lymphoma
CEPRATE stem-cell concentrator 199
Cerebral atrophy 792
Cerebrospinal fluid for MRD detection 663
Champlin et al (1989) 249
Chan et al
  MDR 19
Characteristics of class I and class II molecule assembly and peptide presentation (table) 332
Chatterjee et al (1994) 852
Chediak-Higashi syndrome 229, 231
Cheese 817
Chemotherapy 552, 554–55, 572–87
  Adriamycin 200
  alkylating agents used for autografting 582
  BEP 220
  BMT and
    children in 84, 90
    high dose 18–27
  breast cancer and 192–201
    new regimens 200–201
  CAF 192, 192
  carboplatin 194, 200
  CPA/cDDP/BCNU 192, 193, 194, 201
  ChlVPP 131
  drug pharmacology 572
  empirical antimicrobial 692–94
  epithelial ovarian cancer and 206–10
  haematological malignancies for 558–59
  high dose prior to transplant
    acute leukaemias in 573–76
    dose effect 581–82
    dose intensity 18–19
    drug combinations 584

drug resistance 19
dose response and dose and toxicity 20, 21
drugs used 18
interpatient pharmacokinetic variability and 20
isobologram approach to evaluation 21–23
lymphomas in 578–82
oncologist's role 20
outcome and 18
pharmacodynamics 20, 21
solid tumours in 581–86
schedule of administration 21–23
tumour factors affecting response 19
Hodgkin's lymphoma and 131
ifosfamide 200
LOMAC 192
malignant melanoma and 209
MDS and 101–102
mobilization of PBSC with 455
MOPP 131
multiple myeloma and 112
MVPP 131
nutrition and 813
PBSC and
  high dose 18–27
principles of 572
radiation based preparative regimens compared 559–60
relapse and 679–80
RAEB and 101–102
side effects 555–58, 575–76
single cycle and metastatic breast cancer 193–94
small-cell lung cancer and 209
solid tumours
  in adults and 205–10
  in children and 174–86
sAML 103–104
thiotepa 193, 194
Chest
  infections post stem-cell transplant (figure) 719
  radiograph of a young woman post stem-cell transplant with parainfluenza virus type 3 pneumonia (figure) 717
  X-ray showing some of the features of pulmonary aspergillosis (figure) 729
Children 840–46
  cardiovascular system and 843
  dental problems and 844–45
  gastrointestinal system and 844
  growth and 15, 94, 272, 544, 841–42, 861
  hair loss and 927–29
  infertility and ethnic considerations 928–29
  neurological problems and 843–44
  neuropsychological problems and 843–44
  opthalmological problems and 844
  organ toxicity and 840–41
  osteopena and 845
  osteoporosis and 845
  premenarchial females 861
  renal system and 843
  respiratory system and 843
  second malignancies and 845
Children's Cancer Group 178
  AML and allogeneic BMT trials 34
Chinese communities 922
  hair loss and 927
Chlorambucil 153, 159, 241, 298, 300, 788
Chloramphenicol 651
ChlVPP 131
Choi et al (1989) 24
CHOP 153, 156, 164, 300
Chopra et al (1993) 135, 138, 142

Christian Scientists 933
Christianity 932–33
  Brethern
    hair loss and 933
    sperm banking 933
Chromosome abberations as major PCR targets for MRD detection in acute leukaemias (table) 670
Chronic graft-versus-host disease of the skin (figure) 625
Chronic granulomatosis disease 230
Chronic lymphocitic lymphoma (CLL) 298–302
  allogeneic BMT 298–302
    donors 300
    patients 300
    PBPC and 300
    purged 300
    pretransplant therapy 300
    probability of survival after 301
    results 300–301
  autologous BMT 298–301, 300–302
    probability of survival after 301
    results 300–301
  choice of therapy for 298
  immune modulation and 123
  small lymphocytic lymphoma and 158
Chronic myelomonocytic leukaemia (CMML) 100
  BMT and 103, 105
Cimetidine 651
Circumcision
  female 925, 935
  male 925
Cisplatin 18, 22, 193, 206, 209, 214, 215, 218, 219, 582, 788
  administration 25
Civin et al (1996) 198
Class I antigen-processing pathway (figure) 393
Classification of chronic GcHD (table) 621
Classification of mismatches (table) 338
Clift et al (1994) 545
Clindamycin-primaquine 736, 792
Clinical grading of acute graft-versus-host disease (table) 603
Clinical manifestations of chronic GvHD (table) 622–23
CML
  allogeneic BMT 49, 51–57
    age limits for 376–77
    children in 93
    cytoreductive regimens 52
    donors other than HLA-identical siblings 55–57
    survival rates 51
    unrelated donor transplants 375–77
  atypical forms 49
    allogeneic BMT and 49
  autografting 57–58
  children in 92–93
    allogeneic BMT 93
    busulfan 92
    hydroxyurea 92
    interferon alpha 92
  cyclophosphamide 52
  cytoreductive regimens 52
    Baltimore Group 52
    busulfan 52
    Hammersmith Hospital 52
    Sloan Kettering Cancer Center 52
  definition 48
  donor lymphocyte infusions and 32
  graft-versus-host disease 52, 55–56, 59, 376
  graft-versus-leukaemia effect and 52–53
  Hammersmith Hospital studies 52, 376

immune modulation and 123
integrated approach to management 58
PH-positive
  biological aspects of 49–50
  chromosomal and molecular features of 48–49
  purging the graft 512
  relapse 52–55
    allogeneic BMT and 53–54
    cells of donor origin 54
    cytogenetic 53
    rtPCR studies 53
    total body irradiation 52
  treatment
    busulfan 50, 58, 92
    hydroxyurea 50, 58, 92
    interferon-alpha 50–51, 55, 58, 92
    radiotherapy 50
CMML see Chronic myelomonocytic leukaemia
CNS toxicity
  cytosine arabinoside and 22, 65
  paclitaxel and 22
  thiotepa and 22
Coldman and Goldie
  high dose chemotherapy 19
Colistin 758
Colloids 491–92
Colon, cancer of 210
Comeroff (1982) 925
Common HLA-B:DR haplotypes in the British population (table) 329
Common sites for entrance of infection and localized infection (table) 691
Communication between patient and medical staff 922–24
  eye contact 923
  interpreters 923
  language problems 923
Comparison of engraftment kinetics following allogeneic PBSC transplant and historical BMT controls (table) 468
Comparison of G-CSF dose and CD34+ yield in normal donors (table) 464
Comparison of major transplant endpoints using matched siblings and alternative stem-cell donors (table) 402
Comparison of PBSC transplant and BMT for antibiotic and blood product support requirements (table) 463
Comparison of total body irradiation (TBI) versus chemotherapy-based preparative regimens (table) 560
Comparison of two methods of CD34+ cell selection on T-cell content of bone marrow (figure) 494
Compatibility score of stem-cell donors (table) 395
Complement
  mediated cell lysis 517–18
  monocolonal antibodies and 481–82
Complications of percutaneous catheter insertion (table) 426
Complications 15, 94–95, 768–80
  acute renal failure 774–75
  adrenal gland problems 851
  allogeneic BMT of 15
  autologous BMT of 15, 39
  capillary leak syndromes 15
  cardiovascular complications 777–78
    children and 843
  catheters of 426–29
  cholecystitis 770
  delayed puberty 15
  diarrhoea 769–70

  distinguishing original disease from 792–93
  endocrine disturbance 94
  gastroduodenitis 769
  gonadal failure 15, 858–61
  graft-versus-host disease see Graft-versus-host disease
  growth arrest 15, 94, 272, 544, 861
  haemorrhagic cystitis 15
  hepatic failure 15
  immune deficiency 15
  infertility 15, 272, 856–64
  interstitial pneumonitis 773–74
  metabolic 778
  mucositis 769
  nausea 768
  neurological 778–80
    children and 843–44
  oesophagitis 769
  ovaries 851–52
  pancreatitis 770
  pituitary gland 850
  renal failure 15
    children and 843
  respiratory distress 15
    children and 843
  restrictive lung disease 15
  secondary malignancies 15
  suppressed and recovering marrow 789–93
  testis 852–53
  thyroid gland 850–51
  typhlitis 769–70
  unrelated donor 381–82
  veno-occlusive disease 15, 770–73
  vomiting 768
Composition of harvests from normal donors (PBSC) (table) 466
Computed topography head scan showing an acute subdural haematoma (figure) 789
Computed topography scan showing multiple ring-enhancing lesions which were cerebral abscesses (figure) 790
Conditioning regimen for children with MDS (table) 374
Conditioning-related cardiovascular toxicity 777–78
  treatment 777
Confirmation of normal pituitary function (table) 850
Congenital agranulocytosis 233
Considerations for patients when setting up a new BMT unit (table) 872
Considerations for staff when setting up a new BMT unit (table) 875
Contraceptive pill 861
Contrast-enhanced computed tomography scan showing lesion in the thalamus which was thought to represent an abscess (figure) 792
Cook-chill foods 817
Coombes et al (1986) 198
Copelan and McGuire (1995) 65
Cord blood
  biology 444–45
  gene therapy and 447
  graft-versus-host disease and 442, 443–44
  history of use 442–43
  New York Blood Center 442
  stem cells 5, 383–84
    GvHD and 5
    numbers required 444
  T-cell depletion 495
  transplants 14, 88, 91
    broadness of applicability for 442
    disorders used for 443

    Fanconi anaemia and 263
    graft-versus-host disease and 609–610
    immunodeficiency disease and 232–33
    thalassaemia and 273–74
Corradini et al (1995) 122
Correlation between donor type and clinical outcome (allogeneic stem-cell transplantation) (table) 408
Corticosteroid therapy and neurological problems 788–89
Cosset et al (1991) 144
Costimulatory signal blocking 612
Cote et al (1991) 196
Counselling 834
CPA/cDDP/BCNU 192, 193, 194, 201
Criteria for normal gonadal function in men (table) 861
Criteria for normal gonadal function in women (table) 858
Crossing histocompatibitiy barriers using sequential immunomodulation (figure) 403
Cross-reactive groups of HLA-A and HLA-B alleles (table) 329
Crump et al (1993) 138, 140
Cruse and Foord (1980) 872
Crypt of rectal mucosa with acute GvHD (figure) 639
Cryptococcosis 729
Cryptococcus neoformans 791
Crytposporidiosis 742
CT scan of abmomen showing multiple microabscesses throught the liver and spleen in chronic disseminated candidosis (figure) 728
CT scan of chest in chronic disseminated candidosis showing micronodular miliary distribution of lesions (figure) 728
Cultural concepts concerning body image (table) 927
Cultural considerations see Ethnic considerations
CVP 153
Cyclophosphamide 18, 20, 22, 72, 111, 113, 117, 118, 121, 135, 200, 219, 226, 228, 252, 298, 299, 300, 307, 309, 372, 463, 552, 566, 567, 576, 582, 604, 652
  administration 23
  AML in children and 84
  breast cancer and 193, 194, 200, 201
  CML and 52, 375, 376
  conditioning related toxicity and 777
  Fanconi's anaemia and 260, 261, 372
  germ-cell tumours and 217
  growth and endocrine disturbances and 94
  haemorrhagic cystitis and 776
  malignant melanoma 209
  mantle cell lymphoma and 159
  myelodysplastic syndromes in childhood and 374
  neurological problems and 788
  phagocytic cell disorders and 230
  pharmacology 582–83
  preparative regimens 550
  relapse and 678
  small-cell lung cancer and 209
  small lymphocytic lymphoma and 159
  sperm count and 858
  syndrome of inappropriate antidiuretic hormone secretion 778
  TBI and 544–45, 575
  veno-occlusive disease and 22, 771
Cyclosporin 4, 250, 253, 260, 306, 604, 629, 630, 775, 776, 778, 789
  GvHD and 33, 300

GvL and 33
Cyprofloxacin resistance 244
Cyst of cryptosporidium parvum on faeces (figure) 742
Cysts of pneumocystis carinii in bronchoalveolar lavage fluid stained by immunofluorescence (figure) 737
Cytarabine 133, 169, 300
Cytokine activated cells, purging graft 513
Cytokines and relapse 680–81
Cytokines upregulated during acute GvHD (table) 637
Cytomegalovirus (CMV) 632–33, 698–706, 793
  cellular therapy 705
  definition 698
  diagnosis 698–701
    antiviral agents and 701
    autopsy 700–701
    biopsy 700–701
    bronchoalveolar lavage fluid 700
    PCR 700, 705
    saliva 700
    standardization of methods 701
    urine 700
    viraemia 699–700
  platelet transfusion and 804–805
  prevention 701–702
    pre-emptive therapy 702
    prophylaxis 702, 704–705
    suppression 702
  primary 698
  reinfection 698
  secondary 698
  seropositivity 271
  survival 704–705
  treatment 702–704
    pre-emptive therapy 703
    prophylaxis 702–704
    suppression 703
Cytosine arabinoside 18, 22, 552, 582
  administration 26
  ALL and 65
  autografting in CML and 57, 58
  autoimmune disorders and 309
  haemorrhagic cystitis and 776
  Hiddeman et al (1992) 26
Cytoxan see Cyclophosphamide
Cytoxic T-cell precursor (CTLp) 336–37

D

Dairy products 817
Dana Farber Cancer Institute 91, 102, 154, 158
Danorubicin 300, 788
Dausset, Jean 4
Davies et al (1994) 654
Davies et al (1995) 600
Davies et al (1997) 372
Davitz and Samesima (1976) 929
de Wynter et al (1995) 495
Deeg et al (1995) 812
Demuynck et al (1996) 102
Density-gradient centrifugation 511
Dental
  assessment 319
  problems and children 844–45
Deoxycoformycin 298, 481
Depletion of white cells from platelets (table) 801
Dermal features of graft-versus-host disease 599–602, 621–22, 627, 636–38
Detachabead® 198
Devergie et al (1995) 545
DexaBEAM 133, 138, 141, 142, 145

Dexamethasone 792
Diagnosis of herpes simplex virus infection post stem-cell transplant (table) 714
Diagnostic criteria for hepatic veno-occlusive disease (table) 770
Diagnosis of varicella-zoster virus infection post stem-cell transplant 715
Diagrammatic representation of an implantable device (figure) 422
Diarrhoea 769–70, 812, 814, 823
Dietary restrictions 815–17
  cook-chill foods 817
  dairy products 816–17
  eggs 817
  fruit 816
  low microbial diet 761, 815–16
  microwave oven cooking 817
  modified ward diets 816
  seasoning 817
  sterile diets 815
  vegetables 816
  water 761, 816, 873
Dietrich et al (1973) 870
Dietrich et al (1992, 1994) 596
Differences in graft characteristics and clinical outcome following T-cell depletion with T10B9 versus OKT3 (table) 398
Differential diagnosis of hepatic veno-occlusive disease (table) 772
Dimopoulos et al (1993) 121
Dinh and Ganesan (1990) 932
Diptheria toxoid vaccination 746–49
Disease-free survival (DFS)
  BMT and 14
Disgeusia 813–14
Disproportionate growth in a young woman, showing shortening of the spine and normal growth of limbs (figure) 841
DNA typing 337, 341–45
  MRD detection by 663–70
  PCR-AFLP 342
  PCR fingerprinting 342
  PCR-SSP 343–44
  PCR-SSOP 342–43
    and reverse-hybridization dot-blotting 343
  purged bone marrow 508–509
  SBT 345
Donor availability (stem-cell) (figure) 395
Donor information topics (table) 357
Donor lymphocyte transfusions 32
  ALL in 73
  relapse and 681–84
Donors for BMT 17
  age 320
  autologous blood donation 321
  blood group 320
  consent 321–22
  cytomegalovirus serology 319–20
  cytoxic T-cell precursor (CTLp) 336–37
  Europdonor 4, 353
  functional histocompatibility tests 336
  helper T-cell precursor (HTLp) as predictor 337
  HLA-identical siblings 36, 74–77, 102–104, 225, 260–65, 269, 287, 300, 335, 364, 375
    graft-versus-host disease incidence 597
  HLA matching 336–39
  information topics (table) 357
  international 354–55
  lymphocyte cross-match 336
  lymphocyte infusions 32
  North American Marrow Donor Pool (NAMDP) 4

other than HLA-identical siblings 55–57, 70, 76, 104–105, 225–27, 231–33, 261–62, 269, 287, 335–36
  factors affecting success rates with 56–57
  graft-versus-host disease and 598–99
  success rates using ANBMT donors 355–57
panels 7
parity 320
percentage of transplant recipients whose donor was identified on the initial search of the Anthony Nolan Register (table) 359
psychological aspects of donation 321
recruitment of 357–58
  National Association of Round Tables of Great Britain and Ireland 357
searching registry 352–60
selection 319, 335–45, 366
  guidelines for 339
  unrelated donors 336
sensitization against antigens by patient 336
sex 320
source of cells 320
typing strategies 359
unrelated 55, 352–60, 364–86
  adults and 375–80
  alternative stem cell sources 383–86
  complications of 381–82
  disease relapse treatment 383
  errors of metabolism 380
  graft failure 381
  immunodeficiencies 380
  indications for 380–81
  myeloma 380
  non-Hodgkin's lymphoma 380
  paediatrics and 364–75
  success rates 355–57, 375–76
  venous access 320–21
Downie et al (1992) 288
Doxorubicin 118, 300, 776, 788
DTIC 209
Dunbar et al (1995) 123
Dunphy et al (1990, 1992) 193
Dusenbury et al (1995) 545
Dynabeads-CD34 198

E

Eastern Co-operative Oncology Group 220, 898
Education of patients 884–85
Effect of CD34+ cell dose on post-PBSC transplant support therapy requirement (table) 459
Effect of different previous regimens of chemotherapy on yield of CD34+ cells following subsequent stem-cell mobilization (figure) 460
Effect of immunomagnetic CD34+ cell selection on residual lymphocyte subpopulations (figure) 493
Effect of number of CD34+ cells on haematologic reconstitution following high-dose therapy (table) 457
Effect of T-cell depletion on the probablity of graft failure or death due to complications of pancytopenia (figure) 647
Effect of the total leukocyte count on day 16 after bone-marrow transplantation on the probability of graft failure or death due to complications of pancytopenia (figure) 648
Effect of the type of donor on the probability of graft failure or death due to pancytopenia (figure) 648

Effects of agents used in the preparative regimen overlap (figure) 550
Effects of growth hormone administration on growth after total body irradiation showing no catch up (figure) 842
Effects of total body irradiation on 49 patients after TBI for BMT (figure) 842
Eggs 817
Endocarditis 778
Endocrine disturbance, complication of BMT 94
Endogenous viral reactivations (table) 712
Endogenous flora 758–62
  catheters and 758
  suppressive regimens 758
Endothelialitis of the portal vein in acute GvHD (figure) 641
Endoxan see Cyclophosphamide
Energy requirements and nutrition 818
Engel (1980) 929
Engelhard et al (1991) 752
Engraftment following infusion of CD34+- selected PBSC: results of selected studies (table) 462
Engraftment 397–99, 407–408, 456–62, 468
  donor factors determining 551–52
  factors affecting 12
  recipient factors determining 551
Enhanced immunoablative conditioning regimen (figure) 401
Enrichment of CD34+ cells by immunoadherence using the GenCell CELLector' system (figure) 520
Enrichment of CD34+ cells on the CellPro biotin avidin affinity column (figure) 521
Enteroviruses 718
Environmentally acquired virus infections post stem-cell transplant (table) 711
EORTC trial 42, 43, 102
EORTC/GIMIMA
  allogeneic BMT study 35
  autologous BMT study 42, 43
Epidermis in acute GvHD (figure) 638
Epithelial ovarian cancer 206–208
  autologous BMT 208
  high dose chemotherapy and 206–208
    carboplatin 206, 208
    cyclophosphamide 208
    doxorubicin 208
    melphalan 206
    mitoxantrone 206
  peripheral stem-cell transplants 206
Epstein-Barr virus 94, 169, 229, 272
  clinical aspects 716
  diagnosis 716
  management 716
Ergorin et al 21
E-rosetting 478–77
Ethnic considerations 922–38
  blood tests and 932
  Buddhists 930
  Chinese patients 922, 927, 929
  children 927–29
  Christian Scientists 933
  Christianity 932–33
  circumcision
    female 925, 935
    male 925
  Hinduism 933–34
  Indian communities
    hair loss and 927
  infertility 928–29
    sperm banking 928–29
  Islam 935–36

Jainism 937
Japanese 929
Jehovah's Witnesses 936
Judaism 936–37
  pain and 929–31
  Rastafarians 937
    background 927
    hair loss and 927
    scarring 928
  Sikhs 937–38
    hair loss and 927
  Vietnamese 932
Etoposide 18, 22, 117, 131, 133, 193, 200, 214, 215, 217, 218, 219, 230, 568, 581, 582, 776, 788
  administration 25
  children and 25, 180
  autografting in CML and 57, 58
  pharmacology 583
  relapse and 678
Etretinate 631
Europdonor 4, 353, 355
European Bone Marrow Transplant Group 4, 67, 87–88, 102, 103, 104, 110, 114, 130, 142, 143, 144, 154, 155, 176, 179, 181, 208, 270, 287, 299, 367, 376, 454, 596, 651
  database information 14, 41
European League Against Rheumatism and 306, 310
  evaluation of pre-autografting regimens for acute leukaemias 577
  evaluation of pre-autografting regimens for lymphomas 581
  guidelines for staff numbers 880
  Immunology Working Party 353
European Bone Marrow Transplant leukaemia working party
  AML and allogeneic BMT trials 35
European Donor Secretariat 353
European League Against Rheumatism and 306, 310
European Marrow Donor Infomation System 353
European Neuroblastoma Study Group 178
European Working Group on Myelodysplastic Syndrome in Childhood 374
EVAP 133
Ewing's sarcoma 182, 183, 208
Example of pretransplant critical pathway (table) 886
Examples of high-dose therapy followed by stem-cell transplantation in leukaemia (table) 574
Examples of high-dose therapy followed by stem-cell transplantation in lymphomas and myelomas (table) 579
Examples of high-dose therapy followed by stem-cell transplantation for breast cancer (table) 585
Examples of high-dose therapy followed by stem-cell transplantation in solid tumours (other than breast cancer) (table) 586
Examples of leukaemia-associated immunophenotypes in acute leukaemia (figure) 661
Examples of malignant and non-malignant disorders for which cord-blood transplantation has been utilized (table) 443
Exercise 834
Exogenous flora acquisition 759
  air filtration 760
  low microbial diet 761

  protective isolation 760
  reverse barrier nursing 760
  room hygiene 760–61
Eye contact between patient and medical staff 923

F

Fabrega and Tyma (1976) 929
Factors affecting adaptation to normal life after BMT (table) 828
Factors affecting outcome of UD transplantation (table) 385
Factors associated with acute GvHD (figure) 598
Factors associated with predisposition to graft failure (table) 646
Factors contributing to pregnancy problems (table) 857
Factors determining marrow engraftment (table) 551
Factors encouraging outpatient autologous transplantation (table) 891
Factors involved in immunosuppression in bone-marrow transplantation (table) 690
Factors worsening long-term effects of BMT (table) 843
Fanconi anaemia 241, 242, 248, 254, 260–65
BMT
  alternative donor transplants 261–62
  children in 372–73
  cord blood transplants 263
  HLA-identical sibling transplants 260–61
  gene therapy 263–64
  preparative regimens 556–57
  principal causes of death 262
  secondary tumours 233
Farber's disease 290
Features of chronic disseminated candidosis (table) 727
Features of cord blood cells (table) 610
Feldman et al (1993) 25, 117
Fermand et al (1989) 117
Ferrant et al (1995) 37
Ferribee 3
Ferster et al (1995) 280
Fertility see Infertility
Field size on dedicated TBI unit (figure) 541
Fields et al (1995) 200
Filopovich et al (1992) 231
Five core concepts contributing to provisional practice (table) 871
Flow cytometry 510
Flucytosine 734
Fludarabine 153, 159, 298, 300, 569
Fluid requirements and nutrition 818
  parenteral nutrition and overload 821
Fluorouracil 788
Focal lesions 790–92
Follicular lymphoma
  adriamycin 153
  anti-CD20 153
  BEAM 155
  chlorambucil 153
  CHOP 153, 154
  CVP 153
  description of 152
  fludarabine 153
  interferon-alpha 153
  molecular biology 152
  myeloablative therapy 153
    allogeneic BMT and 158
    lymphoma at molecular level following 158
    with ABMT 153–54

with peripheral blood progenitor cells 155–56
myelodisplasia and secondary AML 157
radiation therapy and 152
remission
  myeloablative therapy and ABMT 154–55
transformation
  myeloablative therapy and ABMT following 155
Follow-up investigations post-BMT (table) 846
Food poisoning causes 815
Foodborne infections 815–16
Foods *see* nutrition
Foods to be avoided by immunocompromised patients (table) 822
Foroozonfar *et al* (1977) 364
Fractionated irradiation and AML 32
France Greffe de Moelle 353, 355
Freedman (1994) 927
Freezing, purging graft 512
Frei and Cannellos 18
Frei *et al* (1985) 192
French Registry (1995) 118
Frequencies of Ig and TCR gene rearrangements and deletions in precursor B-ALL and T-ALL (table) 665
Frequency distribution of T-cells and T-cell subpopulations in peripheral blood and bone-marrow (figure) 478
Fruit 816
Functional histocompatibility tests 336
Functional tests for optimizing unrelated donor selection (table) 337
Fungal infections 724–37
  aspergillus 724, 725, 728–29, 762
  candida 724, 725, 762
  cryptococcosis 729
  diagnosis 726
  fusariosis 730
  immunosuppressive therapies and 735
  neutropenia and 724–25
    chemoprophylaxis 735
  pneumocystis carinii 724, 725, 736
    diagnosis 736–37
    prevention 736–37
    treatment 736–37
  prevention 735–36
  prophylaxis 735–36, 762
  terbinafine 734
  treatment 730–36
    adjunctive therapy 734–35
    amphotericin B 730, 731–34, 735, 736
    azoles 730–31
    flucytosine 734
    triazoles 730–31
  trichosporinosis 730
  zygomycosis 730
Fungal minimum inhibitory concentrations and minimum fungicidal concentrations (table) 731
Fungal pathogens in BMT patients (table) 724
Fusariosis 730

G

Gahrton *et al* (1991, 1995) 110, 111
Ganciclovir 651, 702, 703, 705
Garvey, Marcus 927
Gastroenteritis 718
Gastrointestinal cancer 210
Gastrointestinal complications 813
  children and 844
  cholecystitis 770
  diarrhoea 769–70
  gastroduodenitis 769
  infections post stem-cell transplant (figure) 719
  mucositis 769
  nausea 768
  oesophagitis 769
  pancreatitis 770
  typhlitis 769–70
  vomiting 768
Gastrointestinal features of graft-versus-host disease 602, 626, 628, 629, 639–41
Gastrointestinal toxicity
  cytosine arabinoside and 22
  melphalan and 22
  mitoxantrone and 22
  thiotepa and 22
Gastrostomy tubes 820
Gatti *et al* (1968) 224, 225
Gaucher's disease 288, 291
Gaxitt *et al* (1995) 122
Gazitt *et al* (1996) 461
G-CSF injections 233
GELA study 167
Gene therapy
  compared with BMT for lysosomal enzyme deficiencies 291
  cord blood and 445–47
  metabolic diseases and 290–93
  congenital disorders affecting stem cells and 5
General principles of vaccination after blood or marrow transplantation (table) 747
Genes
  retroviral marking 123
  transfection into human cells 5
Genetics of histocompatibility (figure) 394
Genoa group 57
German Acute Lymphoblastic Leukaemia Therapy Group 898
German Multicenter Acute Leukaemia Therapy Trials Groups 898
German Testicular Cancer Cooperative Study Group 184, 219
Germ-cell tumours 182–84
  adverse key prognostic factors 214, 215
  autologous BMT and 215, 219
  high dose chemotherapy 214–18
    BEP 220
    bleomycin 214, 215, 218, 219
    carbopec 219
    carboplatin 215–16, 218, 219
    cisplatin 214, 215, 218, 219
    cyclophosphamide 218, 219
    etoposide 214, 215, 217, 218, 219
    ifosfamide 218, 218, 219
    oxazophosphorine 217
    PBSC and 214, 219
    platinum 218
    primary treatment for advanced cancer 219–20
    salvage 214–19
    vinblastine 214, 218, 219
    vincristine 215
  incidence 214
  prognosis 214, 215
    after conventional salvage chemotherapy 216
    factors prior to high-dose chemotherapy 218
Gerritsen *et al* (1994) 753
Glactocerebrosidase deficiency 289
Globoid cell leukodystrophy 289
Gluckman *et al* (1989) 556
Glucksberg GvHD grading system 602
GM1 gangliosidosis 290
GOELAM trial 43
Goldschmidt *et al* (1996) 461
Gonadal failure 543–544
  complication of BMT 15, 858–61
Goodrich *et al* (1991, 1993) 703, 704, 705
Gorin (1995) 71
Gorin *et al* (1986) 41
Gottlieb *et al* (1990) 754
Graft failure 14, 249–52, 646–55
  aplastic anaemia and 651
  autologous transplantation and 652
  blood stem-cell allografts and 651–52
  bone-marrow microenvironment and 650–51
  definition 646–47
  drug induced myelosuppression 651
  growth factors and 652–53
  immunologic 650
  immunosuppression for 251
  preparative regimens and 652
  prevention of 652
  second transplant for 251, 653–54
  therapeutic 654–55
  treatment where high risk 17
  unrelated donor BMT and 381
Graft-versus-host disease (GvHD) 3–4, 5–6, 11–12, 14
  acquired aplastic anaemia and 248
  acute 596–612
    CD 34$^+$ cells 610–16
    clinical features 599–602
    cord blood cells and 609–610
    costimulatory signal blocking 612
    dermal features 599–601, 636–38
    essential elements (Billingham) 596
    future prospects 609
    gastrointestinal features 602
    grading systems 602
    hepatic features 602
    immunosuppressants 611–12
    incidence 597–99
    in vitro predictive tests 599
    pathophysiology of 596–597
    PBSC and 610
    prevention 604–606
    prophylactic treatment 604–606, 611–12
    risk factors 597–99
    T-cell depleted marrow and PBSC in mismatched transplants 611
    treatment 606–609
  acute renal failure and 775
  ALL and 70, 72–73
  allogeneic stem-cell transplantation and 399–401, 404–406
  alloresponse and 9, 14
  AML and 32
  blood transfusion associated 804
  chronic 620–34
    autoimmune disorders 627
    children and 844
    classification of 620–21
    dermal features 621–24, 627, 638
    evaluation 628–29
    eye problems 624, 627, 629, 633
    fungus infections 632
    gastrointestinal problems 626, 628, 629, 844
    gynaecological problems 627, 629
    haematopoietic system problems 627
    hepatic problems 626–27, 628, 629
    immune system problems 627, 629, 632
    mouth problems 624–26, 627–28, 629, 632, 633
    muscle problems 627, 629, 633
    prognosis 628
    respiratory tract problems 626, 628, 629

risk factors 620
Sjögren's syndrome 624
skin manifestations 621–24, 627, 638
sun, protection from 633
thyroid 629
treatment 629–34
vaccinations 633
viruses 632–33
CML and 52, 55–56, 59, 376
cord blood stem cells and 5, 442, 443–44
cyclosporin treatment 4, 33
cytoxic T-cell precursor (CTLp) as predictor 337
gastrointestinal manifestations 602, 626, 628, 629, 639–40, 813
helper T-cell precursor (HTLp) as predictor 337
hepatic features 602, 626–27, 628, 629
immune recovery and 11–12, 746
immunodeficiency diseases and 225, 226, 227
leukocyte adhesion deficiency 231
lichenoid 638
lung features 641–42
lymphoid organ features 642
methotrexate 33
mHag and 334–35
MLC assays as predictor 340
multiple myeloma and 111
neurological complications and 780
nutrition and 814
outcome of BMT 17
non-HLA-identical sibling transplants and 55
oropharynx features 642
PBSC transplant and 468–69, 474–76
protective isolation and 870
red-cell transfusion requirements 796
relapse and 684–85
sclerodermatous 638
sickle cell amaemia 281
T-cells 596–97
 depletion and 381–82
thalassaemia and 270, 272
unrelated donors and 55, 70
 tests to predict with 56
Graft-versus-leukaemia (GvL) effect 5, 16, 382
AML and 32–34
CML and 52
cord blood and 444
lymphokine activated killer cells and 444
natural killer cells and 444
outlook for 684–85
PBSC transplantation and 476
Graft-versus-leukaemia effect of donor lymphocyte transfusions in acute myeloid leukaemia (table) 683
Graft-versus-leukaemia effect of donor lymphocyte transfusions in acute lymphoid leukaemia (table) 683
Graft-versus-leukaemia effect of donor lymphocyte transfusions (table) 682
Graft-versus-lymphoma effect 167, 168
Graft-versus-marrow effect 16
Graft-versus-tumour effect 9, 13
Grandara et al (1991) 25
Griff et al (1995) 464
Grimwade et al (1994) 140
Grinsky et al (1994) 540
Growth arrest and BMT 15, 94, 272, 544, 861
Growth factors 166
graft failure and 652–53
relapse and 680–81
stem cells and 7–8
Gthalie et al (1995) 194

Guidelines for a second infusion of cells in case of delayed or failed engraftment (table) 654
Gynaecological problems with graft-versus-host disease 627, 629

H

H_2-receptor blocking agents 651
Haas et al (1994) 457
Haematoma, acute subdural (figure) 789
Haematopoiesis 3, 8, 166
haematopoietic growth factors 7, 8, 245
haematopoietic stem-cell transplantation 5
Haematopoietic growth factors see Growth factors
Haematopoietic system problems with graft-versus-host disease 627
Haemolytic uraemic syndrome 775–76
Haemophilus influenzae vaccination 749, 759
Haemorrhagic cystitis 15, 776–77
cyclophosphamide and 776
ifosfamide and 22
prevention 776
treatment 777
Haemorrhagic myocarditis 22
Hahn et al (1991, 1995) 421
Hair loss 926–27, 933, 934, 935
Haire et al (1991) 421
Ham's test 240
Hamilton (1895) 2
Hammarstrom et al (1993) 752
Hammersmith Hospital
autografting for CML 57
CML cytoreductive regimens 52
Hansen et al (1980) 364
Harousseau et al (1992, 1995) 117, 119
Hathorn (1994) 871, 873
Haynes et al (1995) 457
HDM 577
Healthcare Telematics Project 353
Heat, purging graft 512
Hebart et al (1995) 608
Helman (1992) 927, 927, 929
Helper T-cell precursor (HTLp) 337
Henner et al (1986) 24
Henner et al (1987) 24
Henon et al (1988) 117
Henslee-Downey et al 406
Hepatic failure 15
Hepatic features of graft-versus-host disease 602, 626–27, 628, 629, 640–41
Hepatic veno-occlusive disease see Veno-occlusive disease
Hepatitis B 718
vaccination 749–50
Hepatitis C 718
Herbs and spices 817
Herpes simplex virus (HSV) 633
aciclovir and 714
clinical aspects 713–14
management 714
Herpes simplex virus antigens in infected cells detected using direct fluorescein-labelled monoclonal antibody to HSV-1 proteins (figure) 714
Hervé et al (1992) 608
Heslop et al (1995) 608
HHV6 716
HHV8 716
Hib see Haemophilus influenzae
Hickman catheter 422
insertion 423–25
Hickman line in its final position (figure) 425

Hiddeman et al (1992) 26
Hiemenz and Green (1993) 870
High-grade malignant lymphoma of the CNS (figure) 791
High-risk ALL patients who are candidates for BMT in CR1 (table) 367
Hinduism 933–34
blood transfusions 934
diet 934
hair loss 934
jewellery 934
medical examination 934
Hinterberger-Fischer et al (1991) 858
Hiroshima 2
Histological changes of acute hepatic GvHD (table) 640
Histopathalogical grading of acute GvHD of the intestine (table) 639
Histopathological grading of acute GvHD of the skin (table) 638
HLA class I molecule assembly and endogenous peptide presentation (figure) 333
HLA class I peptide binding (figure) 334
HLA class II molecule assembly and exogenous peptide presentation (figure) 333
HLA class II peptide binding (figure) 334
HLA system 1996 366
HLA-identical siblings 36, 74–77, 102–104, 225, 260–61, 269, 287, 300, 335, 375
graft-versus-host disease incidence 597–99
identical twin donors 70
other donors 55–57, 70, 76, 225–26, 231–234, 261–62, 269, 287, 335–36, 375–76, 378–80, 560–61
factors affecting success with 56–57
graft-versus-host disease and 598–99
Ho (1990) 932
Hodgkin's lymphoma
adjuvant radiotherapy 142
age and prognosis 134
BMT and 135, 138
allogeneic versus autologous 143
busulfan 135
chemosensitivity and 139–40
compared with PBSC transplant 142–43
conditioning regimen 141–42
CR and risk of progression 140
cyclophosphamide 135
DFS 138
prognostic factors 139–41
radiation therapy 135
relapse after 138
survival rates 137, 139
TBI 135, 141
unrelated donors and 380
bone-marrow purging 143
chemotherapy 131
ABVD 131, 132, 140
ARDIC 132
B-CAVe 132
BCNU 141
BEAM 135, 136, 138, 141, 144
CBV 134, 141
ChlVPP 131
DexaBEAM 133, 138, 141, 142, 145
etoposide 133
EVAP 133
LOPP 133
melphalan 133
MOPP 131, 132, 133, 140
MVPP 131
Stanford V 131
conventional treatment 130–32
double transplants 141

high dose chemotherapy and 18
   adjuvant radiotherapy and 142
   financial considerations 144–45
   first complete remission and 143–44
   indications 132–34
   response rates 135–36
   salvage regimens 140
incidence 130
International Prognostic Factors project 133
interstitial pneumonitis and 134
late procedure-related mortality and morbidity 144
progression 138
Reed-Sternberg cells 130
relapse rates 131
salvage therapy 132, 140
survival 136, 137
   in poor-risk patients 135
   University College London Hospital 134, 136, 138–41
     criteria for transplantation 132
Hospitalization is not directly dependent on neutrophil count (table) 892
HOVON trial 42, 43
HRT 857
   reproduction in patients taking 862
   selection of patients for 861
Hryniuk and Bush (1984) 192
Hryniuk and Levine 20
Human anti-IL-2RA 608
Human antimurine antibodies (HAMA) 587
Human Fertilisation and Embryology Authority 859–61, 864
Human histocompatibility antigen (HLA) 4, 11
   matching 11, 335, 336–39
     guidelines 339
     HLA-Cw 339
     HLA-DP 339
     non-inherited maternal antigens 339
   major
     matching 335
   minor (mHag) 334–35
     graft-versus-host disease and 335
     matching 335
     T-cells and 335
   molecules
     peptide presentation by 332–34
     structure of 331–37
   overview of system 326–35
   sensitization against donor 336
   typing 337
     cellular assays 340
     DNA typing 337, 341–45
     isoelectric focusing (IEF) 340–41
     MLC assays 340
     serology 337
     strategies for donors on ANBMT registry 359–60
Human resource management 880–81
Humanism 934–35
Hunter disease 289
Hurler's disease 288, 289
Hydroxyurea
   CML treatment 50, 58
     children in 92
Hypertension 778
Hypomanaeaemia 778
Hypoplastic bone marrow with peripheral blood pancytopenia, causes 239
Hypothetical graph representing the putative relative frequencies of leukaemic cells in blood or bone marrow of acute leukaemia patients during and after chemotherapy and during development of relapse (figure) 660
Hypothyroidism 543

I

IBMTR allogeneic BMT risk study 37
IBMTR children ≤ 17 years (UK) (table) 366
IBMTR children ≤ 17 years (USA) (table) 365
Ice machines 816
ICE 581
ICSI and IVF assisted conception (table) 863
Idarbuicin
   autografting in CML and 57, 58
   ifosfamide and 22
Ifosfamide 200, 218
Ifosfamide 18, 22, 200, 218, 219, 582
   administration 23
IL-1-RA 608
IL-2, purging graft 513
Immune
   deficiency 15
   modulation 123
   recovery 14, 746
     types of transplantation compared 746
   system problems with graft-versus-host disease 627, 629
     infectious disease prophylaxis 632
   thrombocytopenic purpura 306
Immunmagnetic enrichment of CD34$^+$ cells using paramagnetic nanoparticles (figure) 525
Immunoaffinity columns 520–521
Immunocycochemical staining 510
Immunodeficiency diseases
   allogeneic BMT and 224
   BMT for 227–37
     donors 231–34, 380
   cartilage-hair hypoplasia 229
   conditioning regimen 228
     busulfan 228
     cyclophosphamide 228
     TBI 228
   congenital agranulocytosis 233
   cord blood stem-cell transplantation and 232–33
   DiGeorge's syndrome 224, 225
   G-CSF injections 233
   MHC class II deficiency 229
   Omenn's syndrome 229
   phagocytic cell disorders 229–31
   preparative regimens 556
   primary 227
   purine nucleoside phosphorylase deficiency 229
   severe combined immuodeficiency see Severe combined immuodeficiency
   T-cell immune deficiencies 229, 231
   Wiskott-Aldrich syndrome 238, 228–29, 231
   X-linked hyper IgM syndrome 229
Immunomagnetic enrichment of CD34$^+$ cells using superparamagnetic microspheres (figure) 524
Immunomagnetic separation 521–27
Immunomagnetic separation systems (figure) 522
Immunomagnetic T-cell depletion
   colloids 491–92
   microspheres 489–91
   nanoparticles 491–92
Immunophenotype of CD34$^+$ cells in bone marrow compared to mobilized peripheral blood (table) 455
Immunophenotyping 661–63
   acute myeloid leukaemia 663
   cerebrospinal fluid 663
   precursor B-cell acute lymphoblastic leukaemia 661–62
   T-cell acute lymphoblastic leukaemia 662–63
Immunoreconstitution following allogeneic bone-marrow transplantation from a partially-mismatched related donor (figure) 494
Immunosuppression
   graft-versus-host disease prevention
     combined agent 604–606
     new drugs 611–12
     single-agent 604
   graft-versus-host disease treatment 630
   TBI 538–39
   withdrawal for relapse 679
Immunotherapy
   hit-and-run 655
Immunotoxins 487–89
Implantable devices 422
Improved selective toxicity of lipid preparations of amphotericin B (figure) 733
Indian communities
   hair loss and 927
Indications for reliable venous access (table) 420
Indications for using lipid preparations (table) 734
Indications of blood and marrow transplantation in North America (figure) 900
Infection management 870
Infectious disease prophylaxis (table) 632
Infertility
   children and cultural issues 928–29
   complications of BMT 15, 272, 856–64
   religious issues 931–38
   marriage and 928–29
   ovum donation 859–61
   recovery of gonadal function
     females 858–61
     males 861
   sperm banking 928–29
Influenza
   A and B 717–18
   vaccination 750–51
Intercranial sepsis 790
Interferon-alpha
   CLL treatment 300
   CML treatment 50–51, 55, 58
     children in 92
     autografting and 57, 58
   follicular lymphoma 153
   multiple myeloma 118, 123–24
   relapse and 680
Intergroupe Français du Myeloma (1996) 119
International Bone Marrow Transplant Registry (BMTR) 4, 33, 51, 67, 90, 113, 114, 231, 261, 299, 406, 596
   database information 15
   HLA-identical sibling transplants 36
   institutions participating in 912–15
   transplant and non-transplant comparative analyses 14
   unrelated donors and 365
International Cord Blood Transplant Registry 610
International Prognostic Factors project 133
Interpreters 923
Interstitial pneumonitis 773–74
   Hodgkin's lymphoma and 134
Intracytoplasmic sperm injection 863
Iradubicin 169

Irradiation
  blood products 244
  fractionated 32
  relapse and 680
  total body 32, 552
    acute renal failure and 775
    ALL and 71, 72
    autoimmune disorders and 309
    cateracts 544
    cell kill for 539
    CLL and 299
    CML and 52, 375, 376
    conditioning 542
    dose 573–74
    dose distribution 540
    dosimetry 541
    drugs and 544–45
    equipment 540
    Ewing's sarcoma and 182
    follicular lymphoma and 154
    fractionation 541–42, 573–74
    future of 544–45
    gonadal failure 543–44
    graft failure and 652
    hepatic veno-occlusive disease 543
    high dose regimens in acute leukaemias 573–75
    history 538
    Hodgkin's lymphoma and 135, 141
    hypothyroidism 543
    immunodeficiency diseases and 228
    immunosuppression for 538–39
    lymphoplasmacytoid lymphoma and 159
    mantle cell lymphoma and 159
    multiple myeloma and 116, 117, 121
    neuroblastoma and 179
    nutrition and 813
    patient selection 542
    pneumonitis 543
    pregnancy and 856
    preparation 542
    preparative regimens 554, 559–60
    reduced relapse rates 41
    relapse and 678
    renal impairment 544
    second malignancies 544
    shielding organs 540
    side effects 542–44, 555–59
    small lymphocytic lymphoma and 159
    toxicity 542–44, 558–59
  total lymphoid 631–32
Islam 935–36
  abortion 935
  circumcision 935
  diet 935
  hair loss 935
  jewellery 935
  menstruation 935
  sexual segregation 935
  sperm banking 935
Isobologram 21–23
Isoelectric focusing (IEF) 340–41
Issues of concern for patients from different ethnic backgrounds when undergoing bone-marrow transplantation (table) 931
Issues relating to BMT which may potentially affect nutritional status (table) 812
Italian CML Study Group 898
ITP 307

J

Jackson et al (1994) 166
Jacobsen (1948) 2

Jagannath et al (1992) 117, 141
Jainism 938
  diet 938
jCML 49, 93, 373–75
  BMT and 93
  Sanders et al (1979, 1988) 93
Jehovah's Witnesses 936
  blood transfusions 936
Jejunostomy tubes 820
Jones et al (1990) 143, 192
Jourden et al (1995) 36
Judaism 936–37
  blood transfusions 937
  diet 937
  infertility 937
Junctional regions of Ig or TCR geners as major PCR targets for MRD detection in acute leukaemias (table) 665

K

Kaplan 18
Kaplan-Meier probability of reaching 0.5 x 109/litre neutrophils after high dose chemotherapy (figure) 458
Kaur et al (1996) 769
Keller et al (1990) 818
Keohane et al (1983) 421
Kernan et al (1993) 231, 600
Kessinger et al (1991) 140, 142
Khouri et al (1994) 299
Klein et al (1995) 289
Klumpp et al (1995) 461
Known ovum donation (table) 859
Kodish et al (1991) 281
Korbling et al (1995) 464, 465, 467
Krabbe's disease 289
Kuttah et al (1995) 770

L

Lai and Yue (1990) 932
LAK see Lymphokine activated killer cells
Landy (1977) 930
Language problems 923
Laporte et al (1991) 166
Laporte et al (1993) 102
Late effects of bone-marrow transplantation in childhood (table) 837
Laussaniere and Auzannea (1995) 931
Leach (1968) 927
Leake and Leake (1923) 2
Learner et al (1974) 636
Lectin treatment 478–79
Legionnaires' disease 873
Leukaemia
  acute lymphoblastic see ALL
  acute myeloid see AML
  bone-marrow transplants and 3, 4
  chronic myeloid see CML
  chronic neutrophilic see CNL
  comparison of allogeneic and autologous BMT with chemotherapy 14
  high dose chemotherapy prior to transplant 18, 573–76
  juvenile chronic myeloid see jCML
Leukaemia-associated immunophenotypes in acute leukaemia (table) 662
Leukocyte adhesion deficiency 229, 231
  graft-versus-host disease and 231
Leukopenia 789–90
Levine et al (1973) 870
Lichenoid changes within the mouth seen with advanced chronic GvHD (figure) 626

Lichenoid chronic GvHD 638
Linch et al (1995) 461
Line attached to an introducer and pulled through subcutaneous tissue (catheter insertion) (figure) 424
Lipid-containing preparations (table) 732
Lipton et al (1993) 852
Live vaccines which are contraindicated for immunocompromised patients 746
Liver
  problems and graft-versus-host disease 602
  virus infections post stem-cell transplant (figure) 720
Ljungman et al (1990, 1991) 752, 753
Locatelli et al (1997) 375
Lohri and Connors (1994) 139
LOMAC 192
Longo et al (1992) 132
Long-term tunnelled lines 423
LOPP 133
Lorenz 2
Lorenz et al (1951) 538
Lortan et al (1992) 751
Lotz et al (1993) 206
Low microbial diet 761, 815, 816
Lucarelli et al (1989, 1990) 556
Lum et al (1986) 748
Lumen catheter 421–22
Lung problems with graft-versus-host disease 641–42
Lung shielding blocks (figure) 540
Lymphoblastic lymphoma 168
Lymphocytes
  alloresponse and 8
  cross-match 336
  immune function 8
Lymphoid organ problems with graft-versus-host disease 642
Lymphokine activated killer cells and 444
  purging the graft with 513
Lymphomas
  high dose chemotherapy prior to transplant 18, 578–581
Lymphoplasmacytoid lymphoma 159
  ABMT and 159
  chlorambucil and 159
  fludarabine 159
  myeloablative therapy and 159
  TBI and 159
Lysosomal
  storage diseases 286–93
    allogeneic BMT and 286–90
    Farber's disease 290
    Gaucher's disease 288, 291
    glactocerebrosidase deficiency 289
    globoid cell leukodystrophy 289
    GM1 gangliosidosis 290
    Hunter disease 289
    Hurler's disease 288, 289
    Krabbe's disease 289
    Marateaux-Lamy disease 289
    metachromatic leukodystrophy 289
    Morquio's disease 289
    mucopolysaccharidoses 288
    Niemann-Pick disease 290
    Sandhoff disease 290
    Sanfilippo's disease 289
    stem-cell gene therapy 290–293
    Tay-Sachs disease 290

M

Maculopapular rash becoming more acute in some areas (figure) 601

Mafosfomide 513
Major ABO incompatibility (table) 800
Major and minor ABO incompatibility (table) 800
Major histocompatibility complex (MHC) antigens 10
Malignancies
  bone-marrow transplants and 3–4, 13
  secondary
    children 845
    complication of BMT 15
  solid tumours and high dose chemotherapy prior to transplant 18, 19
Malignant brain tumours in childhood 185
Malignant melanoma 209
  autologous BMT 209
  high-dose chemotherapy 209
    BCNU 209
    cisplatin 209
    cyclophosphamide 209
    DTIC 209
    melphalan 209
    thiotepa 209
Management of herpes simplex and varicella-zoster post stem-cell transplant (table) 715
Management of relapsed ALL according to duration of CR1 and site of relapse (table) 370
Management of relapsed AML in CR2 according to previous treatment (table) 371
Mandelli (1990) 124
Mansi et al (1987) 196
Mantle cell lymphoma 159–60
  cyclophosphamide and 159
  myeloablative therapy and 159–60
  TBI and 159
Marateaux-Lamy disease 289
Mares (1985) 930
Marks et al (1993) 600
Marriage 928–29
Marrow
  see also Bone-marrow
  alternative sources 435
  buffy coat preparations 436–37
  collection 434–38
    problems 435
    risks 434
    technique 434
    timing 434
  cryopreservation 437
  engraftment 12–13
  freezing 437
  infusion 438
  mononuclear cell separation 437
  preservation 437
  quality assurance 438
  red-blood cell depletion 436
    dilution with compatible red-blood cells 436
    starch sedimentation 436
  storage conditions 437
  thawing 437–38
  transporting 435–36
  volume reduction 436
Marsh et al (1989) 650
Martin et al (1990, 1991) 607
Maruta et al (1995) 856
Mathé et al (1965) 678
Mathé, George 5
McCarthy and Goldman (1984) 117
MCF7 (breast cancer) in vitro dose-response curves (figure) 582
McGlave et al (1993) 600
McQuaker et al (1996) 461

MDS see Myelodysplastic syndromes (MDS)
Measles 717
  vaccination 751
MEC 180
Medical examination, attitudes to 924–25
Mellstedt et al (1995) 123
Melphalan 18, 22, 552, 568, 581, 582
  administration 24
  autoimmune disorders and 309
  breast cancer and 193
  Choi et al (1989) 24
  CLL and 300
  epithelial ovarian cancer and 206
  Ewing's sarcoma 182
  graft failure and 652
  Hodgkin's lymphoma and 133
  malignant melanoma 209
  multiple myeloma 110, 115, 116, 117, 118, 119, 121
  myelodysplastic syndromes in childhood and 374
  neuroblastoma 180
  neurological problems and 788
  thalassaemia and 270
Meningeal infiltration by acute myeloblastic leukaemia (figure) 793
Meningoencephalitis 742
Menopause, post 862
Menstruation
  amenhorroeic patients 861
  cultural attitudes to 925, 935
  monitoring menstruating patients 862
Merocyanine (MC540) 514–15
Metabolic
  complications 778
  disorders 16
Metachromatic leukodystrophy 289
Metallic taste 823
Metastatic breast cancer 192–93
Methods for T-cell depletion of allogeneic stem-cell grafts (table) 478
Methods of nutrition support used in bone-marrow transplantation (table) 819
Methods of reducing infection in bone-marrow transplantation patients (table) 758
Methotrexate 18, 22, 169, 300, 374, 604, 775
  administration 26
  children and 26
  GvHD and 33
  GvL and 33
Meyers et al (1988) 702, 704
MHC class II deficiency 229
MHC 326
  genetic structure 330–31
Microassisted fertilisation techniques 863
Microassisted fertilization (MAF) techniques (figure) 864
Microorganisms isolated in proven catheter-related infections (table) 427
Microscopic polyangiitis 307
Microspheres 489–91
Microwave ovens 817
Miflin et al (1996) 464, 467
Miltenyi/Amgen large-scale separator for immunomagnetic enrichment of CD34+ cells using paramagnetic nanoparticles (figure) 526
Miltenyi Biotech immunomagnetic device 198, 199
Mineral
  requirements 819
  water 816

Minimal residual disease (MRD)
  methods of detection 660–72
    immunophenotyping 661–62
    PCR techniques 663–64
Minor ABO incompatibility (table) 798
Minor histocompatibility antigens (mHag) 10, 334–35
Mirabell et al (1996) 775
Mitomycin C 775
Mitoxantrone 22, 206, 582
  administration 24–25
  Canal et al (1993) 25
  Feldman et al (1993) 25
  Grandara et al (1991) 25
  Henner et al (1986) 24
  pharmacology 583
Mixed known/unknown ovum donation (table) 860
MLC assays 340
  graft-versus-host disease and 340
Modified ward diets 816
Molrine et al (1996) 751
Monoclonal antibodies 481
  anti-ab 486–87
  anti-CD2 485, 608
  anti-CD3 484, 608
  anti-CD5 608
  anti-CD6 485–86
  anti-CD25 608
  anti-IL-2R 608
  anti TNFa 608
  CAMPATH 481, 482–84
  CBL1 608
  complement and 481–82
  Human anti-IL-2RA 608
  IL-1-RA 608
  pan T-cell antibody combinations 487
  purging the graft 517–18
  ricin A 608
  TCRab 608
  toxin conjugate 198
  treatment of graft-versus-host disease 606–609
Mononuclear cell separation 437
Monozygotic twins 248–49
MOPP 131, 132, 133, 140
Morquio's disease 289
Mouth blindness 823
Mouth problems with graft-versus-host disease 624–26, 627–28, 629, 633
  topical treatment of 632
MRD see Minimal residual disease
MTX 604, 605, 607
Mucopolysaccharidoses 288
Mucormycosis 730
Mucosal toxicity
  cystosine arabinoside and 22
  mitoxantrone and 22
Mucositis 823
  etoposide and 22
  methotrexate and 22
Mullen et al (1993) 232
Multicentre observational databases 896–910
  alternative treatment comparison 897–99
  Autologous Blood and Marrow Transplant Registry – North America 896
  British Medical Research Council 898
  comparison of regimes 897
  current use and outcomes of transplantation 898–910
  descriptive studies 897
  Eastern Cooperative Oncology Group 898

European Group for Blood and Marrow Transplantation 4, 14, 41, 67, 88, 102, 103, 104, 110, 114, 130, 142, 143, 144, 154, 155, 176, 179, 181, 208, 306, 310, 367, 376, 455, 577, 596, 651, 880
German Acute Lymphoblastic Leukaemia Therapy Group 898
German Multicenter Acute Leukaemia Therapy Trials Groups 898
International Bone Marrow Transplant Registry 4, 14, 15, 33, 36, 51, 67, 90, 113, 114, 231, 261, 299, 365, 406, 596
late consequences determination 898
need for 896–97
Italian CML Study Group 898
Pediatric Oncology Group 898
prognostic factors identification 897
transplant outcome statistical methodology development 898
Multiple moles following chemoradiotherapy (figure) 846
Multiple myeloma
allogeneic BMT 110–15
stem cells 113
survival rates 111–13
unrelated donors and 380
autologous BMT 115–22
carmustine 117
cyclophosphamide 117
doxorubicin 118
etoposide 117
immune modulation and 123
interferon-alpha 118, 123–24
melphalan and 115, 116, 117, 118, 119, 121
PBSC transplant compared 119–20
peripheral blood stem-cell 117–21
purged 116–17
relapse after 124–25
TBI 116, 117, 121
thiotepa 121
VAD 115
VAMP 115, 119
vincristine 118
busulfan 111, 113, 117, 119, 121
chemotherapy 110
complete remission in 110, 116
contamination of PBSC harvested cells 460–61
cyclophosphamide 111, 113, 117, 121
graft-versus-host disease and 111
positive stem-cell selection 122–23
post-transplantation maintenance therapy 123–24
retroviral gene marking 123
standard treatment 110
Mumps 751
Murakami et al (1994) 207–208
Muscle problems
graft-versus-host disease and 627, 629, 633
parenteral nutrition and 821
Muslims see Islam
Mustine 131
MVPP 131
Myelodysplastic syndromes (MDS) 100–104
allogeneic BMT and 102–105, 379–80
Dana Farber study 102
AML and 100, 379–80
autologous bone-marrow transplant and 102
Demuynck et al (1996) 102
Laporte et al (1993) 102
BMT and 93–94, 102–105
chemotherapy and 101–102
children in 373–75
cytogenetic abnormalities and 104

DFS 104
cytogenetic abnormalities and 104
European Working Group on Myelodysplastic Syndrome in Childhood 374
French-American-British (FAB) classification 100, 373
juvenile chronic myeloid leukaemia 373
myelofibrosis and 104
prognosis 100–101
Myleran see Busulfan

N

Nademanee et al (1995) 140
Nagasaki 2
Nanoparticles 491–92
Nash et al (1992) 598
Nasogastric feeding 820
National Association of Round Tables of Great Britain and Ireland 357
National Marrow Donor Program (USA) 353, 355, 364
Natural killer cells 444
Nausea 768, 812, 814, 823
Nemunaitis et al (1990) 652
Neomycin 758
Nephrotoxicity and cisplatin 22
Neuberger (1987) 931
Neuroblastoma 175–81
autologous BMT and 175
Children's Cancer Group 178
double autograft procedures 179
European Neuroblastoma Study Group 178
MEC 180
OMEC 180
survival rates 175–76, 178
TBI versus high-dose chemotherapy 179
Neurological complications post-BMT (table) 779
Neurological complications 65–66, 778–80, 788–93
children and 843–44
drug related 788–89
graft-versus-host disease and 780
tolerance of adults to treatment
Neurotoxicity and ifosfamide 22
Neutropenia 690, 724–25
antibiotic prophylaxis 758–59
blood transfusion and 805–806
chemoprophylaxis 735
gut decontamination 758–59
reducing length 762
New York Blood Center 442
Nicholls (1975) 934, 935
Niemann-Pick disease 290
Nitrogen
balance 818
mustard
autologous BMT in children and 174–86
requirements and nutrition 818
Nobel Prize for Physiology or Medicine 5
Nocardia 743
Non-alkylating agents 18
Non-continuous confinement of patients see Outpatient care
Non-haematological effects of perparative regimens (table) 555
Non-Hodgkin's lymphoma
contamination of PBSC after harvesting 461–65
high grade 164–70
allogeneic BMT 167–68
autologous BMT 164–67
BEAM 166, 167
chemotherapy regimens 165

CHOP 164
CNS of 168
dose escalation 167
GELA study 167
graft-versus-lymphoma effect 167, 168
haemopoietic growth factors and autologous BMT 166
high-dose chemotherapy 169
radiotherapy after high-dose chemotherapy 169
intermediate 164–70
Kiel classification 152
lymphoblastic lymphoma 168
purging the graft 508
see also Follicular lymphoma, Small lymphocytic lymphoma, Lymphoplasmacytoid lymphoma, Mantle cell lymphoma
Non-tunnelled central venous catheters 422
Normal life
readaption to 830–34
interventions to facilitate 834–35
North American Marrow Donor Pool (NAMDP) 4
Northern Regional Haematology Group AML and allogeneic BMT trials 34–35
Nuclear weapons and bone marrow failure syndrome 2
Number of transplants using ANBMT donors (table) 356
Number of UK recipients of bone marrow from international registries (table) 355
Nurse transplant coordinator 317
Nursing staff 875, 880–87
administration 880–82
human resource management 880–81
strategic planning 880
ambulatory care 885
development of 881–82
documentation of care 885
education of 881–82
orientation of 881–82
patient education 884–83
planning patient care 882–83
policies and procedures 884
role 881
stress 882
transplant coordinator 317
Nutrition
anorexia 812
assessment 319, 817–18
bioelectrical impedance and 818
calories 823
chemotherapy and 812–13
diarrhoea and 814, 823
dietary restrictions 815–17
discharge planning 821–22
disgeusia and 813–14
energy requirements 818
fluid requirements 818–19
gastrointestinal problems and 813
gastrostomy tubes 820
graft-versus-host disease and 814
jejunostomy tubes 820
mineral requirements 819
nasogastric feeding 820
nausea and 814, 823
nitrogen
balance and 818
requirements and 818
nutritionally complete supplements 820
oesophagitis and 813
oral 819–24
infections and 814

Index

mucositis and 813
parenteral nutrition 820–21
protein 823
requirements pre-transplant 812
support during BMT 812–23
taste changes 823
TBI and 812–13
underlying disease and 812
vitamin requirements 819
vomiting and 814, 823
xerostomia and 813, 823
Nystatin 758

O

Oesophagitis and nutrition 813
Officially recognized HLA loci within the human MHC (table) 327
OMEC 180
Omenn's syndrome 229
Omeprazole 651
Oncologist, high dose chemotherapy prior to transplant 20
Opthalmological problems in children 844
Oral
   infections 814
   mucositis 813
Orientation programme (nursing staff) (table) 881
Oropharynx problems with graft-versus-host disease 642
Osteoporosis in children 845
Ostepena in children 845
Other monoclonal antibodies and complement used in graft manipulation (table) 484
Ototoxicity and cisplatin 22
Ouaknin (1992) 931
Outpatient care 870–71, 885, 890–93
   allogeneic transplants
      long-term follow up 893
      peritransplant 891–93
      pretransplant 891
   autologous transplants
      long-term follow up 891
      peritransplant 890–91
      pretransplant 890
Ovarian
   problems 851–52
   recovery 862–63
Ovum donation 859–61
   (table) 859
Owen et al (1996) 461
Oxazophorine 217

P

Paclitaxel 18, 22, 582, 788
   administration 26–27
   pharmacology 584
   Stemmer et al (1996) 27
Paediatric Haematology Forum 281
Pain, cultural attitudes to 929–31
   Buddhists 932
Pan T-cell antibody combinations 487
Pancytopenia 646–55
Panning 479–80, 519–20
Papadopoulou et al (1994) 813
Papovaviruses 717
Parainfluenza 1–3 717–18
Parasitic infections and bone-marrow treatment 2
Parenteral nutrition 820–21
   complications
      fluid overload 821

muscle wasting 821
Parsi see Zoroastrianism
Parsons, Talcott 828
Parvovirus B19 718
Patient
   adaption to illness 828–30
   adaption to normal life 830–34
   appetite 820
   assuming role of 828
   care
      ambulatory 885
      BMT 17
      documentation of 885
      planning 882–83
      policies and procedures 884
   Chinese 922
   communication with 922–24
   counselling
      for TBI 542
      post transplant 834
   drilling 863
   education 884–85
   fitness for transplantation 318–20
   isolation 870–71
   language problems 922
   non-continuous confinement 870–71
   nutrition 812–823
   overseas
      food and 819
   pretransplant
      consultation 316–18
      dental assessment 319
      investigations 318–20
      nutritional assessment 319, 817–19
   selection
      BMT 13–14, 245–46, 316
      TBI 542
   sensitization against donor antigens 336
   time off work 318
   transplant talk 317–18
   venous access 320
Patients who should not be considered eligible for live vaccination after blood or marrow transplantation (table) 747
PCR 508–509, 510
   CMV detection 700, 705
   fingerprinting 342
   MRD detection and 663–64
      chromosome aberrations as PCR targets for 669–70
      junctional regions as targets for 664–70
PCR-AFLP 342
PCR-based HLA typing methods, main features of common (table) 341
PCR-SSOP 342–43
   and reverse-hybridization dot-blotting 343
   outline of and various detection techniques (figure) 343
PCR-SSP 343–44
   outline of technique (figure) 344
Peak incidence of herpesvirus reactivations post stem-cell transplantation (figure) 713
Pediatric Oncology Group 898
Pegg 3
Pentamidine 736
Pentostatin 481
Percentage of allogeneic transplants from unrelated donors (figure) 900
Percentage of BMT respondents reporting current status was not normal, almost normal or normal (table) 831
Percentage of patients searches referred from UK transplant centres finding 6/6 antigen-matching donors (table) 354

Percentage of transplant recipients whose donor was identified on the initial search of the Anthony Nolan Register (table) 359
Pericarditis 778
Peripheral blood progenitor cells 384–86
   breast cancer and 196
   myeloablative therapy and 155–56
Peripheral blood stem cell transplantation. Data reviewed (table) 611
Peripheral blood stem cells (PBSC)
   characteristics of 454
   contamination by tumour cells 460
      myeloma 460–61
      non-Hodgkin's lymphoma 461–62
   graft-versus-host disease and 610
   mobilization 463–67
      chemotherapy with 455
      factors affecting 459
      growth factors with 455–60
      kinetics of 456
   positive selection 122–23
   stem cell rescue in paediatric oncology 186
   T-cell depletion 474–504
      mismatched transplants 611
   allogeneic 463–69, 492–96
   autologous 454–63
   acquired aplastic anaemia and 239
   $CD34^+$ cells 462–63
   engraftment following 456–62
   graft failure 476–77
   graft-versus-host disease and 399–401, 407–408, 468–69, 474–76
   graft-versus-leukaemia and 476
   Hodgkin's lymphoma and 142–43
   multiple myeloma in 117–21
   high dose chemotherapy and 18–27
   venous access for harvesting 420–25
Peripheral nervous system see Neurological complications
Peripheral venous cannulation 421
Pernicious anaemia 2
Pesaro classification of transplantation risk 269
Petersdorf et al (1995) 600
Pettengell et al (1993) 456
P-glycoprotein (Ppg)-mediated multidrug resistance (MDR) 19
Phagocytic cell disorders 229–31
   Chediak-Higashi syndrome 229, 231
   chronic granulomatosis disease 230
   conditioning regimen 230
   leukocyte adhesion deficiency 229, 231
      graft-versus-host disease and 231
   severe congenital neutropenias 230
Pharmacokinetics 21
Pharmacodynamics
   high dose chemotherapy 20, 21
Phase I–II studies of monoclonal antibodies for the treatment of acute GvHD (table) 608
PH-chromosome 48
   ALL and 49, 64, 367
   BCR gene and 48
   CML and 48, 49–51
   CNL and 49
   generation of 48
   jCML and 49
   Rowley (1973) 48
Pheripheral neuropathy and cisplatin 22
Philadelphia chromosome see PH-chromosome
Philips et al (1991) 134, 142
Photoactive agents
   purging graft 514
      merocyanine (MC540) 514–15
Physical sequelae 828
Pituitary gland problems 850

955

Platelet storage (table) 801
Platelet
  post transplant problems 789
  transfusion 801–804
    apheresis platelets 804
    cytomegalovirus and 804–805
    filtration 803
    HLA immunization 802–803
    immunological refractoriness 803–804
    leukodepletion 803
    major histocompatibility complex and 802–803
    monitoring outcome 801
    quality of concentrates 801
    single donor platelets 804
    trigger 802
Platinum 218
Pneumococcal prophylaxis 632
Pneumococcus vaccination 751–52, 759
Pneumocystis carinii 632, 724, 725
  diagnosis 736
  prevention 736–37
  treatment 736–37
Pneumonitis 543
Poe et al (1994) 870
POG trial 42, 43, 87
Pokeweed antiviral protein (PAP) 519
Poliakoff (1995) 922
Policies and procedures for BMT unit (table) 884
Poliovirus vaccination 752
Polycystic ovaries 862
Porro et al (1988) 196
Portal tract in chronic GvHD showing absent interlobular bile duct (figure) 641
Possible sites of entry of infection with central venous catheters (table) 690
Post BMT problems in females (table) 852
Post-BMT findings in males (table) 853
Precursor B-ALL patient with a Vd-Dd3 rearrangement as PCR target for MRD detection (figure) 666
Predisposing factors for infection after bone-marrow transplant (table) 758
Prednisolone 66, 307
  multiple myeloma 110
Prednisone 131, 300, 604, 605, 629, 630
Pregnancy
  see also Infertility
  acquired aplastic anaemia and 254
  TBI and 856
Prentice et al (1994) 702, 704
Preparative regimens for immune deficiencies and congenital disorders (table) 557
Preparative regimens for severe aplastic anaemia [SAA and Fanconi anaemia (FA)] (table) 558
Preparative regimens 12, 15, 550–61
  antibodies 552
  anti-leukaemic effect 553–54
  antitumour regimens 554–55
  bone marrow disorders 556
  chemotherapy 552, 554–55
    compared with radiation 559–60
  common agents used 567–70
  Fanconi anaemia 556–57
  function 550
  graft failure and 652
  haematological malignancies 558, 566
    chemotherapy only 558–59
  high risk transplants in 552–57
  history 550
  immunodeficiency diseases 556
  immunosuppression 550–53
  inborn errors 556
  mismatched donors 560–61
  myeloablation 553–54
  radiation 553
  secondary malignancies and 584–87
  severe aplastic anaemia 557–58
  side effects 555–59
  TBI-based regimens 554
  unrelated donors 560–61
Preparative regimens used in allgeneic BMT for malignant disorders (table) 559
Pretransplant arragements (allogeneic patients) (table) 891
Pretransplant arrangement autolgous transplant patients (table) 890
Pretransplant investigations (table) 318
Pretransplant investigations for the donor (table) 319
Preventing Legionella infection (table) 873
Prevention of graft failure: approach to a high-risk autograft recipient (table) 653
Prevention of graft rejection: approach to a high-risk allograft recipient (table) 649
Probability of leukaemia-free survival after allogeneic BMT for acute lymphoblasitic leukaemia (figure) 903
Probability of leukaemia-free survival after allogeneic BMT for acute myelogenous leukaemia (figure) 904
Probability of leukaemia-free survival after autotransplants for acute lymphoblastic leukaemia (figure) 903
Probability of leukaemia-free survival after autotransplants for acute myelogenous leukaemia (figure) 904
Probability of survival after autotransplants for Hodgkin's disease (figure) 908
Probability of leukaemia-free survival after BMT for chronic myelogenous leukaemia in chronic phase (figure) 904
Probability of leukaemia-free survival after HLA-identical sibling BMT for chronic myelogenous leukaemia (figure) 903
Probability of leukaemia-free survival after HLA-identical sibling and unrelated BMT for severe aplastic anaemia (figure) 905
Probability of survival after autotransplants for breast cancer (figure) 909
Probability of survival after autotransplants for intermediate grade or immunblastic non-Hodgkin's lymphoma (figure) 909
Probability of survival after autotransplants for low-grade non-Hodgkin's lymphoma (figure) 908
Probability of survival after autotransplants for metastatic breast cancer (figure) 910
Probability of survival after HLA-identical sibling BMT for chronic myelogenous leukaemia (figure) 903
Problems associated with bone-marrow harvest (table) 435
Problems in the acute phase post-BMT (table) 883
Problems reported after BMT (table) 833
Procarbazine 604
Prognostic factors identification 897
Progressive multifocal leukoencephalopathy (figure) 791
Prophylactic treatment for general infection post transplant 758–63
  endogonous flora 758–62
Proposal indications for transplant procedures in children 1997 (table) 368

Protective isolation units 750, 870–71
  psychosocial impact on patients 871
Protozoan infections 742
Przepiorka et al (1995) 24
Psoralen with ultra violet light 630
Psychological aspects of donation 321
Psychosocial sequelae 828
Psychotherapy 834
Puberty 15
Pulmonary injury and cyclophosphamide 22
Purging graft 508–28
  4-hydroperoxycyclophosphamide 198
  ALL and 512
  AML and 508–509
  breast cancer and 196–200
  childhood solid tumours 185–86
  CD34 198
  CellPro column 200
  CML and 512
  CEPRATE stem-cell concentrator 199
  Detachabead" 198
  Dynabeads-CD34 198
  Hodgkin's lymphoma and 143
  monoclonal antibody-toxin conjugate 198
  Miltenyi Biotech immunomagnetic device 198, 199
  multiple myeloma and 116–17
  negative 198
  non-Hodgkin's lymphoma 508
  PCR and 508–509, 510
  positive selection 198–200
  techniques 510–27
    4-hydroperoxycyclophosphamide 514
    alkyl-lysophospholipids 515–16
    antibody targeted purging 517–18
    antisense oligonucleotides 516
    autologous bone marrow cells and IL-2 513
    centrifugal elutration 511–12
    culture purging 512–13
    cytokine activated cells 513
    density-gradient centrifugation 511
    freezing 512
    heat 512
    immunoaffinity columns 520–21
    immunomagnetic separation 521–27
    lymphokine activated killer cells 513
    mafosfomide 513
    panning 519–20
    photoactive agents 514–15
    unit gravity sedimentation 511
  tumour detection 509–10
    flow cytometry 510
    immunocyochemical staining 510
  WR-2721 198
Purine nucleoside phosphorylase deficiency 229
Pyrimethamine 792

Q

Quality of life 830–34
Qureshi (1994) 922, 934

R

Raaf catheter 423
Rabinowe et al (1993) 299
Racadot et al (1995) 608
Radiotherapy, targetted 545
  see also Total body irradiation
Randomised studies comparing conditioning with BuCY and CyTBI (table) 545
Ranitidine 651
Rapoport et al (1993) 134, 138
Rastafarians 937

background 927
diet 937
hair loss and 927
Recommendations for patients without matched siblings (allogeneic stem-cell transplantation) (figure) 409
Recommended immunization schedule in blood or marrow transplant recipients excluding those with chronic graft-versus-host disease (table) 748
Recommended immunization schedule in patients with chronic graft-versus-host disease (table) 749
Rectal mucosa with grade III GvHD changes (figure) 639
Red-cell transfusion (table) 797
Red-cell transfusions 796–801
Reducing acquisition of exogenous flora (table) 760
Reece and Philips (1994) 140
Reece et al (1993) 117, 134, 140, 142
Reed-Sternberg cells 130
Refractory anaemia (RA) 100
    BMT and 103, 105
  with excess of blasts (RAEB) 100
    BMT and 103, 105
    chemotherapy and 101
  with excess of blasts in transformation (RAEBt) 100
    BMT and 105
  with ring sideroblasts (RARS) 100
    BMT and 102
Regime comparison 897
Registry of bone marrow donors
  Anthony Nolan Bone Marrow Trust 352
    maintenance of register 358–59
    number of transplants using donors from (table) 356
    world distribution of transplants performed using donors from (table) 356
  Autologous Blood and Marrow Transplant Registry
    institutions participating in 915–17
  Blood Transfusion Service Register 352
  Bone Marrow Donors Worldwide 353
  British Bone Marrow and Platelet Donor Panel 352
  Europdonor 4, 353, 355
  France Greffe de Moelle 353, 355
  Healthcare Telematics Project 353
  International Bone Marrow Transplant Registry
    institutions particicipating in 912–15
  National Marrow Donor Program (USA) 353, 355, 364
  number of UK recipients of bone marrow from international registries (table) 355
  registering a search 352
  search results 353
  search statistics 352
  transmission of search requests 353
  Unrelated Bone Marrow Donor Register (Canadian) 355
  world-wide-web 353
  Zentrales Knochenmark-spenderregister 353, 355
Reimmunization 746–54, 761
  adoptive transfer of protective immunity 753–54, 762
  childhood immunizations 746
  graft-versus-host disease and 746
  passive immunization 754, 761
    white blood cells and 804
  vaccination 746–53

measurement of immune response to 753
Reisner et al (1983) 226
Relapse 678–85
  autograft as primary treatment 40
  BMT and
    treatment of 15
  CML and 52–57
  donor lymphocyte transfusions 681–84
  forms 679
  graft-versus-host disease 681–85
  graft-versus-leukaemia effect 682–94
  nature of 678–79
  risk factors 678–79
  total body irradiation and 41
  transient cytogenetic 53
  treatment of
    chemotherapy 679–80
    cytokines 680–81
    growth factors 680–81
    immunosuppression withdrawal 679
    radiotherapy 680
    second marrow transplants 681
Related disciplines (to nursing) (table) 880
Relationship between CD34+ cells measured in the peripheral blood and CD34+ cells subsequently collected in leukapheresis product shows a good correlation (figure) 457
Religious considerations 931–38
  Baha'i 931–32
  Buddhist 932
  Christian Science 933
  Christianity 932–33
  Hinduism 933–34
  Humanism 934–35
  Islam 935–36
  Jainism 938
  Jehovah's Witnesses 938
  Judaism 938–39
  Rastafarian 927, 937
  Sikhism 937–38
  Zoroastrianism 938
Renal failure
  complication of BMT 15
  children and 843
Renal impairment 544, 777
  acute renal failure 774–75
  acute tumour lysis syndrome 776
  children and 843
  haemolytic uraemic syndrome 775–76
  haemorrhagic cystitis 776–77
Renal toxicity
  ifosfamide and 22
  methotrexate and 22
  paclitaxel and 22
Requirements for an outpatient autologous transplant unit (table) 891
Resources 882
  human see Nursing staff
Respiratory distress
  complication of BMT 15
  children and 843
Respiratory tract
  infections 717–18
  problems of graft-versus-host disease 626, 628, 629
Responses in CML patients treated for cytogenetic or haematological relapse (figure) 682
Restrictive lung disease 15
Results from the only two randomised trials of TBI dose escalation by Clift et al from Seattle (table) 539

Results of randomized trials of growth factors following autologous PBSC transplantations (table) 461
Results of UD BMT in acute leukaemia (table) 379
Reticular dysgeneses see Severe combined immunodeficiency
Retroviral gene marking 123
Retrovirus vectors 292
Reverse barrier nursing 760
Rh blood groups in transfusions 798, 800–801
Rhabdomyosarcoma see Sarcoma
Rheumatoid arthritis 306
Ribas-Mundo et al (1981) 870
Ricin A 519, 608
Ringden et al (1994) 545
Risk factors for psychosocial morbidity (table) 835
Risk factors for the development of chronic GvHD (table) 620
Rodenhuis et al (1996) 194
Rowley (1973) 48
rtPCR studies 53
Rubella vaccination 752
Rummelhart et al (1990) 232
Russell and Miflin 468
Russell et al (1992) 870
Russell et al (1996) 463, 467, 468

S

Salooja et al (1994) 852
sAML 102
  BMT and 103–104, 105
  chemotherapy 103–104
Sanders (1991) 858
Sanders et al (1979) 93
Sanders et al (1988) 93, 851, 856
Sanders et al (1996) 858
Sandhoff disease 290
Sanfilippo's disease 289
Sarcoma 181, 208–209
  autologous BMT and 208
  high-dose chemotherapy and 208
SBT 345
Scanning electron micrograph of an antibody-sensitized lymphoma cell rosetted with Dynal M450' (figure) 523
Scanning electron micrograph of target-cell coated with Miltenyi paramagnetic nanoparticles (figure) 526
Scarring and ethnic considerations 928
Schematic representation of a CD4+ T-cell (figure) 392
Schiller et al (1994) 600
Schiller et al (1995) 462
Schirmer's test 629
Schmidt et al (1991) 703
Schmitz et al (1995) 467, 468
Schouten et al 155
Schretzenmeyer (1937) 2
Schwartzberg et al (1993) 457
SCID see Severe combined immuodeficiency
Sclerodermatous chronic GvHD 638
Sclerodermatous form of chronic graft-versus-host disease (figure) 625
Scott (1995) 928
Searches for bone marrow donors
  Anthony Nolan Bone Marrow Trust (ANBMT) 352
    maintenance of register 358
    number of transplants using donors from (table) 356

world distribution of transplants using donors from (table) 356
Blood Transfusion Service Register 352
Bone Marrow Donors Worldwide 353
British Bone Marrow and Platelet Donor Panel 352
Europdonor 4, 353, 355
European Donor Secretariat 353
European Marrow Donor Information System 353
France Greffe de Moelle 353, 355
Healthcare Telematics Project 353
National Marrow Donor Program (USA) 353, 355, 364
percentage of patients referred from UK finding antigen-matching donors (table) 354
registering a search 352
search results 353
success rate using ANBMT donors 355–57
statistics 352
transmission of search requests 353
Unrelated Bone Marrow Donor Register (Canadian) 355
world-wide-web 353
Zentrales Knochenmark-spenderregister 353, 355
Seasoning 817
Seattle transplant team 84
Secondary infections in the mouth afflicted by cGvHD (figure) 626
Secondary malignancies
  children and 845
  complication of BMT 15
Selassie, Haile 927
Selection of blood products after BMT with major ABO incompatibility (table) 800
Selection of Rh blood group (table) 800
Semiconductor diodes in position for *in vivo* dosimetry (figure) 541
Sen (1967) 933
Sensitive IGK target for MRD monitoring (figure) 668
Septicaemia (complication of catheters) 427–28
Sequence dependency in drugs 27
Serology 337, 339–40
Severe acute GvHD of the skin, showing desquamation and blister formation (figure) 601
Severe aplastic anaemia
  preparative regimens 557–58
Severe combined immuodeficiency 238
  adenosine deaminase negative 233
  BMT and 225
    alternative donors 225–27
    busulfan and 226
    conditioning regimen and 226
    cyclophosphamide and 226
    factors influencing outcome 227
    graft failure 227
    graft-versus-host disease 225, 226, 227
    HLA-donors 225, 226
    recovery of immune function 227–28
    sources of donors 226
    T-cell depletion methods 226
  fetal liver transplants and 226
  graft-versus-host disease 225, 226, 227
  main syndromes 224
Severe congenital neutropenias 230
Severe osteoporosis of the spine secondary to growth hormone deficiency and radiation (figure) 845
Shapiro *et al* (1991) 289
Shciller *et al* (1995) 122

Sheath separated from line by pulling the sides gently apart (catheter insertion) (figure) 425
Sheridan *et al* (1992) 455
Shiobara *et al* (1992) 858
Shpall *et al* (1991) 198
Shpall *et al* (1994) 462
Sick role 828
Sickle-cell disease
  BMT and 14, 15, 278–83
    aims 280
    benefits 280
    donors 280
    graft-versus-host disease 280
    medical problems 280
    patient selection 281, 282
    results 279–80
Sikhs 937–38
  diet 938
  five symbols 938
  hair loss and 927, 937–38
Simplified genetic map of current major histocompatibility complex (figure) 326
Singer (1993) 924
Singh, Guru Gobind 927
Sjögren's syndrome 624, 627, 629, 633
  Schirmer's test 629
Skin and graft-versus-host disease 599–602, 621–24, 627, 636–38
Skin in chronic GvHD showing scleroderma-like changes (figure) 639
Skin with acute GvHD showing lymphocytes attached to surrounding individual necrotic epithelial cells (figure) 638
Slattery *et al* (1995) 652
Sloan Kettering Cancer Center
  CML cytoreductive regimens 52
Small lymphocytic lymphoma 158
  allogeneic BMT 159
  CLL and 158
  cyclophosphamide and 159
  myeboablative therapy 158–59
  TBI and 159
Small-cell lung cancer 209
  autologous BMT 209
  high-dose chemotherapy 209
    carmustine 209
    cisplatin 209
    cyclophosphamide 209
Socié *et al* (1990) 631
Solid tumours in adults 206–10
  autologous BMT and 206
  epithelial ovarian cancer 206–208
  gastrointestinal cancer 210
  high-dose chemotherapy and 206, 581–86
  malignant melanoma 209
  peripheral stem-cell transplant 206
  sarcoma 208–209
  small-cell lung cancer 209
Solid tumours in children 174–86
  autologous BMT and 174
  bone marrow purging and 185–86
  CECC regimen 186, 187
  chemotherapy for 174, 186
  distribution by age 174
  Ewing's sarcoma 182, 183
  germ-cell tumours 182–84
  malignant brain tumours 185
  neuroblastoma 175–81
    autologous BMT and 175
    Children's Cancer Group 178
    double autograft procedures 179
    European Neuroblastoma Study Group 178
    MEC 180

OMEC 180
  survival rates 175–76, 178
  TBI versus high-dose chemotherapy 179
  PBSC and 186
  rhabdomyosarcoma 181
  Wilms' tumour 182, 184
Somolo *et al* (1994) 200
Soyinka (1992) 927
Spector (1991) 927
Spectrum of fungal infections (table) 725
Spencer *et al* (1995) 600
Spitzer *et al* (1994) 461
Spleen
  bone-marrow failure syndrome and 2
  bone-marrow repopulation and 3
Staff *see* Nursing staff
Standard systemic treatment of chronic GvHD (table) 630
Stanford V 131
Statistical information on transplantation 898–910
Stem cells
  see also Peripheral blood stem cells (PBSC)
  allogeneic in multiple myeloma transplants 113
  cord blood 5, 383–84, 442–47
  defective in transplants 15
  gene therapy
    metabolic diseases and 290–93
  peripheral blood 5, 142–43
  positive selection 122–23
  progeny and 8
Stem-cell sources (figure) 899
Stemmer *et al* 27
Sterile diets 815
Stiff *et al* (1994, 1995) 206
Stomach, cancer of 210
Strathern (1982) 927, 928
Subdural empyema 790
Subspecialists in follow-up of allogeneic bone-marrow and blood cell transplant patients (table) 893
Subspecialists in management of allogeneic bone-marrow and blood cell transplant patients (table) 893
Subzonal sperm injection 863
Sucralfate 651
Suggested approach to heatitis B immunization in BMT where unspecified (table) 750
Sullivan *et al* (1981) 620
Sullivan *et al* (1988) 629
Sulphadiazine 792
Summary of results of prophylactic studies at 100 days post-transplant (CMV) (table) 702
Supertypic groups of HLA-B and HLA-DR alleles (table) 329
Survival after unrelated donor BMT for severe aplastic anaemia (table) 373
Survival and event-free survival of 18 patients, AML in CR post-unrelated donor BMT (table) 380
Susceptibility of organs to treatment-related damage (table) 837
Swerdlow and Stjernsward (1982) 930
Syndrome of inappropriate antidiuretic hormone secretion 778
Syngeneic twins 248–49
  outcome of transplants 249
Systemic lupus erythematosus 306, 307
Systemic necrotizing vasculitis 307
Systemic sclerosis 306, 307
Szasz (1961) 923

Index

T

Tacrolimus 630, 789
Tain bo Cuailnge 2
Tannock *et al* 20
Targetted radiotherapy 545
Taste changes 823
Taylor, E.B. (1871) 922
Tay-Sachs disease 290
TBI using a conventional linear accelerator (figure) 540
T-cell depletion balance (figure) 475
T-cells 6, 10–11, 14, 17, 229, 231, 309
  antigen recognition 332
  depletion 400
    allogeneic PBSC grafts 492–96
    allogeneic stem-cell grafts 474–504
    centrifugal elutriation 480
    CML relapse after allogeneic BMT 53–55
    PBSC and, in mismatched transplants 611
  depletion of donor bone marrow 251
    CML in 376
    paediatrics in 369
    drug-mediated techniques 481
    e-rosetting 478–79
    immunomagnetic 489–91
    immunotoxins 487–89
    laboratory evaluation of 495–96
    lectin treatment 478–79
    monoclonal antibodies 481–87
    panning 479–80
  immune deficiencies 229, 231
    BMT for 229
  positive selection by 495
  graft-versus-host disease and 11, 382, 596–97
  immune reconstitution 496–97
  mHag and 334–35
  receptor and peptide antigen interaction 9
  ways to prevent activation (figure) 613
TCRab 608
Terasaki 4
Terbinafine 734
Testis
  function 863
  microassisted fertilisation 863–64
  problems 852–53, 857
  semen quality 863
Tetanus toxoid vaccination 752–53
Thalassaemia major 268–74
  age distribution 268
  clinical forms of a 268
  clinical forms of b 268
  BMT and 13, 15, 268–74
    conditioning regimens 270
    cord blood transplants 273–74
    cost 274
    donors 269, 381
    fertility problems 272
    graft-versus-host disease and 270, 272
    growth retardation 272
    in utero transplants 274
    iron depletion 273
    rejection 271
    second transplants 272
    survival rates 270
  cytomegalovirus seropositivity 271
  gene therapy 274
  secondary malignancy 272–73
  treatment 268
Thalidomide 631
Thiotepa 18, 22, 121, 193, 194, 209, 270, 552, 568, 582, 652
  administration 24
  pharmacology 583

Thomas and Storb (1970) 434
Thomas *et al* (1979) 538
Thomas GvHD grading system 602, 603
Thomas, E Donnell 5
Thrombocytopenia 789
Thrombosis (complication of catheters) 428
Thrombotic thrombocytopenic purpura *see* Haemolytic uraemic syndrome
Thyroid gland problems 850–51
Tiley *et al* (1993) 92
Till and McCulloch (1961) 3
Topical therapy for oral GvHD (table) 632
Total body irradiation 32, 552
  acute renal failure and 775
  ALL and 71, 72
  autoimmune disorders and 309
  cateracts 544
  cell kill for 539
  CLL and 299
  CML and 52, 375, 376
  conditioning 542
  dose 541
  dose 573–74
    distribution 540
  dosimetry 540
  drugs and 544–45
  equipment 539–40
  Ewing's sarcoma 182
  follicular lymphoma and 154
  fractionation 541–42, 573–74
  future of 544–45
  gonadal failure 543–44
  graft failure and 652
  hepatic veno-occlusive disease 543
  high dose regimens in acute leukaemias 573–75
  history 538
  Hodgkin's lymphoma and 135, 141
  hypothyroidism 543
  immunodeficiency diseases and 228
  immunosuppression for 538–39
  lymphoplasmacytoid lymphoma and 159
  mantle cell lymphoma and 159
  multiple myeloma and 116, 117, 121
  neuroblastoma and 179
  nutrition and 813
  patient selection 542
  pneumonitis 543
  pregnancy and 856
  preparation 542
  preparative regimens 554
    chemotherapy compared with radiation-based 559–60
  relapse and 678
  reduced relapse rates 41
  renal impairment 544
  second malignancies 544
  shielding organs 540
  side-effects 542–44, 555–59
  small lymphocytic lymphoma and 159
  toxicity 542–44, 555–56
Total lymphoid irradiation 631–32, 652
Toxicity of bone-marrow transplantation (table) 544
Toxoplasma gondii 742–43, 790
Toxoplasmosis 779–80
  (figure) 790
Tranfusion/donor related infections (table) 711
Transplant
  outcome statistical methodology development 898
  related mortality 17
  talk 317–18
  unit
    accommodation 872

    air-conditioning 873
    capital costs 873
    catering facilities 874
    equipment 874
    infection and 870–71
    nursing staff 875, 880–87
    resources 882
    running costs 873
    setting up 870–75
    staff accommodation 875
    visitors' accommodation 875
    waste disposal 874
    water supply 873, 874
Transplantation of bone-marrow 2–15
  history 2–4
Triazoles 730–31
Trichosporinosis 730
Tricot *et al* (1995, 1996) 113, 118, 124
Trimethoprim-sulphamethoxazole 736, 743, 759
Trophozoites of toxoplasma gondii (figure) 743
Tsuruo and Fiedler 1981) 192
Tuberculomas 791
Tuberculous meningitis (figure) 791
Tumour purging *see* Purging graft
Tumour purging techniques (table) 511
Twins
  bone-marrow transplants and 3
  syngeneic 248–49
Types of food restrictions used with patients undergoing bone-marrow transplantation (table) 815
Types of ovum donation (table) 859
Typical maculopapular rash of early acute graft-versus-host disease (figure) 601
Typical patchy pigmentation changes of chronic graft-versus-host disease (figure) 625

U

Uberoi (1992) 927, 937
UK MRC AML-10 trial
  allogeneic transplants 37
  autologous transplants 42
UK Paediatric MDS Register 375
Umbilical cord *see* Cord blood
Unit gravity sedimentation 511
University College London Hospital 134, 136
  criteria for transplantation 132
University of Colorado Bone Marrow Transplant Program 201
Unknown fertile ovum donation (table) 859
Unkown infertile ovum donation (table) 860
Unrelated Bone Marrow Donor Register (Canadian) 355
Unrelated donor BMT distribution throughout Europe as registered to the EBMT group (table) 365
Uppsala group 57
Uptake and release of amphotericin B from liposomes (figure) 733

V

Vγ3–Jγ2.3 rearrangement used as MRD target to monitor precursor B-ALL (figure) 667
Vaccinations 633, 746
  diptheria toxoid 748
  haemophilus influenzae 748–9, 759
  hepatitis B 749–50
  influenza 750
  measles 750
  measurement of immune response to 753
  pneumococcus 752–54, 759

poliovirus 752
rubella vaccination 752
tetanus toxoid vaccination 752–53
VAD 115–16
Vahdat *et al* (1995) 194
VAMP 115–16
Varicella zoster virus (VZV) 633
  management 716
  primary 714–15
  reactivation 715–16
Vegetables 816
Vellodi *et al* (1995) 290
Veno-occlusive disease 543, 770–73
  aetiology 771
  busulfan and 22, 771
  clinical features 770–71
  complication of BMT 15
  cyclophosphamide and 22, 771
  diagnosis 770, 771–72
    doppler ultrasound 772
    liver histology 771
    serological virus detection 772
    transjugular liver biopsy 772
  management 772–73
  pathogenesis 771
  prevention 772
Venous access 320–21
  indwelling vascular catheter 320–21
Venous access
  arteriovenous fistulae and grafts 421
  catheters 420
    central venous 421–22
  indications for reliable 420
  peripheral blood stem-cell harvesting 420–25
  peripheral venous cannulation 421
Vesole *et al* (1993) 113
Vesole *et al* (1996) 119
Vietnamese 932
Vinblastine 131, 214, 218, 219, 788
Vinca alkaloids 788
  vinblastine 131, 214, 218, 219, 788
  vincristine 66, 118, 131, 180, 215, 300, 788
Vinca nuclear power plant 5
Vincristine 66, 118, 131, 180, 215, 300, 788
Viral infections 710–20

adenoviruses 716–17
brain infections (figure) 719
chest infections (figure) 719
cytomegalovirus *see* Cytomegalovirus
endogenous viral reactivation 710–13
enteroviruses 718
Epstein-Barr virus (EBV) 94, 169, 229, 272, 716
gastroenteritis 718
gastrointestinal tract (figure) 719
hepatitis B 718
hepatitis C 718
herpes simplex virus (HSV) 633, 713–14
HHV6 716
HHV8 716
liver infections (figure) 720
measles 717
papovaviruses 717
parvovirus B19 718
respiratory tract infections 717–18
sources of infection
  blood products 710
  donor tissue 710
  environmental 710
  transfusion 710
varicella-zoster virus (VZV) 633, 714–16
Virus infections of the brain post stem-cell transplant (figure) 719
Virus infections of the chest post stem-cell transplant (figure) 719
Virus infections of the gastrointestinal tract post stem-cell transplant (figure) 719
Virus infections of the liver post stem-cell transplant (figure) 719
Virus infections of the skin post stem-cell transplant (figure) 719
Vitimin requirements 819
Volosinov (1976) 923
Vomiting 768, 812, 814, 823
Von Bueltzingsloewen *et al* (1993) 703

W

Wade and Schimpff (1987) 871, 872
Water
quality following transplant 761, 816, 874
supply in transplant unit 873
Watson (1994) 928
Wegener's granulomatosis 307
Weight *see* Body weight
Weisdorf *et al* (1984, 1987) 821
Weisdorf *et al* (1995) 652
Whitley *et al* (1993) 288
Wilms' tumour 182, 184
Wilson (1995) 872
Wingard *et al* (1989) 628
Winston *et al* (1983) 751
Winston *et al* (1993) 703, 705
Wiskott-Aldrich syndrome 224, 228–29, 231
Work, time off 318
World distribution of transplants performed using ANBMT donors (table) 356
World-wide-web donor registry homepages 353
WR-2721 198
Wulff *et al* (1983) 796

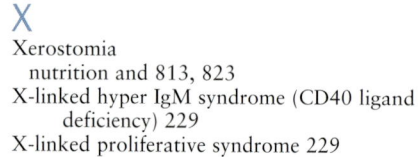

X

Xerostomia
  nutrition and 813, 823
X-linked hyper IgM syndrome (CD40 ligand deficiency) 229
X-linked proliferative syndrome 229

Y

Yahalom *et al* (1993) 134
Yates and Holland (1973) 870
Young and Rubin (1987) 870

Z

Zaehner (1979) 938
Zbrowski (1952) 930
Zentrales Knochenmark-spenderregister 353
Zoroastrianism 938
  blood transfusion 938
  diet 938
Zulian *et al* (1989) 134
Zygomycosis 730